# Idiopathic Scoliosis

## The Harms Study Group Treatment Guide

Thieme

# Idiopathic Scoliosis

## The Harms Study Group Treatment Guide

Peter O. Newton, MD
Clinical Associate Professor
Department of Orthopaedic Surgery
University of California–San Diego
Division of Orthopaedic Surgery
Rady Children's Hospital
San Diego, California

Randal R. Betz, MD
Chief of Staff
Medical Director
Spinal Cord Injury Unit
Shriners Hospital for Children
Philadelphia, Pennsylvania

Michael F. O'Brien, MD
Director of Research
Baylor Spine Center
Spinal Surgeon
Southwest Scoliosis Institute
Plano, Texas

Robert A. Dickson
Emeritus Professor
Orthopaedic Surgery/Consultant
Spine Surgeon
University of Leeds and Leeds General Infirmary
Leeds, United Kingdom

Harry L. Shufflebarger, MD
Director
Department of Orthopaedic Surgery
Miami Children's Hospital
Miami, Florida

Jürgen Harms, MD
Professor and Chief
Department of Orthopaedics and Traumatology
Klinikum Karlsbad–Langensteinbach
Karlsbad, Germany

Thieme
New York • Stuttgart

Thieme Medical Publishers, Inc.
333 Seventh Ave.
New York, NY 10001

Editorial Director: Michael Wachinger
Executive Editor: Kay D. Conerly
Managing Editor: J. Owen Zurhellen IV
Editorial Assistant: Emma Lassiter
International Production Director: Andreas Schabert
Production Editor: Kenneth L. Chumbley, Publication Services
Vice President, International Marketing and Sales: Cornelia Schulze
Chief Financial Officer: James W. Mitos
President: Brian D. Scanlan
Illustrator: James Millerick
Compositor: Thomson Digital
Printer: Replika Press Pvt Ltd.

Library of Congress Cataloging-in-Publication Data

Idiopathic scoliosis : the Harms Study Group treatment guide / [edited by] Peter O. Newton ... [et al.].
p. ; cm.
Includes bibliographical references.
ISBN 978-1-60406-024-9 (alk. paper)
1. Scoliosis. I. Newton, Peter O. II. Harms Study Group.
[DNLM: 1. Scoliosis—therapy. 2. Adolescent. 3. Braces. 4. Orthopedic Procedures—methods. 5. Spine—surgery. WE 735 I19 2010]
RD771.S3I35 2010
616.7'3—dc22

2010007751



**Important note:** Medical knowledge is ever-changing. As new research and clinical experience broaden our knowledge, changes in treatment and drug therapy may be required. The authors and editors of the material herein have consulted sources believed to be reliable in their efforts to provide information that is complete and in accord with the standards accepted at the time of publication. However, in view of the possibility of human error by the authors, editors, or publisher of the work herein or changes in medical knowledge, neither the authors, editors, nor publisher, nor any other party who has been involved in the preparation of this work, warrants that the information contained herein is in every respect accurate or complete, and they are not responsible for any errors or omissions or for the results obtained from use of such information. Readers are encouraged to confirm the information contained herein with other sources. For example, readers are advised to check the product information sheet included in the package of each drug they plan to administer to be certain that the information contained in this publication is accurate and that changes have not been made in the recommended dose or in the contraindications for administration. This recommendation is of particular importance in connection with new or infrequently used drugs.



Printed in India

5 4 3 2

ISBN 978-1-60406-024-9

We dedicate this book to our respective families

# Contents

# Foreword

The diagnosis and treatment of idiopathic scoliosis, as well as more complex types of spinal deformity, has experienced revolutionary advances since Paul Harrington of Houston introduced the concept of Harrington rod instrumentation and then instrumentation plus fusion (Moe) in about 1960. Prior to that, surgical correction of scoliosis was unpredictable and difficult, depending on in situ posterior spinal fusions (Hibbs, 1911), followed by prolonged periods of casting in large, often grotesque body casts (LeMesurier et al., "fishnet" cast).

Following Paul Harrington's revolutionary introduction, instrumented surgical correction of scoliosis made evolutionary gains, including Luque spinal instrumentation (laminar wiring), the segmental attachment of spinal instrumentation including derotation (Cotrel and Dubousset), and the more revolutionary concept of pedicle screw attachment to the spine (Roy and Camille ) that provided an even better grasp for segmental control and correction.

As these advances were evolving, spine treatment centers of excellence evolved throughout the world (United States, France, United Kingdom, Germany, and elsewhere). The German school of scoliosis surgery became internationally recognized in the 1970s and 1980s through the work of Klaus Zielke in Bad Wildungen, where I gained first-hand exposure to German thinking while attending an international scoliosis instructional course in the mid-1980s. At that time, a dynamic, energetic, and relatively *junior-level* professor, Jürgen Harms, presented his work. Despite his young age, whispered conversations in the teaching auditorium and operating rooms concluded that Harms represented the future of German spine and scoliosis surgery. This new and important text represents to a great extent the accuracy of that prophecy.

Other developments in the 1970s and 1980s included major advances in the management of scoliosis and spinal disorders by brilliant surgeons who worked in regional centers, including Kenton Leatherman at the Kosair Children's Hospital in Louisville, Kentucky, and Robert Dickson, a prior fellow with Dr. Leatherman, who then became professor and head of the orthopedic department at the University of Leeds in the United Kingdom. Their landmark 1988 textbook, *The Management of Spinal Deformities*, synthesized a global understanding of scoliosis, but was never revised to a second edition. Instead, that classic text provided the basic model for this new Harms Study Group book. In fact, the first four chapters are written by Dickson.

The dynamic, innovative, and often complex methods for correcting spinal deformity developed by Harms and colleagues in Germany quickly spread throughout much of Europe and then to the United States—first, via Harry Shufflebarger (Miami), and then to other North American centers dedicated to the concepts of Harms' treatment methods, including Randy Betz (Philadelphia), Peter Newton (San Diego), and Michael O'Brien (Dallas). The international multicenter Harms Study Group was then developed. This organization, which in some ways resembles the long-term patient follow-up program set up by the A-O documentation center in Bern and Davos, Switzerland, was established to study the efficacy of scoliosis treatment methods.

The Harms Study Group database has become a world-class information source regarding scoliosis treatment outcomes, which has led to hundreds of publications and presentations (Scoliosis Research Society and other conferences). The result has been a synthesis of current knowledge and thinking about the treatment of spinal deformity, both in children and adolescents, as well as adults.

*Idiopathic Scoliosis: The Harms Study Group Treatment Guide*, edited by Peter Newton and colleagues, with multiple authors from the Harms Study Group, as well as other recognized experts from throughout the scoliosis world, provides state-of-the-art information on the natural history, etiology, and nonoperative treatment, as well as both basic and extremely advanced concepts for surgical correction of spine deformity.

Scoliosis fellows, young surgeons, and even experienced scoliosis surgeons, will find much that is new and important in this book. Just reading Robert Dickson on the history, pathogenesis, epidemiology, and basic principals of scoliosis treatment justifies owning this book, while at the same time correcting the intellectual deficit of not having read or had access to the original *The Management of Spinal Deformities* by Leatherman and Dickson.

This book provides a strong basis for understanding scoliosis as we enter the second decade of the twenty-first century and will likely remain a landmark work throughout the century—a period which promises unrivaled further advances in understanding and treating the still somewhat mysterious condition know as idiopathic scoliosis.

*Dennis R. Wenger, MD*
Director, Pediatric Orthopedic Training Program
Rady Children's Hospital-San Diego
Clinical Professor of Orthopedic Surgery
University of California–San Diego

# Preface

The concept for this complete and current book, addressed entirely to the disorder known as idiopathic scoliosis at all stages of life, had its origin in the experience of the Harms Study Group. The Harms Study Group was initiated in 1995 to investigate questions relating to idiopathic spinal deformity. The Group has prospectively collected data for patients treated surgically for idiopathic deformities of the spine in adolescence, which included more than 2300 patients as of 2010. It was felt that the experience gained from this group of patients would serve as a sound foundation for this textbook, and many of the facts addressed in the book come from an analysis of this database.

All of the contributors to this work are recognized experts in the evaluation and treatment of spinal deformity. This book presents all aspects of the evaluation and treatment of idiopathic spinal deformity. Specific surgical approaches to the several types of adolescent deformity are presented, with the rationale, techniques, and results for each. And because the database of the Harms Study Group covers the past 15 years, this book provides details of changes in and the evolution of current techniques in surgery for adolescent idiopathic deformities of the spine.

This state-of-the-art work on idiopathic spinal deformity should be most useful to those who treat this problem. It should also be valuable to all practitioners of nonsurgical care for spinal deformities and to all who work with patients who have such deformities.

## Acknowledgments

The processes of writing and publishing this first book specifically dedicated to adolescent idiopathic scoliosis and its lifelong ramifications could not have been accomplished without contributions from many sources. We hope to give all of them the credit that is their due for helping to make this book possible.

The idea for this book began with the core members of the Harms Study Group, particularly Jürgen Harms, Peter Newton, and Randy Betz. Without the initiative and constant input of these surgeons, this book would never have been begun or completed.

Lutz Biedermann provided the initial funding for starting the project of writing. Without him, this book would never have been begun. Our thanks to Lutz.

Thieme Publishers and its managing editor, J. Owen Zurhellen IV, have continually supported the publication of this book. We thank Thieme for their support.

Michael F. O'Brien undertook the enormous task of editing this project, which required vast amounts of time, knowledge, and energy.

Many assistant editors brought the peer review of the book to fruition and spent uncounted hours completing its editing. The text would not have been finished without the diligent efforts of all, including Fran Faro, Burt Yaszay, Pat Cahill, and William Lavelle. We thank the many authors involved in writing the chapters for this book and express our gratitude for their contributions to the finished product.

We thank Michelle Marks, multisite coordinator for the Harms Study Group, for her vital contributions, which included coordinating all inquiries related to the study group database, assisting in the analysis of these inquiries, and providing invaluable insight into interpretation of the necessary data.

Raymarla Pinteric has been the driving force in pushing this text to completion. Without her devotion to the task and her firmly guiding hand in dealing with all of the editors and authors involved in it, the project would not have been completed. Our thanks to Ray.

# Contributors

**Mark F. Abel, MD**
Lillian Pratt Distinguished Professor and Chair
Department of Orthopaedic Surgery
Professor of Pediatrics
University of Virginia
Charlottesville, Virginia

**Jahangir Asghar, MD**
Surgeon
Department of Orthopaedics
Shriners Hospital for Children
Philadelphia, Pennsylvania

**Joshua D. Auerbach, MD**
Chief of Spine Surgery
Department of Orthopaedics
Bronx-Lebanon Hospital Center
Albert Einstein College of Medicine
Bronx, New York

**Tracey P. Bastrom, MA**
Clinical Research Director
Department of Orthopedics
Rady Children's Hospital
San Diego, California

**Shay Bess, MD**
Rocky Mountain Scoliosis and Spine
Rocky Mountain Hospital for Children
Denver, Colorado

**Randal R. Betz, MD**
Chief of Staff
Medical Director
Spinal Cord Injury Unit
Shriners Hospital for Children
Philadelphia, Pennsylvania

**John T. Braun, MD**
Associate Professor
Department of Orthopaedics and Rehabilitation
University of Vermont
Burlington, Vermont

**Patrick J. Cahill, MD**
Attending Spine Surgeon
Shriners Hospital for Children
Philadelphia, Pennsylvania

**David H. Clements III, MD**
Associate Professor
Department of Orthopaedic Surgery
Robert Wood Johnson Medical School
Co-director
Cooper Spine Program
Cooper University Hospital
Camden, New Jersey
Shriners Hospital for Children
Philadelphia, Pennsylvania

**Alvin H Crawford, MD, FACS**
Professor of Orthopaedics and Pediatrics
Director of the Spine Center
Department of Pediatric Orthopaedic Surgery
Cincinnati Children's Hospital Medical Center
Cincinnati, Ohio

**Linda P. D'Andrea, MD**
Co-director
Division of Spinal Disorders
Brandywine Institute of Orthopaedics
Pottstown, Pennsylvania

**Robert A. Dickson**
Emeritus Professor
Orthopaedic Surgery/Consultant
Spine Surgeon
University of Leeds and Leeds General Infirmary
Leeds, United Kingdom

**John P. Dormans, MD, FACS**
Chief of Orthopaedic Surgery
Department of Orthopaedic Surgery
The Children's Hospital of Philadelphia
Philadelphia, Pennsylvania

**Frances D. Faro, MD**
Fellow
Department of Orthopaedics
Union Memorial Hospital
Baltimore, Maryland

**James T. Guille, MD**
Co-director
Division of Spinal Disorders
Brandywine Institute of Orthopaedics
Pottstown, Pennsylvania
Consult Spine Surgeon
Shriners Hospital for Children
St. Christopher's Hospital for Children
Philadelphia, Pennsylvania

**Munish C. Gupta, MD**
Professor
Chief of Spine
Co-director of Spine Center
Department of Othopaedic Surgery
University of California–Davis Medical Center
Sacramento, California

**Thomas R. Haher, MD**
Syracuse Orthopaedic Specialists
Syracuse, New York

**Jürgen Harms, MD**
Professor and Chief
Department of Orthopaedics and Traumatology
Klinikum Karlsbad–Langensteinbach
Karlsbad, Germany

**Joshua E. Heller, MD**
Chief Neurosurgery Resident
Temple University Hospital
Philadelphia, Pennsylvania

**HoSun Hwang, MD**
Assistant Clinical Professor
Department of Orthopedic Surgery
Baylor College of Medicine
Memorial Bone and Joint Clinic
Houston, Texas

**Rubens G. Jensen, MD**
Spine Surgeon
Department of Orthopaedics and Traumatology
Klinikum Karlsbad–Langensteinbach
Karlsbad, Germany

**Safdar N. Khan, MD**
Chief Resident
Department of Orthopaedic Surgery
University of California–Davis Medical Center
Sacramento, California

**Virginie Lafage, PhD**
Director of Spine Research
Department of Orthopaedics
Hospital for Joint Diseases
New York University
New York, New York

**Loren Latta, PE, PhD**
Professor and Director of Biomechanics Research
Department of Orthpaedics
Miller School of Medicine
Professor
Department of Industrial Engineering
Department of Biomedical Engineering
University of Miami
Director of the Max Biedermann Institute
for Biomechanics
Mount Sinai Medical Center
Miami Beach, Florida

**Elizabeth Demers Lavelle, MD**
Assistant Professor
Department of Anesthesia and Pediatrics
Upstate Medical University
Syracuse, New York

**William F. Lavelle, MD**
Assistant Professor
Department of Orthopaedic Surgery
Upstate Medical University
Syracuse, New York

**Lawrence G. Lenke, MD**
The Jerome J. Gilden Endowed Professor
of Orthopaedic Surgery
Co-chief Adult/Pediatric Scoliosis & Reconstructive
Spinal Surgery
Professor of Neurological Surgery
Washington University School of Medicine
St. Louis, Missouri

**Lynn J. Letko, MD**
Spine Surgeon
Department of Orthopaedics and Traumatology
Klinikum Karlsbad–Langensteinbahc
Karlsbad, Germany

**Baron S. Lonner, MD**
Director
Scoliosis and Spine Associates
Clinical Associate Professor
Department of Orthopaedic Surgery
New York University Hospital for Joint Diseases
New York, New York

**Thomas G. Lowe, MD**
Clinical Professor
Department of Orthopaedics
University of Colorado Health Sciences Center
Denver, Colorado
(deceased)

**Sara P. Lozano, MD**
Department of Pediatric Anesthesiology
Cleveland Clinic
Cleveland, Ohio

**Angel Macagno, MD**
Department of Orthopedic Surgery
Downstate Medical Center
Brooklyn, New York

**Mohamed Mahmoud, MD**
Assistant Professor of Clinical Anesthesia and Pediatrics
Director
Department of Radiology Anesthesia and Sedation
Cincinnati Children's Hospital Medical Center
Cincinnati, Ohio

**Michelle C. Marks, PT, MA**
Spine Deformity Research Director
Harms Study Group Foundation
San Diego, California

**Daniel S. Mulconrey, MD**
Assistant Clinical Professor of Surgery
Department of Surgery
Midwest Orthopaedic Center
University of Illinois College of Medicine
Peoria, Illinois

**Peter O. Newton, MD**
Clinical Associate Professor
Department of Orthopaedic Surgery
University of California–San Diego
Division of Orthopaedic Surgery
Rady Children's Hospital
San Diego, California

**Michael F. O'Brien, MD**
Director of Research
Baylor Spine Center
Spinal Surgeon
Southwest Scoliosis Institute
Plano Texas

**Alan E. Oestreich, MD, FACR**
Emeritus Pediatric Radiologist
Department of Radiology
Cincinnati Children's Hospital Medical Center
Cincinnati, Ohio

**James W. Ogilvie, MD**
Professor
Department of Orthopaedic Surgery
University of Utah School of Medicine
Staff Surgeon
Shriners Hospital for Children
Chief Medical Advisor
Axial Biotech, Inc.
Salt Lake City, Utah

**Rod J. Oskouian Jr, MD**
Surgeon
Department of Neurosurgery
Swedish Neuroscience Institute
Seattle, Washington

**Joshua M. Pahys, MD**
Adult and Pediatric Spine Fellow
Department of Orthopaedic Surgery
Washington University School of Medicine
St. Louis, Missouri

**Ashish Patel, MD**
Research Fellow
Department of Orthopaedics
Hospital for Joint Diseases
New York University
New York, New York

**Amer Samdani, MD**
Director, Pediatric Spine Surgery
Department of Orthopedic Surgery
Shriners Hospital for Children
Philadelphia, Pennsylvania

**Charles A. Sansur, MD, MHSc**
Assistant Professor
Department of Neurosurgery
University of Maryland School of Medicine
Baltimore, Maryland

**Frank Schwab, MD**
Clinical Assistant Professor
Chief of the Spinal Deformity Service
Department of Orthopaedics
Hospital for Joint Diseases
New York University
New York, New York

**Christopher I. Shaffrey, MD**
Professor
Department of Neurological Surgery
University of Virginia
Charlottesville, Virginia

**Suken A. Shah, MD**
Co-director
Spine and Scoliosis Center
Alfred I. duPont Hospital for Children
Nemours Children's Clinic
Wilmington, Delaware
Associate Professor
Department of Orthopaedic Surgery
Jefferson Medical College of Thomas Jefferson University
Philadelphia, Pennsylvania

**Harry L. Shufflebarger, MD**
Director
Department of Orthopaedic Surgery
Miami Children's Hospital
Miami, Florida

**Paul D. Sponseller, MD**
Riley Professor and Head
Department of Pediatric Orthopaedics
Johns Hopkins Medical Institutions
Baltimore, Maryland

**Daniel J. Sucato, MD, MS**
Staff Orthopaedic Surgeon
Director
Sarah M. And Charles Seay/Martha and Pat Beard Center of Excellence in Spine Research
Texas Scottish Rite Hospital for Children
Associate Professor
Department of Orthopaedic Surgery
University of Texas Southwestern Medical Center
Dallas, Texas

**Ryan Takenaga, MD**
Resident
Department of Orthopaedics and Rehabilitation
University of Iowa Hospitals and Clinics
Iowa City, Iowa

**See Wan Tham, MBBS**
Pediatric Anesthesia Fellow
Seattle Children's Hospital
Seattle, Washington

**Vidyadhar V. Upasani, MD**
Resident
Department of Orthopaedic Surgery
University of California–San Diego
San Diego, California

**Mark Vadney, DO**
Chief Resident
Department of Anesthesiology
Upstate Medical University
Syracuse, New York

**Burt Yaszay, MD**
Rady Children's Hospital
Voluntary Faculty
Department of Orthopaedics
University of California–San Diego
San Diego, California

# 1 History of the Treatment of Scoliosis

*Robert A. Dickson*

Images and writings about people with spinal deformities go back to prehistoric times. These severely disfigured individuals were stigmatized, ridiculed, and often feared and hated.[1] In the fifth century BC, Hippocrates described scoliosis for the first time, and designed a distraction apparatus for correction of the deformity.[2] In the second century AD, Galen coined the terms *scoliosis*, *kyphosis*, and *lordosis*, and described their treatment by chest binding and the application of spinal jackets.[3] The Dark Ages (ca. 500 to 1000 A.D.) saw little further advancement in the knowledge and treatment of spinal deformities; these were then thought to result from divine retribution and consequently such patients were regarded as heretics. The treatment for these patients and the punishment due to criminals was the same—to put them on the rack.[4]

Then, in the mid-sixteenth century in France, Ambroise Paré first described congenital scoliosis and understood spinal cord compression as a cause of paralysis.[3] He also described the management of open fractures consequent upon the treatment of his own compound tibial fracture, which went on to union without residual disability.[5] During the next 30 years Paré went on to appreciate the progression of spinal deformities with growth, and recommended new external breastplates to be made every 3 months or so (**Fig. 1.1**).[6]

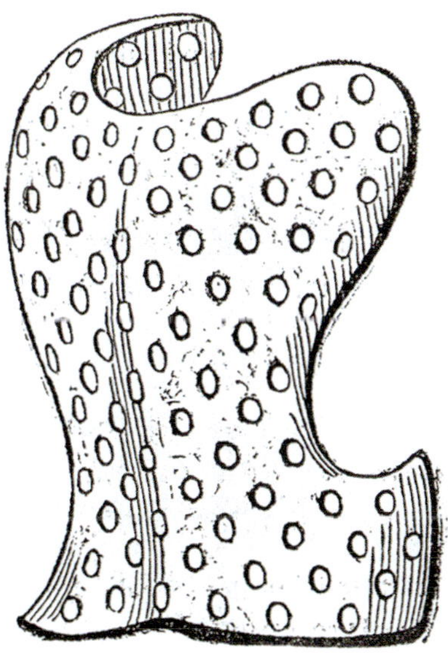

**Fig. 1.1** The first brace for scoliosis, developed in 1564. The metalwork and leather padding were designed by Paré.

It is alleged that in 1741, Nicholas André first coined the word *orthopaedia*. At this time André was a grumpy 80-year-old Parisian pediatrician, and his book *Orthopaedia* was a self-help book written for parents of children with orthopedic disorders.[7] The full title of the book was *Orthopaedia: Or the Art of Correcting and Preventing Deformities in Children: By Such Means as May Easily be Put in Practice by Parents Themselves and All Such as Are Employed in Educating Children*. Thus, orthopedics literally means "correcting and preventing deformities in children."

André felt that scoliosis was the result of muscle imbalance and poor sitting posture. Accordingly, he believed that proper tables and chairs were important in preventing scoliosis.[6] He also recommended periods of recumbency as well as braces and corsets for treating the disorder, and advised that persons with scoliosis carry books on their highshoulder side.[8]

Both of the Le Vacher brothers contributed to the treatment of spinal deformities.[9] Francois-Guillaume invented the jury mast and the Minerva cast for the treatment of tuberculosis of the spine, and Thomas wrote a book about scoliosis and invented an extension chair with vertical traction and lateral pressure straps (halter-antigravity–wheelchair traction).

Jean-André Venel bought an old abbey in 1780 and started the first orthopedic hospital specializing in the treatment of skeletal deformities.[10] He developed a day brace for scoliosis, the removal of which was followed by the patient's entering an orthopedic bed to relax with traction at night. The idea of an orthopedic bed then became very popular. Venel achieved much in treating skeletal deformities, and rivals André for the title of "Father of Orthopaedics."

## The Introduction of Surgery

The first surgical attempts to treat scoliosis were reported in the mid- to late nineteenth century. Delpech "recorded" surface shape by making plaster casts of his patients,[11] and introduced tenotomy in 1818.[12] Delpech was the father of French orthopedics. Guerin then became an enthusiast for Delpech's method and applied it to scoliosis.[13] Some thought he carried this to excess. Guerin published his results of 740 patients treated with tenotomy, of whom 358 were completely cured, 287 benefited, 77 did not benefit, and 18 died.[13] Malgaigne wrote an editorial on "orthopaedic illusion"[14] and Guerin sued him. Malgaigne wrote of Guerin that "It is important to know what to do but no less important to know what not to do." A fairly vindictive critic, Malgaigne wrote in the *Gazette Medical de Paris* that "the work of Dr X contains many things both new and good. Unfortunately the good things are not new and the new things are not good."[15]

In 1889 Volkman attempted to resect rib deformities, and this is thought to have been the first known scoliosis surgery on bony structures.[16] Maas also favored rib resection.[17] However, the nineteenth century saw a continued majority opinion that scoliosis was caused by poor posture and therefore could be treated accordingly.[18] Lewis Sayre wrote a book on spinal disease and spinal curvature in 1877, describing his methods of suspension and casting—a forerunner of the Boston brace.[19] He was also known for the immediate closure of myelomeningocele, and was President of the American Medical Association in 1880 and founder of the *Journal of the American Medical Association*.

William Adams, apart from realizing that the rotational prominence in scoliosis was made worse by forward bending (the Adams forward-bend test), carefully dissected cadavers with idiopathic scoliosis, and recognized the important lordosis at the curve apex.[20] In 1876 he went to the United States with Lister to watch Sayre and was made a Fellow of the American Orthopaedic Association (AOA) in 1898.[21]

In 1895 Bradford and Brackett developed a horizontal distraction frame that had a "localiser" attachment for curve correction.[3] Cast application was then performed.

In 1895 Roentgen discovered X-rays, and they were first used for imaging in surgery in March of 1896.[22] Roentgen won the Nobel Prize in 1901. However, it could well be argued that although radiographs of the spine produced beautiful novel pictures, their two-dimensional nature would frustrate further developments in understanding the pathogenesis of idiopathic scoliosis consequent upon Adams's original dissections and his subsequent statement that "lordosis + rotation = lateral flexion."[20]

## The Use of Surgical Implants

In the half century after Bradford and Brackett's work, little progress was made in the nonoperative treatment of spinal deformities, whereas much progress was made in their surgical treatment. Berthold Hadra first applied implants to the spine in the nature of spinous process wiring in 1891.[23] Then, in 1902, Fritz Lange implanted metal rods attached to the spinous processes with double slings of silk.[24] Both of these early implants were attempts to prevent tuberculous spinal deformity and promote healing.

It would appear that Wreden, in Germany, was the first to apply metal implants to the spine in the treatment of scoliosis.[25] He first resected the ribs on each side of the apex, put the patient in an extension bed (the forerunner of halter or halo-extension), and then fixed metal plates to the spinous processes.

For nearly three centuries, osseous defects had been replaced by bone grafts. Perhaps the first surgeon to do so was Meekren in Holland, who in 1682 repaired a defect in the cranium of a soldier with a piece of a dog's skull.[26] The advent of antiseptic surgery allowed William McEwen in 1878 to successfully rebuild a boy's humeral shaft with bone grafts.[27] However, it was not until 1911 that bone grafting was applied to the spine, by Fred Albee[28] in the United States and by DeQuervain in Europe.[29] Both applied cortical struts to the spine for treating tuberculosis, Albee using a piece of tibial autograft placed between split spinous processes and DeQuervain using the scapular spine instead of the tibia.

Albee, and his colleague Kusher, went on to describe his spinal fusion operation in the treatment of scoliosis.[30] He used his tibial strut graft on the curve concavity and anchored the apical vertebrae transversely with bone keys (**Fig. 1.2**). He also propped up the lower ribs on the concave side of the pelvis with graft material. Albee carpentered grafts with his newly developed power saw, and likened callus to cabinetmaker's glue.[31]

## Spinal Fusion

Russell Hibbs, in New York, changed the face of fusion surgery, using his fusion procedure between 1914 and 1919 to treat 59 patients, most of whom were polio patients who had undergone preoperative correction through head–pelvic traction.[32] He dissected subperiosteally right out to the facet joints and base of the transverse processes, and excised the facet joints. Using a gouge and bone forceps, he then raised flaps that he turned up and down so that adjacent vertebrae would be conjoined with bone graft. He next closed the periosteum over the fusion area. His operative technique is precisely the same as that used today. As Hibbs stated, "the dissection may be made in a practically dry field without injury to the muscles if it is sub-periosteal and if free use is made of gauze packs. Only in an operative wound that is free from hemorrhage can the operator see to exercise the care necessary for thorough work. Not only the baring of the bones may be complete, but the periosteum may be separated from them in a practically unbroken sheet and without disturbance of its relation to the surrounding tissues and blood supply. The greatest care should be exercised in the dissection as by its extent and thoroughness the area of fusion is measured." This was an extraordinary concept of a real biological approach to surgery for scoliosis, and not surprisingly there was only a 2% mortality rate.

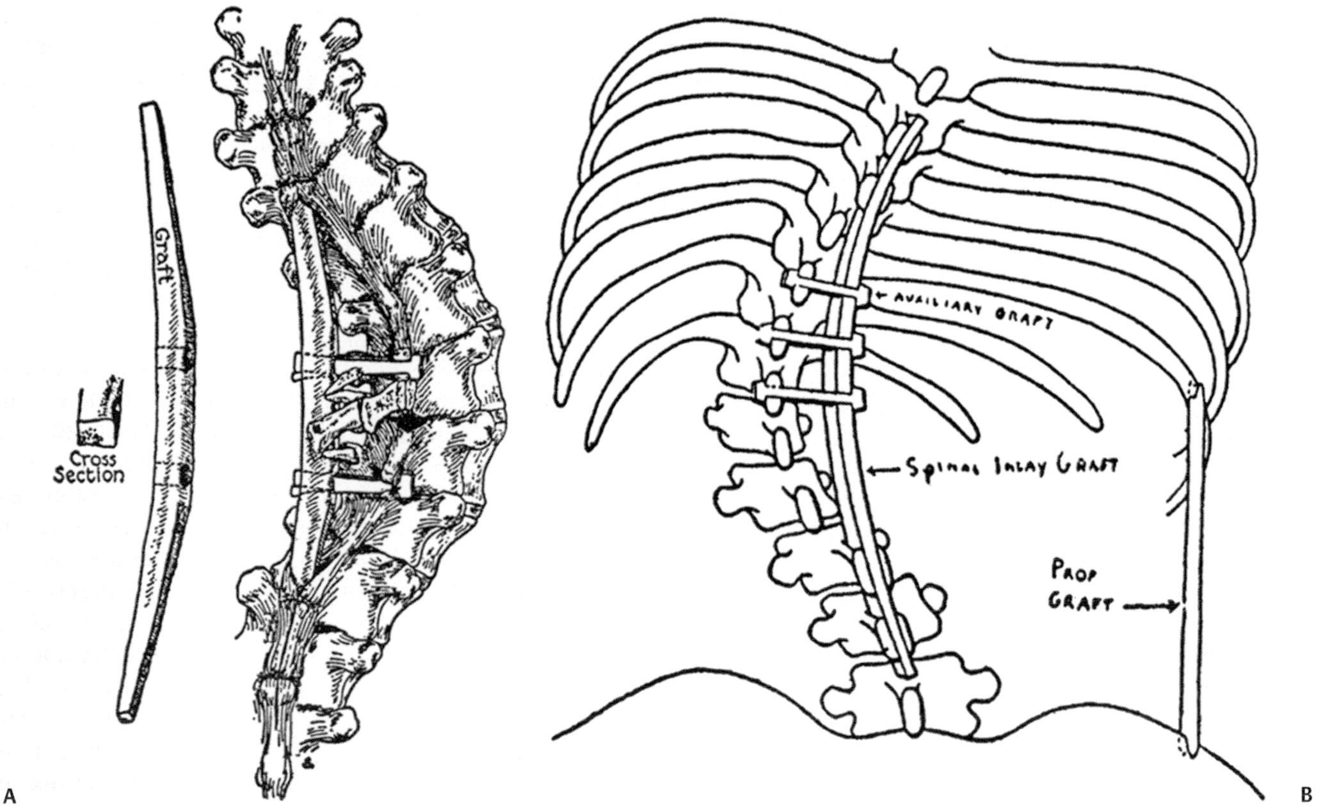


**Fig. 1.2** Albee's spinal operation. **(A)** A bone-distracting cortical graft on the concave side acts like a distraction rod attached to the spine by horizontal bone keys. **(B)** The 10th rib on the concave side is distracted from the pelvis through use of a prop graft.

In 1931, Hibbs, along with Joe Risser and Albert Ferguson, went on to report on 360 cases treated surgically over a 13-year period.[33] The purpose of the surgery was to prevent progression, and this was achieved in almost 50% of the cases, with about 30% having an increase in deformity because of too short a fusion or inaccurately selected fusion areas. Notwithstanding, the 50% rate of good results was encouraging, and occurred in association with meticulous preoperative and postoperative care. Risser, along with Hibbs, designed a turnbuckle cast, which they began using in 1920 with traction and bending forces applied over the 2 to 4 weeks before fusion. Disadvantages included the obligatory prolonged bed rest along with the possibility of pressure sores.

During this early part of the twentieth century, mixed results were reported for spinal fusion, with Arthur Steindler in 1929 giving up spinal fusion in the face of a 60% rate of pseudarthrosis or failure to obtain or maintain correction.[34] However, Howorth, in 1943, reported 600 cases with only a 14% pseudarthrosis rate.[24]

In the early 1950s Risser developed his localizer cast, which was applied using a special head and pelvic traction frame, and exerted pressure over the back of the rotational prominence.[35] In some cases three casts were used before surgery. As was standard practice, a window was cut out in the back of whatever form of preoperative immobilization device had been applied, so that the fusion operation could be performed and the position maintained postoperatively for a minimum of 6 months. Risser also noted that spinal growth appeared to correlate with the development, migration, and fusion of the apophysis of the iliac crest, and this is referred to as the Risser sign.[36] Unfortunately, the spine often grows until the late teens or early twenties, when the vertebral endplate epiphyses eventually fuse.[37] Not surprisingly, 2 cm of spinal growth (seen as an increase in sitting height) occurs after the apophysis of the iliac crest has fused.[38]

Meanwhile, in 1941 the AOA conducted a multicenter review of the treatment of scoliosis, and 425 cases were examined, half of which were treated with spinal fusion.[39] The rate of pseudarthrosis was 28%, with an even greater rate of complete loss of correction. Among those treated nonoperatively, 60% had an increase in their deformity. The overall end results were a discouraging figure of almost 70% of outcomes rated as fair or poor, with only 30% rated as good or excellent. It was concluded that correction with a cast or turnbuckle followed by fusion produced better results.

The great polio epidemics of the 1940s and 1950s motivated further development of scoliosis treatment. John Cobb was an active proponent of spinal fusion and in 1952 reported on 672 cases treated over a 15-year period, with only a 4% rate of pseudarthrosis.[40] He emphasized the need for additional bone graft material to supplement Hibbs type fusions, and used autologous, donor, or cadaveric bone. Cobb insisted on a 6- to 9-month period of bed rest postoperatively.

Cobb also devised, in 1948, the method of measuring the size of a curve on a frontal X-ray film, which is still widely used today.[41]

## The Introduction of Bracing

Walter Blount in Milwaukee developed his brace, which was designed for postoperative support of the collapsing spine in poliomyelitis.[42,43] It initially sought to prop up the occiput and chin against the pelvis by distraction, but dental problems[44] led to the use of a choker and then to the realization that superstructure wasn't required, and that scoliosis could be treated nonoperatively with an underarm brace originally devised by John Hall in Boston.[45]

Notwithstanding the good results with spinal fusion reported by Cobb and Risser, these were not the norm, and indeed, Blount and colleagues, among 87 patients treated with spinal fusion and immobilization in a brace, reported a pseudarthrosis rate of almost 40%.[46] However, he did not routinely use facet joint fusions or an adequate period of immobilization.

Subsequently, John Moe, who developed the world-famous Twin Cities Scoliosis Treatment Center in Minneapolis, reported performing 266 spinal fusions in 1958, replicating Hibbs' method of careful dissection and facet joint fusion augmented with supplemental bone grafting.[47] Moe advocated fusion from neutral vertebra above to neutral vertebra below the scoliotic curve in the spine as his fusion levels, and with this the proportion of failed fusions fell to only 14%. However, cast correction and spinal fusion continued to mean 6 to 9 months of bed rest and hospitalization approaching a year, still without insignificant rates of fusion failure, infection, and loss of correction. In response to this, various attempts at using internal fixation methods were reported.

Allan in 1955 reported using an expandable jack-type device placed between the transverse processes,[48] and Gruca implanted springs on the convex side of the scoliotic curve fastened to the transverse processes at the end of the curve.[49]

## The Harrington Revolution

The development in 1955 by Paul Harrington in Houston, Texas, of his distraction and compression instrumentation was the most significant milestone in the development of effective scoliosis surgery.[50] For the first time there was a reliable means of obtaining and maintaining maximal deformity correction (**Fig. 1.3**). The driver for this was again the growing polio population, which did not well tolerate cast correction. Harrington conceived of his instrumentation as a means of halting curve progression, and regarded this as "dynamic correction" unaccompanied by spinal fusion. However, the early results were disappointing, with metalwork cut out and failure prompting the routine addition of spinal fusion to this procedure.

In 1966 Moe and Valuska published the results for 173 scoliosis patients treated by Harrington instrumentation and posterior fusion as compared with those for 100 patients treated with Risser localizer casting and fusion.[51] The instrumented group had greater correction (61% vs. 54%), was ambulatory sooner (2 $^1/_2$ months vs. 5 $^1/_2$ months), and was immobilized for a shorter period (7 months vs. 10 months). The pseudarthrosis rate in the two groups was similar (17% vs. 13%), but the instrumented group had more complications, with metalwork displacement occurring in 15%, and a greater rate of infection. Despite the apparent advantages of Harrington instrumentation, Moe said at the 1966 Paris meeting of the Société Internationale de Chirurgie Orthopédique et de Traumatologie (SICOT) that the general conclusion was that a good result of surgical treatment was an identical degree of curvature at the end of growth as when treatment had begun.

Harrington continued to improve his results, and this was demonstrated in a report of almost 600 cases in 1973.[52] He recommended a long fusion, from one vertebra above to two below the upper and lower end-vertebrae of the scoliotic region of spine, respectively. It was important that these levels fell within what Harrington described as the "stable zone" when parallel lines were drawn upward from the lumbosacral facet joints. Interestingly, despite Harrington's enormous improvement in spinal instrumentation, his early reports were published in the local writings of the Texas Institute of Rehabilitation and Research[53] because his articles were often turned down by the leading orthopedic journals, presumably because it was felt that his treatment was still somewhat revolutionary.

In 1973, Paul Harrington, then President of the Scoliosis Research Society (SRS) in Gothenburg, Sweden, recommended a common database or registry of all scoliosis surgeons to document their treatment results.[6] His lead was not followed by this group, but was taken up enthusiastically by surgeons who implanted hip and knee replacements.[54]

Some modifications were made of Harrington's original instrumentation, and so as to maintain a lumbar lordosis, Moe developed the square-ended rod-and-hook configuration for a better sagittal contour.[55] However, it was Harrington's original design that the distraction rod on the concave side be complemented by a compression system on the convex side that conferred considerable stability to

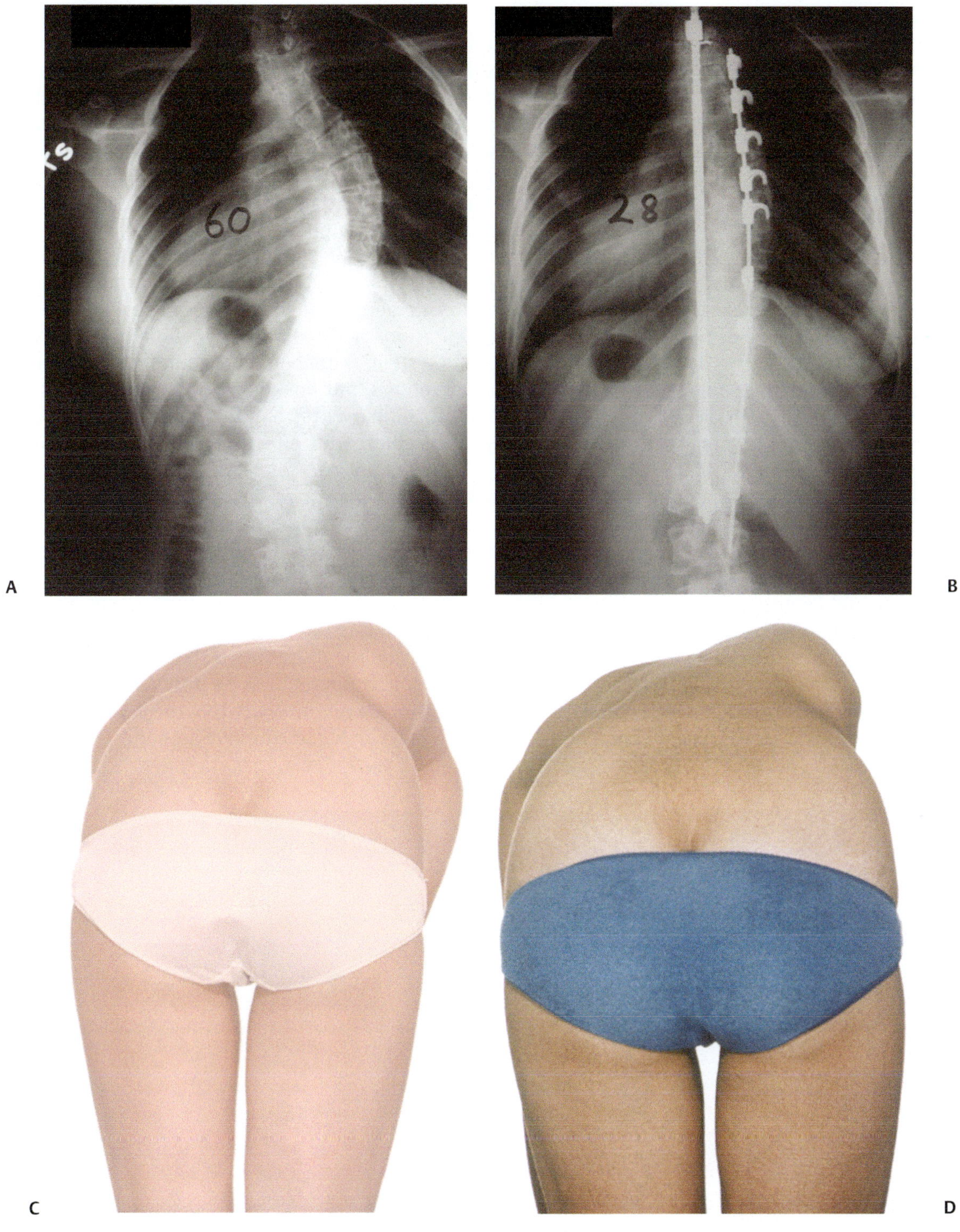


**Fig. 1.3** Harrington's operation. **(A)** Preoperative posteroanterior (PA) X-ray film of a thoracic curve. **(B)** Appearance after use of instrumentation for distraction and compression, showing a significant improvement in the frontal plane. **(C)** Rib hump before surgery. **(D)** Rib hump 2 years after surgery, showing that the deformity in the transverse plane has remained unaltered.

the construct.[56,57] Nevertheless, many practitioners ignored the compression system, which was one reason for the greater pseudarthrosis rates among their patients than among Harrington's.

Clearly, greater curves tended to be instrumented more often than lesser ones in the early years, and there was concern over neurological injury being caused by the rapid stretching of these rigid curves, which in turn led to the development of preoperative distraction devices. In 1959 Nickel and Perry designed the halo,[58] and various halo-traction devices were then developed, including those for halo-femoral traction by Moe,[55] halo-pelvic traction by DeWald,[59] and halo-wheelchair traction by Stagnara.[60]

## Segmental Instrumentation

In the late 1970s Resina and Alves in Portugal added wiring to the Harrington rod construct to provide better fixation and correction without the need for external immobilization.[61] This was followed in 1982 by the description by Eduardo Luque in Mexico of his system of two L-rods to which segmental sublaminar wires pulled the spine transversely to effect an improved correction with better stability (**Fig. 1.4**).[62] He also added cross-links to spread the load on the spine. Luque first used his system for neuromuscular curves, there being a high prevalence of poliomyelitis in Mexico at the time, but it soon became utilized for idiopathic curvatures of the spine.

To fix Luque's segmental instrumentation more solidly in paralytic curves, Allan and Ferguson devised the technique known as the Galveston technique, whereby the bottom short L of the L-rod construct could be passed across the posterior pelvis.[63]

However, although this improved frontal-plane correction with the instrumentation, there was no alteration in the size of the rib hump, which is what patients with idiopathic scoliosis most want to have treated. At the time it was still perceived that idiopathic thoracic scoliosis of adolescent onset was the potential cause of cardiopulmonary compromise in early adulthood,[64] and stabilizing the curve or obtaining modest correction were therefore the goal of treatment in this patient population. But in both France[65] and England[66] it was appreciated that the transverse-plane component of the deformity was secondary to the buckling of a lordosis in the sagittal plane, and thus that what the spine required was not so much distraction as derotation. Rather than developing new instrumentation, the Leeds Group modified the Harrington–Luque system by deliberately bending the Harrington rod into kyphosis and not distracting the rod until the concave sublaminar wires had lifted the depressed concavity in the spine, thus effecting significant derotation (**Fig. 1.5**). So as not to stretch the spinal canal and to render the middle portion of the curve more flexible, preliminary anterior multiple transthoracic discectomy was performed in a first stage of treatment.[67] This anterior discectomy procedure is sometimes called an anterior release, but this is not the case because it is the anterior spinal column that is too long in idiopathic scoliosis (as Adams knew), and the procedure is therefore not a release but a space-making operation with simultaneous removal of the growth plates anteriorly so that the excessively long anterior column would not continue growing.

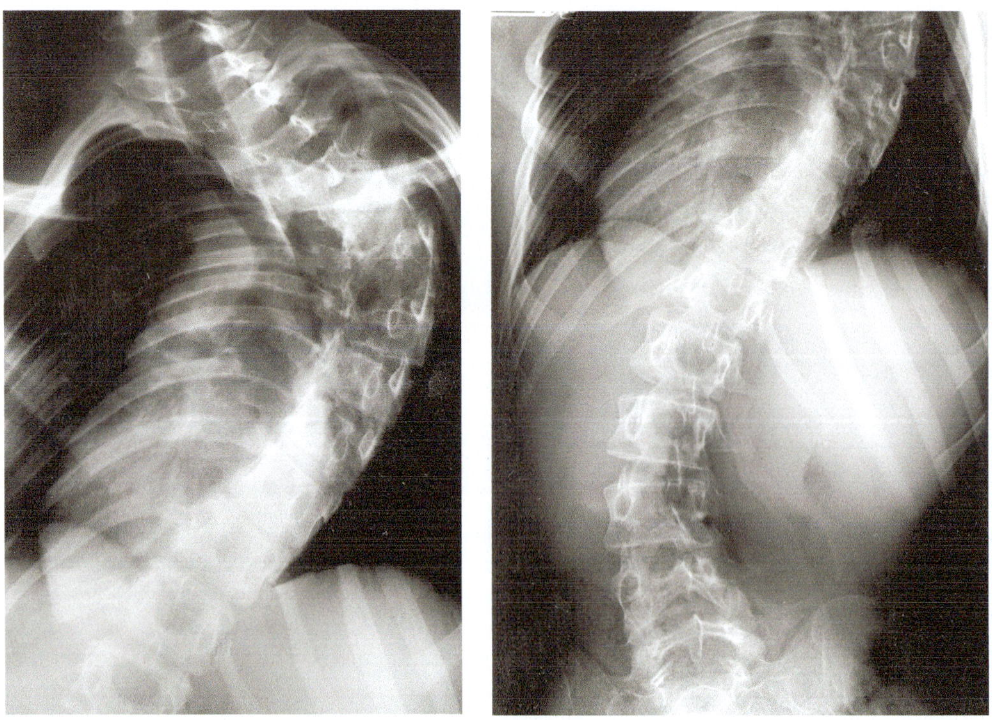
A B

**Fig. 1.4** Luque segmental L-rod instrumentation for a child with Friedreich's ataxia. **(A,B)** PA X-ray films before surgery.

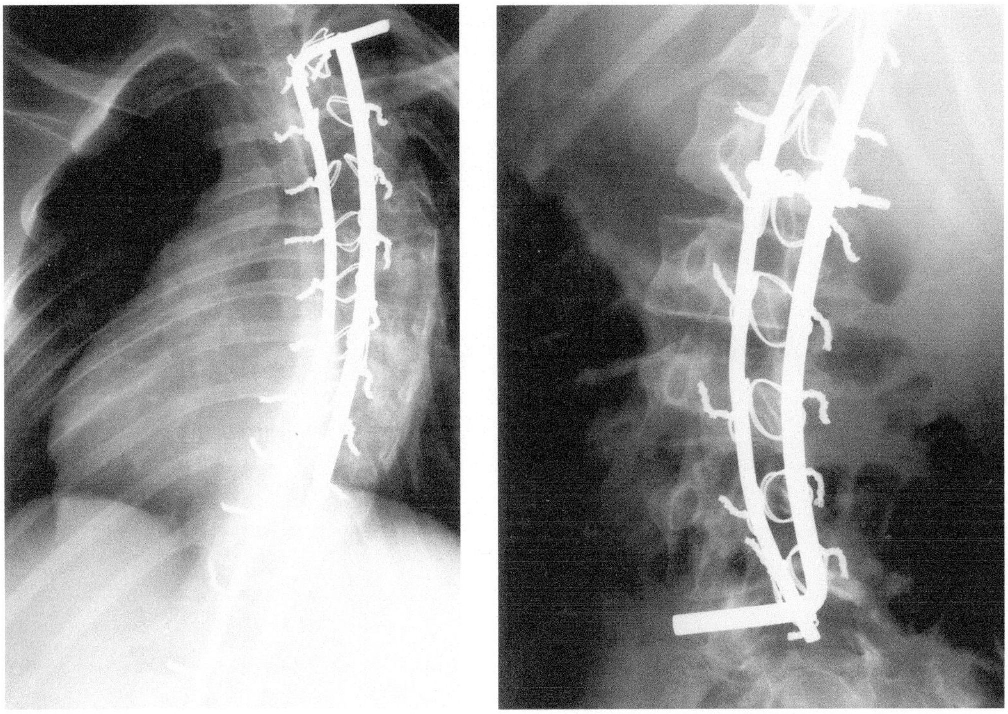

C D

**Fig. 1.4** (*Continued*) **(C,D)** PA X-ray films after instrumentation.

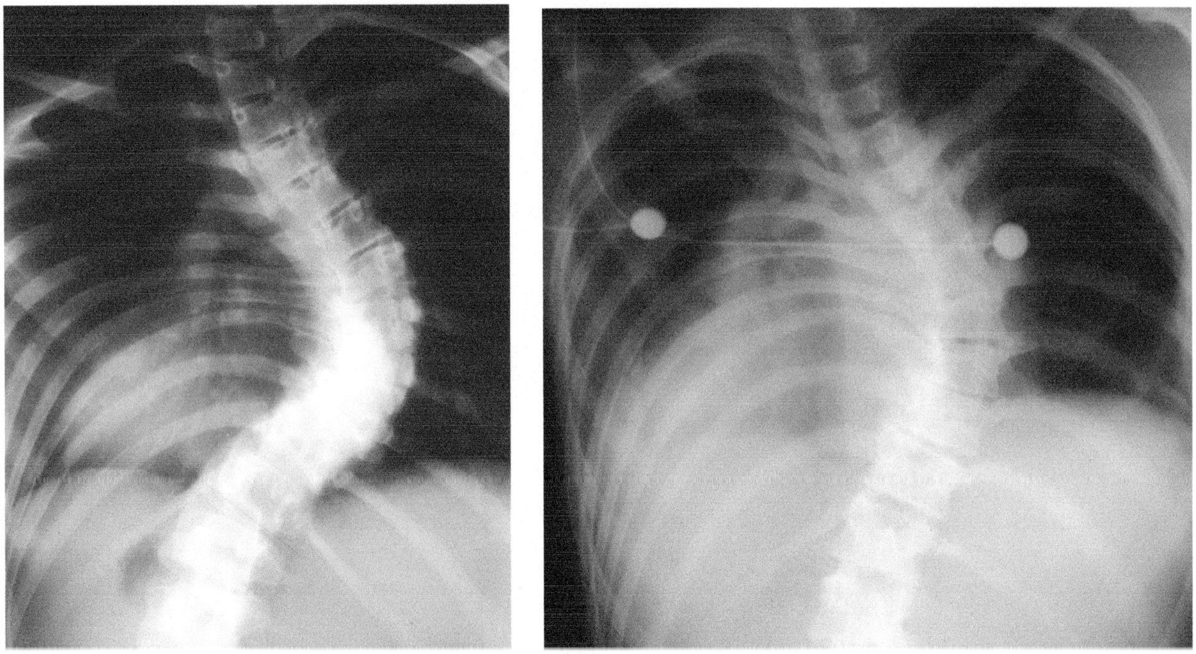

A B

**Fig. 1.5** The "Leeds Procedure." **(A)** PA X-ray film of a rigid 90-degree idiopathic thoracic curve. **(B)** PA X-ray film in recovery after anterior multiple discectomy (five discs removed). There has already been a 70% correction of the Cobb angle simply from shortening of the leading edge of the spinal deformity and allowing it to collapse into itself.

(*Continued on page 8*)

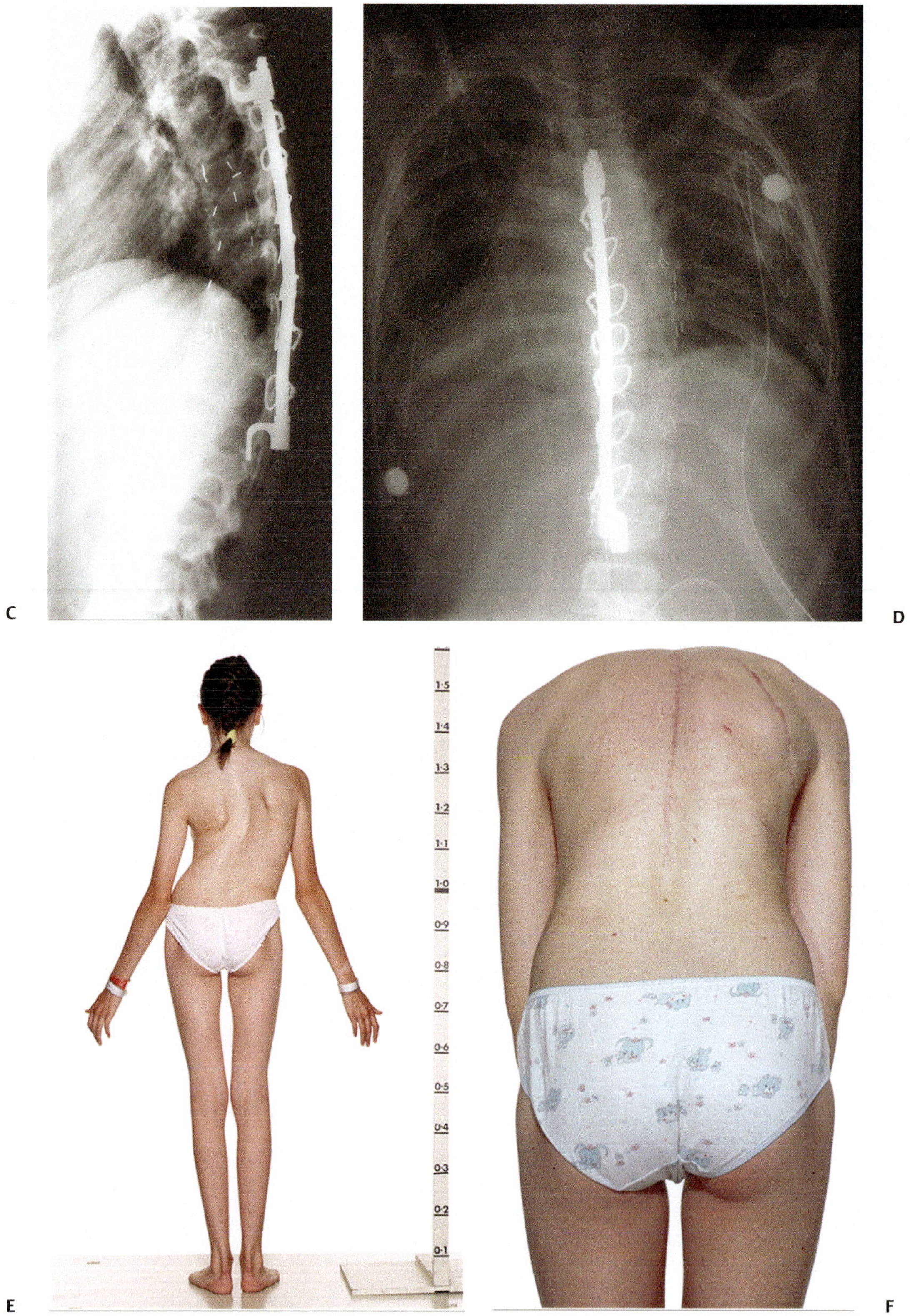


**Fig. 1.5** (*Continued*) The "Leeds Procedure." **(C)** In the second stage of instrumentation, the rod has been pre-bent to restore kyphosis, and the concave sublaminar wires now pull backward to derotate the spine. **(D)** PA view after instrumentation, showing almost complete restoration of rotation and rib asymmetry. **(E)** Preoperative PA view of the patient's severe deformity. **(F)** Postoperative appearance, showing virtually complete correction.

In France, Cotrel and Dubousset devised a revolutionary new system of spinal instrumentation[68] (known as the "French Revolution"), upon which all third-generation posterior constructs are based (**Fig. 1.6**). This was a two-rod system, with one rod for the concave side and one for the convex side of the scoliotic curve, with multiple hooks on each rod so that segments of the spine could be compressed or distracted on the same rod. Importantly, before final tightening the concave rod was turned from the frontal to the sagittal plane, thus producing derotation and restoration of apical thoracic kyphosis.

Modern two-rod systems continue to make use of the ability to compress and distract different segments of the spine, but do not involve the concave-rod rotational maneuver originally described by Cotrel and Dubousset.

Improved fixation of treatment devices to bone has been achieved with multiple transpedicular screws, and it is possible, by using screws bilaterally at each level, to correct deformities of appreciable size without recourse to anterior discectomies, and by going only from one end-vertebra to the other; so powerful is the system that it will drag into line the vertebrae above and below the end-vertebrae (**Fig. 1.7**).[69]

## The Development of Anterior Surgical Procedures

The twentieth century also saw the development of anterior spinal surgical techniques. In 1934 Ito described anterior surgery for tuberculosis of the spine,[70] which was then popularized by Arthur Hodgson in Hong Kong, again initially for treating tuberculosis of the spine.[71] By resecting diseased bone and other necrotic material, Hodgson effectively excised the disease, correcting the deficit by strut grafting from the iliac crest. This was particularly important because many patients were not compliant in taking their medications. In 1965 Hodgson turned his surgical expertise with the anterior spine to the problems of congenital scoliosis,[72] but his opening wedge osteotomy caused a high incidence of paralysis by stretching the spinal cord.

Anterior resection of congenital vertebral anomalies goes back to Royle in 1928,[73] whose work was followed by Compere,[74] Von Lackum and Smith,[75] and Wiles.[76] These had only varying degrees of success, and also had high complication rates. However, in 1973 Leatherman published his classic paper on closing wedge osteotomy for rigid spinal curves,[77] whereby a suitably sized wedge of bone was excised at the

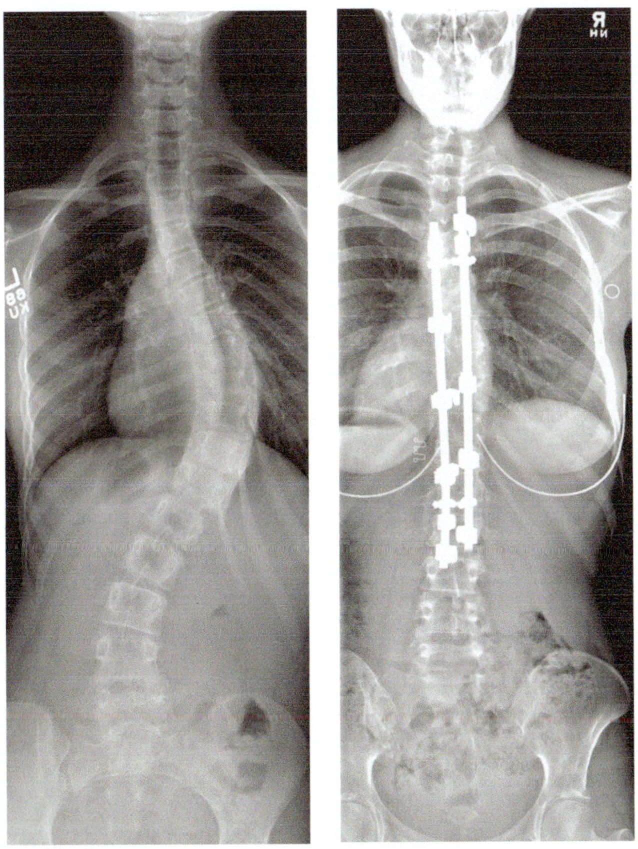

A,B

**Fig. 1.6** Cotrel–Dubousset instrumentation. **(A)** PA X-ray film of a thoracic curve. **(B)** PA X-ray film after Cotrel–Dubousset instrumentation.

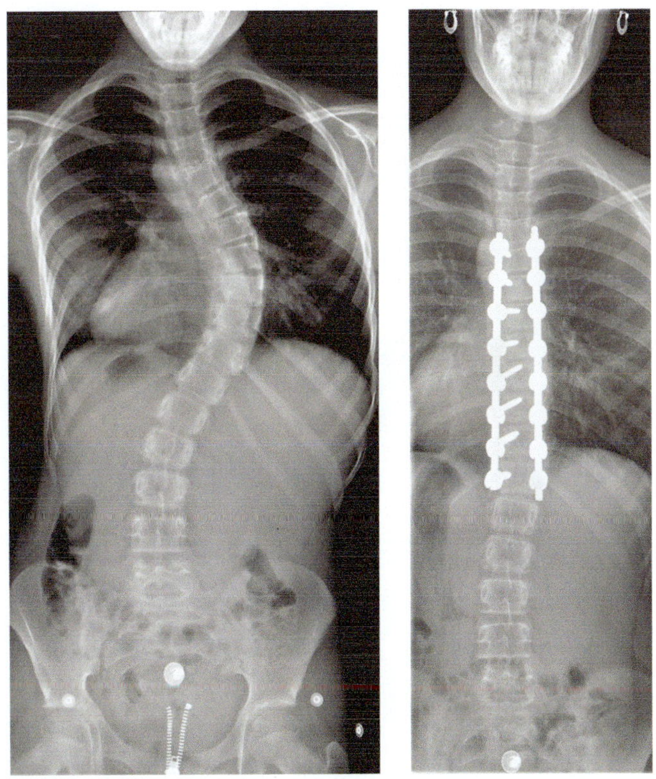

A,B

**Fig. 1.7** **(A)** PA X-ray film of a thoracic curve. **(B)** Appearance after use of end-vertebra-to-end-vertebra bilateral transpedicular screw instrumentation.

curve apex based on the convex side, the anterior vertebral body being excised in the first stage, and the back of the wedge then being excised in a second stage, followed by closure of the wedge. Initially, without Harrington instrumentation, Leatherman had difficulty closing his wedges and had to use unsatisfactory constructs such as staples. The advent of the Harrington compression system solved his problems, and permitted the wedge to be closed in a controlled manner, followed by the insertion of a Harrington distraction rod on the concave side of the curve for increased stability (**Fig. 1.8**).[78]

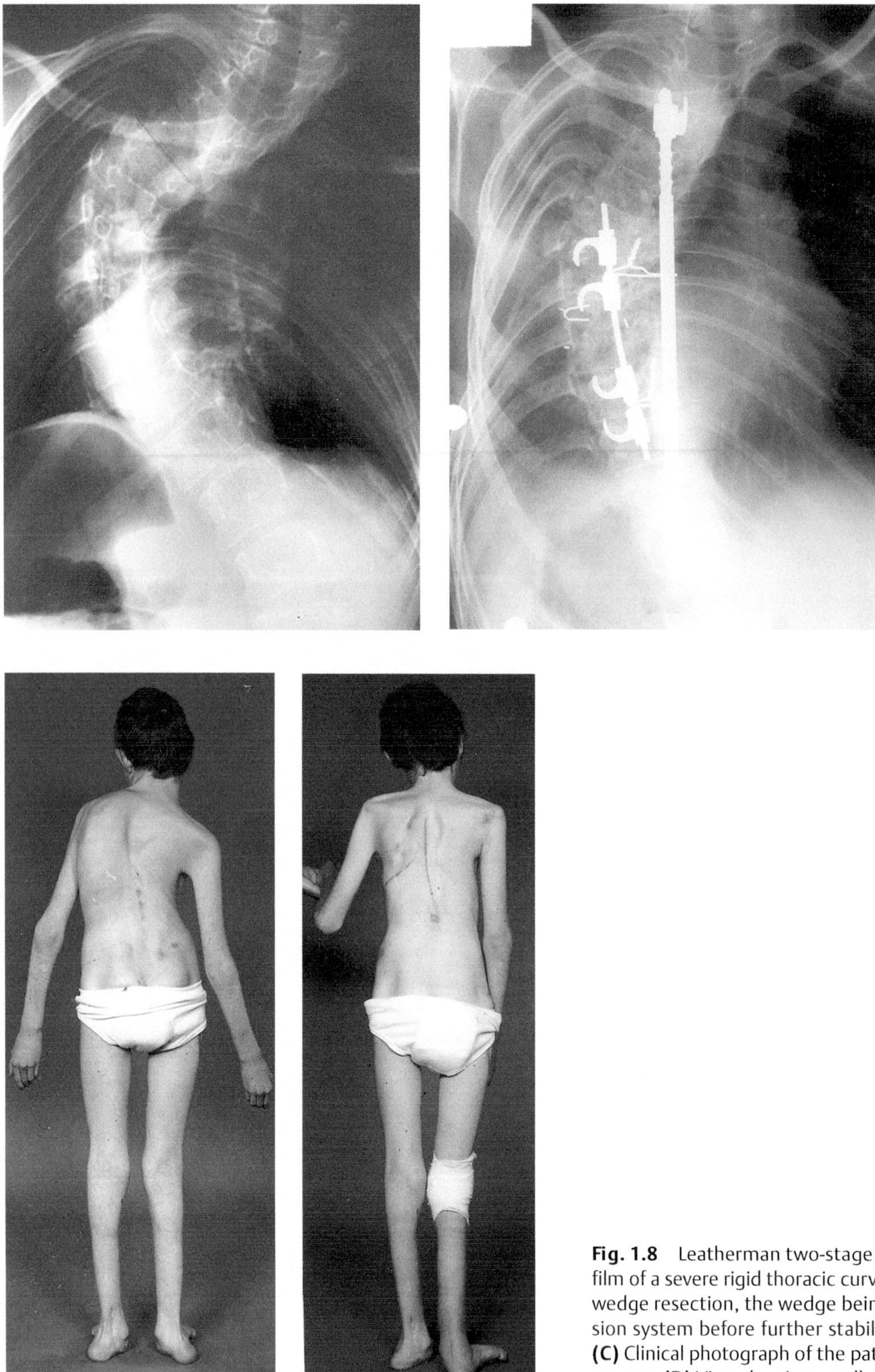

A B C,D

**Fig. 1.8** Leatherman two-stage wedge resection. **(A)** PA X-ray film of a severe rigid thoracic curve. **(B)** PA X-ray film after apical wedge resection, the wedge being first closed by the compression system before further stabilization with a distraction rod. **(C)** Clinical photograph of the patient's severe deformity before surgery. **(D)** View showing excellent correction after surgery.

Today, osteotomies can be performed posteriorly by subtraction techniques[79] based on Heinig's description of his decancellation egg-shell procedure in 1984.[80]

## The Introduction of Anterior Instrumentation

Anterior instrumentation for idiopathic scoliosis was first described by Dwyer et al in Australia in the 1960s (**Fig. 1.9**).[81] He passed screws transversely across the apical vertebral bodies, having resected the intervertebral discs and growth plates down to endplate bone. The screws had holes in their heads through which was passed a braided metal cable. At each level of the scoliotic curve the screw heads were compressed to shorten the curve convexity, and were then crimped over the cable to maintain correction. Dwyer and Schaefer described this particularly for idiopathic scoliosis, but scoliosis[82] surgeons in many countries worldwide initially adopted this instrumentation for patients with paralytic scoliosis because they felt that it might constitute dangerous overtreatment for idiopathic deformities. Because the intervertebral discs were removed in Dwyer's technique, the area of instrumentation was reduced, and this was a very safe procedure with regard to neurological complications. It also produced excellent corrections for thoracolumbar and lumbar curves without requiring extensive posterior instrumentation. This allowed the retention of mobile segments below the construct, as well as the ability to maintain lumbar lordosis.

In Germany, Klaus Zielke modified the Dwyer system, using a threaded compression rod in place of the braided cable (**Fig. 1.10**).[83] This was an excellent design and was a forerunner of modern anterior smooth-rod systems for treating scoliosis. Although Zielke's technique of lordosation worked well for the lumbar spine, it did not work in the thoracic spine, in which the anterior column is already lordotic. Jurgen Harms promoted the concept of kyphosing the thoracic spine with anterior instrumentation.[84]

## The Young Scoliosis Patient

One of the most difficult scoliotic deformities to treat is the infantile idiopathic progressive curve, and Mehta[85] in England and Morrell[86] in France first devised and used serial plaster cast treatment for this under light general anesthesia, with the casts changed every 2 or 3 months with growth, until the end of the third year of life if necessary (**Fig. 1.11**). This capitalized on the infantile growth spurt and the ability of the plaster cast to mold the more malleable infantile skeleton. Such casts are still used today, and if referral to a

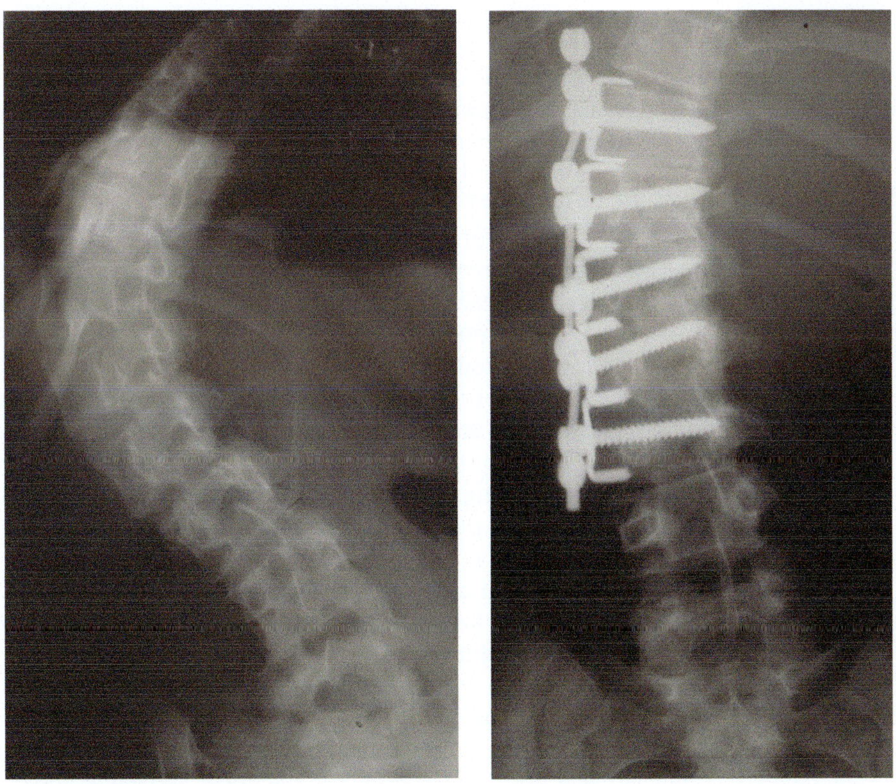

A B

**Fig. 1.9** The Dwyer procedure. **(A)** PA X-ray film of a 90-degree thoracolumbar curve. **(B)** PA X-ray film 2 years later, showing excellent correction with only four inter-vertebral joints fused.

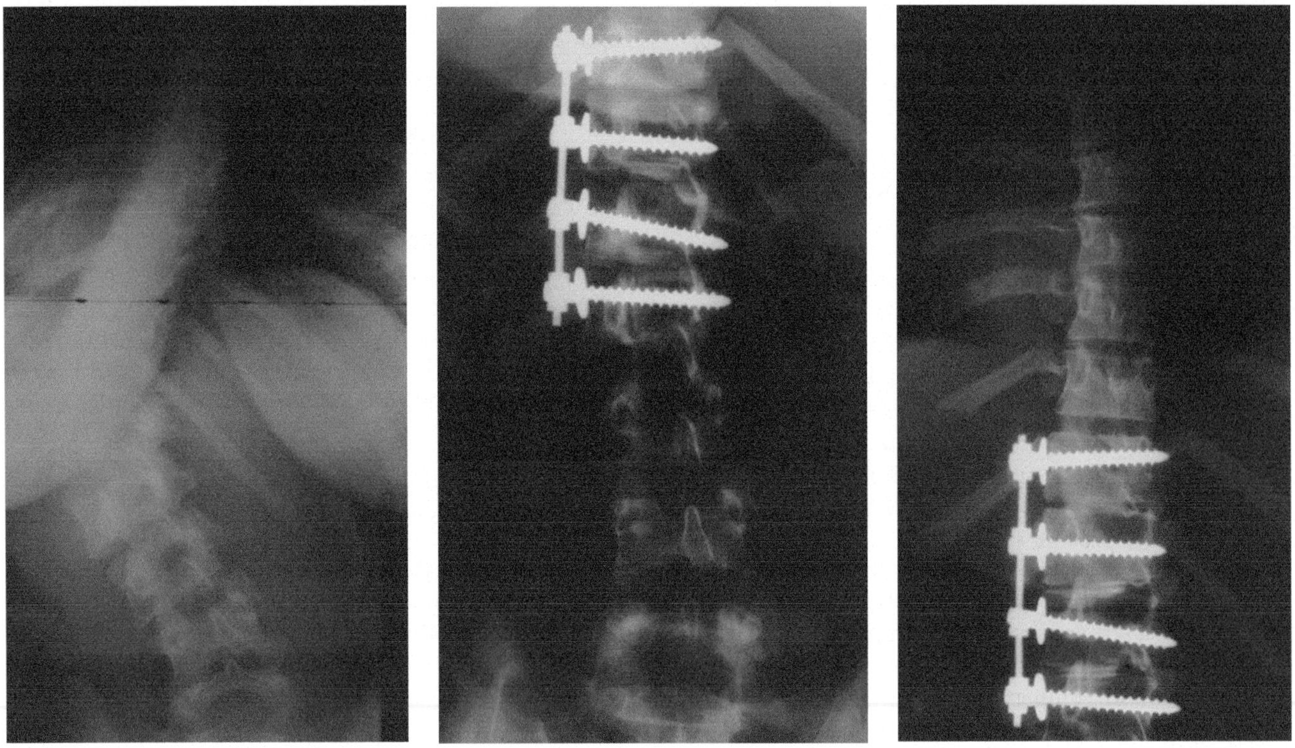
A–C

**Fig. 1.10** The Zielke procedure. **(A)** PA X-ray film of a 70-degree thoracolumbar curve. **(B,C)** PA X-ray films 2 years postoperatively. The entire thoracolumbar spine has been restacked with the use of only four screws and fusion of only three inter-vertebral joints.

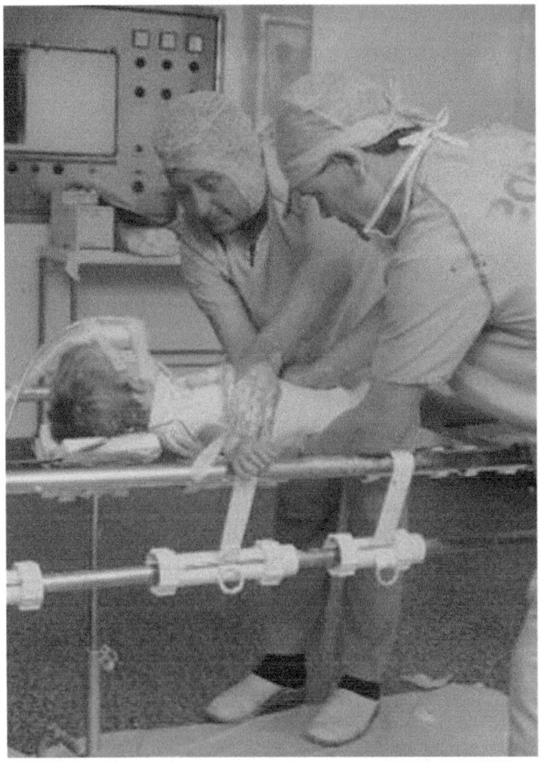

**Fig. 1.11** Applying an elongation–derotation–flexion (EDF) cast to an infant with progressive idiopathic scoliosis: an essential form of treatment. This treatment may need to be repeated every 2 or 3 months until the patient reaches the age of 4 years.

scoliosis center is not delayed, this treatment can be very effective in correcting deformities or at least preventing their progression. This is important because only deformities beginning before the age of 5 years militate against good cardiopulmonary health in adulthood. Mehta described measurement of the the rib–vertebra angle difference (RVAD), and if this was more than 20 degrees, progression was likely.[87]

For deformities that do not respond to cast treatment, surgical treatment is necessary, and because the essential lesion in early-onset scoliosis is, like that in late-onset disease, a lordosis in the sagittal plane, it would be extremely counterproductive to do a posterior fusion, which would further tether the back of the spine and induce what is described as the crankshaft phenomenon, whereby anterior growth continues against a posterior tether, thus actually accelerating progression of the deformity. Roaf in Liverpool tried to halt the growth of the antero-convex side of the spine by way of convex hemi-epiphysiodesis,[88] but by the time the biology caught up with fusion, the biomechanics of the buckling lordosis in early-onset scoliosis had led to unacceptable progression.[89,90]

Moe in 1984 described the use of a subcutaneous Harrington rod for the treatment of progressive curves in very young children while allowing growth to continue.[91] This was possible because only the upper and lower hooks were subperiosteal, the rest of the rod running extraperiosteally through or superficial to the paraspinal muscle. At repeated

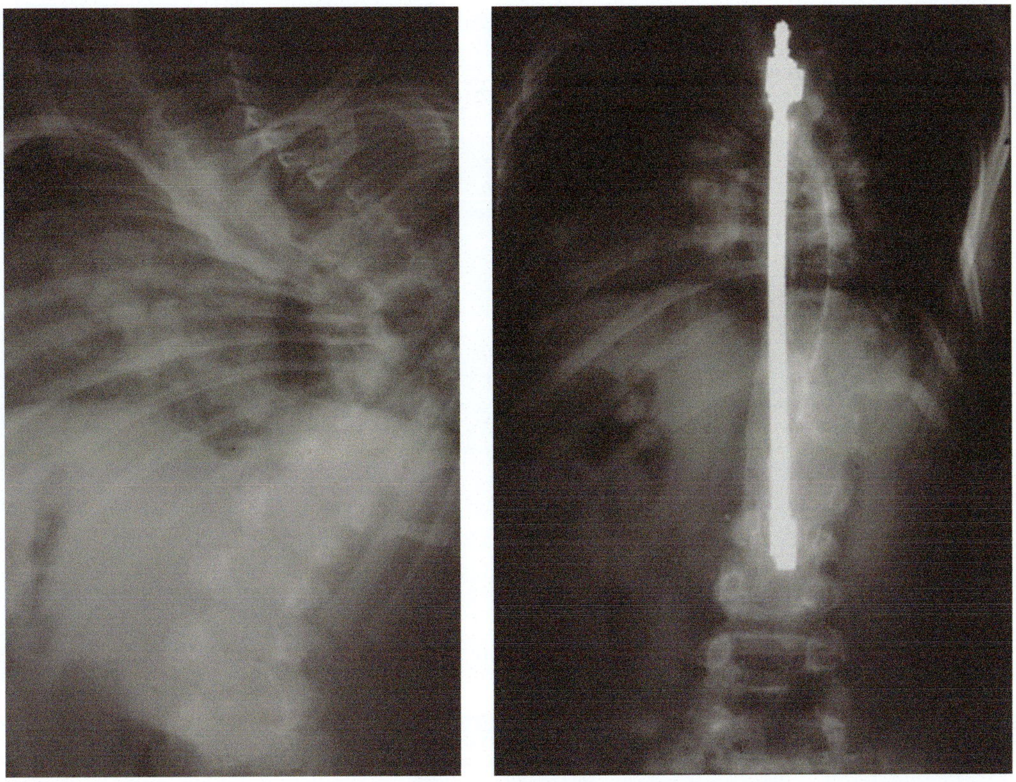

A B

**Fig. 1.12** The use of a subcutaneous growing rod. **(A)** PA X-ray film showing a 100-degree thoracic curve in a boy aged 6 years. **(B)** PA X-ray film 10 years after anterior multiple thoracic discectomy and the insertion of a growing rod, which was lengthened or exchanged 12 times.

intervals of 6 months to a year, the rod could be extended as the child grew (**Fig. 1.12**). Leatherman popularized the Luque trolley procedure (L-rods with sublaminar wires without fusion) to allow continued spinal growth. This can be done with one rod and wires (**Fig. 1.13**). The same principle of allowing posterior spinal growth can be achieved with modern third-generation spinal instrumentation systems.

More recently, Roaf's principles have been recycled in the form of epiphyseal stapling,[92] and attention has also been directed to using rib distractors to prevent progression of scoliosis in the young patient.[93]

What is important in treating scoliosis of early onset, apart from not tethering the posterior part of the spine, is to stop anterior growth of the lordosis by multiple anterior discectomy and growth-plate removal followed by use of a stable posterior construct.

## Conclusion

Both Hippocrates in the fifth century BC and Galen in the second century AD described scoliosis and devices for treating it. In France in the sixteenth century, Paré described congenital scoliosis, and in 1780 Venel developed a brace for scoliosis. In the late noneteenth century Volkman was the first to describe costoplasty. William Adams in England, at the same time, dissected cadavers with structural scoliosis and noted that through the apex of the deformity the front of the spine was longer than the back. He described the pathogenesis of idiopathic scoliosis by saying that "lordosis plus rotation equals lateral flexion."

In the late nineteenth and early twentieth centuries, Harda, Lange, and Wreden used metal implants to treat scoliosis. In 1911 Albee described bone grafting to the spine using a tibial strut, and Hibbs in New York treated scoliosis with his subperiosteal fusion procedure. Then Risser, along with Hibbs, described the preoperative turnbuckle cast. In the early 1950s Risser described the preoperative localizer cast, and 1952 John Cobb reported 672 cases of spinal fusion with only a 1% pseudarthrosis rate.

In 1958 Blount described the Milwaukee brace, which was refined by Hall in Boston into an underarm variant.

The first meaningful instrumentation for correcting scoliosis was described by Paul Harrington in Texas in 1955, and revolutionized the surgical management of scoliosis. In Minneapolis John Moe soon adopted Harrington instrumentation. Following this, Resina in Portugal and Luque in Mexico described using segmental wiring to rods. In 1986, the importance of the lordotic component of the scoliotic deformity was confirmed in both France and England, and treatment strategies were designed to primarily derotate the spine. This led to the development of Cotrel–Dubousett

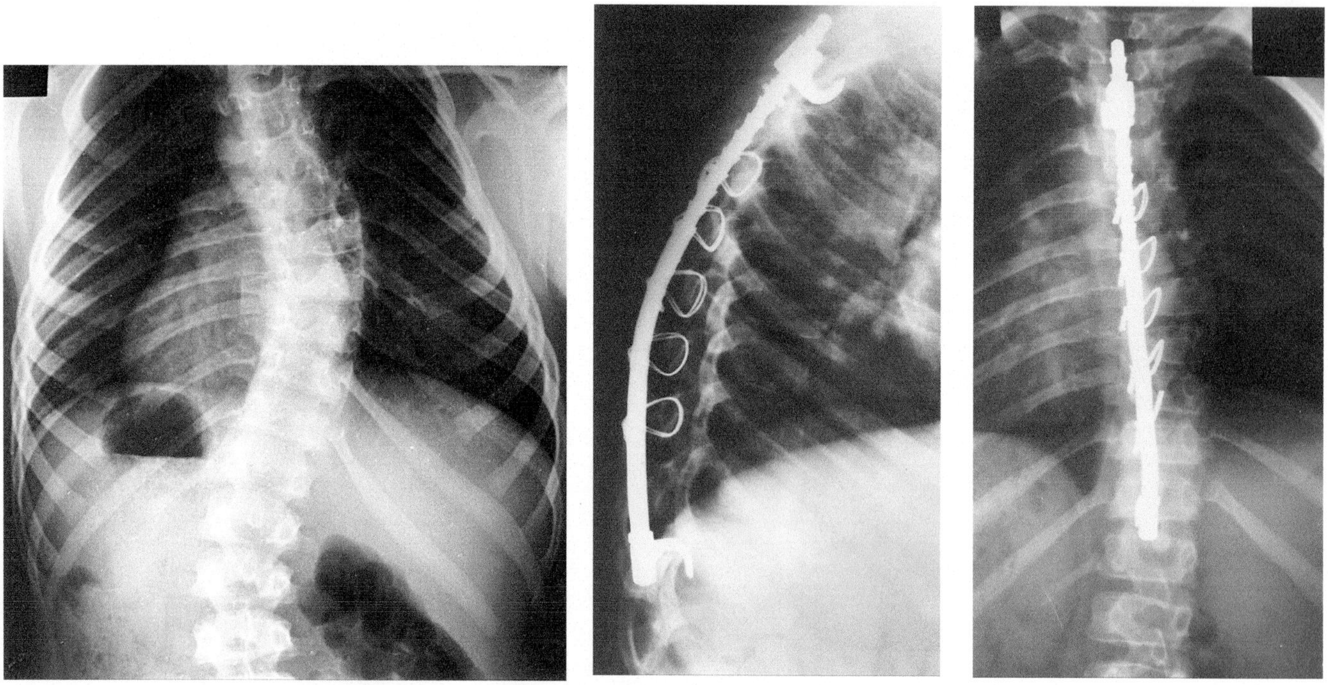

A–C

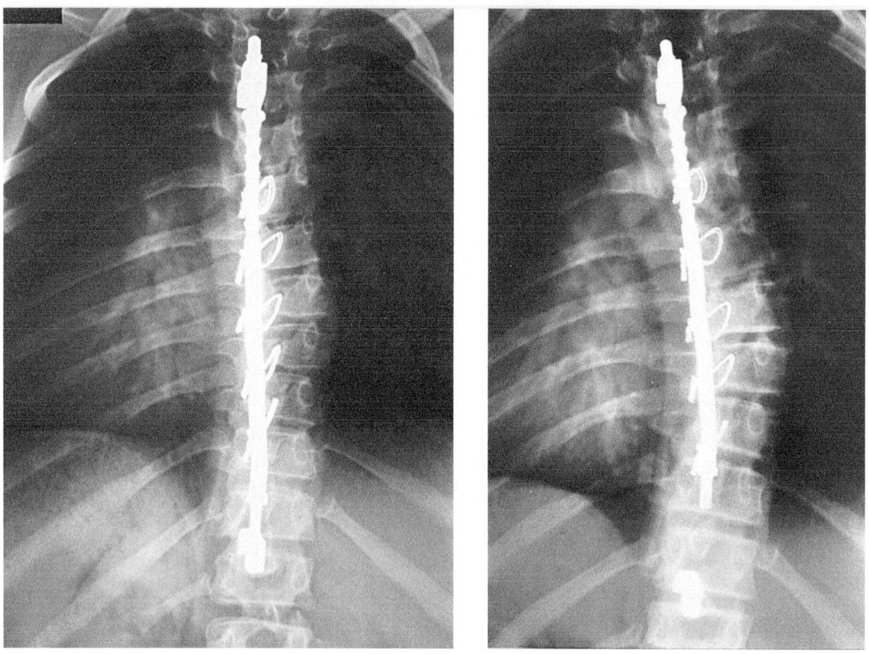

D,E

**Fig. 1.13** PA X-ray films of a patient with infantile idiopathic scoliosis treated with serial EDF casting but whose scoliosis was still progressing at the age of 5 years. **(A)** PA X-ray film before surgery. **(B)** Lateral X-ray film after segmental instrumentation without fusion. **(C)** PA X-ray film after surgery, showing that the kyphosis has been restored so as to stop subsequent buckling. **(D)** PA X-ray film made 3 years after surgery, showing that the lower end of the rod has come out of the lower hook, indicating growth. **(E)** PA X-ray film made when the patient was a teenager, showing very considerable growth of the affected part of the spine, and that elevation of the periosteum for insertion of the sublaminar wires did not prevent spinal growth. At maturity, the metalwork was removed and the correction was maintained.

instrumentation, on which modern two-rod instrumentation systems are based. Attention was turned to instrumentation of the anterior side of the spine by Dwyer in Australia in the 1960s. His instrumentation system was refined by Zielke in Germany and applied by Harms in the thoracic region to deliberately kyphose the spine.

For the dangerous early-onset idiopathic form of scoliosis, Mehta in London and Morrell in France devised the application of small plaster jackets to mold the infantile spine. Because posterior fusion is illogical for early-onset scoliosis, Roaf in Liverpool described hemi-epiphysiodesis in an effort to restrict growth at the leading edge of the deformity in scoliosis, and this has more recently been used to provide support through stapling. To stop posterior fusion, Moe developed the subcutaneous posterior rod, which can be lengthened with childhood growth.

If more was known about the natural history of idiopathic scoliosis throughout growth, it might be possible to devise even more truly biological approaches to the management of this complex three-dimensional deformity.

## References


1. Halter U, Krödel A. [Praying for the hunchback man. On the cultural history of scoliosis and kyphosis]. Z Orthop Ihre Grenzgeb 1997;135:557–562
2. Jones WHS. Hippocrates (4 vols). London: Heinemann; 1922–1931.
3. Huebert HT. Scoliosis. A brief history. Manit Med Rev 1967;47: 452–456
4. Kumar K. Spinal deformity and axial traction. Spine 1996;21: 653–655
5. Rang M. The Story of Orthopaedics. Philadelphia: WB Saunders; 2000:381–382
6. Moen KY, Nachemson AL. Treatment of scoliosis. An historical perspective. Spine 1999;24:2570–2575
7. Rang M. The Story of Orthopaedics. Philadelphia: WB Saunders; 2000:8–9
8. Rang M. The Story of Orthopaedics. Philadelphia: WB Saunders; 2000:161
9. Rang M. The Story of Orthopaedics. Philadelphia: WB Saunders; 2000:199
10. Böni T, Rüttimann B, Dvorak J, Sandler A. Historical perspectives: Jean-André Venel. Spine 1994;19:2007–2011
11. Rang M. The Story of Orthopaedics. Philadelphia: WB Saunders; 2000:154
12. Rang M. The Story of Orthopaedics. Philadelphia: WB Saunders, 2000:334
13. Rang M. The Story of Orthopaedics. Philadelphia: WB Saunders, 2000:160
14. Malgaigne JF. De quelques illusions orthopédiques, a l'occasion du rélève general du service orthopédique de MJ Guerin. J Chir (Paris) 1843;1:256–265
15. Rang M. The Story of Orthopaedics. Philadelphia: WB Saunders; 2000:377
16. Hall JE. Spinal surgery before and after Paul Harrington. Spine 1998;23:1356–1361
17. Maas R. Verhandlung Deutsche Orthopädische Gesellschaft 1914; 13:376
18. Tolo VT. Progression in scoliosis. A 360 degree change in 75 years. Spine 1983;8:373–377
19. Sayre JW. Lewis Albert Sayre. Spine 1995;20: 1091–1096
20. Adams W. Lectures on the Pathology and Treatment of Lateral and Other Forms of Curvature of the Spine. London: Churchill and Sons; 1865
21. Rang M. The Story of Orthopaedics. Philadelphia: WB Saunders; 2000:153
22. Rang M. The Story of Orthopaedics. Philadelphia: WB Saunders; 2000:22–23
23. Rang M. The Story of Orthopaedics. Philadelphia: WB Saunders; 2000:417–421
24. Howorth MB. Evolution of spinal fusion. Ann Surg 1943;117: 278–289
25. Wreden. Zentralorgan der gesellschaft der gesamten chirurgie und ihrer grenzgebiete, 1923:434
26. Rang M. The Story of Orthopaedics. Philadelphia: WB Saunders; 2000:318
27. Rang M. The Story of Orthopaedics. Philadelphia: WB Saunders; 2000:319–321
28. Albee F. Transplantation of a portion of the tibia into the spine for Potti disease: A preliminary report. JAMA 1911;57:885–886
29. DeQuervain F, Hoessly H. Operative immobilisation of the spine. Surg Gynecol Obstet 1917;24:428–436
30. Albee FH, Kuscher R. The Albee spine fusion operation in the treatment of scoliosis surgery. Gynecol Obstet 1938;66:797–803
31. Rang M. The Story of Orthopaedics. Philadelphia: WB Saunders; 2000.
32. Hibbs RA. A report of fifty-nine cases of scoliosis treated by fusion operation. J Bone Joint Surg 1924;6:3–19. (Reprinted from Clin Orthop 1988;229:4–20)
33. Hibbs RA, Risser JC, Ferguson AB. Scoliosis treated by the fusion operation. End-result study of three hundred and sixty cases. J Bone Joint Surg 1931;13:91–104
34. Steindler A. Diseases and Deformities of the Spine and Thorax. St Louis: CV Mosby; 1929
35. Risser JC, Lauder CH, Norquist DM, Cruis WA. Three types of body casts. Instr Course Lect 1953;10:131–142
36. Risser JC. The iliac apophysis: An invaluable sign in the management of scoliosis. Clin Orthop Rel Res 1958;11:111–119
37. Bernick S, Cailliet R. Vertebral end-plate changes with aging of human vertebrae. Spine 1982;7:97–102
38. Howell FR, Mahood JK, Dickson RA. Growth beyond skeletal maturity. Spine 1992;17:437–440
39. Research Committee of the American Orthopaedic Association. End result study of the treatment of idiopathic scoliosis. J Bone Joint SurgAm 1941;23:963–977
40. Cobb JR. Technique, after-treatment, and results of spine fusion for scoliosis. In: Edwards JW, ed. Instructional Course Lectures. Ann Arbor: American Academy of Orthopaedic Surgeons, 1952; vol 9:65–70
41. Cobb JR. Outline for the study of scoliosis. Instr Course Lect 1948;5:261
42. Blount WP. Scoliosis and the Milwaukee brace. Bull Hosp Joint Dis 1958;19:152–165
43. Blount WP, Moe JH. The Milwaukee Brace. Baltimore: Williams & Wilkins; 1973
44. Alexander RG. The effects on tooth position and maxillofacial vertical growth during treatment of scoliosis with the Milwaukee brace. Am J Orthod 1966;52:161–189
45. Watts HG, Hall JE, Stanish W. The Boston brace system for the treatment of low thoracic and lumbar scoliosis by the use of a girdle without superstructure. Clin Orthop Relat Res 1977;126: 87–92
46. Blount WP, Schmidt AC, Keever ED, Leonard ET. The Milwaukee brace in the operative treatment of scoliosis. J Bone Joint Surg Am 1958;40A:511–525
47. Moe JH. A critical analysis of methods of fusion for scoliosis; An evaluation in two hundred and sixty-six patients. J Bone Joint Surg Am 1958;40A:529–554, passim
48. Allan FG. Scoliosis: Operative correction of fixed curves. J Bone Joint Surg Br 1955;37-B:92–96
49. Gruca A. The pathogenesis and treatment of idiopathic scoliosis; a preliminary report. J Bone Joint Surg Am 1958;40A:570–584
50. Harrington PR. Treatment of scoliosis. Correction and internal fixation by spine instrumentation. J Bone Joint Surg Am 1962;44A: 591–610
51. Moe JH, Valuska JW. Evaluation of treatment of scoliosis by Harrington instrumentation. J Bone Joint Surg Am 1966;48A:1656–1657

52. Dickson JH, Dickson SH. An eleven-year clinical investigation of Harrington instrumentation. A preliminary report on 578 cases. Clin Orthop Relat Res 1973;93:113–130
53. Harrington PR. Scoliosis 1972. Summary 1962–1971. Report of the Texas Institute for Rehabilitation and Research. Houston, TX
54. Herberts P, Malchau H. How outcome studies have changed total hip arthroplasty practices in Sweden. Clin Orthop Relat Res 1997;344:44–60
55. Moe JH. Modern concepts of treatment of spinal deformities in children and adults. Clin Orthop Relat Res 1980;150:137–153
56. Harrington PR. Technical details in relation to the successful use of instrumentation in scoliosis. Orthop Clin North Am 1972;3:49–67
57. Gaines RW, Leatherman KD. Benefits of the Harrington compression system in lumbar and thoracolumbar idiopathic scoliosis in adolescents and adults. Spine 1981;6:483–488
58. Nickel VL, Perry J, Garrett A, Heppenstall M. The halo. A spinal skeletal traction fixation device. J Bone Joint Surg Am 1968;50:1400–1409
59. Dewald RL, Ray RD. Skeletal traction for the treatment of severe scoliosis. The University of Illinois halo-hoop apparatus. J Bone Joint Surg Am 1970;52:233–238
60. Stagnara P, Mauroy JC, Gonon GP, et al. Scolioses cyphosantes de L'adulte et greffes antérieures. Int Orthop 1978;2:149–165
61. Resina J, Alves AF. A technique of correction and internal fixation for scoliosis. J Bone Joint Surg Br 1977;59:159–165
62. Luque ER. Segmental spinal instrumentation for correction of scoliosis. Clin Orthop Relat Res 1982;163:192–198
63. Allen BL Jr, Ferguson RL. The Galveston technique for L rod instrumentation of the scoliotic spine. Spine 1982;7:276–284
64. Nachemson AL. A long term follow-up study of non-treated scoliosis. Acta Orthop Scand 1968;39:466–476
65. Dubousset J, Graf H, Miladi L, et al. Spinal and thoracic derotation with CD instrumentation. Orthop Trans 1986;10:36
66. Archer IA, Deacon P, Dickson RA. Idiopathic scoliosis in Leeds: A management philosophy. J Bone Joint Surg Br 1986;68B:670
67. Dickson RA. Idiopathic scoliosis: Foundation for physiological treatment. Ann R Coll Surg Engl 1987;69:89–96
68. Cotrel Y, Dubousset J, Guillaumat M. New universal instrumentation in spinal surgery. Clin Orthop Relat Res 1988;227:10–23
69. Newton PO, Faro FD, Lenke LG, et al. Factors involved in the decision to perform a selective versus nonselective fusion of Lenke 1B and 1C (King-Moe II) curves in adolescent idiopathic scoliosis. Spine 2003;28:S217–S223
70. Ito H, Tsuchiya J, Asami GA. A new radical operation for Pott's disease. J Bone Joint Surg 1934;16:499–515
71. Hodgson AR, Stock FE. Anterior spinal fusion a preliminary communication on the radical treatment of Pott's disease and Pott's paraplegia. Br J Surg 1956;44:266–275
72. Hodgson AR. Correction of fixed spinal curves. J Bone Joint Surg Am1965;47:1221–1227
73. Royle ND. The operative removal of an accessory vertebra. Med J Aust 1928;1:467
74. Compere EL. Excision of hemivertebrae for correction of congenital scoliosis. J Bone Joint Surg 1932;14:555–562
75. Von Lackum HL, Smith A de F. Removal of vertebral bodies in the treatment of scoliosis. Surg Gynecol Obstet 1933;53:250–256
76. Wiles P. Resection of dorsal vertebrae in congenital scoliosis. J Bone Joint SurgAm 1951; 33A, 151–154
77. Leatherman KD. The management of rigid spinal curves. Clin Orthop Relat Res 1973;93:215–224
78. Leatherman KD, Dickson RA. Two stage corrective surgery for congenital spine deformities. J Bone Joint SurgBr 1977;59B:497
79. Ondra SL, Marzouk S, Koski T, Silva F, Salehi S. Mathematical calculation of pedicle subtraction osteotomy size to allow precision correction of fixed sagittal deformity. Spine 2006; 31:E973–E979
80. Heinig CF. Eggshell procedure. In: Luque ER, ed. Segmental Spinal Instrumentation. Thorofare, NJ: Slack Inc.; 1984
81. Dwyer AF, Newton NC, Sherwood AA. An anterior approach to scoliosis. A preliminary report. Clin Orthop Relat Res 1969;62: 192–202
82. Dwyer AF, Schafer MF. Anterior approach to scoliosis. Results of treatment in fifty-one cases. J Bone Joint Surg Br 1974;56: 218–224
83. Zielke K, Berthet A. [VDS—ventral derotation spondylodesis: Preliminary report on 58 cases]. Beitr Orthop Traumatol 1978;25: 85–103
84. Betz RR, Harms J, Clements DH III, et al. Comparison of anterior and posterior instrumentation for correction of adolescent thoracic idiopathic scoliosis. Spine 1999;24:225–239
85. Mehta MH. The natural history of infantile idiopathic scoliosis. In: Zorab PA, ed. Scoliosis: Proceedings of the Fifth Symposium. London: Academic Press; 1977:103–122
86. Mehta MH, Morel G. The non-operative treatment of infantile idiopathic scoliosis. In: Zorab PA, Siegler D, eds. Scoliosis: Proceedings of the Fifth Symposium. London: Academic Press; 1979:71–84
87. Mehta MH. The rib-vertebra angle in the early diagnosis between resolving and progressive infantile scoliosis. J Bone Joint Surg Br 1972;54:230–243
88. Roaf R. The treatment of progressive scoliosis by unilateral growth arrest. J Bone Joint Surg Br 1963;45:637–651
89. Andrew T, Piggott H. Growth arrest for progressive scoliosis. Combined anterior and posterior fusion of the convexity. J Bone Joint Surg Br 1985;67:193–197
90. Millner PA, Dickson RA. Idiopathic scoliosis: Biomechanics and biology. Eur Spine J 1996;5:362–373
91. Moe JH, Kharrat K, Winter RB, Cummine JL. Harrington instrumentation without fusion plus external orthotic support for the treatment of difficult curvature problems in young children. Clin Orthop Relat Res 1984;185:35–45
92. Betz RR, D'Andrea LP, Mulcahey MJ, Chafetz RS. Vertebral body stapling procedure for the treatment of scoliosis in the growing child. Clin Orthop Relat Res 2005;434:55–60
93. Waldhausen JH, Redding GJ, Song KM. Vertical expandable prosthetic titanium rib for thoracic insufficiency syndrome: A new method to treat an old problem. J Pediatr Surg 2007;42:76–80

# 2 Basic Principles of Scoliosis Treatment

*Robert A. Dickson*

## Definitions and Terminology[1]

### Planes and Deformities

Spinal deformities are described according to the three planes of the body (**Fig. 2.1**). In the *coronal* (frontal) *plane* the spine should be straight, and any lateral curvature is referred to as *scoliosis*. In the *sagittal* (lateral) *plane*, once a child has achieved head control and started walking, there are four natural spinal curvatures, two convex anteriorly (*lordoses*), in the cervical and lumbar regions, respectively, and two curvatures convex posteriorly (*kyphoses*), in the thoracic and sacral regions, respectively (**Fig. 2.2**). Only when these lateral curvatures are excessive or reduced do they assume clinical significance.

### Nonstructural and Structural Scolioses

To differentiate between relatively unimportant scolioses and important ones, the terms *nonstructural* and *structural* are applied, the former comprising purely lateral curvatures, whereas the latter have a rotational component in the *transverse plane*. Nonstructural curvatures are nonprogressive and secondary to some other problem (e.g., a pelvic tilt secondary to leg-length inequality or muscle spasm in association with back pain) (**Fig. 2.3**). Structural scolioses are important and often progressive. The rotational component is clearly seen on X-ray films, with the spinous processes rotating toward the curve concavity (**Fig. 2.4**), and is seen clinically by the presence of a rib or loin hump as the attached ribs and transverse processes rotate with the spine (**Fig. 2.5**). Structural curves are primary or intrinsic to the spine itself.

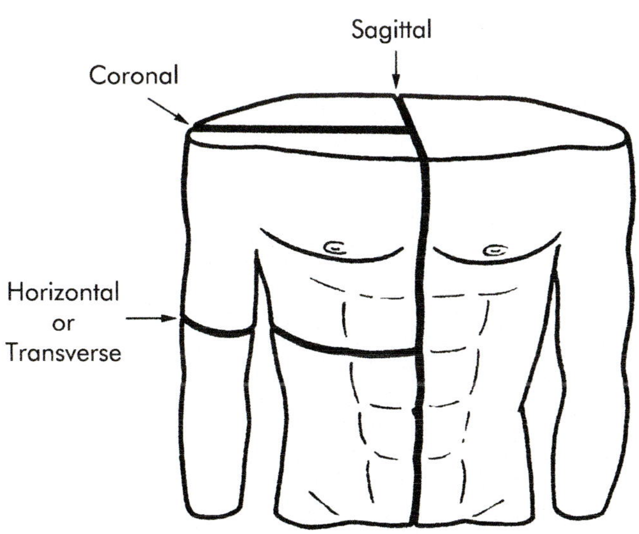


**Fig. 2.1** The planes of the body.

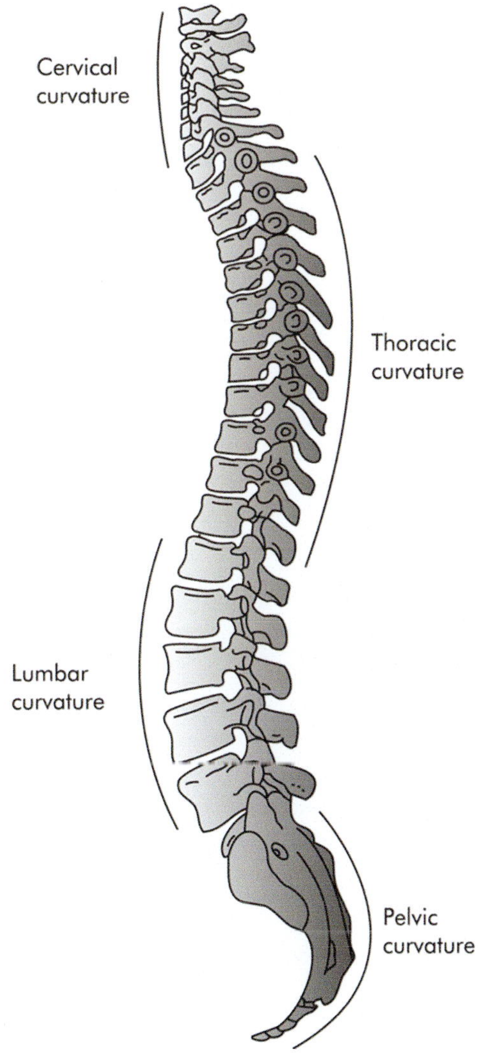


**Fig. 2.2** The four natural curvatures of the spine in the sagittal plane: cervical and lumbar lordoses and thoracic and pelvic kyphoses.

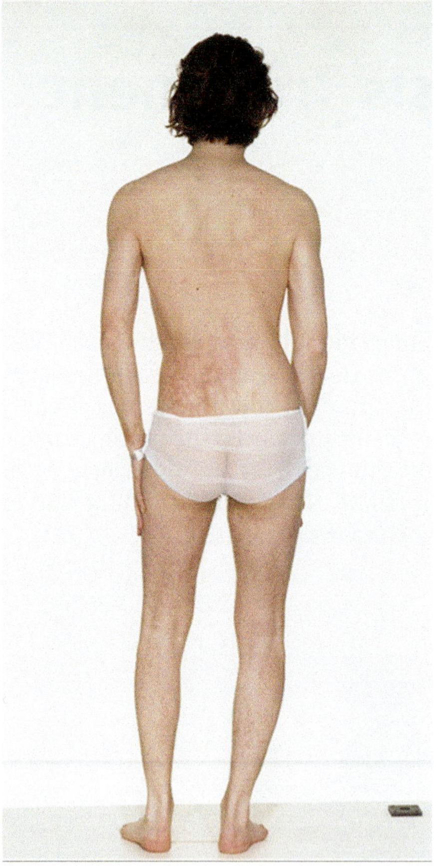

A

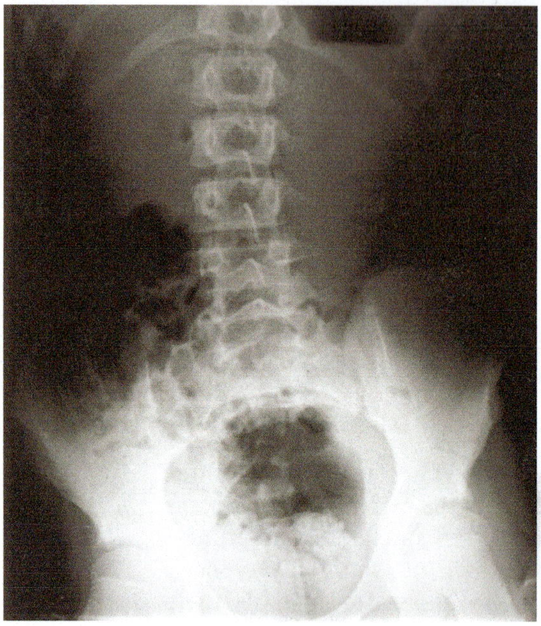

B

**Fig. 2.3** **(A)** A teenage boy with a nonstructural lumbar scoliosis caused by muscle spasm from an adolescent disc hernia. **(B)** PA X-ray film of a nonstructural lumbar curve secondary to a leg- length inequality.

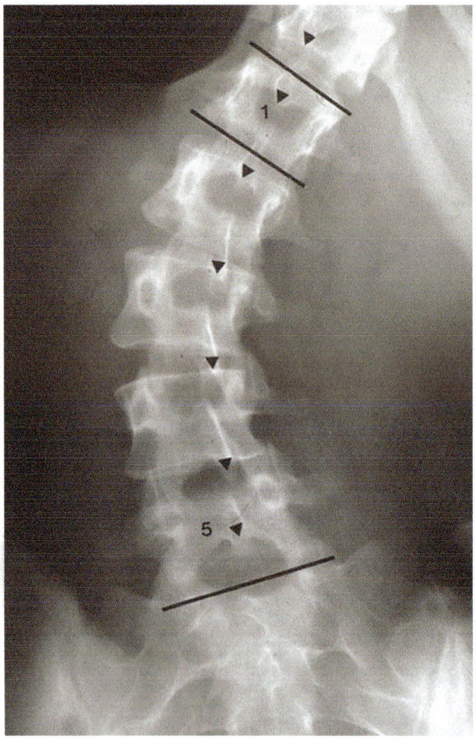


**Fig. 2.4** PA X-ray film of a lumbar curve. The spinous processes have been labeled with *black triangles*, and it can be clearly seen that they rotate toward the concavity of the curve, as is always the case with structural scoliosis.

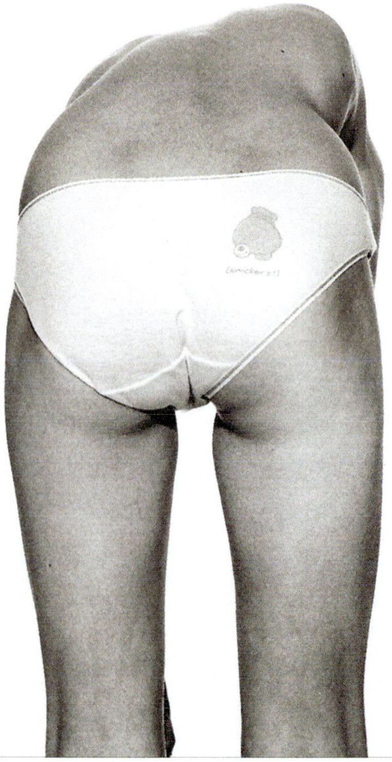

**Fig. 2.5** The rib hump associated with an idiopathic thoracic curve, which results from twisting of the attached ribs when the spine twists.

# Curve Characteristics

## Named Vertebrae

The *apical vertebra* or vertebrae are those at the center of the scoliotic curve (**Fig. 2.6**). These are the most rotated vertebrae in the transverse plane. The upper and lower *neutral vertebrae* are the first nonrotated vertebrae above and below the scoliotic curve. The *end-vertebrae* are those maximally tilted above and below the apex of the curve. By convention, the extent of a scoliotic curve is described from neutral vertebra to neutral vertebra (e.g., T4 to L1), whereas the end-vertebrae are the reference points for measurement of the magnitude of the curve.

## Curve Size

The usual method of measuring curve size is that of Cobb (**Fig. 2.6**).[2] In this method, lines are drawn along the upper endplate of the upper end-vertebra and the lower endplate of the lower end-vertebra, with the angle subtended by these lines being the Cobb angle. The case of large curves these lines intersect on the X-ray film, whereas for smaller curves perpendiculars have to be dropped for the measurement to be made. However, use of the Oxford Orthopaedic Engineering Centre Cobbometer obviates these problems and reduces the measurement error to much less than half of what it would otherwise be (**Fig. 2.7**).[3]

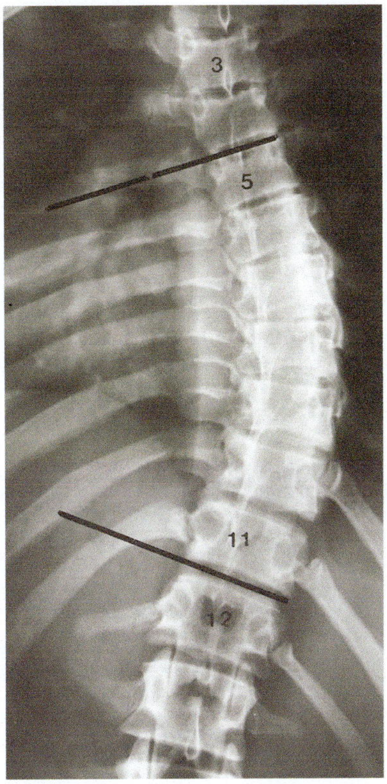


**Fig. 2.6** PA X-ray film of a thoracic curve. The end-vertebrae for Cobb angle measurement (the most tilted vertebrae at the top and bottom of the curve) are T5 above and T11 below. The first neutral vertebra above is T3, two above the upper end-vertebra; T12 is the lower neutral vertebra.

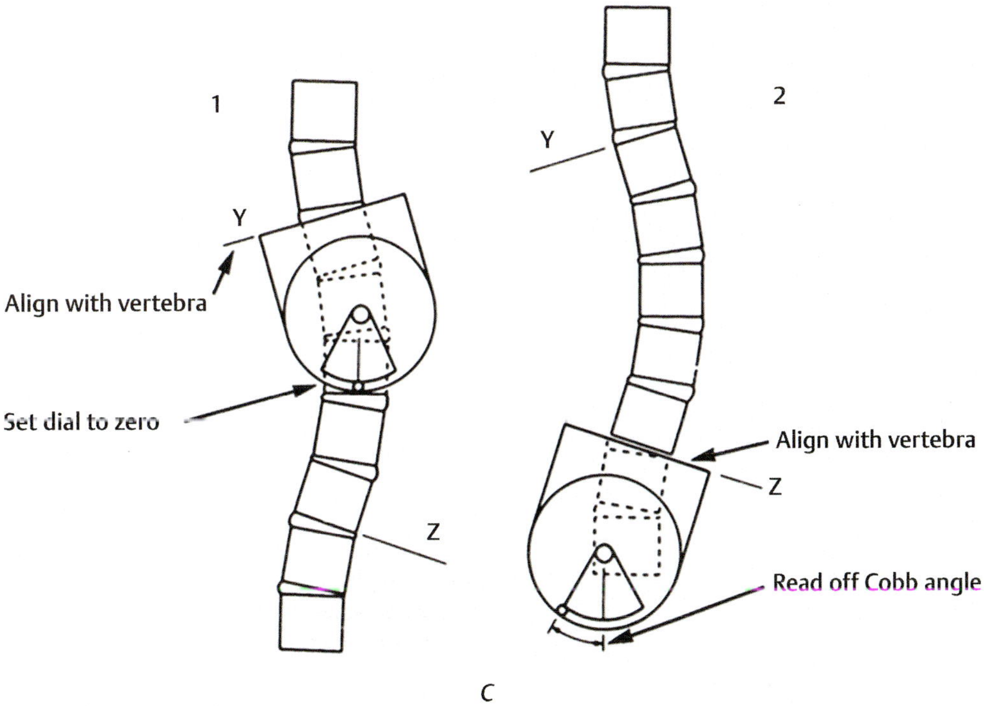


**Fig. 2.7** Measuring the Cobb angle with the Oxford Cobbometer (a protractor with a vertically free hanging needle). The upper border of the instrument is first aligned with the upper surface of the upper end-vertebra, and the protractor dial is set to zero. When the upper border of the instrument is then aligned with the lower surface of the lower end-vertebra, the needle gives the Cobb angle.

It should be remembered that these measurements are made on an anteroposterior (AP) radiograph of the patient, and that the vertebrae within the curve are rotated out of the frontal plane of the patient, the apical vertebra being the most rotated. Accordingly, bigger curves are progressively rotated further away from the plane of the patient and thus, for example, a curve of 60 degrees is much more than twice as big as a curve of 30 degrees because the 60 degree curve is seen less *en face* (**Fig. 2.8**). For this reason Stagnara favored taking radiographs of the scoliotic spine with respect to the amount of apical rotation, and he called these *plan d'election* views.[5] If, for instance, the apical vertebra is rotated 30 degrees from the frontal plane of the patient, the patient or X-ray beam is turned 30 degrees from the frontal plane, so that a true AP plan d'election view is obtained. Necessarily, the size of the scoliotic curve on the plan d'election AP view is larger than on the AP view of the patient. So as to understand this point more clearly it is useful, for example, to examine a coat hanger in different planes of projection (**Fig. 2.9**). When the coat hanger is at right angles to the plane of projection (Stagnara's AP plan d'election view), the angle measures 60 degrees. If the coat hanger is rotated 90 degrees from this, then no angle is subtended, or the angle is 0 degrees and represents the

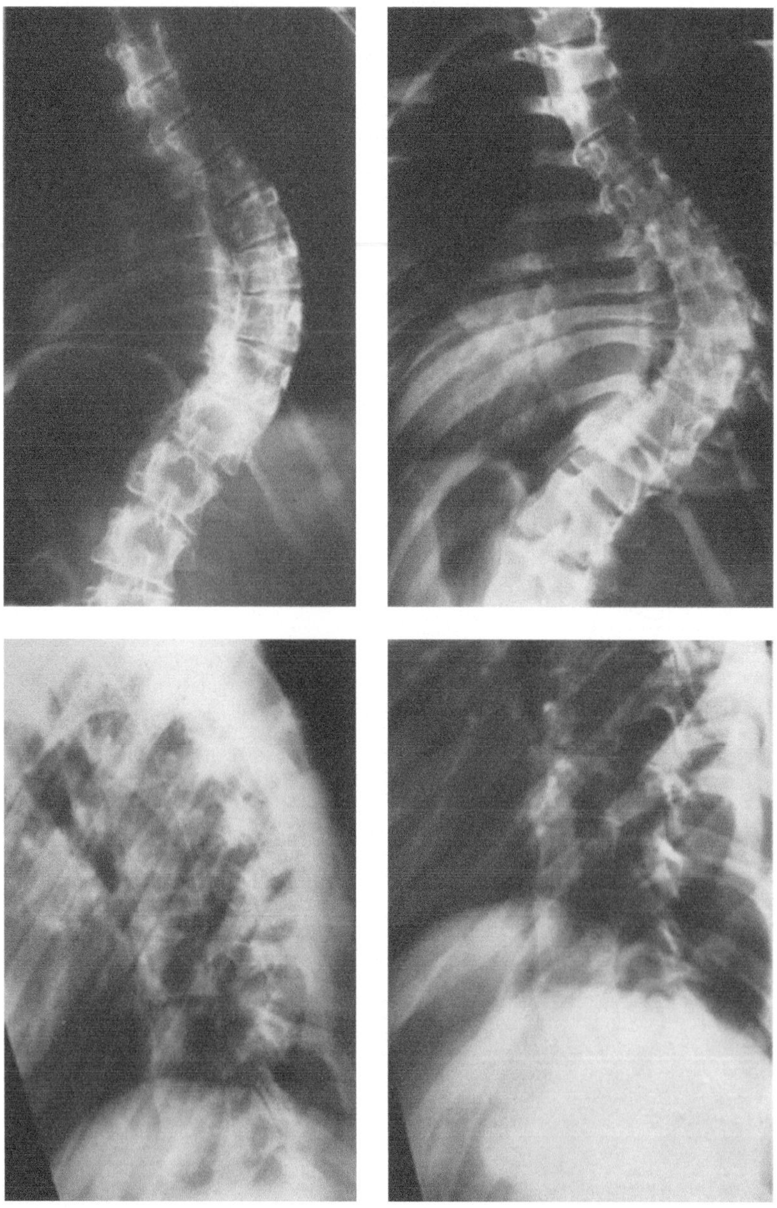

A B C D

**Fig. 2.8** **(A)** PA view of the patient; **(B)** a true PA view; **(C)** a lateral view of the patient; **(D)** a true lateral view.

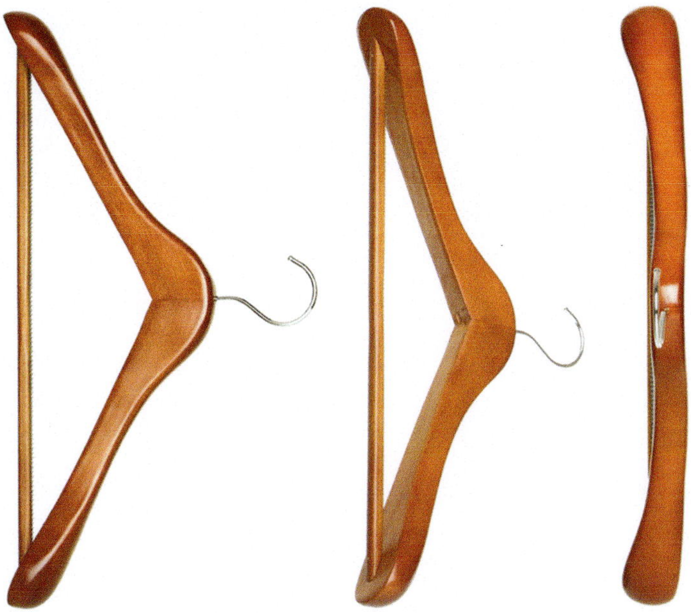

A–C

**Fig. 2.9** **(A)** Lateral view of a coat hanger, showing an angle of 60 degrees. **(B)** The coat hanger has been rotated 45 degrees and now the Cobb angle registers only 30 degrees because the coat hanger is not being seen *en face* as it is in **(A)**. **(C)** When the coat hanger is turned a further 45 degrees there is no angle at all.

true lateral projection. As the coat hanger is rotated from this true lateral projection to the true AP projection, the angle increases, so that the angle subtended halfway between the true lateral and AP planes is 30 degrees.

For both the coat hanger and the patient, the Cobb angle changes magnitude simply in terms of the plane of projection.

Although publications about scoliotic curve size before and after treatment compare mean Cobb angles, these are clearly not arithmetic data, because a curve correction from 60 degrees to 30 degrees as the result of treatment represents much more than a 50% improvement.

## Vertebral Rotation

The extent to which the apical vertebra is rotated from the frontal plane in a patient with scoliosis can be measured with Perdriolle's protractor[6] (**Fig. 2.10**) or by the method of Nash and Moe,[7] which measures the displacement of the convex pedicle from the convex side of the vertebral body. With these techniques the amount of vertebral rotation does relate linearly to the size of the spinal deformity, but they are much less popular measurements than measurement of the Cobb angle. Moreover, obvious limitations to these other techniques are the inability to determine pedicular landmarks after instrumentation.

Another index of rotation, in addition to the position of the pedicles, is the angular appearance of the ribs on each side of the scoliotic curve. This is of particular significance for idiopathic deformities of early onset (infantile idiopathic scoliosis), which are common in the United Kingdom but much less prevalent in the United States. Fortunately, the

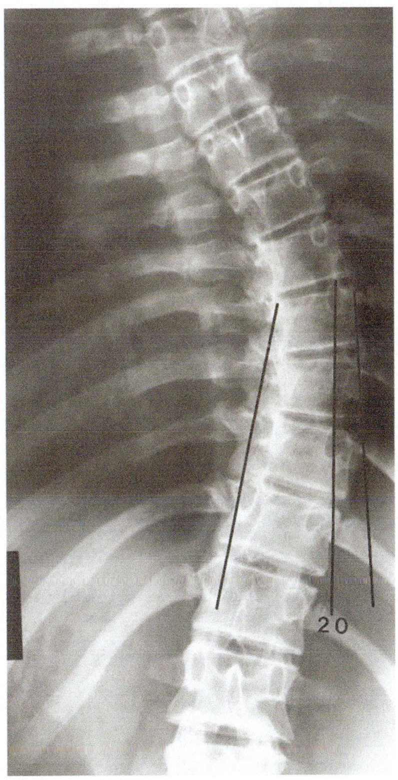


**Fig. 2.10** Measuring rotation using Perdriolle's protractor. The protractor comprises diverging lines and is laid over the PA radiograph, with the side lines of the projector aligned with the sides of the vertebral body. The line that bisects the convex pedicle indicates the degree of rotation of that vertebra.

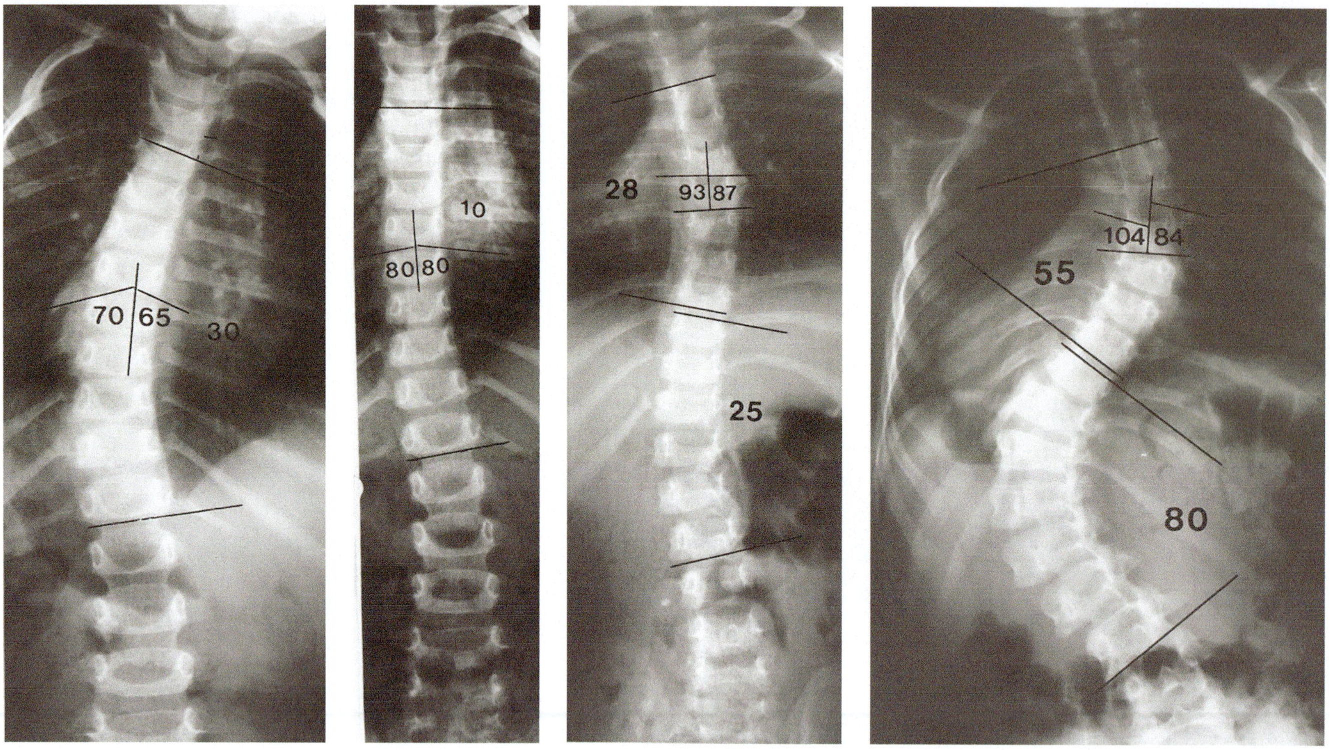


A–D

**Fig. 2.11** **(A)** Infantile idiopathic thoracic scoliosis. Although the Cobb angle is 30 degrees the RVAD is only 5 degrees. **(B)** Two years later, the deformity has almost resolved. **(C)** Infantile idiopathic double-structural scoliosis to the right in the thoracic region and to the left in the thoracolumbar region. Although the Cobb angles measure only 28 and 25 degrees, respectively, and the RVAD of the thoracic curve measures only 6 degrees, infantile double-structural curves are always progressive unless treated. **(D)** One year later both curves have increased significantly, particularly the lower one. Unfortunately, no therapeutic action was taken in the interim.

majority of such deformities resolve, but some progress and can cause cardiopulmonary dysfunction. It is therefore critically important to identify those that need immediate treatment and those that can be monitored.

Thirty years ago, Min Mehta studied a large number of infants with scoliosis, and one of the important measures he used was the rib–vertebra angle difference (RVAD) (**Fig. 2.11**).[8] In this procedure the angle that the neck of the rib makes with the vertical axis of the apical vertebra (the rib–vertebra angle [RVA]) is measured on each side of the vertebra, and if the difference (the RVAD) is 20 degrees or more, there is a strong likelihood of progression of scoliosis. Therefore, this radiographic measure is particularly important in addition to the clinical assessment of such infants.

## Curve Patterns

Patterns of scoliotic curvature are described according to the location of the apical vertebra (**Fig. 2.12**). Thus, *thoracic curves* have an apex between T2 and T11 inclusive, whereas *lumbar curves* have an apex between L2 and L4. *Thoracolumbar curves* have an apex between T12 and L1. Curves above and below these regions of the spine are unusual, but are defined according to the same principles, with *cervicothoracic curves* apical at C7/T1; *cervical curves* apical above this; and *lumbosacral curves* having an apex at L5/S1.

The direction of a scoliotic curve is described according to its *convexity*. Curves can also be *single* or *multiple*, and a single right thoracic and left lumbar curve are common patterns of scoliosis. Because there can be more than one curve in the spine, a right thoracic combined with a left lumbar *double curve* pattern is also common, as indeed are *triple curve* patterns.

## Spinal Balance (Compensation)

If there is a single structural curve in the spine then *compensatory curves* above and below it bring the head and pelvis into straight alignment. These curves are not rotated and are therefore nonstructural. If there is a double or triple structural curve pattern, the nonrotated compensatory curves are above and below these.

For clinical purposes, spinal balance *(compensation)* can be demonstrated if a plumb line suspended from the vertebra prominens bisects the gluteal cleft. If such a line passes to the right of the gluteal cleft for a right-sided curve, then the spine is termed *decompensated*. Balance

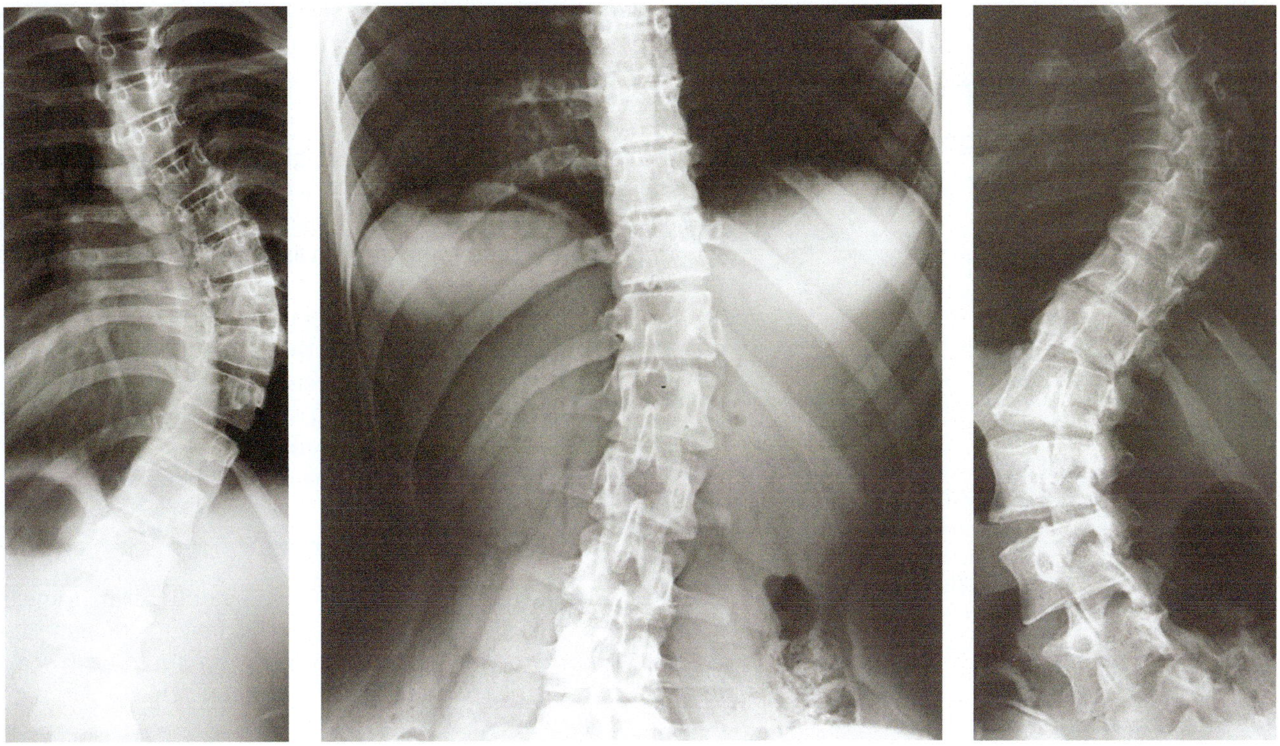
A–C

**Fig. 2.12** A selection of common curve patterns in infantile idiopathic scoliosis. **(A)** Right thoracic curves: these are always apical between T7 and T9. **(B)** Right thoracolumbar curves: these are apical at T12 or L1. **(C)** In cases of right thoracic and left lumbar double-structural curves, the lumbar curves are always apical at L2.

can, however, be assessed more accurately by measuring the size of the compensatory curves: if the compensatory curves are of equal magnitude, then the spine is in balance, whereas if the lower compensatory curve is larger than the upper curve, the spine is decompensated (**Fig. 2.13**).

Why some deformities are nicely balanced and others badly imbalanced is unknown. Decompensation markedly worsens a patient's appearance, and achieving balance is therefore an important consideration in treating scoliosis.

## Biological Growth

Because scoliotic deformities in children have the potential to progress during growth, it is very important to assess this risk accurately and to repeat measurements regularly to see how children travel through their adolescence.

### Indices of Maturity

Most patients with scoliosis require assessment and treatment during adolescence, and as with other skeletal deformities, their condition worsens during phases of rapid growth and ceases to worsen at the attainment of skeletal maturity. The two popular methods for assessing progression of scoliosis are to determine the status of ossification of the *iliac crest* and *vertebral ring apophyses*. Unfortunately, the vertebral ring apophyses are progressively less conspicuous

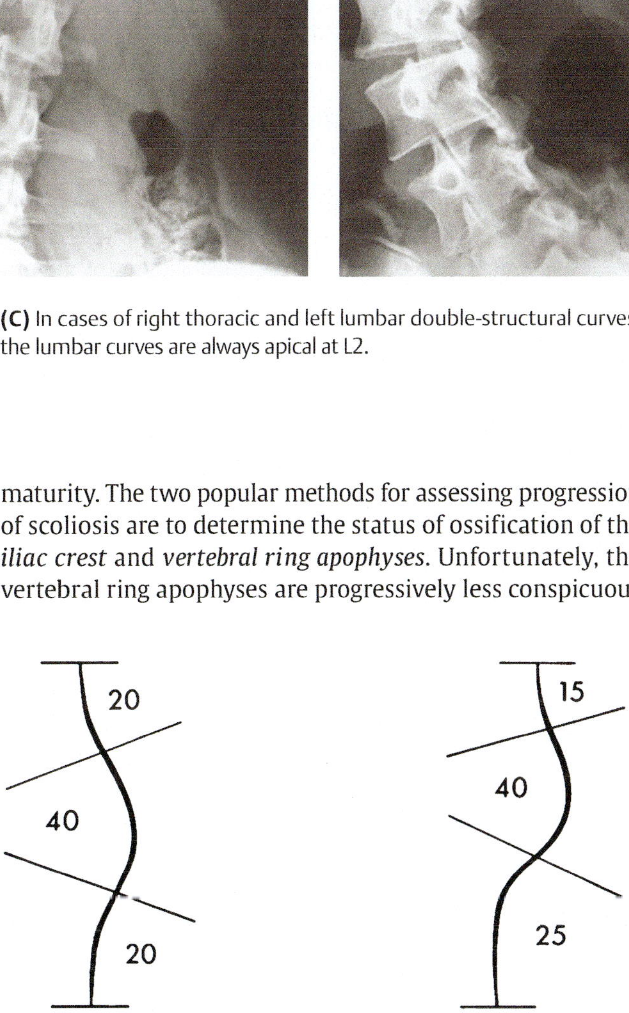


**Fig. 2.13** Measuring spinal balance (compensation). The sum of the upper and lower compensatory curves is always equal to the size of the structural curve. (*Left*) When the spine is in perfect balance, the upper and lower compensatory curves are of equal magnitude. (*Right*) When the spine lists to the side of the convexity of the curve (decompensation), it does so, because the lower compensatory curve is bigger than the upper compensatory curve. In this case the spine is decompensated by 10 degrees.

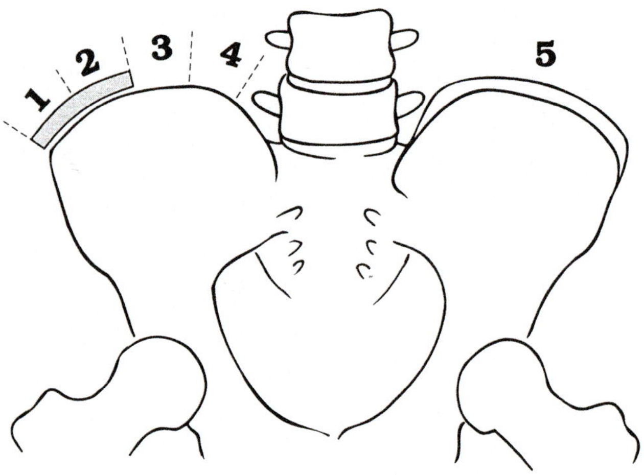


**Fig. 2.14** The Risser sign. The iliac crest apophysis appears first anteriorly and then moves round the iliac crest to end posteriorly. This excursion is divided into quarters, with Risser 5 occurring when the iliac crest apophysis fuses with the pelvis. Accordingly, patients' maturity can be rated from Risser 0 through Risser 5.

and thus more difficult to identify the closer the patient comes to maturity. Risser first described the migration and subsequent ossification and fusion of the iliac crest apophysis, dividing it into quarters as its ossification progresses posteriorly (Risser 0 [no apophysis] to Risser 5 [fused apophysis]) (**Fig. 2.14**).[9] Unfortunately, this is not particularly useful, because spinal growth continues for at least a further 2 years after the attainment of general skeletal maturity.

The Leeds Group demonstrated that adolescents grew all of 2 cm after maturation of the pelvis,[10] and although this has little import for the straight spine, it does provide a mechanism for curve progression after Risser 5.

### Measurement of Bone Age

Measurement of bone age from radiographs of the left hand and wrist is a long-standing convention in pediatrics, particularly in relation to children with systemic growth disorders involving stature. The size of the carpal bones can be measured and the status of ossification of the epiphyses in the wrist and hand can also be assessed to provide a measure of bone age when radiographs of these structures are compared with standard skeletal atlases.

The original Greulich and Pyle atlas[11] was based on well-advanced, upper-class children in Cleveland, Ohio, in the 1930s. A more up-to-date and precise atlas is that by Tanner and Whitehouse (Second Method[12]), which can permit measurement of bone age to one decimal place. A girl of age 12 years chronologically is commonly 11 or 13 years of age skeletally, and it is much more important to know skeletal age than chronological age. A posteroanterior (PA) X-ray film of the left hand and wrist, made on an annual basis, is quite safe and describes how a child is progressing sequentially through his or her growth phase.

### Centile Charts

For assessing standing height and sitting height, there are *centile charts* against which these anthropometric measurements can be plotted. A phase of increased growth velocity (i.e., acceleration) is often associated with progression of a scoliotic curve (**Fig. 2.15**).

There are also photographic standards for breast and pubic hair development through adolescence, but use of these is probably too precise and intrusive for the assessment of the patient with scoliosis. However, the time of menarche is very important because it heralds the beginning of the adolescent growth spurt in females.

### Assessing the Scoliosis Patient

With the resources that have been described, measurements of standing height, sitting height, and bone age can easily be made on each visit by a patient with scoliosis, and titrated against the characteristics of the patient's deformity.

## Etiological Classification

The Scoliosis Research Society in 1973 described a simple classification of spinal deformity according to etiology.[1] **Table 2.1** shows this classification, which is memorable and simple to apply. With the exception of the first category, of *idiopathic scoliosis*, a definable pathological process deforms the spine in all categories of scoliosis. Thus, idiopathic scoliosis occurs in children who are by definition otherwise entirely normal, which is the reason for the Greek word *idiopathic* (self-generating) being applied to this category of the condition.

### Idiopathic Scoliosis

Idiopathic scoliosis is defined as a lateral curvature of the spine with rotation in the absence of any congenital spinal anomaly or associated musculoskeletal condition. The geometry of this deformity is easy to appreciate from plain radiographs. There is always a lateral curvature of the spine with rotation such that the posterior elements turn toward the curve concavity (*concordant rotation*) (see **Fig. 2.4**). This is confirmed by clinical examination of the patient with the rotational prominence on the convex side of the scoliotic curve and a corresponding depression on the concave side (see **Fig. 2.5**).

Although James, in Edinburgh, divided the onset of idiopathic scoliosis into the three categories[13] of infantile (0 to 3 years of age), juvenile (4 to 9 years of age), and adolescent

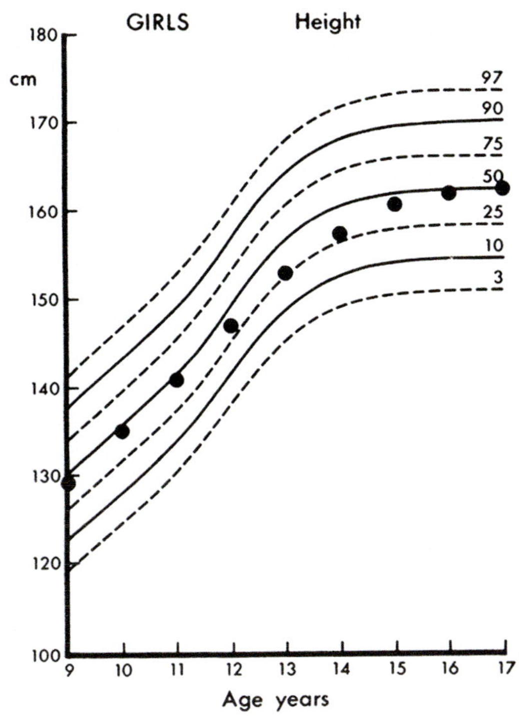


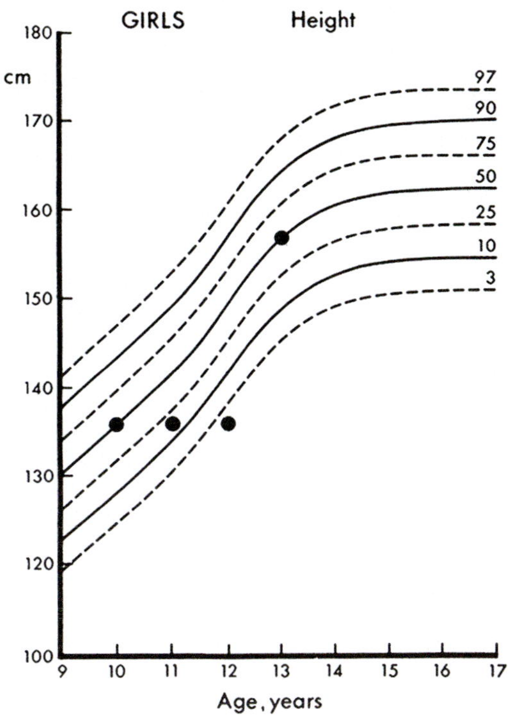


**Fig. 2.15** The 1975 Tanner and Whitehouse centile chart for the height of girls. **(A)** On this chart the 50th centile of the 1959 standard is plotted, showing how "normal" girls today will appear taller without any growth abnormality. **(B)** On this chart is plotted the height of a 10-year-old girl who does not grow for the next 2 years. However, between the ages of 12 and 13 years she has experienced 3 years worth of growth, to re-enter the 50th centile, and during this period her growth velocity is therefore excessive.

(age 10 years to maturity), what is really important is the threshold of 5 years of age.[14] Before this, and particularly in the first year of life, a scoliosis in the thoracic region can compromise the development of the heart and lungs, leading to cardiopulmonary problems in adulthood (**Fig. 2.16**).[15] Beyond the age of 5 years no such organic health risks apply,[16] and the problem is one of appearance and deformity only, albeit with attendant psychosocial distress. Therefore, idiopathic scoliosis is better divided into the two categories of *early-onset* (before the age of 5 years) and *late-onset* (after the age of 5 years) (**Fig. 2.17**).[14]

**Table 2.1 Etiological Classification of Spinal Deformities**

| |
|---|
| Idiopathic deformities |
| Congenital deformities |
| Neuromuscular deformities |
| Deformities caused by neurofibromatosis |
| Deformities caused by mesencyhmal disorders |
| Traumatic deformities |
| Deformities caused by infection |
| Deformities caused by tumors |
| Miscellaneous conditions in which a spinal deformity is common |

## Early-onset Idiopathic Scoliosis

Early-onset idiopathic scoliosis is almost certainly a problem of postnatal body pressure molding, because the convexity of the scoliosis is associated with the side affected by plagiocephaly, plagiopelvy, bat ear, and wry neck, all of

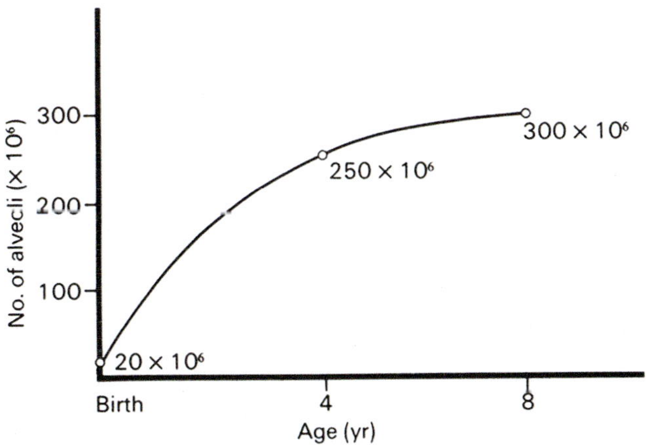


**Fig. 2.16** Graph demonstrating the rate of development of pulmonary alveoli. A maximum is reached at the age of 8 years, with five-sixths of alveoli being developed by the age of 4 years and half by the age of 1 year.

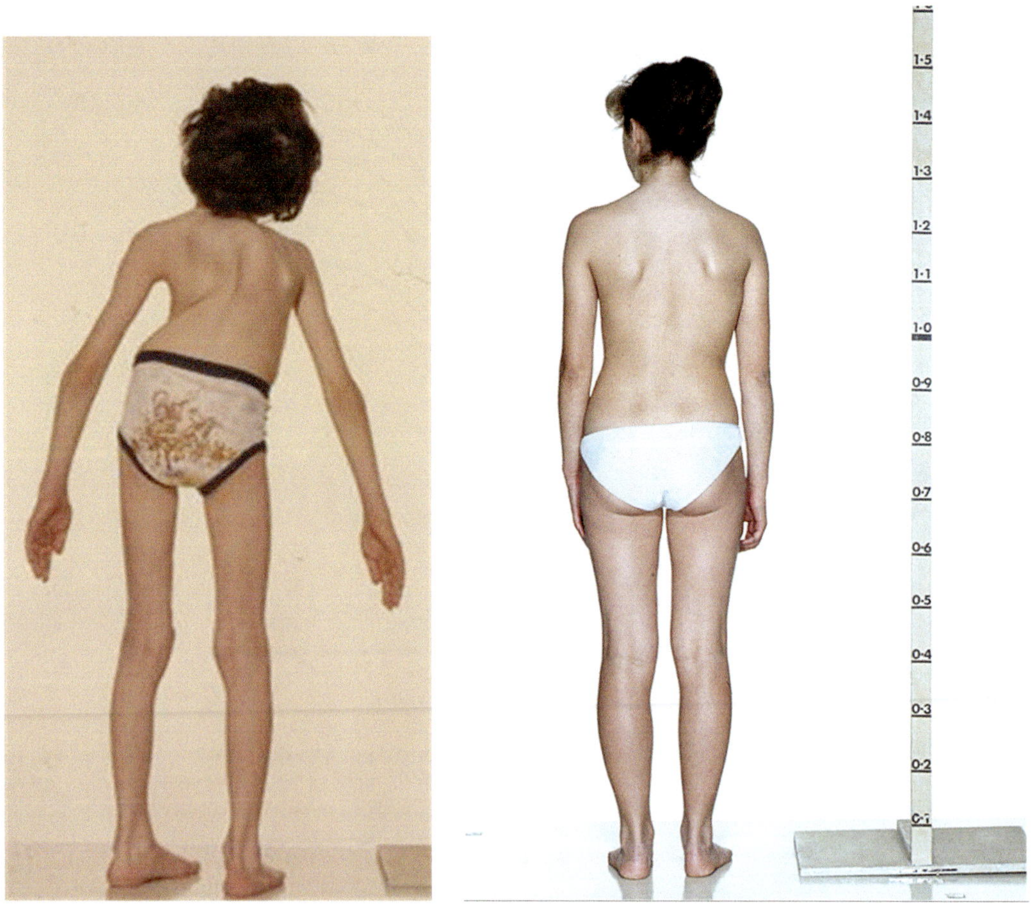


A B

**Fig. 2.17** The two fundamental types of idiopathic scoliosis according to age of onset: **(A)** early onset and **(B)** late onset.

which deformities are associated with early-onset scoliosis and all of which develop after birth.[17] Fortunately, 90% of early-onset scolioses resolve, but 10% are static or progressive. Mehta studied early-onset scoliosis and noted certain factors indicative of progression.[8] Boys are affected more often than girls, and thoracic and thoracolumbar curves tend to resolve whereas double-structural curves have a definite progression potential. Initial curve size at presentation and the amount of apical rotation (RVAD) are also important determinants of the course of the condition. A small initial curve size and RVAD of less than 20 degrees suggest a benign prognosis. A stiff curve and hypotonicity in an infant are notorious predictors of progression.

## Late-onset Scoliosis

Late-onset scoliosis is by far the most prevalent type of idiopathic scoliosis, and the age of its onset implies a more benign course, without the cardiopulmonary consequences of early-onset scoliosis. The earlier the onset of scoliosis during this phase of growth, the greater is the progression potential and therefore the greater the need to monitor the growth and skeletal age of the patient.

## References

1. Goldstein LA, Waugh TR. Classification and terminology of scoliosis. Clin Orthop Relat Res 1973;93:10–22
2. Cobb JR. Outline for the study of scoliosis. Instr Course Lect 1948; 5:261–275
3. Whittle MW, Evans M. Instrument for measuring the Cobb angle in scoliosis. Lancet 1979;1:414
4. Ferguson AB. The study and treatment of scoliosis. South Med J 1930;23:116–120
5. Péloux J, Fauchet R, Foucon B, Stagnara P. Le plan d'election pour l'examen radiologique des cyphoscolioses. Rev Chir Orthop Reparatrice Appar Mot 1965;51:517–524

6. Perdriolle R. La Scoliose: Son Étude Tridimensionnelle. Paris: Maloine; 1979.
7. Nash CL Jr, Moe JH. A study of vertebral rotation. J Bone Joint Surg Am 1969;51:223–229
8. Mehta MH. The rib-vertebra angle in the early diagnosis between resolving and progressive infantile scoliosis. J Bone Joint Surg Br 1972;54:230–243
9. Risser JC. The iliac apophysis; an invaluable sign in the management of scoliosis. Clin Orthop Relat Res 1958;11:111–119
10. Howell FR, Mahood JK, Dickson RA. Growth beyond skeletal maturity. Spine 1992;17:437–440
11. Gruelich WW, Pyle SI. Radiographic Atlas of Skeletal Development of the Hand and Wrist, ed. 2. Stanford: Stanford University Press; London: Oxford University Press; 1959
12. Tanner JM, Whitehouse RH. Height Standard Chart. Hounslow, UK: Printwell; 1959
13. James JIP. Idiopathic scoliosis; the prognosis, diagnosis, and operative indications related to curve patterns and the age at onset. J Bone Joint Surg Br 1954;36B:36–49
14. Dickson RA. Conservative treatment for idiopathic scoliosis. J Bone Joint Surg Br 1985;67:176–181
15. Davies G, Reid L. Effect of scoliosis on growth of alveoli and pulmonary arteries and on right ventricle. Arch Dis Child 1971;46: 623–632
16. Branthwaite MA. Cardiorespiratory consequences of unfused idiopathic scoliosis. Br J Dis Chest 1986;80:360–369
17. Wynne-Davies R. Infantile idiopathic scoliosis. Causative factors, particularly in the first six months of life. J Bone Joint Surg Br 1975; 57:138–141

# 3 Pathogenesis of Idiopathic Scoliosis

*Robert A. Dickson*

A clear understanding of the pathogenesis of idiopathic scoliosis is essential to appreciating its clinical behavior. Although epidemiological surveys have shown an enormous number of children with minor coronal-plane deformities of the spine, only a relatively small number show evidence of progressive idiopathic scoliosis, which means that other factors must be superimposed to make a deformity idiopathic and progressive. The environment of growth is clearly important, as with other progressive skeletal deformities. The prevalence rate of minor curves in boys is about half that for each age in girls, and the difference is progressively more obvious the greater the size of the curve. Boys are therefore in some way protected from idiopathic scoliosis, but their spines are going to be subjected to much the same neuromuscular, metabolic, and endocrine processes during growth as those of girls. On a commonsense basis it would seem unlikely that pointing the finger of suspicion, for instance, at the paravertebral musculature, brain, eyes, ears, spinal cord, nerve roots, muscles, collagen, and even platelets would not be a profitable line of research into the cause of idiopathic scoliosis. Notwithstanding, this path has largely been the focus of research activity in the etiology of idiopathic scoliosis over the past half century.

## Muscular Theories

Most hypotheses and speculations put forward about the cause of idiopathic scoliosis concern neuromuscular theories, although idiopathic scoliosis is defined as a spinal curvature in the absence of any associated musculoskeletal condition. Since Lerique and Le Coeur first demonstated electromyographic asymmetry in the paraspinal muscles of patients with the condition,[1] much work on the paraspinal musculature has been performed, including studies of muscle fiber type and ultrastructural differences,[2–11] although Zetterberg and colleagues showed that these abnormalities resembled the sort of changes encountered after endurance training, indicating a secondary or adaptive process (i.e., secondary to the presence of a spinal curvature) in their occurrence.[12] Saartok et al went even further, stating that "a neuromuscular imbalance has not been shown to be an etiological factor for the idiopathic form of scoliosis."[13] The histological specimens were obtained during scoliosis surgery from a highly selected group of patients with larger curves, focusing on the difference between the right and left sides, when the geometric problem is instead a front-to-back buckling lordosis (vide infra).

Platelets contain actin and myosin, and because of their resemblance to those in skeletal muscle, these structures have also been examined in idiopathic scoliosis. Early studies reporting abnormal morphology and function of platelets in patients with idiopathic scoliosis[14–16] were not confirmed in subsequent studies, which showed no difference between patients with idiopathic scoliosis and controls.[17,18] Platelet aggregation abnormalities were shown to be more prevalent in those with larger scoliotic curves, again indicating a secondary effect.[19,20] Calmodulin regulates the contractile properties of muscles and platelets through changes in calcium concentration, and higher platelet calmodulin levels have been demonstrated in patients with progressive curves,[21] as have lower levels of melatonin, a calmodulin antagonist.[22] It is unclear what these changes reflect other than the biochemistry of growth in general.

## Neurological Theories

Because scoliosis is associated with many neurological diseases, from those affecting the brain to those of peripheral nerves, several neurological abnormalities have been described in association with idiopathic scoliosis.

Electroencephalography, proprioception, and vibration sense have been examined in idiopathic scoliosis, as well as balance and electronystagmography.[23–26] Recently, abnormal somatosensory function has been demonstrated in patients with adolescent idiopathic scoliosis,[27,28] but its relationship to curve severity again suggests changes secondary to the presence of a deformity. Forty years ago it was thought that idiopathic scoliosis could be caused by a short spinal cord,[29] and more recently Porter has shown that in patients with the condition the spinal canal is shorter than the spine itself.[30–32] This theory has been fancifully called "uncoupled neuro-osseous growth,"[32] and the concept of this difference in length has also been supported through screening with magnetic resonance imaging (MRI).[33] Thirty years ago in Oxford, cadaver spines with idiopathic scoliosis were measured and it was shown that the spinal canal takes the shortest route down the spine.[34]

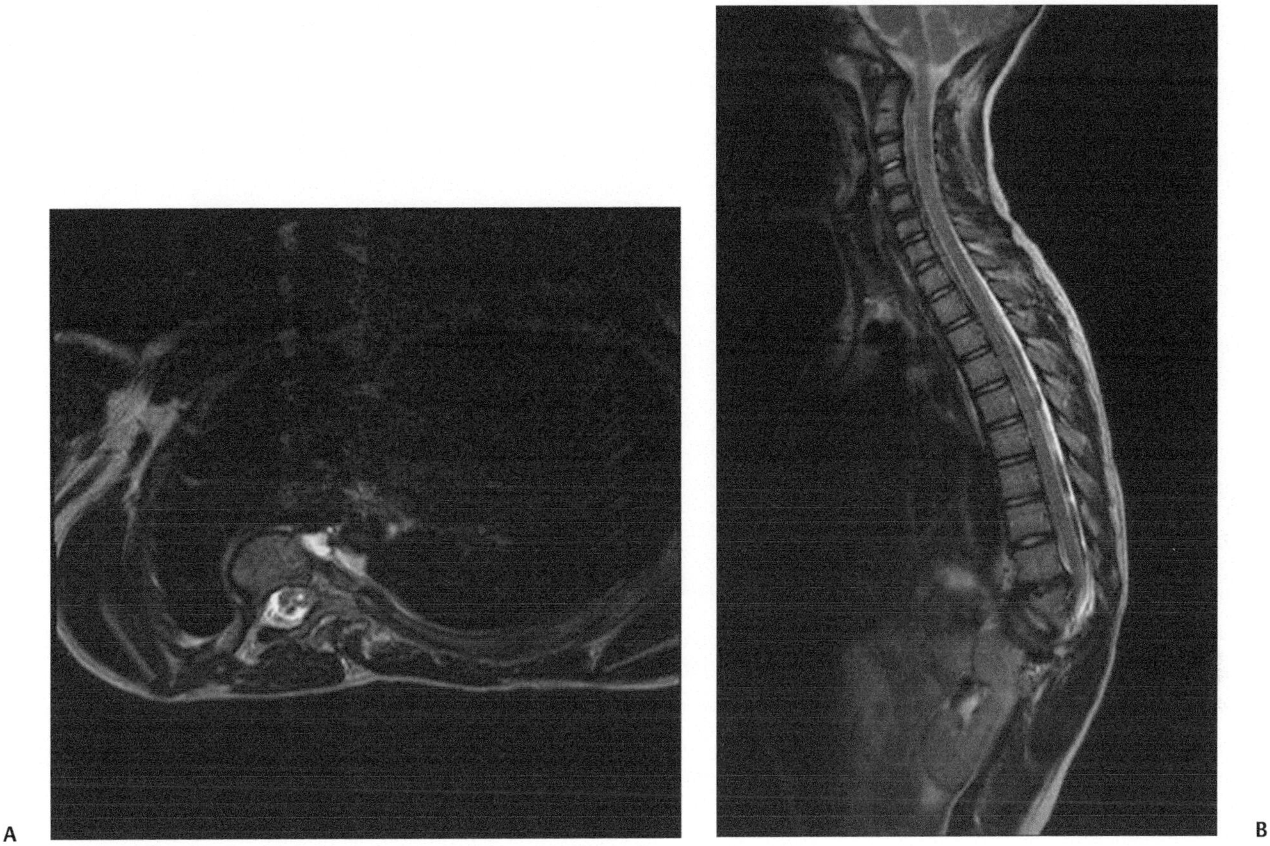

Fig. 3.1 **(A)** Axial MRI scan through the apex of an idiopathic thoracic scoliosis, showing that the spinal cord lies close to the posterolateral elements on the concave side. **(B)** Sagittal MRI scan of a post-traumatic kyphosis, showing the spinal cord applied to, and indeed stretched over, the back of the kyphosis.

The Leeds Study Group looked at the same specimens in more detail and confirmed the findings that the postero-concave canal distance was the shortest spinal route.[35] Since MRI scanning first became available, the Leeds Group has looked at patients with idiopathic spinal deformities. Whereas in Scheuermann's thoracic hyperkyphosis the spinal cord hugs the back of the vertebral bodies at the apex of the curve, the spinal cord also takes the shortest route in the opposite deformity of idiopathic lordoscoliosis, being close to the back of the vertebral body/pedicle on the concave side of the curve (**Fig. 3.1**). Patients with idiopathic scoliosis do not have any known clinical neurological abnormality, nor does MRI scanning show any tethering effect in this condition, such as a low conus or a secondary Arnold–Chiari malformation. A spinal canal proportionately shorter than the rest of the axial skeleton in idiopathic scoliosis merely reflects what one would expect of the geometry of a lordoscoliosis.

The advent of MRI scanning demonstrated a greater prevalence of a syrinx in the spinal cord than had previously been found, particularly for less common curve patterns such as a left thoracic curve, a stiff curve, a very painful curve, or a progressive curve in a boy (**Fig. 3.2**).[36] These unusual curves do have a neuromuscular basis, and syrinx drainage or shunting usually leads to curve stabilization or improvement.

Experimental animal models of root or cord damage have produced nonidiopathic curves, usually instantly upon awakening of the animal from anesthesia.[37–40] Interestingly, Langenskiold and Michaelsson produced scoliosis in rabbits by dividing the costotransverse ligament,[41] but the resulting curves again turned out to be neuromuscular curves. De Salis and colleagues showed that the segmental artery to the spinal cord in rabbits runs just under the costotransverse ligament,[42] and that damage to this segmental blood supply produced a neuromuscular type of deformity. In rabbits, the spinal cord depends upon a segmental feeding vessel at each level (**Fig. 3.3**). Not surprisingly, when the costotransverse ligament was divided in primates with an Adamkiewicz type of cord blood supply, the spine remained straight.[43] Thermal coagulation of the facet joint capsules in rabbits also produces a spinal deformity from ischemic cord damage.[44]

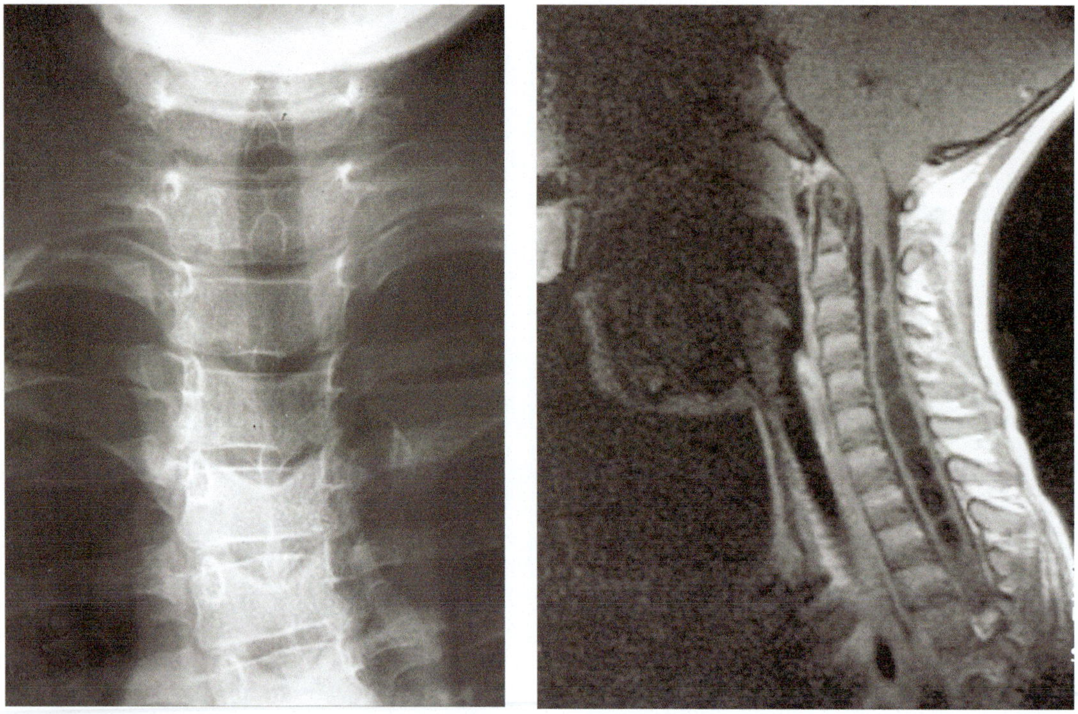


**Fig. 3.2** **(A)** PA view of the lower cervical/upper thoracic spine of a boy with a painful thoracic "idiopathic" scoliosis, showing the typical gross interpedicular widening of a syrinx. **(B)** Sagittal MRI scan of the same region, showing a very large syrinx.

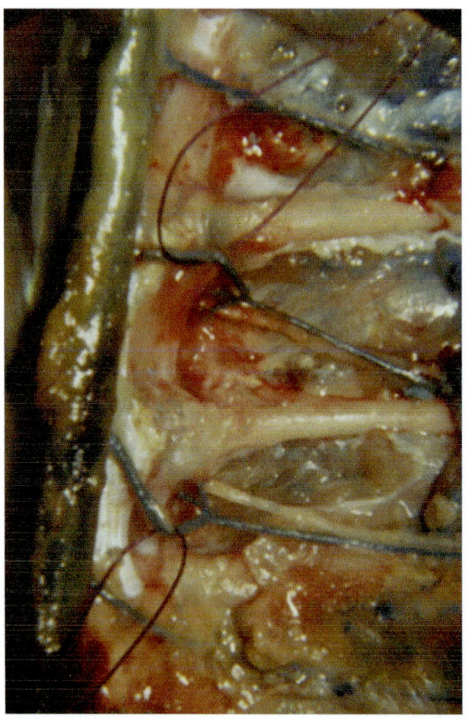

**Fig. 3.3** Dissection of the segmental blood supply to the spinal cord in the rabbit. The blood supply depends upon a feeding vessel at each level.

## Connective-tissue Abnormalities

Because connective tissue disorders such as Marfan or Ehlers–Danlos syndrome are associated with an increased prevalence of spinal deformity collagen structure and metabolism have been extensively investigated both in the skin and in the intervertebral discs in idiopathic scoliosis.[45–50] Again the findings were thought to be secondary to the presence of a spinal deformity, and indeed, recent research has excluded collagen abnormalities as potential genetic causes of idiopathic scoliosis.[51,52]

## Genetic Theories

In the late 1960s and early 1970s, the familial nature of idiopathic scoliosis was clearly demonstrated in both Scotland[53] and the United States.[54] It was thought that idiopathic scoliosis might be inherited in a sex-linked dominant mode, but with variable expressivity and incomplete penetrance. Genomic screening and chromosome studies have suggested chromosome 19 as a possible candidate for a genetic source of the disorder,[55,56] but idiopathic scoliosis is so multifactorial that it is extremely unlikely that only a single gene is responsible for it.

Longitudinal studies of growth in relation to idiopathic scoliosis show that early reports of children with the condition having been taller and having advanced earlier in adolescent growth, while later experiencing growth retardation, were not strictly correct because they relied upon historical controls already shown to be unreliable.[57] When compared with contemporaneous controls, these children showed no differences in comparison with straight-backed counterparts. However, children with bigger curves are significantly taller at each age, but do not grow faster, indicating that a genetically tall stature may be related to the progression potential of idiopathic scoliosis.[57] In such families one would expect to find a high prevalence rate of idiopathic scoliosis, and the concept of a gene for idiopathic scoliosis therefore loses credibility when the familial nature of the disorder can be explained in part on the basis of stature. Moreover, the whole pattern of growth during adolescence is strongly familial,[58] with, for instance, girls and their mothers having their menarches at similar chronological ages.

If idiopathic scoliosis is a matter of abnormal spinal shape that runs in families, then how that shape is achieved must also be genetically determined. Delmas[59] and Stagnara et al[60] both put forward the notion that children have a spinal physiognomy just as they have, for instance, a facial one, and suggested that lateral profile may be governed genetically just as are many other aspects of body shape.

Recently, the familial nature of sagittal spinal shape has been investigated in schools, using the Quantec surface-shape scanning technique, which can noninvasively register the lateral spinal profile.[61] We were particularly interested in the mid-lower thoracic spine, where idiopathic thoracic scoliosis is apical. We compared unrelated children of the same age and sex, opposite-sex siblings, and same-sex siblings, and then went to the Society of Twins meeting in the United Kingdom (Twins and Multiple Births Association) and examined both nonidentical and identical twins. With progression up the hierarchy from unrelated children to identical twins, the lateral profile of the lower thoracic spine steadily increasingly correlated with kinship, with identical twins having the same thoracic spinal shape (**Fig. 3.4**).

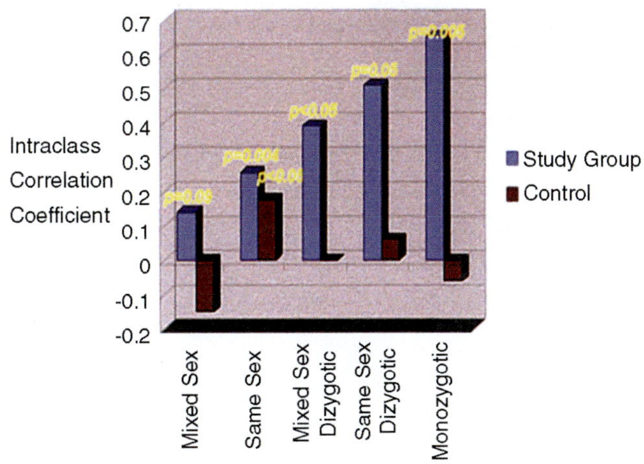


**Fig. 3.4** Lateral spinal profile measured in children in a school screening program with a surface-shape computer. This histogram of correlation coefficients demonstrates that as one passes from mixed-sex siblings through same-sex, mixed-sex dizygotic, and same-sex dizygotic to monozyotic siblings (from left to right), the correlation coefficients steadily increase in magnitude, indicating ever closer correspondence between lateral spinal profiles until with identical twins the lateral spinal profiles are virtually the same. This is a very important genetic element in the pathogenesis of idiopathic scoliosis.

## How the Three-Dimensional Deformity Develops

In trying to understand the pathogenesis of idiopathic scoliosis, it is useful to consider how the deformity develops and to start with some basic clinical and radiological observations. Considering thoracic scoliosis, in which the changes in spinal shape are most obvious, the deformity looks much less impressive in the erect position than on forward bending, when the rib hump is maximized (**Fig. 3.5**). This was observed by Adams 160 years ago,[62] but its importance was not appreciated by others for many years. Clearly, something mechanical is happening to the spinal column from the erect to the forward-bend position.

When posteroanterior (PA) X-ray films of idiopathic scoliosis are inspected, it can be observed that the direction of rotation of the spine is constant, with the posterior elements turning toward the curve concavity, and with this rotation being maximal at the curve apex. (**Fig. 3.6;** see also **Fig. 2.4**) The posterior elements of the spine are therefore running, as it were, the shorter, inside lane of the “running track,” as this appearance clearly indicates that the back of the spine must be shorter than the front. The PA X-ray view of the patient’s spine is, however, a PA view of everything except the structural curve, because from the neutral vertebra above down to the apex of the scoliotic curve, each vertebra is progressively more rotated out of the frontal plane before recovering from the apical vertebra to the lower neutral vertebra. If the apical vertebra is, for instance, rotated by 30 degrees, then to make a true anteroposterior (AP) film, either the patient or the X-ray beam has to be rotated by 30 degrees from the frontal plane, in which case the size of the deformity is maximized. Stagnara devised this AP view and termed it the *plan d’election* view (see **Figs. 2.9** and **2.10**).[63] If a true lateral X-ray film of the curve apex is to be made, the X-ray beam has to be rotated 90 degrees with reference to the AP plan d’election view (**Fig. 3.7**) When this is done, the essential lordosis is visualized.

The Leeds Group studied articulated skeletons with idiopathic scoliosis at the Royal College of Surgeons of Edinburgh Museum, which helped to visualize the lordosis and the nature of the seemingly complex three-dimensional deformity in the disorder.[35,64] **Figure 3.8** shows one such specimen. The PA view shows a significant deformity, with

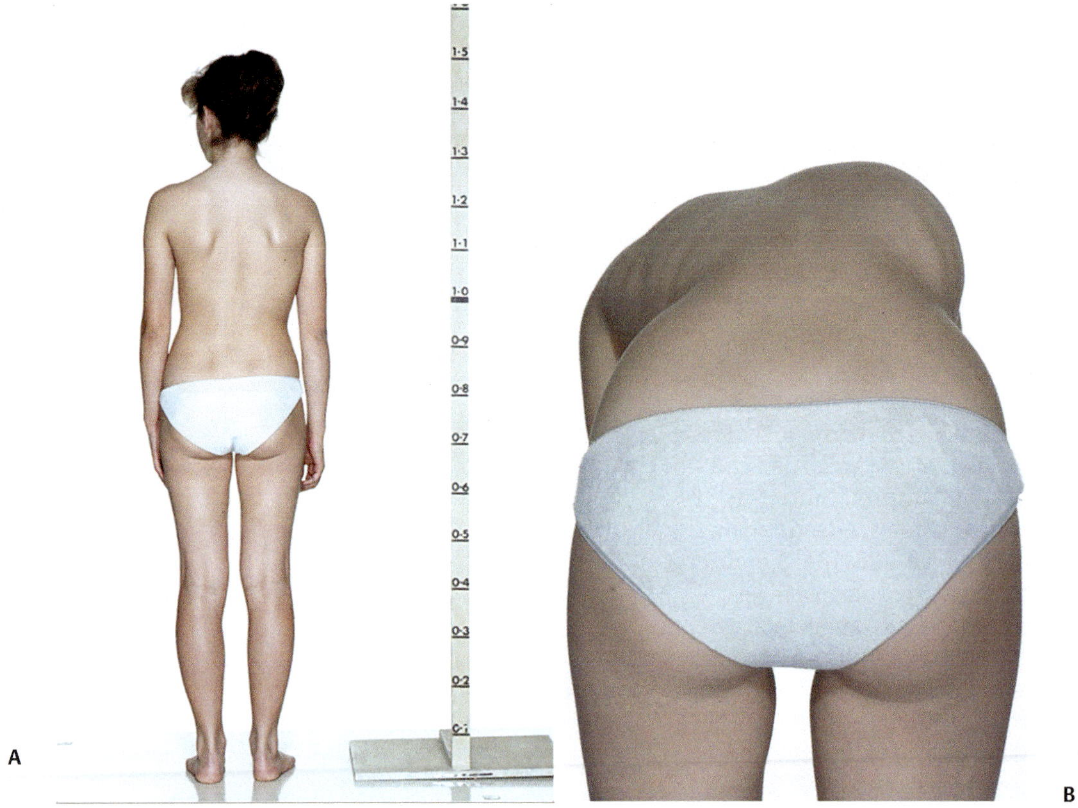


**Fig. 3.5** A 14-year-old girl with a 45-degree spinal curve. In the erect position **(A)** the deformity is much less obvious than **(B)** on forward bending, in which the rib hump is maximized.

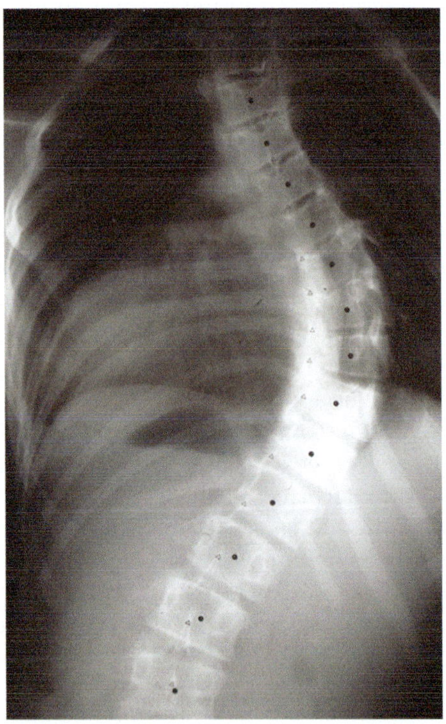

**Fig. 3.6** PA X-ray film of a thoracic idiopathic scoliosis with the tips of the spinous processes marked with triangles and the middle of the vertebral bodies with dots. It can be seen that the distance down the back of the spine is shorter than the distance down the front, confirming that all structural scolioses are lordotic.

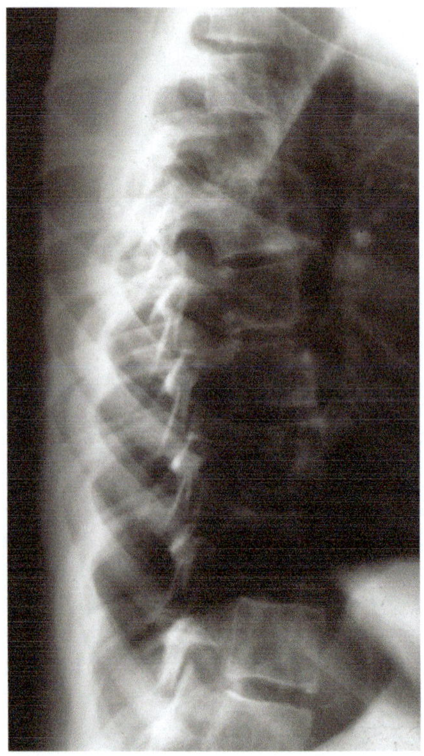

**Fig. 3.7** A true lateral view of the apex of the curvature shown in Fig. 3.6, demonstrating the lordosis.

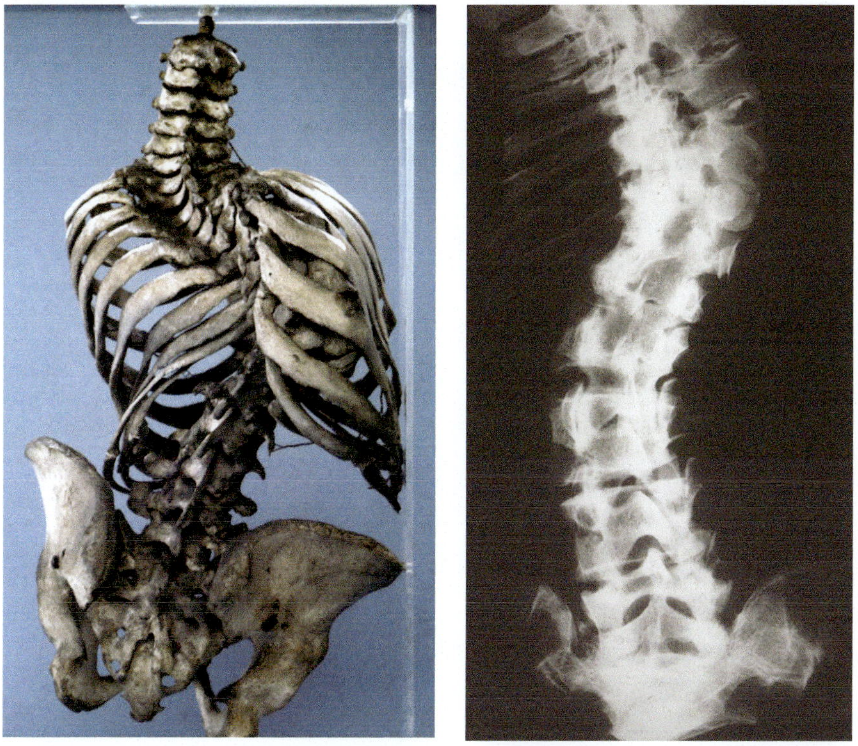

A,B

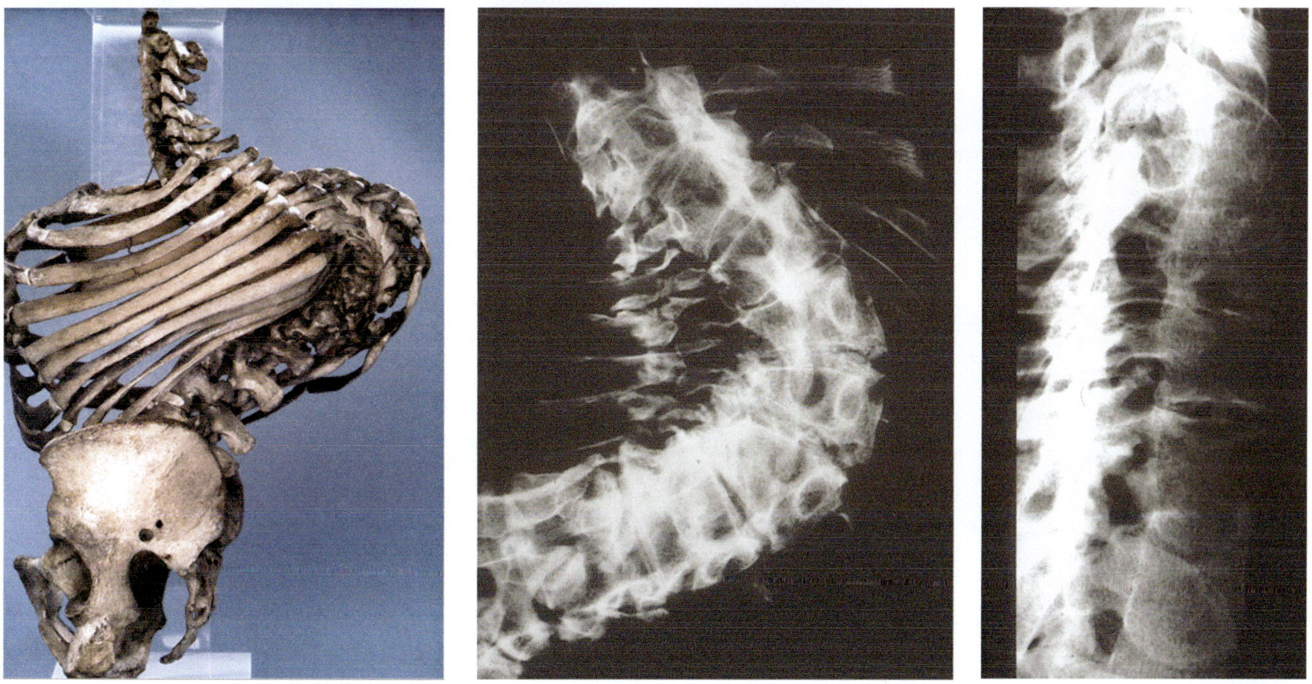

C–E

**Fig. 3.8** **(A)** Museum specimen of a severe idiopathic thoracic scoliosis. Back view showing the right thoracic curve with a lot of rotation. **(B)** PA X-ray film of the specimen, showing so much rotation that it is almost a lateral view of the curve apex. **(C)** Side view of the specimen, showing the spurious appearance of kyphosis, but it is not the back of the spine pointing backward. **(D)** Lateral X-ray film of the specimen, showing almost a PA view of the curve apex. **(E)** True lateral X-ray view showing the essential lordosis.

considerable rotation, and the PA X-ray film demonstrates almost 90 degrees of rotation, with the apical vertebra being seen in an almost lateral projection. The lateral view of the specimen would appear to show the presence of a kyphosis, but it can be seen at the curve apex that the spinous processes are pointing almost directly backward. The lateral X-ray film of the specimen now looks more like an AP view of the curve apex, again confirming a rotation of almost 90 degrees. A true lateral view of the apex thus unmasks the essential lordosis.

Going back to the clinical inspection of patients, it is possible to see the lordosis in idiopathic scoliosis if one knows where to look. **Figure 3.9A** shows a young man with a 30-degree right thoracic curve. His whole thoracic

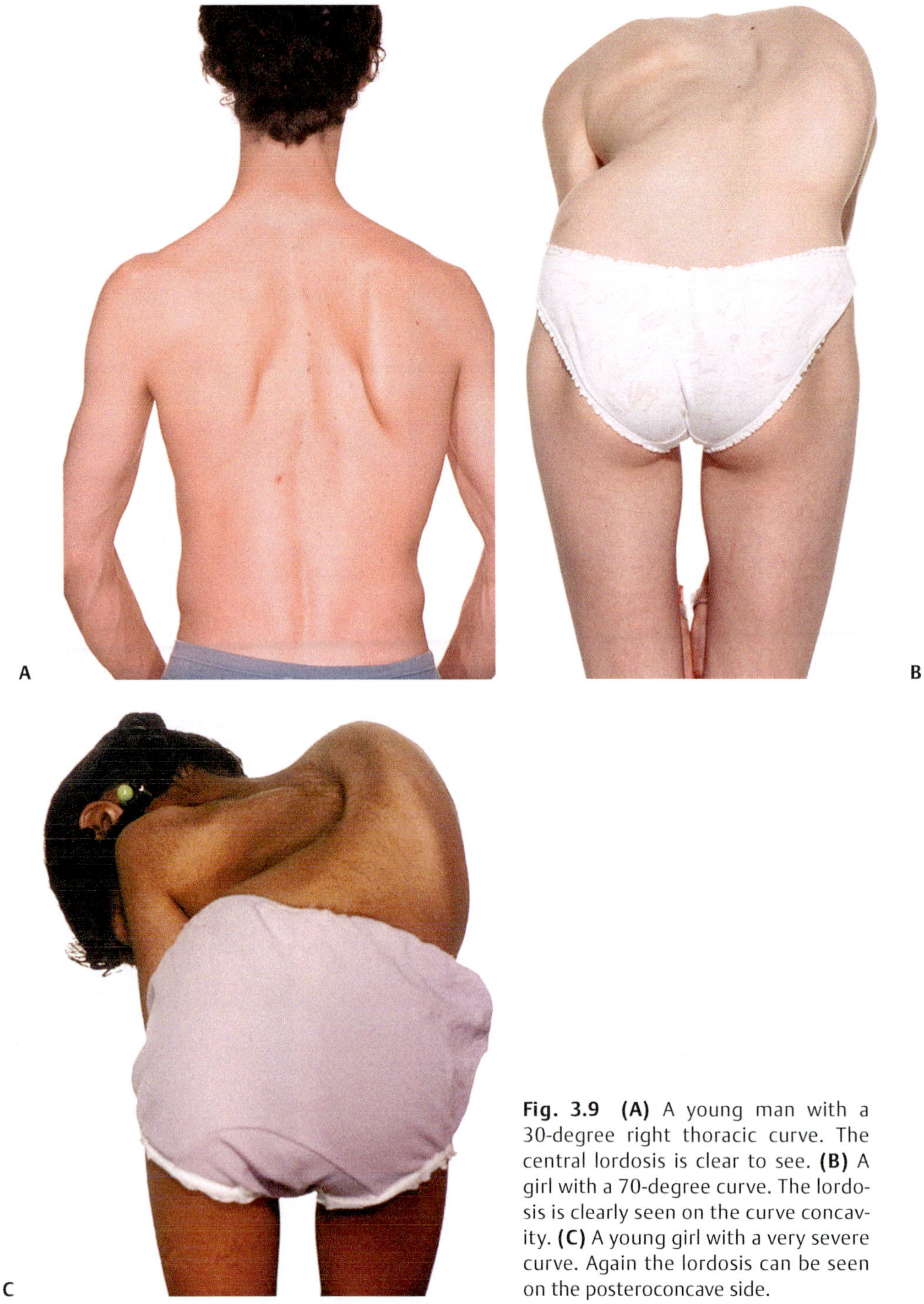

Fig. 3.9 **(A)** A young man with a 30-degree right thoracic curve. The central lordosis is clear to see. **(B)** A girl with a 70-degree curve. The lordosis is clearly seen on the curve concavity. **(C)** A young girl with a very severe curve. Again the lordosis can be seen on the posteroconcave side.

kyphosis is flattened, and there is clearly a lordosis in the middle. **Figure 3.9B** shows a girl with a 70-degree curve. Again looking at the concavity at the curve apex, there is clearly a lordosis. **Figure 3.9C** shows an extreme degree of infantile progressive scoliosis. The structure bulging backward underneath the convex ribs is in fact the front of the spine, with the vertebral bodies, whereas looking toward the concave side of the curve apex clearly shows the lordosis.

Returning to the biomechanics of forward bending, the axis of spinal-column rotation normally passes in front of the thoracic kyphosis and behind the cervical and lumbar lordoses (**Fig. 3.10**). This confers protection to the thoracic spine against buckling, because this region of the spine is normally under tension. With the development of a thoracic lordosis, however (**Fig. 3.11**), the vertebral bodies move progressively further forward, toward and in front of

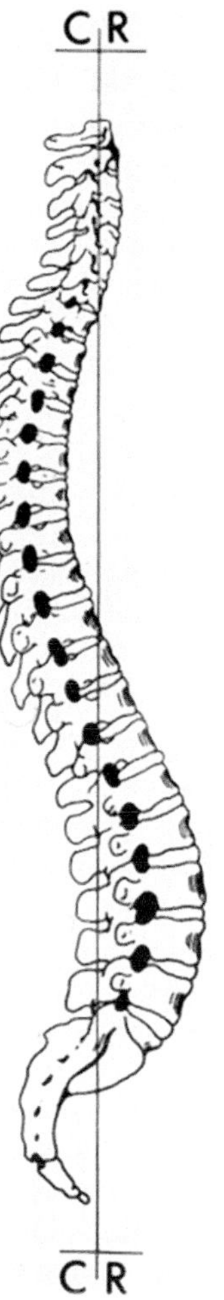


**Fig. 3.10** The axis of spinal column rotation. This is determined by the orientation of the posterior facet joints at each level.

this axis of rotation, making them very vulnerable to buckling and explaining the increased rotational prominence seen on forward bending in idiopathic scoliosis (**Fig. 3.9**).[65]

If one compares the true lateral view of the apex of the idiopathic thoracic scoliotic curve with a lateral view of Scheuermann's kyphosis, they would appear to be opposite directional deformities in the sagittal plane (**Fig. 3.12**). Thoracic hyperkyphosis is, however, progressively further behind the axis of spinal-column rotation, and therefore progresses solely in the sagittal plane (**Fig. 3.13**). However, it is well known that more than two-thirds of patients with Scheuermann's idiopathic thoracic hyperkyphosis have an idiopathic scoliosis below this deformity, and this is where the lumbar hyperlordosis, which exists to balance the thoracic hyperkyphosis above, buckles to produce Scheuermann's disease and idiopathic scoliosis in the same spine (**Fig. 3.14**).[66]

The distribution of thoracic kyphosis is probably Gaussian, with patients at the flat end of the spectrum in danger of developing idiopathic scoliosis and those at the round end of the spectrum in danger of developing Scheuermann's disease. The nature of the distribution would be confirmed by idiopathic scoliosis and Scheuermann's disease having similar familial relationships and community prevalence rates.[67]

Considering the spine as the engineer's beam or column, it can be confirmed that the column is subject to only two primary modes of failure: angular collapse (kyphosis) and beam buckling (lordoscoliosis) (**Fig. 3.15**). Furthermore, engineers have established laws of the behavior of flexible columns, the critical load being decreased by: (1) increased curvature; (2) increased length; and (3) increased intrinsic load.[65] The greater the curve becomes, the more likely it will progress, as studies of the natural history of idiopathic scoliosis have clearly shown[68] (the further the Leaning Tower of Pisa leans, the more it will be likely to fall down). Girls with idiopathic scoliosis are significantly taller than age-matched counterparts even when their spinal deformity has not been "uncoiled."[69,70] The concept of an increased intrinsic load refers to a situation in which the spinal column is weakened, and here one can bring in some of the other parts of the classification of spinal deformities. Thus, for instance, neuromuscular scoliosis occurs because the neuromuscular support to the spine is inadequate (**Fig. 3.16A**), whereas in neurofibromatosis or osteogenesis imperfecta, the more dystrophic the bone the greater the prevalence of structural scoliosis and the earlier its onset (**Fig. 3.16B**). With Marfan syndrome or Ehlers–Danlos syndrome the spine fails at the soft-tissue level (**Fig. 3.16C**).

The differences between scoliosis and kyphosis would appear to be very obvious, particularly with the established clinical conditions of, for example, 60 degrees of thoracic scoliosis and 60 degrees of thoracic hyperkyphosis, but the changes are much more subtle than that. The upper and lower thoracic vertebrae are either straight or are parts of the cervical or lumbar lordoses, leaving about eight real thoracic vertebrae. A figure of ~24 degrees would be reasonable for the thoracic kyphosis in early adolescence, and each of the eight vertebrae would therefore be kyphotically wedged by something of the order of 3 degrees. It is necessary to lose only a little more than 3 degrees of kyphosis to create lordosis and the danger of buckling into a lordoscoliosis (**Fig. 3.17**).[65] Because these changes are so subtle, it should not be any wonder that school screening programs have demonstrated that 2.2% of girls aged 12 to 14 years have idiopathic scoliosis (a lateral curvature in excess of 10 degrees with rotation).[71]

Both Willner and Johnson in Sweden[72] and the Leeds Group[61] have shown that the thoracic kyphosis changes considerably during growth. It is at a minimum at about the age of 10 years before going up to its maximum of 30 to 40 degrees or so at the age of 15 years. Girls grow fastest between the ages of 10 or 11 years, when the thoracic kyphosis is at its minimum, and if they overgrow (a feature of the development of spinal deformities), they will therefore

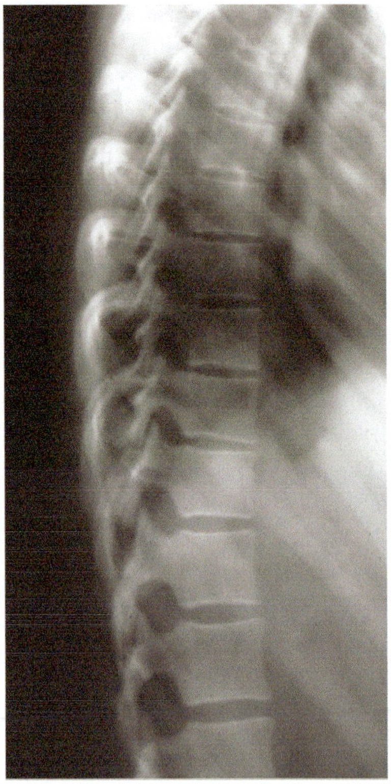

A

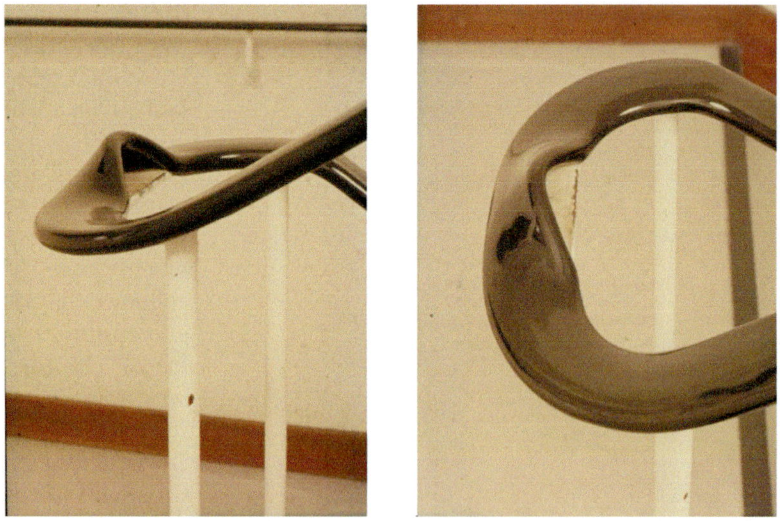

B

**Fig. 3.11** **(A)** A lateral view of a growing spine with a biomechanically unstable lordosis. **(B)** The banister rail outside the operating theater in St. James's University Hospital, Leeds. The banister rail makes a lordosis at each floor level, causing the black plastic handrail to buckle.

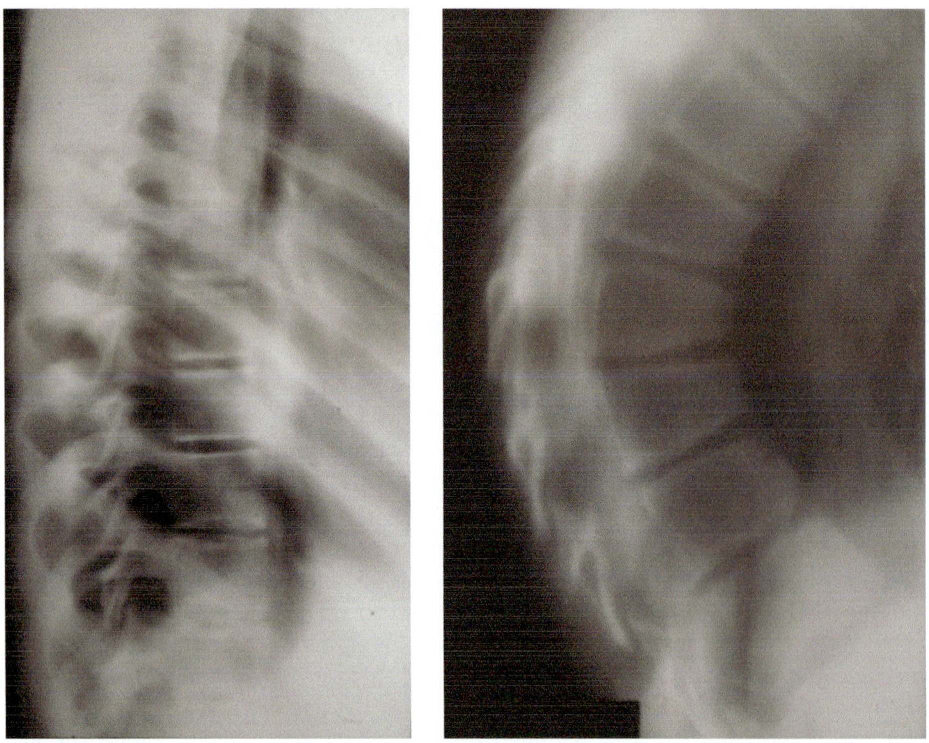

A B

**Fig. 3.12** **(A)** True lateral X-ray view of an idiopathic thoracic curve. **(B)** Lateral X-ray view of Scheuermann's idiopathic thoracic hyperkyphosis. These are opposite deformities in the sagittal plane.

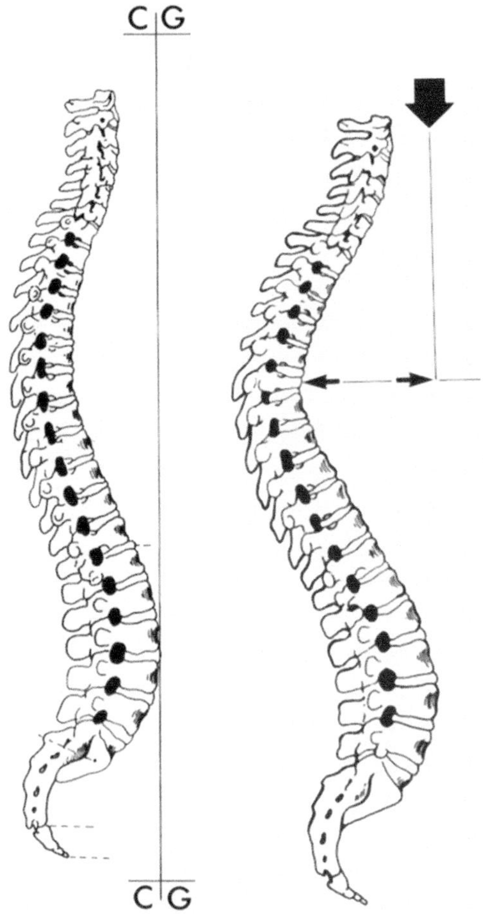


A B

**Fig. 3.13** **(A)** The center of gravity of the body lies just in front of the lumbar spine, and with hyperkyphosis the thoracic spine is therefore progressively behind the axis of spinal column rotation. **(B)** Consequently, the deformity progresses solely in the sagittal plane, with no buckling potential.

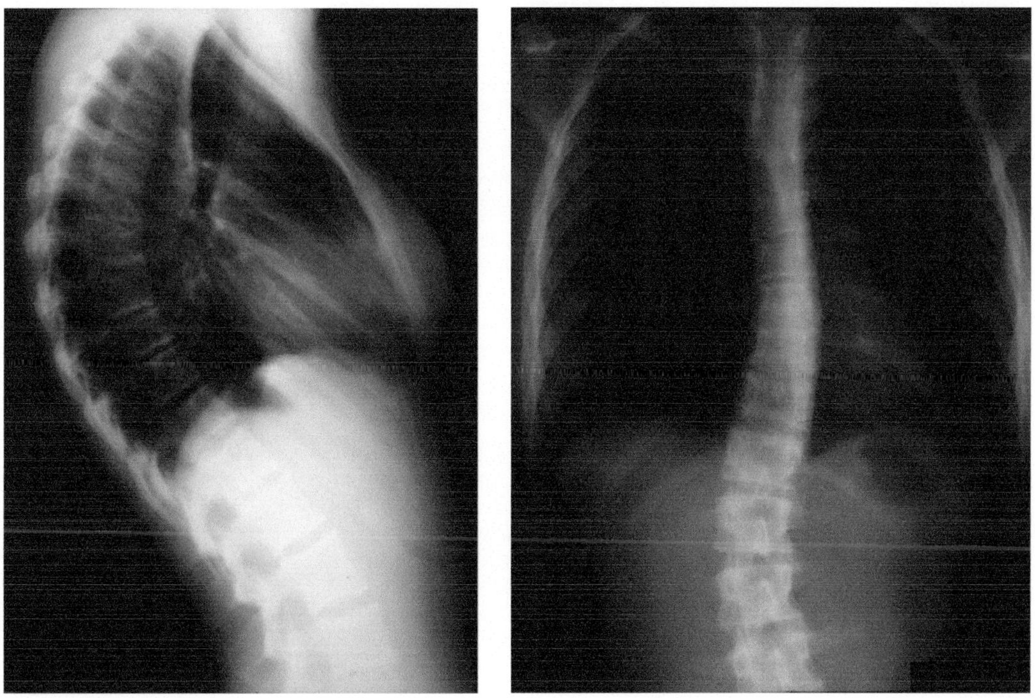

A B

**Fig. 3.14** **(A)** Lateral X-ray film of a boy with Scheuermann's disease. **(B)** PA X-ray film showing that the compensatory lumbar hyperlordosis has buckled to produce idiopathic scoliosis below the area of Scheuermann's disease.

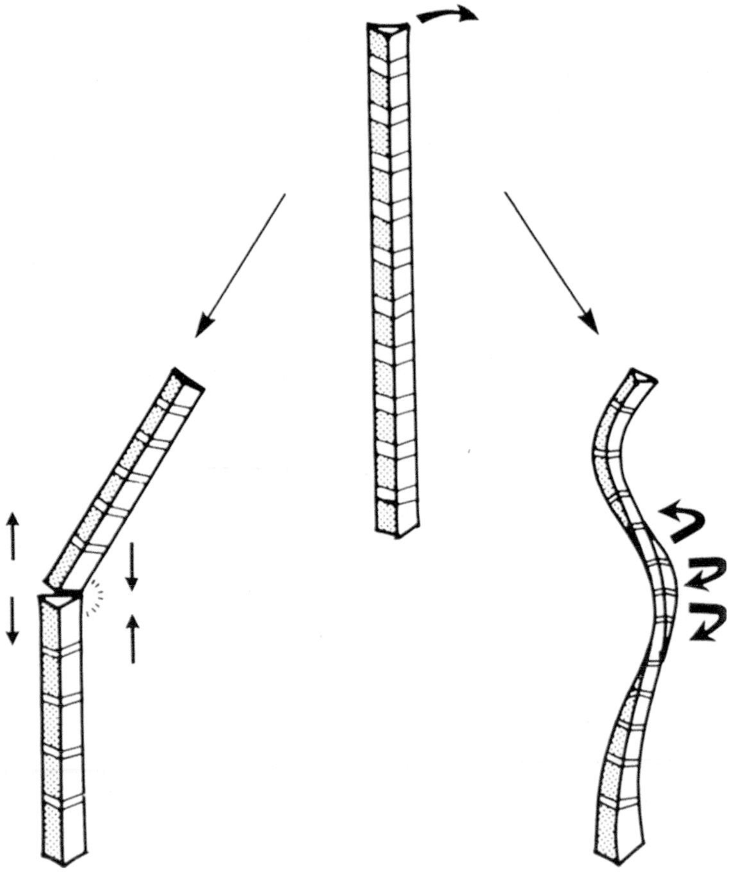

**Fig. 3.15** A column or beam can fail in only two ways: angular collapse (kyphosis) or beam buckling (lordoscoliosis).

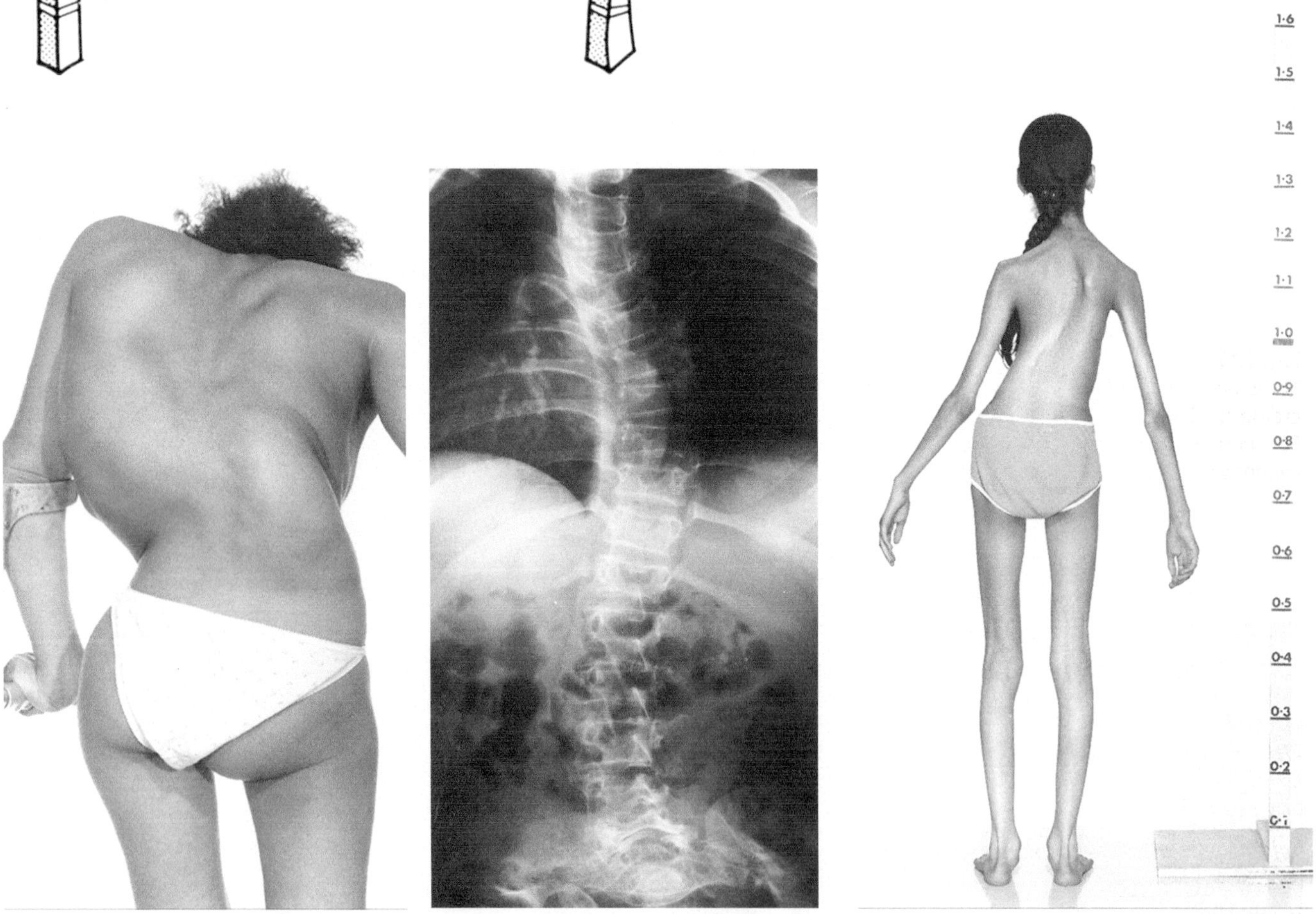


A–C

**Fig. 3.16** **(A)** Scoliosis in association with poliomyelitis. The spine has failed at the neuromuscular level. **(B)** Scoliosis in association with osteogenesis imperfecta. The spine has failed at the bone level. **(C)** Scoliosis in association with Marfan syndrome. The spine has failed at the soft-tissue level.

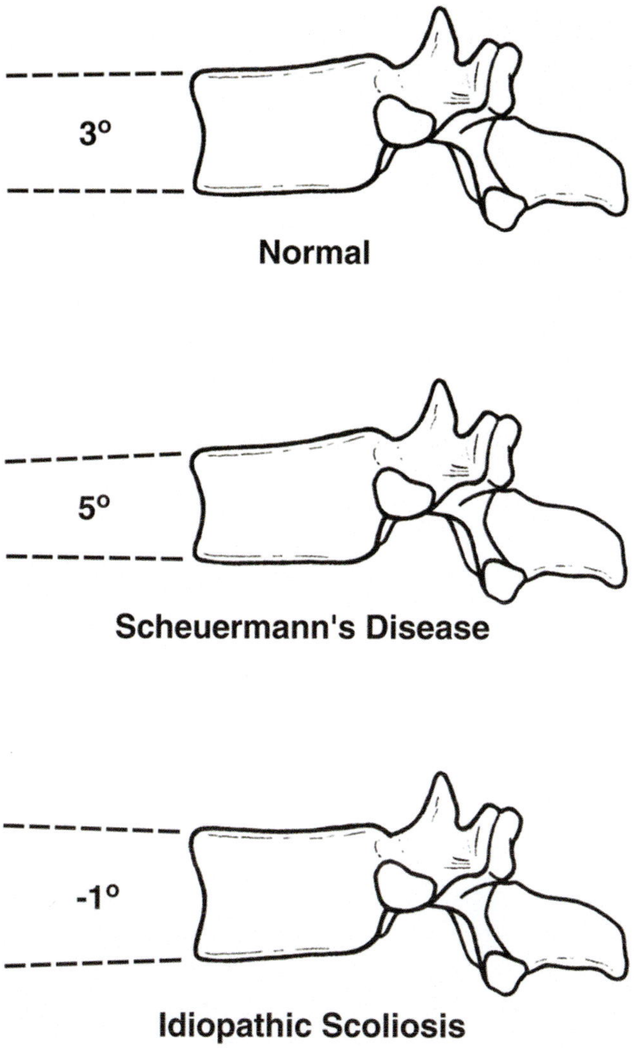


**Fig. 3.17** Sagittal vertebral body shape is a delicate matter. (Top) Three degrees of kyphosis would be about normal. (Middle) An increase by 2 degrees over three levels is Sorenson's definition of Scheuermann's disease. (Bottom) Loss of just over 3 degrees of kyphosis renders the spinal column vulnerable to buckling.

be vulnerable to the development of idiopathic scoliosis (**Fig. 3.18**). Boys do not go through their growth spurt until much later, when the thoracic kyphosis is maximizing, which is why boys are more vulnerable to the opposite condition of idiopathic thoracic hyperkyphosis (Scheuermann's disease) (**Fig. 3.19**).

That a thoracic lordosis is the primary event in the generation of idiopathic thoracic scoliosis was conclusively shown in the Leeds epidemiological survey.[71] A sensitive positive test of an angle of trunk inclination of 5 degrees or more was the criterion for admission to the study, and of the 16,000 Leeds schoolchildren surveyed, 1000 were harvested and subsequently radiographed on an annual basis for 6 years with AP and lateral low dose films. With such a sensitive entry criterion many children had straight backs to begin with, but some developed true idiopathic scoliosis during the course of the study. This afforded the opportunity of going back to look at the lateral profile when the spine was straight in the frontal plane, and children who developed idiopathic scoliosis already had a flat thoracic spine with an apical lordosis (**Fig. 3.20**).

Transverse plane geometry is also important in the normal as well as the scoliotic spine. This became apparent when the specimens of idiopathic scoliosis in the Royal College of Surgeons of Edinburgh Museum were first examined.[34] More detailed studies of the same specimens confirmed this.[35,64] In the cervical and lumbar regions, where the spine is naturally lordotic, the cross-sectional vertebral shape is prismatic, with the base pointing anteriorly. This is most obvious in the lumbar region where the vertebrae in cross-section are typically described as broad and kidney-shaped (**Fig. 3.21**). When prisms are flexed toward their bases, they are much more stable because of the second moment of area, and the potentially vulnerable cervical and lumbar lordoses are therefore countered by having a stable transverse-planar shape. By contrast, vertebrae in the thoracic region are typically heart-shaped in the transverse plane, with the apex of the prism pointing anteriorly. This is

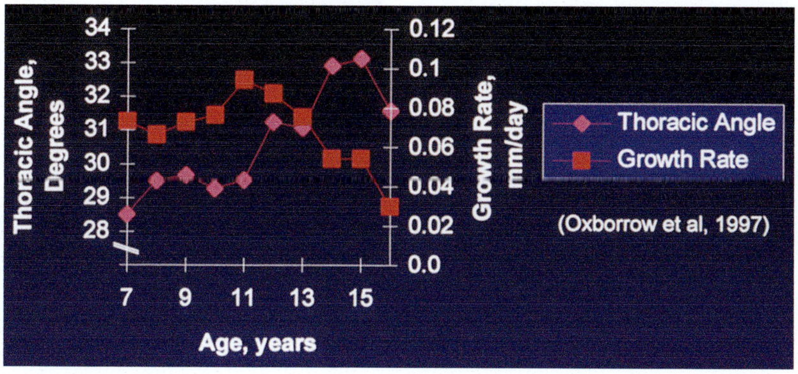


**Fig. 3.18** The thoracic kyphosis is at its minimum when girls grow fastest.

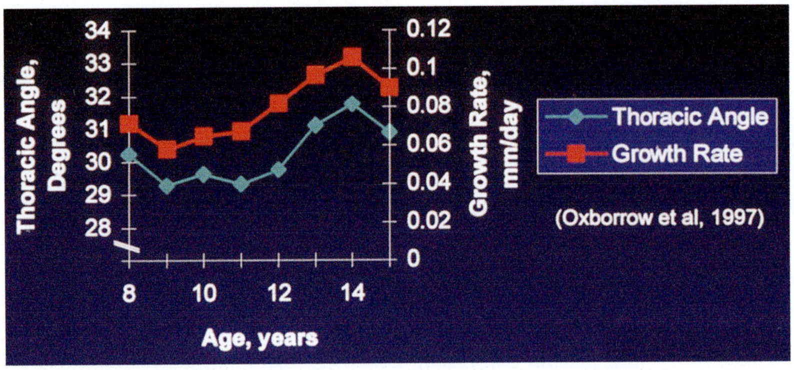


**Fig. 3.19** Boys don't grow fastest until toward the end of growth, when the thoracic kyphosis is maximal.

a dangerous configuration, favoring buckling with flexion, and the thoracic spine is therefore protected by having a safe kyphosis in the sagittal plane.

However, more thoracic curves are convex to the right and more lumbar curves convex to the left, and this is because of a pre-existing asymmetry of vertebral shape in the transverse plane. Anatomists have shown that in the thoracic spine, the T4 to T9 vertebrae are constantly deformed on the left side by the descending thoracic aorta[73] (**Figs. 3.21C and 3.22**), whereas a dynamic form of transverse-planar asymmetry exists in the lumbar region, where the left-sided abdominal aorta provides a restraint on curves tending to go to the right (**Fig. 3.23**).[65] This has been confirmed more recently with axial computed tomography (CT) scans of normal human spines.[74] Not surprisingly, the situation was opposite this in individuals with situs inversus.[75]

Clearly, however, the preponderance of right-sided thoracic curves and left-sided lumbar curves does not equate with the prevalence rate of situs inversus. This is because among small thoracic curves (< 20 degrees), more are left-sided than right-sided, and because lumbar curves do not really have a left predominance until they reach or exceed 15 degrees, according to data of the Oxford School Screening Study (**Table 3.1**).[76]

A–C

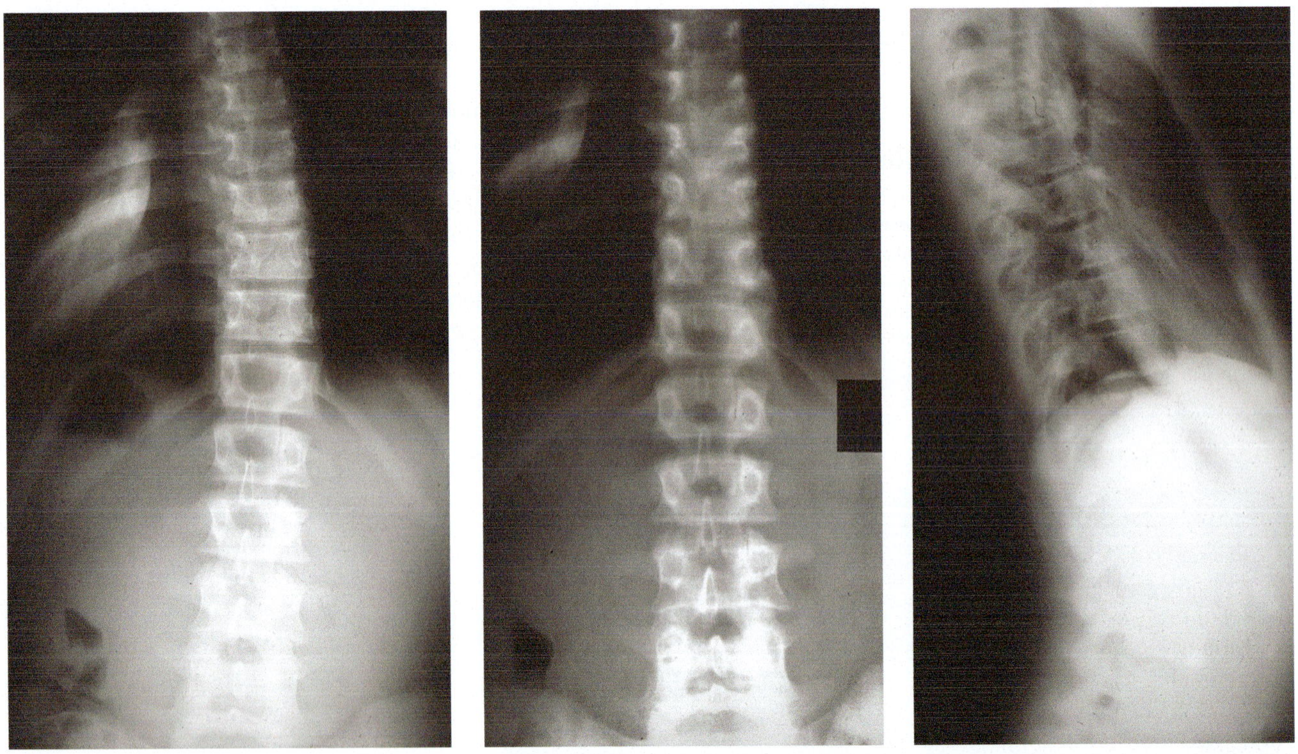

**Fig. 3.20** **(A)** PA X-ray film of a 14-year-old girl with a mild right thoracic idiopathic scoliosis. She was part of the Leeds longitudinal epidemiological survey. **(B)** PA X-ray film made years earlier, when the patient's spine was straight. **(C)** Lateral X-ray film made years earlier, showing the dangerous lateral profile that preceded the development of the patient's curve.

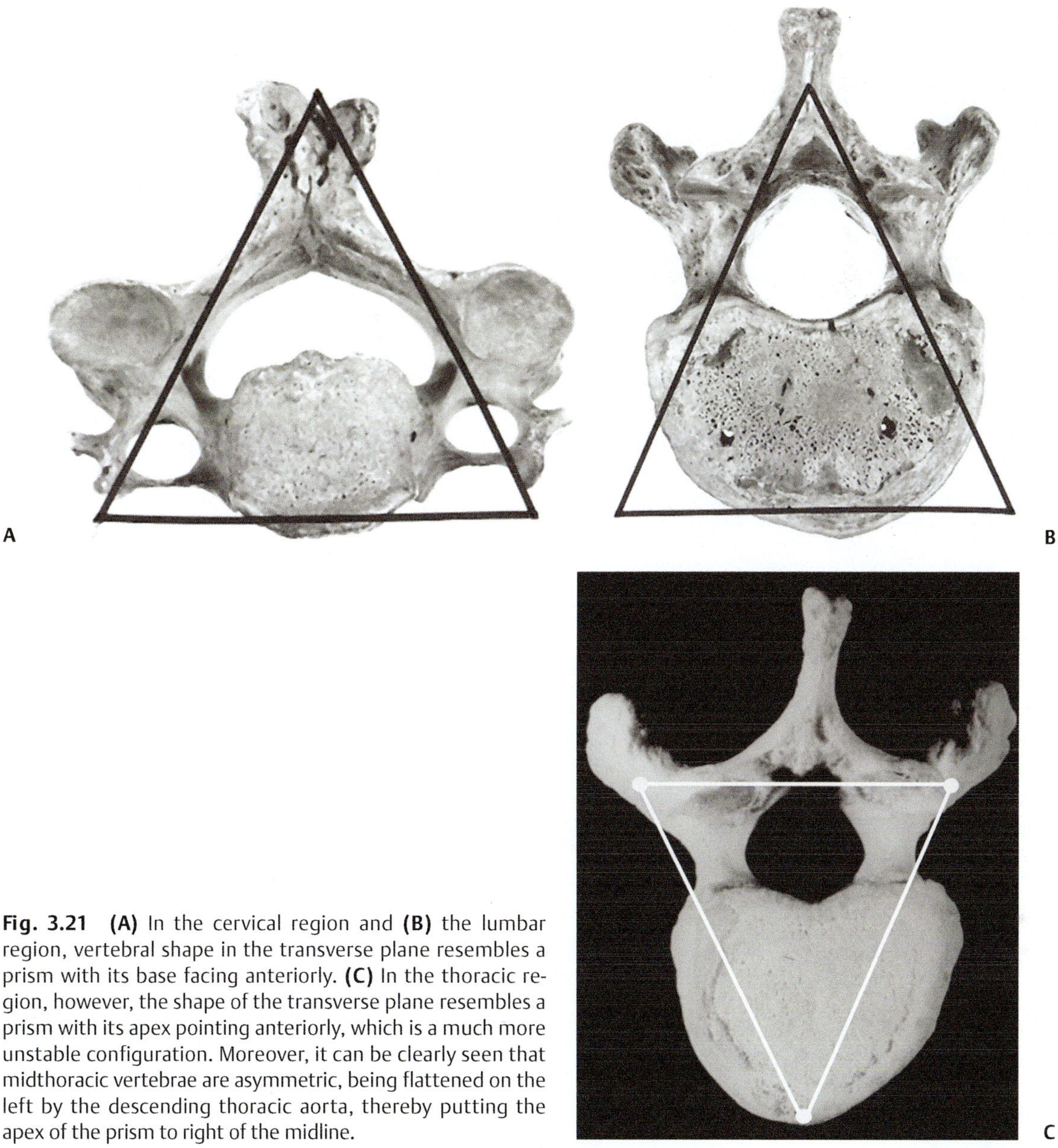


**Fig. 3.21** **(A)** In the cervical region and **(B)** the lumbar region, vertebral shape in the transverse plane resembles a prism with its base facing anteriorly. **(C)** In the thoracic region, however, the shape of the transverse plane resembles a prism with its apex pointing anteriorly, which is a much more unstable configuration. Moreover, it can be clearly seen that midthoracic vertebrae are asymmetric, being flattened on the left by the descending thoracic aorta, thereby putting the apex of the prism to right of the midline.

## Experimental Scoliosis

Following Adams's original dissections of cadavers with idiopathic scoliosis, showing the essential lordosis at the curve apex,[62] Somerville in Oxford produced an experimental model of progressive idiopathic-type scoliosis in the growing rabbit.[44] He tethered the back of the spine into lordosis and then performed a soft-tissue release posteriorly on one side to direct subsequent buckling that would cause the typical lordoscoliotic deformity seen in patients with idiopathic scoliosis. Our group in Leeds conducted extensive experimental work that consistently caused an idiopathic-type deformity in rabbits by producing an asymmetrical lordosis similar to what Somerville achieved with his methods (**Fig. 3.24**).[77–79] Importantly, no buckling occurred if the lordosis wasn't given directional instability. Moreover, if the lordosis was released before the end of spinal growth, and the deformity had not progressed beyond approximately 20 to 30 degrees, the spine grew straight again, suggesting that addressing the sagittal-plane component of the scoliotic deformity in children might be beneficial.[80] If, however, the tether is not released, the deformity progresses relentlessly (**Fig. 3.25**).

We also extensively studied the three-dimensional nature of the deformity in idiopathic scoliosis and in particular its transverse-plane component[81] in both animals

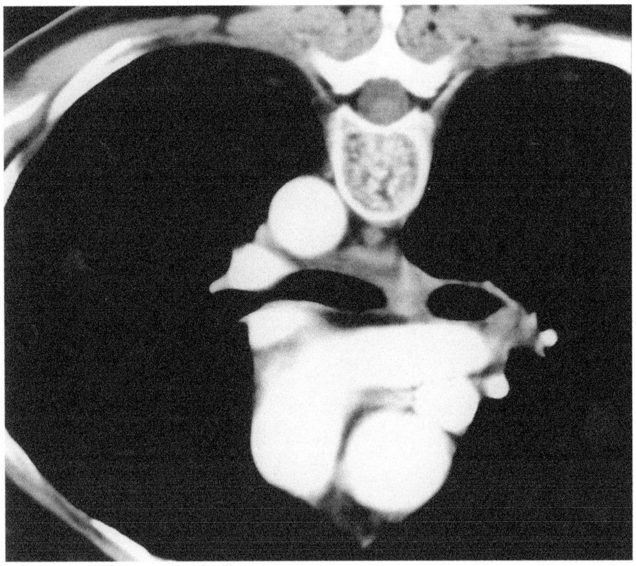

Fig. 3.22 CT scan at the T8 level, showing transverse-plane asymmetry caused by the descending thoracic aorta.

**Table 3.1 Direction of Idiopathic Curves with Curve Size**

| Curve Size | No. of Curves | Direction (%) R | Direction (%) L |
|---|---|---|---|
| **Thoracic** | | | |
| 5–9 | 93 | 38 | 62 |
| 10–14 | 36 | 47 | 53 |
| 15–19 | 9 | 33 | 67 |
| 20+ | 6 | 67 | 33 |
| Total | 144 | 41 | 59 |
| **Lumbar** | | | |
| 5–9 | 50 | 28 | 72 |
| 10–14 | 30 | 43 | 57 |
| 15–19 | 8 | - | 100 |
| 20+ | 6 | - | 100 |
| Total | 94 | 29 | 71 |

and humans. We clearly found the most asymmetrical vertebra at the curve apex, where the pedicle on the convex side was short and stout and that on the concave side was long and slender (**Fig. 3.26**). The transverse-plane geometry changed above and below the apex of the curve, first becoming neutral before becoming the opposite in the compensatory kyphoses that balance the central lordotic

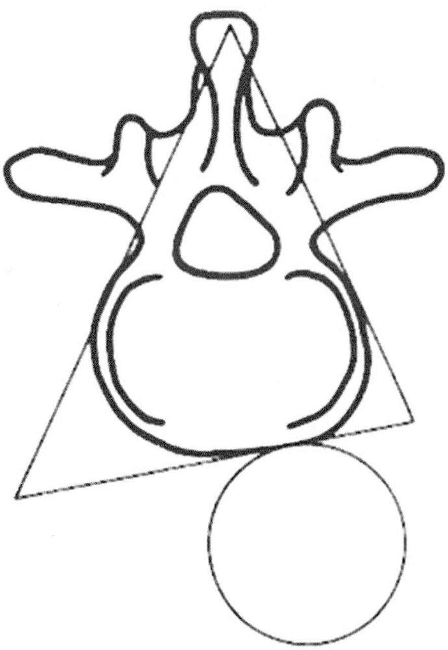

Fig. 3.23 In the lumbar region the abdominal aorta is to the left of the midline and thus rests against the left side of the base of the lumbar prism, favoring left-sided rotation in the lumbar spine.

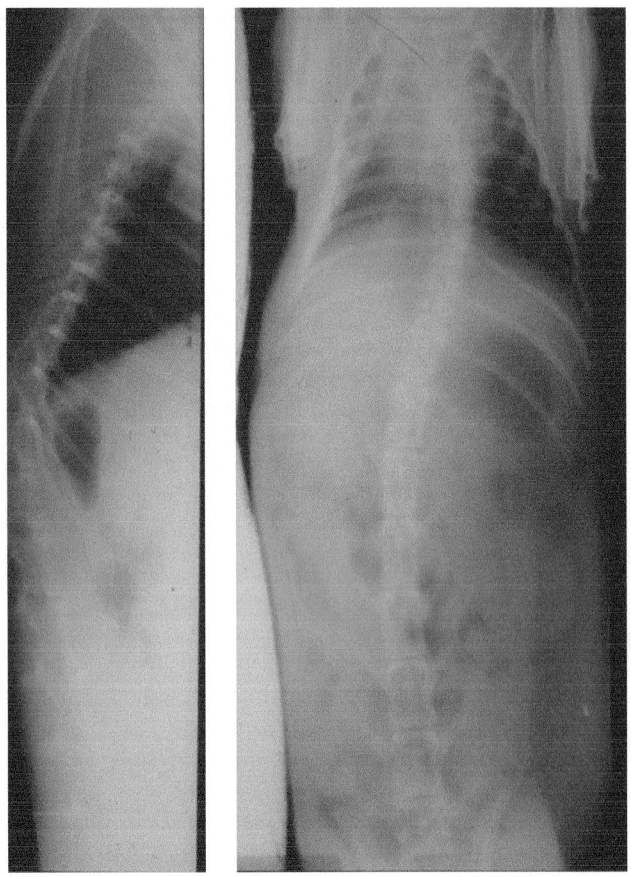

A,B

Fig. 3.24 When the growing rabbit spine is tethered into lordosis **(A)**, a progressive lordoscoliosis develops over the next few weeks **(B)**. If the tether is released at this stage, in which there is a mild curve, the spine will subsequently straighten with growth because the Heueter–Volkmann Law has not irreversibly deformed the apical vertebrae.

A,B

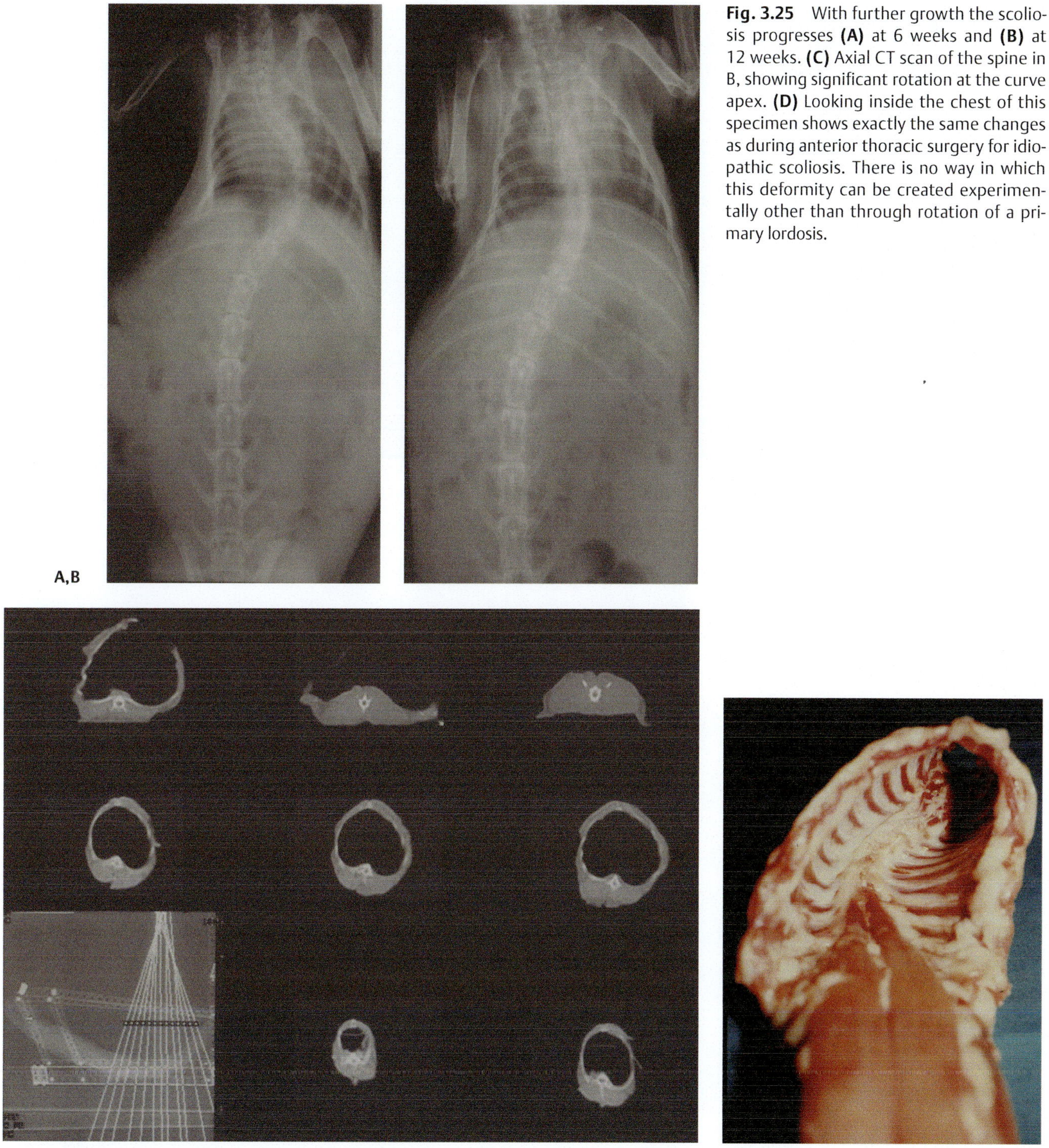

C D

**Fig. 3.25** With further growth the scoliosis progresses **(A)** at 6 weeks and **(B)** at 12 weeks. **(C)** Axial CT scan of the spine in B, showing significant rotation at the curve apex. **(D)** Looking inside the chest of this specimen shows exactly the same changes as during anterior thoracic surgery for idiopathic scoliosis. There is no way in which this deformity can be created experimentally other than through rotation of a primary lordosis.

area. In these regions the pedicle on the convex side was long and slender and that on the concave side short and stout.

The same pattern of apical vertebral-body deformation was seen in the rabbit as in the human, and by labeling areas of active vertebral growth with a dye similar to tetracycline, we observed bone drift toward the curve concavity, indicating that the spine was trying to correct the deformity imposed upon it (**Fig. 3.27**).[81]

When the segmental blood supply to the spinal cord was occluded at the curve apex, a cord infarct was produced, and this led to a significant deformity, in excess of 40 degrees, as soon as the procedure was completed, resembling what was observed in experimental neuromuscular scoliosis

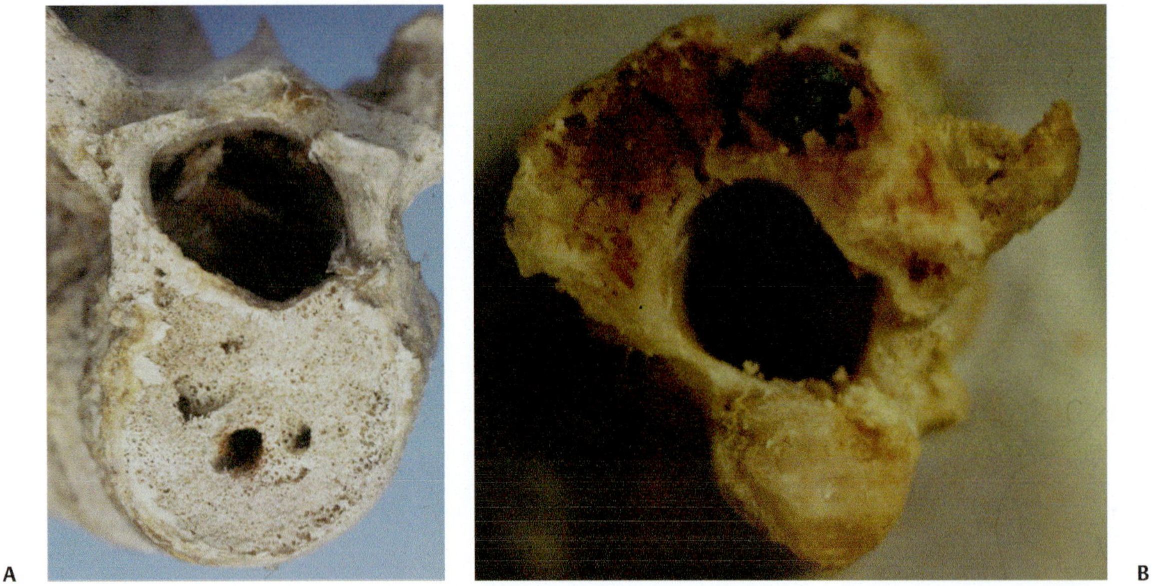

Fig. 3.26 Transverse-plane asymmetry at the curve apex, with a short, stout pedicle on the convex side and a longer, thinner pedicle on the concave side. (A) Human, (B) rabbit.

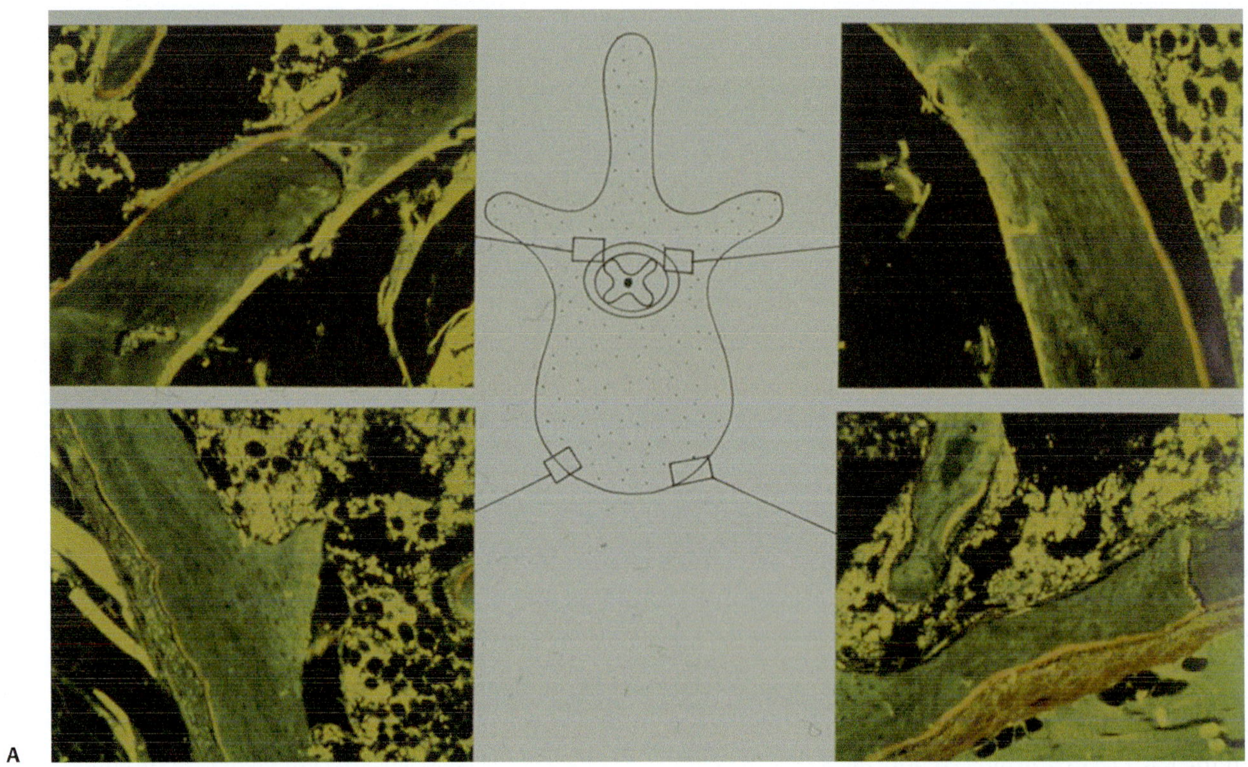

Fig. 3.27 (A) The diagram in the center shows that growth of a normal vertebra in terms of the spinal canal and the vertebral body is outward. Consequently, the orange-stained growth area in the canal above and the vertebral body below is facing outward.

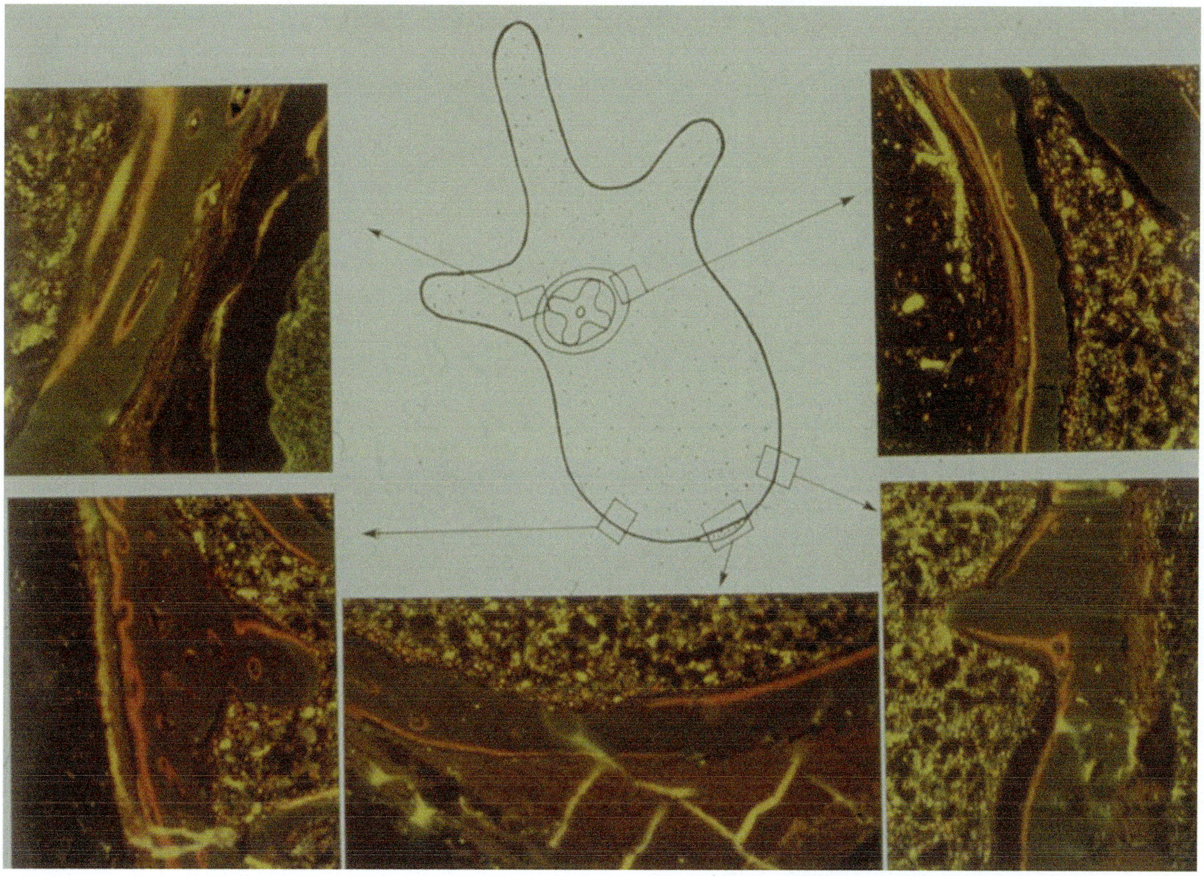

B

**Fig. 3.27** *(Continued)* **(B)** With the apical scoliotic vertebra, the spinal canal and the vertebral body grow toward the concavity, as the orange-stained growth zones indicate. Thus, the transverse plane is trying to correct and not cause the deformity. The transverse plane is therefore not an etiological factor in idiopathic scoliosis.

(**Fig. 3.28**).[82] This is how Langenskiold and Michelsson[41] accidentally produced scoliosis by dividing the costotransverse ligament, because they damaged the segmental blood supply to the spinal cord, as De Salis and colleagues[42] demonstrated. Interestingly, growth and pulmonary function were considerably impaired with a rapidly progressive thoracic deformity, rather like the situation in progressive infantile idiopathic thoracic scoliosis (**Fig. 3.29**).[82]

Much interest in experimental scoliosis was rekindled by observations of pinealectomized chickens and rats popularized by Dubousset et al[83] and Machida et al.[84] The pineal gland produces melatonin from tryptophan through a series of enzyme reactions, and serotonin is intermediary in this pathway. In 1959 Thillard first produced scoliosis in pinealectomized chickens to assess the role of melatonin and its associated compounds in the disorder.[85] If chickens are pinealectomized shortly after they hatch, a scoliosis similar to human idiopathic scoliosis is consistently produced. If melatonin supplements are given after pinealectomy, a scoliosis does not develop.[84] The precise reason why pinealectomy produces this deformity is uncertain, and research translated to the human situation has shown conflicting results with regard to melatonin levels in patients with idiopathic scoliosis and those in controls, with some careful studies involving diurnal variation showing no differences in the two groups.[86,87] It is thought that melatonin activity may be mediated by growth hormone as the common denominator.[88]

However, the biomechanics of this experimental model are also interesting. Even with the pinealectomized animal model it is accepted that the "primary abnormality is a lordosis," which subsequently buckles to produce the typical three-dimensional lordoscoliotic deformity, as confirmed by Machida.[88] This does not occur spontaneously in quadrupeds, and chickens are bipedal. Consequently, Dubousset and Machida and colleagues went on to investigate the effects of pinealectomy in rats.[89] If rats were initially rendered bipedal and then pinealectomiaed, they developed a scoliosis comparable to that in chickens, whereas the spine remained straight in rats that underwent a sham operation after being rendered bipedal (**Fig. 3.30**). Quadrupedal rats when pinealectomized did not develop a spinal deformity.

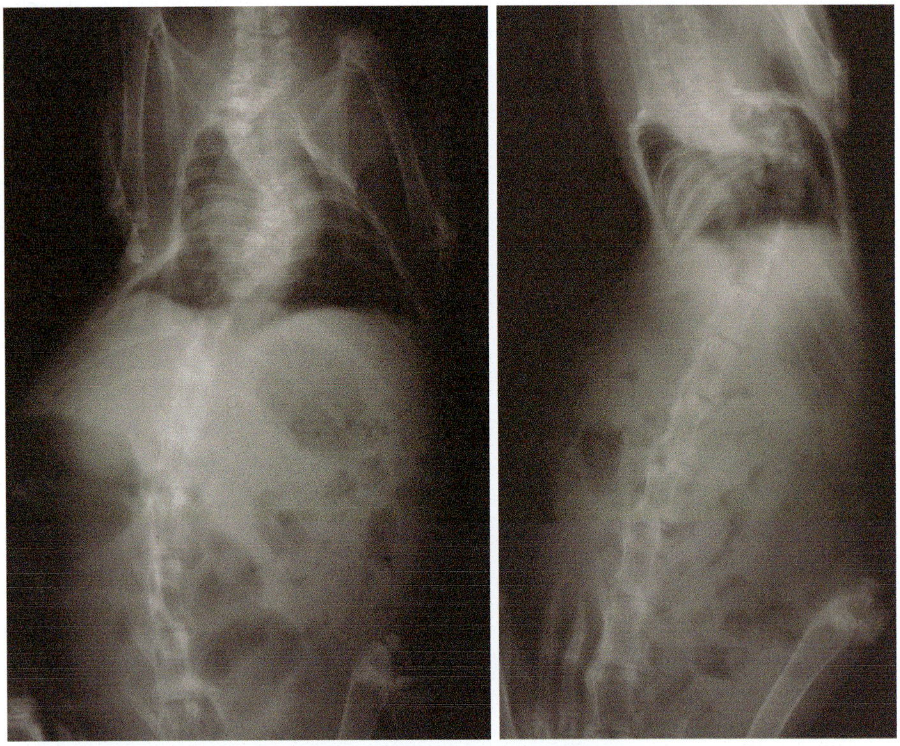

A B

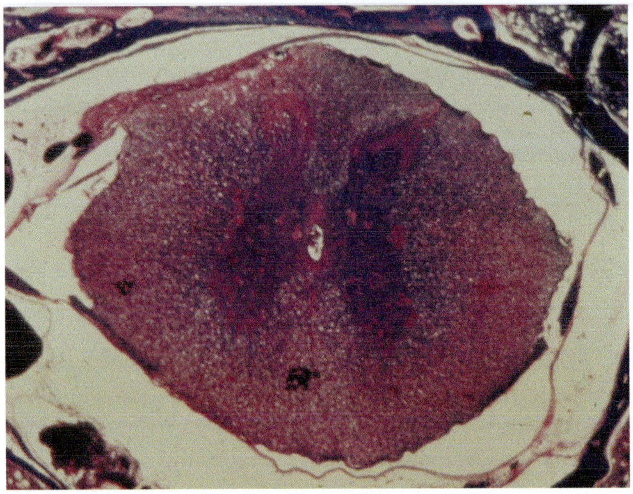

C

**Fig. 3.28** **(A)** Experimental scoliosis. PA radiograph of a rabbit spine. The spine has been tethered into lordosis and the spinal cord damaged by thermal ablation of the facet joints. There was a curvature of 70 degrees immediately after the animal awakened from anesthesia. **(B)** Within a couple of weeks the deformity was gross, as in progressive infantile malignant idiopathic scoliosis. **(C)** Transverse section of the spinal cord at this level showing a dorso-lateral infarct.

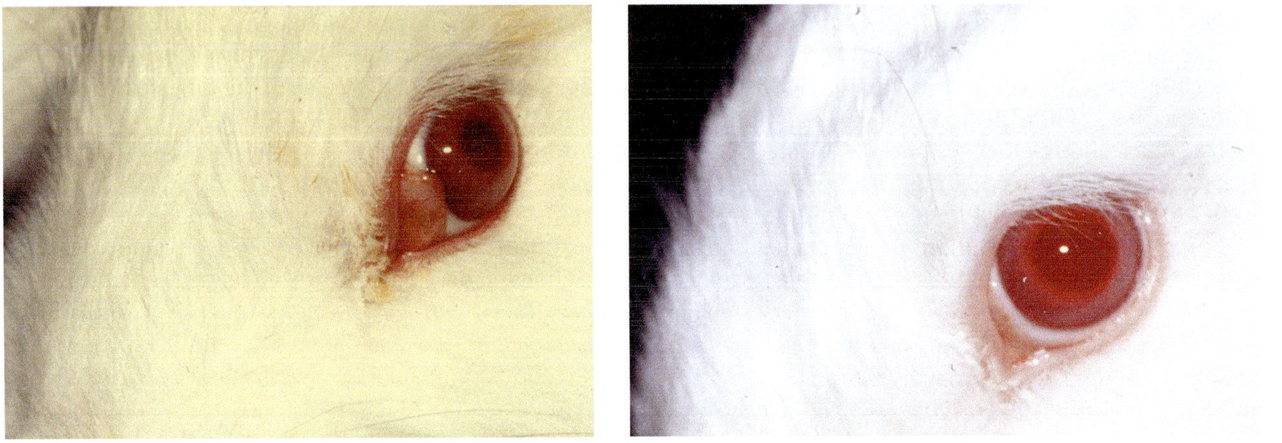

A B

**Fig. 3.29** Two rabbits, one with experimental idiopathic scoliosis (normal eye) **(A)** and the other **(B)** with experimental neuromuscular scoliosis, resembling progressive infantile idiopathic malignant scoliosis with respiratory malfunction and cyanosis (cyanotic eye).

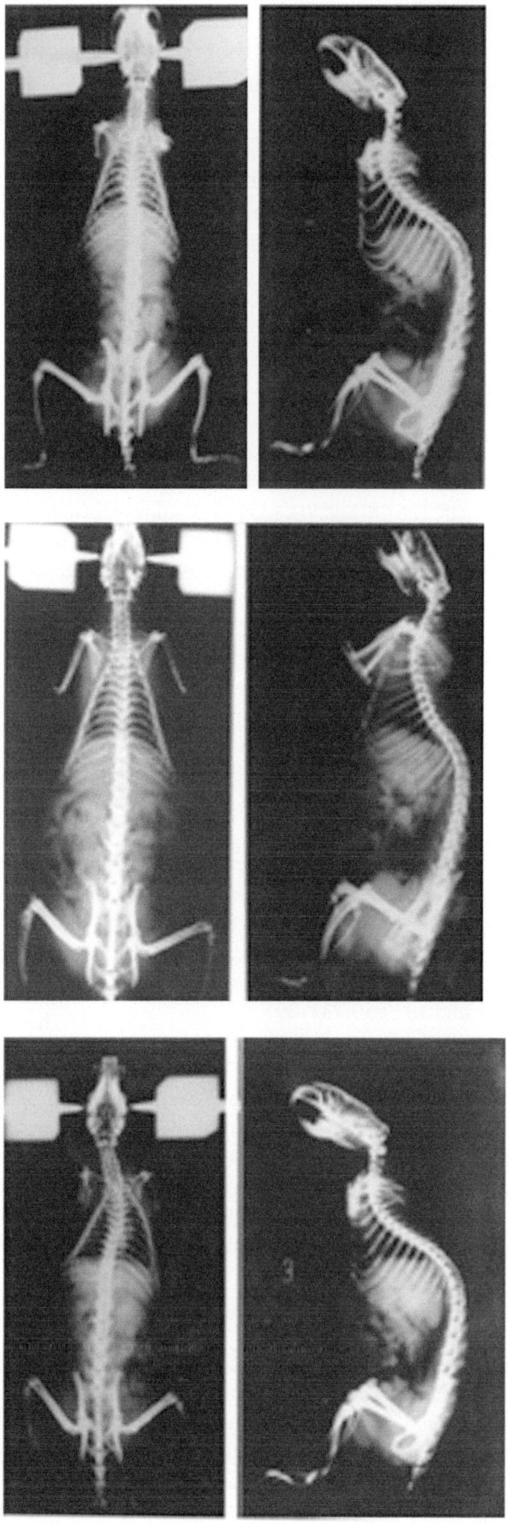

A

B

C

**Fig. 3.30** A pinealectomized quadrupedal rat. **(A)** Sham operation on a bipedal rat. An AP radiograph of the spine revealed a straight spine (*left*), and a lateral view revealed a thoracic hyperlordosis of −43 degrees between C2 and T7 (*right*). **(B)** Pinealectomized quadrupedal rat. An AP radiograph of the spine revealed a straight spine (*left*), and a lateral view revealed a physiological thoracic lordosis of −15 degrees between C2 and T7 (*right*). **(C)** Pinealectomized bipedal rat. An AP radiograph of the spine revealed thoracic scoliosis of 29 degrees (*left*), and a lateral view revealed thoracic hyperlordosis of −48 degrees between C2 and T7 (*right*). (Courtesy of Masafumi Machida, MD)

Furthermore, a scoliosis was more easily produced when the tails of bipedal rats were removed, allowing them to have a more upright posture. The sagittal profiles of these rats showed that the pinealectomized quadrupedal rat had a physiological thoracic lordosis, whereas a thoracic hyperlordosis was produced in both the sham-operated and pinealectomized bipedal rats. In other words, the effect of being bipedal was to exaggerate the existing thoracic lordosis, but no buckling into a lordoscoliosis was produced unless the bipedal rat was pinealectomized, suggesting that the hyperlordosis rendered by the upright posture was destabilized by pinealectomy to produce the scoliosis.

Interestingly, having tethered rabbits' spines into a lordosis, neither Somerville[77] nor the Leeds Group[78–80] could make it buckle unless the lordosis was rendered asymmetrical by producing a few degrees of scoliosis as well. Perhaps pinealectomy would have done the same. In the bipedal chickens and rats that developed scoliosis, there was no preferentiality in its developing either on the right or the left side.

There doesn't seem to be any other explanation for the effect of the pinealectomy performed on rats, because the rats were of much the same weight at the end of the experiment and were not constitutionally disadvantaged.[89] However, scoliosis was also noted in the thoracolumbar region, and this is where the lateral radiographs clearly showed a kyphosis of the order of 40 or 50 degrees. Perhaps these were the slightly asymmetrical kyphoses seen with severe Scheuermann's disease, in which there is a concomitant mild coronal-plane deformity with the opposite direction of rotation to that in idiopathic scoliosis, with the vertebral bodies turning into the curve concavity.[66] This is simple right–left growth asymmetry rather than mechanical buckling.

## References


1. Le Febvre J, Triboulet-Chassevant A, Missirliu MF. Electromyographic data in idiopathic scoliosis. Arch Phys Med Rehabil 1961;42:710–711
2. Gorynski T, Bojkowa M. [Histological changes of spinal muscles in dystonic scoliosis.]. Chir Narzadow Ruchu Ortop Pol 1957;22: 139–142
3. Kaneko T. [Histopathological and histochemical studies on the back muscles in scoliosis]. Nippon Seikeigeka Gakkai Zasshi 1968;42:13–28
4. Hirano S. Electron microscopic studies on back muscles in scoliosis. Nippon Seikeigeka Gakkai Zasshi 1972;46:47–62
5. Fidler MW, Jowett RL, Troup JDG. Histochemical study of the function of multifidus in scoliosis. In: Zorab PA, ed. Scoliosis and Muscle. London: William Heinemann Medical Books; 1974:184–192
6. Fidler MW, Jowett RL. Muscle imbalance in the aetiology of scoliosis. J Bone Joint Surg Br 1976;58:200–201
7. Spencer GSG, Zorab PA. Spinal muscle in scoliosis. Comparison of normal and scoliotic rabbits. J Neurol Sci 1976;30:405–410
8. Spencer GSG, Eccles MJ. Spinal muscle in scoliosis. Part 2. The proportion and size of type 1 and type 2 skeletal muscle fibres measured using a computer-controlled microscope. J Neurol Sci 1976; 30:143–154
9. Wong YC, Yau ACMC, Low WD, et al. Ultrastructural changes of the back muscles of idiopathic scoliosis. Spine 1977;2:251–260
10. Yarom R, Robin GC. Studies on spinal and peripheral muscles from patients with scoliosis. Spine 1979;4:12–21
11. Khosla S, Tredwell SJ, Day B, Shinn SL, Ovalle WK Jr. An ultrastructural study of multifidus muscle in progressive idiopathic scoliosis. Changes resulting from a sarcolemmal defect at the myotendinous junction. J Neurol Sci 1980;46:13–31
12. Zetterberg C, Aniansson A, Grimby G. Morphology of the paravertebral muscles in adolescent idiopathic scoliosis. Spine 1983;8: 457–462
13. Saatok T, Dahlberg E, Bylund P, Eriksson E, Gustafsson JA. Steroid hormone receptors, protein, and DNA in erector spinae muscle from scoliotic patients. Clin Orthop Relat Res 1984;183:197–207
14. Liebergall M, Floman Y, Eldor A. Functional, biochemical, and structural anomalies in platelets of patients with idiopathic scoliosis. J Spinal Disord 1989;2:126–130
15. Yarom R, Muhlrad A, Hodges S, Robin GC. Platelet pathology in patients with idiopathic scoliosis: Ultrastructural morphometry, agrregations, X-ray spectrometry, and biochemical analysis. Lab Invest 1980;43:208–216
16. Yarom R, Blatt J, Gorodetsky R, Robin GC. Microanalysis and X-ray fluorescence spectrometry of platelets in diseases with elevated muscle calcium. Eur J Clin Invest 1980;10(2 Pt 1):143–147
17. Kahmann RD, Donohue JM, Bradford DS, White JG, Rao GH. Platelet function in adolescent idiopathic scoliosis. Spine 1992;17:145–148
18. Suk SI, Kim IK, Lee CK, Koh YD, Yeom JS. A study on platelet function in idiopathic scoliosis. Orthopedics 1991;14:1079–1083
19. Sabato S, Rotman A, Robin GC, Floman Y. Platelet aggregation abnormalities in idiopathic scoliosis. J Pediatr Orthop 1985;5:558–563
20. Floman Y, Liebergall M, Robin GC, Eldor A. Abnormalities of aggregation, thromboxane A2 synthesis, and 14C serotonin release in platelets of patients with idiopathic scoliosis. Spine 1983;8: 236–241
21. Kindsfater K, Lowe T, Lawellin D, Weinstein D, Akmakjian J. Levels of platelet calmodulin for the prediction of progression and severity of adolescent idiopathic scoliosis. J Bone Joint Surg Am 1994; 76:1186–1192
22. Machida M, Dubousset J, Imamura Y, Miyashita Y, Yamada T, Kimura J. Melatonin. A possible role in pathogenesis of adolescent idiopathic scoliosis. Spine 1996;21:1147–1152
23. Petersén I, Sahlstrand T, Selldén U. Electroencephalographic investigation of patients with adolescent idiopathic scoliosis. Acta Orthop Scand 1979;50:283–293
24. Sahlstrand T, Ortengren R, Nachemson A. Postural equilibrium in adolescent idiopathic scoliosis. Acta Orthop Scand 1978;49:354–365
25. Sahlstrand T, Petruson B. A study of labyrinthine function in patients with adolescent idiopathic scoliosis. I. An electro-nystagmographic study. Acta Orthop Scand 1979;50(6 Pt 2):759–769
26. Sahlstrand T, Petruson B, Ortengren R. Vestibulospinal reflex activity in patients with adolescent idiopathic scoliosis. Postural effects during caloric labyrinthine stimulation recorded by stabilometry. Acta Orthop Scand 1979;50:275–281
27. Cheng JC, Guo X, Sher AH, Chan YL, Metreweli C. Correlation between curve severity, somatosensory evoked potentials, and magnetic resonance imaging in adolescent idiopathic scoliosis. Spine 1999;24:1679–1684
28. Guo X, Chau WW, Hui-Chan CW, Cheung CS, Tsang WW, Cheng JC. Balance control in adolescents with idiopathic scoliosis and disturbed somatosensory function. Spine 2006;31:E437–E440
29. Roth M. Idiopathic scoliosis caused by a short spinal cord. Acta Radiol Diagn (Stockh) 1968;7:257–271
30. Porter RW. Idiopathic scoliosis: The relation between the vertebral canal and the vertebral bodies. Spine 2000;25:1360–1366
31. Porter RW. Can a short spinal cord produce scoliosis? Eur Spine J 2001;10:2–9
32. Porter RW. The pathogenesis of idiopathic scoliosis: Uncoupled neuro-osseous growth? Eur Spine J 2001;10:473–481

33. Chu WC, Lam WW, Chan YL, et al. Relative shortening and functional tethering of spinal cord in adolescent idiopathic scoliosis?: Study with multiplanar reformat magnetic resonance imaging and somatosensory evoked potential. Spine 2006;31:E19–E25
34. Deane G, Duthie RB. A new projectional look at articulated scoliotic spines. Acta Orthop Scand 1973;44:351–365
35. Deacon P, Flood BM, Dickson RA. Idiopathic scoliosis in three dimensions. A radiographic and morphometric analysis. J Bone Joint Surg Br 1984;66:509–512
36. Inoue M, Minami S, Nakata Y, et al. Preoperative MRI analysis of patients with idiopathic scoliosis: A prospective study. Spine 2005; 30:108–114
37. Bisgard JD. Experimental thoracogenic scoliosis. J Thorac Surg 1934;4:435–442
38. Schwartzmann JR, Miles M. Experimental production of scoliosis in rats and mice. J Bone Joint Surg 1945;27:59–69
39. Liszka O. Spinal cord mechanisms leading to scoliosis in animal experiments. Acta Med Pol 1961;2:45–63
40. MacEwen GD. Experimental scoliosis. In: Zorab PA, ed. Proceedings of a Second Symposium on Scoliosis: Causation. National Fund for Research into Crippling Diseases Monograph. Edinburgh: Livingstone;1968:18–20
41. Langenskiold A, Michelsson JE. Experimental progressive scoliosis in the rabbit. J Bone Joint Surg Br 1961;43B:116–120
42. De Salis J, Beguiristain JL, Cañadell J. The production of experimental scoliosis by selective arterial ablation. Int Orthop 1980;3:311–315
43. Robin GC, Stein H. Experimental scoliosis in primates. Failure of a technique. J Bone Joint Surg Br 1975;57:142–145
44. Somerville EW. Rotational lordosis; the development of single curve. J Bone Joint Surg Br 1952;34B:421–427
45. Francis MJO, Sanderson MC, Smith R. Skin collagen in idiopathic adolescent scoliosis and Marfan's syndrome. Clin Sci Mol Med 1976;51:467–474
46. Bushell GR, Ghosh P, Taylor TKF. Collagen defect in idiopathic scoliosis. Lancet 1978;2:94–95
47. Scapinelli R, Little K. Observations on the mechanically induced differentiation of cartilage from fibrous connective tissue. J Pathol 1970;101:85–91
48. Pedrini VA, Ponseti IV, Dohrman SC. Glycosaminoglycans of intervertebral disc in idiopathic scoliosis. J Lab Clin Med 1973;82:938–950
49. Ghosh P, Bushell GR, Taylor TKF, Pearce RH, Grimmer BJ. Distribution of glycosaminoglycans across the normal and the scoliotic disc. Spine 1980;5:310–317
50. Taylor TKF, Ghosh P, Bushell GR. The contribution of the intervertebral disk to the scoliotic deformity. Clin Orthop Relat Res 1981;156:79–90
51. Miller NH, Mims B, Child A, Milewicz DM, Sponseller P, Blanton SH. Genetic analysis of structural elastic fiber and collagen genes in familial adolescent idiopathic scoliosis. J Orthop Res 1996;14:994–999
52. Marosy B, Justice CM, Nzegwu N, Kumar G, Wilson AF, Miller NH. Lack of association between the aggrecan gene and familial idiopathic scoliosis. Spine 2006;31:1420–1425
53. Wynne Davies R. Familial (idiopathic) scoliosis. A family survey. J Bone Joint Surg Br 1968;50:24–30
54. Cowell HR, Hall JN, MacEwen GD. Genetic aspects of idiopathic scoliosis. A Nicholas Andry Award Essay, 1970. Clin Orthop Relat Res 1972;86:121–131
55. Alden KJ, Marosy B, Nzegwu N, Justice CM, Wilson AF, Miller NH. Idiopathic scoliosis: identification of candidate regions on chromosome 19p13. Spine 2006;31:1815–1819
56. Chan V, Fong GC, Luk KD, et al. A genetic locus for adolescent idiopathic scoliosis linked to chromosome 19p13.3. Am J Hum Genet 2002;71:401–406
57. Archer IA, Dickson RA. Stature and idiopathic scoliosis. A prospective study. J Bone Joint Surg Br 1985;67:185–188
58. Tanner JM. Growth at Adolescence, ed. 2. Oxford: Blackwell Scientific; 1962
59. Delmas A. Types rachidiens de statique corporelle. Rev Morphophysiol Hum 1951;4:26–32
60. Stagnara P, De Mauroy JC, Dran G, et al. Reciprocal angulation of vertebral bodies in a sagittal plane: approach to references for the evaluation of kyphosis and lordosis. Spine 1982; 7:335–342
61. Oxborrow N, Gopal S, Walder A, et al. A new surface topographical measure of spinal shape in scoliosis. J Bone Joint Surg Br 1998; 80(Supp III):276–277
62. Adams W. Lectures on the Pathology and Treatment of Lateral and other Forms of Curvature of the Spine. London: Churchill and Sons; 1865
63. Stagnara P. Le plan d'election pour l'examen radiologique des cyphoscolioses. Rev Chir Orthop Reparatrice Appar Mot 1965;51: 517–524
64. Deacon P, Archer IA, Dickson RA. The anatomy of spinal deformity: A biomechanical analysis. Orthopedics 1987;10:897–903
65. Millner PA, Dickson RA. Idiopathic scoliosis: Biomechanics and biology. Eur Spine J 1996;5:362–373
66. Deacon P, Berkin CR, Dickson RA. Combined idiopathic kyphosis and scoliosis. An analysis of the lateral spinal curvatures associated with Scheuermann's disease. J Bone Joint Surg Br 1985;67: 189–192
67. Sorenson KH. Scheuermann's Kyphosis. Clinical Appearances. Radiography, Aetiology and Prognosis. Copenhagen: Munksgaard; 1964
68. Weinstein SL. Natural history. Spine 1999;24:2592–2600
69. Archer IA, Dickson RA. Stature and idiopathic scoliosis. A prospective study. J Bone Joint Surg Br 1985;67:185–188
70. Willner S. A study of height, weight and menarche in girls with idiopathic structural scoliosis. Acta Orthop Scand 1975;46:71–83
71. Stirling AJ, Howel D, Millner PA, Sadiq S, Sharples D, Dickson RA. Late-onset idiopathic scoliosis in children six to fourteen years old. A cross-sectional prevalence study. J Bone Joint Surg Am 1996;78: 1330–1336
72. Willner S, Johnson B. Thoracic kyphosis and lumbar lordosis during the growth period in children. Acta Paediatr Scand 1983;72: 873–878
73. Farkas A. Physiological scoliosis. J Bone Joint Surg 1941;23: 607–627
74. Kouwenhoven JWM, Vincken KL, Bartels LW, Castelein RM. Analysis of preexistent vertebral rotation in the normal spine. Spine 2006, 31:1467–1472
75. Kouwenhoven JWM, Bartels LW, Vincken KL, et al. The relation between organ anatomy and pre-existent vertebral rotation in the normal spine: Magnetic resonance imaging study in humans with situs inversus totalis. Spine 2007;32:1123–1128
76. Dickson RA. Scoliosis in the community. Br Med J (Clin Res Ed) 1983;286:615–618
77. Dickson RA, Lawton JO, Archer IA, Butt WP. The pathogenesis of idiopathic scoliosis. Biplanar spinal asymmetry. J Bone Joint Surg Br 1984;66:8–15
78. Smith RM, Dickson RA. Experimental structural scoliosis. J Bone Joint Surg Br 1987;69:576–581

79. Lawton JO, Dickson RA. The experimental basis of idiopathic scoliosis. Clin Orthop Relat Res 1986;210:9–17
80. Dickson RA. Idiopathic scoliosis: Foundation for physiological treatment. Ann R Coll Surg Engl 1987;69:89–96
81. Smith RM, Pool RD, Butt WP, Dickson RA. The transverse plane deformity of structural scoliosis. Spine 1991;16:1126–1129
82. Smith RM, Hamlin GW, Dickson RA. Respiratory deficiency in experimental idiopathic scoliosis. Spine 1991;16:94–99
83. Dubousset J, Queneau P, Thillard MJ. Experimental scoliosis induced by pineal and diencephalic lesions in young chickens: Its relation with clinical findings. Orthop Trans 1983;7:7
84. Machida M, Dubousset J, Imamura Y, Iwaya T, Yamada T, Kimura J. An experimental study in chickens for the pathogenesis of idiopathic scoliosis. Spine 1993;18:1609–1615
85. Thillard MJ. Deformations de la colonne vertebrale consecutives a l'epiphysectomie chez le possin. Extrat des comptes Rendus de l'Association Anatomistes; 1959:751–758
86. Hilibrand AS, Blakemore LC, Loder RT, et al. The role of melatonin in the pathogenesis of adolescent idiopathic scoliosis. Spine 1996;21:1140–1146
87. Fagan AB, Kennaway DJ, Sutherland AD. Total 24-hour melatonin secretion in adolescent idiopathic scoliosis. A case-control study. Spine 1998;23:41–46
88. Machida M. Cause of idiopathic scoliosis. Spine 1999;24:2576–2583
89. Machida M, Saito M, Dubousset J, Yamada T, Kimura J, Shibasaki K. Pathological mechanism of idiopathic scoliosis: Experimental scoliosis in pinealectomized rats. Eur Spine J 2005;14:843–848

# 4 Epidemiology of Idiopathic Scoliosis

*Robert A. Dickson*

Orthopedists who underwent their training three or four decades ago were taught by the scoliosis surgical doyens of the time to treat growing children with idiopathic scoliosis according to a fairly strict protocol (**Table 4.1**). This was relaxed a bit over the early years thereafter.[1]

The rationale for this paradigm was that not many small spinal curves progressed, and that most could therefore merely be watched, whereas large curves should not be allowed to go beyond 60 degrees lest patients succumb to cardiopulmonary dysfunction in adulthood. The principal aim of treatment was to prevent progression by bracing moderate curves and by operating on bigger ones. Before the advent of instrumentation for scoliosis, patients underwent preoperative traction and localizer casting,[2] a fusion being performed through a window in the back of the cast, which had to be worn for at least 3 months.

With the advent of Harrington instrumentation,[3] which provided intraoperative correction and markedly reduced pseudarthrosis rates, surgery for idiopathic scoliosis was enthusiastically prescribed.[4,5] Although it was known that not all curves of 20 degrees or more progressed (four-fifths do not), pioneers of brace treatment dictated that braces should be worn (for up to 23 hours a day) because of : (1) unquestioning faith in brace treatment; and (2) because allowing progression to 60 degrees or more would possibly endanger their patients' lives.[6,7]

Therefore, the perceived wisdom of the day was to inform patients and families that without bracing, idiopathic scoliosis would worsen, and that without surgery serious heart and lung problems could militate against a healthy adulthood. Moreover, wearing a brace would mitigate the likelihood of having to go through a difficult and dangerous operation not without potentially serious complications (which were real concerns four decades ago). Not surprisingly, both providers and recipients of healthcare happily endorsed this treatment program.

Patients often presented, and still do, with curves of 30 or 40 degrees, and on this premise and those described earlier, it seemed perfectly reasonable to try to identify less severe cases in the community. As a result, school screening programs for idiopathic scoliosis were adopted in many parts of the world. Furthermore, because nothing was known about the natural history of idiopathic scoliosis (and not much more is known today), these screening programs might shed some light on its epidemiology.

**Table 4.1 Treatment of Idiopathic Scoliosis**

| | | | | |
|---|---|---|---|---|
| Under 20 degrees | – | Observe | → | 25 Degrees |
| 20–60 degrees | – | Brace | → | 45–50 Degrees |
| 60+ degrees | – | Operate | → | 50+ Degrees |

These were the rules of the game: bracing is effective, and you might die of idiopathic scoliosis if untreated. Belief in bracing was so strong[8–14] that it would have been deemed quite unethical to conduct a trial of it, and indeed, heart and lung dysfunction had been widely reported in particularly severe cases of thoracic idiopathic scoliosis.[15–18] As evidence-based medicine has become more fashionable, the past 20 years has seen both of these premises challenged. Clearly, the "retrospectoscope" is a powerful instrument, but looking back, it wasn't clear from the protagonists how a brace might control this complex three-dimensional deformity from the outside, other than in accord with the simplistic concept of three-point fixation.[19]

What the designers of the brace did point out, however, was that if it did obliterate the lumbar lordosis (and thus pitch the patient forward), it would hyperextend the spine above the lumber lordosis, and that they observed some degree of improvement when the patient was radiographed with the brace applied. This was because the thoracic lordosis was being encouraged to return toward the sagittal plane: the opposite effect, it might be said, to the forward bend test (**Fig. 4.1**).[20] However, a child with a 30-degree curve without the brace might have a 20-degree curve in the brace and be imprisoned in that position for hours on end, whereas the unbraced patient would be able to move through to 10 degrees or less by the side bending of normal activities of daily living. Not surprisingly, it wasn't long before evidence of inefficacy of bracing, from the Gothenburg databank, was published by way of a retrospective trial showing no difference between braced patients and unbraced controls.[21]

Similarly, the evidence for the organic health consequences of untreated idiopathic thoracic scoliosis was seriously misjudged.[20] Data on cardiopulmonary dysfunction came from cases of early-onset idiopathic scoliosis, rather than cases of adolescent idiopathic scoliosis (AIS), in which the curves were well in excess of 100 degrees.[16,17] Davies and Reid showed that pulmonary alveolar reduplication occurs in the main in the first 2 or 3 years of life and certainly

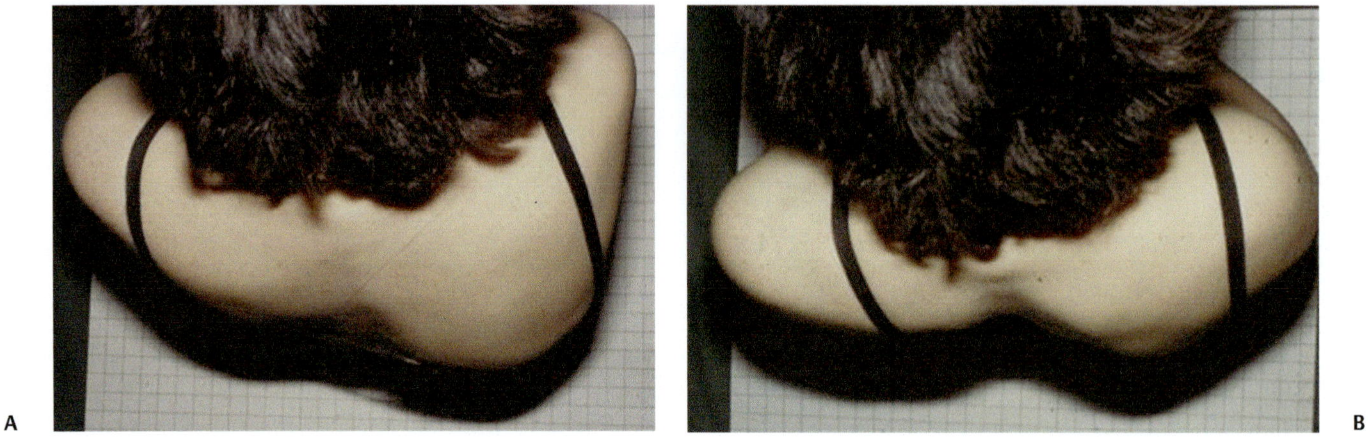

Fig. 4.1 **(A)** Overhead view of a girl with a right thoracic idiopathic scoliosis. **(B)** Overhead view with a lumbar lordosis obliterated, producing thoracic hyperextension and returning the lordosis closer to the midline.

ends by the age of 7 years (see **Fig. 2.16**).[22] If during the early years a significant thoracic deformity is imposed upon this process, it can lead to the hypoplastic lungs encountered in, for example, congenital diaphragmatic hernia, in which the abdominal contents severely compress lung space. This was known as early as 1965 and Reid, the distinguished cardiopulmonary pathologist at the Brompton Hospital in London, presented her findings in this regard at one of the Zorab Scoliosis conferences.[15]

The benign nature of idiopathic thoracic scoliosis of later onset was confirmed by Branthwaite, who succeeded Philip Zorab at the Brompton Hospital. Her study of untreated idiopathic scoliosis demonstrated that the age of 5 years was the crucial threshold of onset.[23] With an onset earlier than this, cardiopulmonary compromise could occur in severe cases; beyond this age idiopathic scoliosis did not have any organic consequences for health.

Notwithstanding this, screening for scoliosis was championed, and the late 1970s and the early 1980s saw reports supporting its use from North America,[24-26] Britain,[27] Europe,[28-30] Australia,[31] and Japan.[32]

## Screening for Scoliosis

### Definitions and Criteria

Screening is defined as the presumptive identification of an unrecognized disease or defect through the application of tests, examinations, or other procedures that can be applied rapidly.[33] A number of authorities, including the World Health Organization, have defined several criteria that should be met for effectively informing an unwitting individual that he or she has a problem (**Table 4.2**).[34] One of these prerequisites is that the natural history of the condition for which screening is to be done is adequately understood, which is manifestly not the case with idiopathic scoliosis. Other criteria are that it should be an important health

**Table 4.2 World Health Organization Criteria for Screening**

| | |
|---|---|
| 1. | The condition sought should be an important health problem for the individual and community. |
| 2. | There should be an accepted treatment or useful intervention for patients with the disease. |
| 3. | The natural history of the disease should be adequately understood. |
| 4. | There should be a latent or early symptomatic stage of the disease. |
| 5. | There should be a suitable and acceptable screening test or examination. |
| 6. | Facilities for diagnosis and treatment should be available. |
| 7. | There should be an agreed policy on whom to treat as patients. |
| 8. | Treatment started at an early stage should be of more benefit than treatment started later. |
| 9. | The cost of screening should be economically balanced in relation to possible expenditure on medical care as a whole. |
| 10. | Case finding should be a continuing process rather than a one-time project. |

problem, that there should be a recognizable latent stage of the disease to identify, and that an effective treatment for the disease can be applied. If these conditions are met, the screening test for the disease should be valid, meaning that it can sort out those with the disease from those without it. In the case of idiopathic scoliosis, the Adams forward bend test or the scoliometer are clearly far too sensitive in this regard.[35] Financial effects should also be taken into consideration, and in the presence of a health service with finite resources, screening for scoliosis should be put on a par with other screening programs, such as for breast or cervical cancer. If the natural history of a disease is not understood, screening may have merit if it is in the nature of an epidemiological survey that elucidates the prevalence and incidence rates and the natural history of the variable being studied.

Screening of selected subgroups of the population selected as being relatively high risk for a disease is called "selective screening," and the selection process is expected to be based on sound epidemiological research,[34] which is clearly not the case with regard to idiopathic scoliosis. That the 10- to 14-year-old age group (the sort of age group most commonly selected) is particularly vulnerable is merely conjectured. There is no doubt that this age selection does produce an enormous harvest, but when the reasons for screening are scrutinized it can be seen that adolescent idiopathic scoliosis is a relatively benign condition.[20] When looking at the results of epidemiological surveys it is often impossible to compare these, because the words *prevalence* and *incidence* are often used interchangeably, and the class intervals of curve magnitude are not the same. The survey that has class intervals from, for example, 0 degrees to 4 degrees, 5 degrees to 9 degrees of curvature, 10 degrees to 14 degrees, and so forth is clearly not comparable to one that has intervals of 5 degrees or less, 6 degrees to 10 degrees, 11 degrees to 15 degrees, and beyond. This is particularly relevant in that the Scoliosis Research Society defines a scoliosis as being present if it measures at least 11 degrees.[36]

## Screening Methods

The forward-bend test is the most commonly used test for scoliosis (**Fig. 4.2**). An alternative is the scoliometer, which measures the angle of trunk rotation in the forward-bend position.[35] Both of these tests, by using forward bending, compress the lordotic component of the deformity and thus enhance spinal buckling. This has the effect of causing overestimation of the deformity. An alternative is to use surface-shape measurements with the patient in the erect position. This is done with computer-driven surface-shape maps of the back of the child, and although very sophisticated (the Quantec surface-shape measurement generates 250,000 data points in a fraction of a second), poses a problem of quantification (**Fig. 4.3**).[37] Although Cobb angles, rib

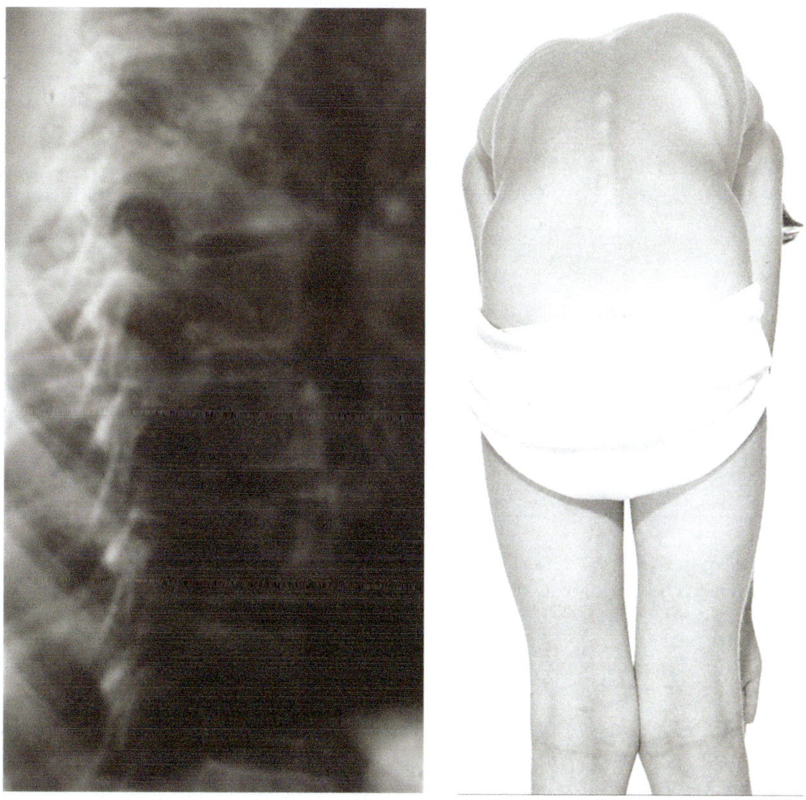

A,B

**Figs. 4.2** The forward-bend test. **(A)** A true lateral radiograph showing the essential lordosis. **(B)** On forward bending this lordosis is compressed and the spine therefore buckles, enhancing the rib hump.

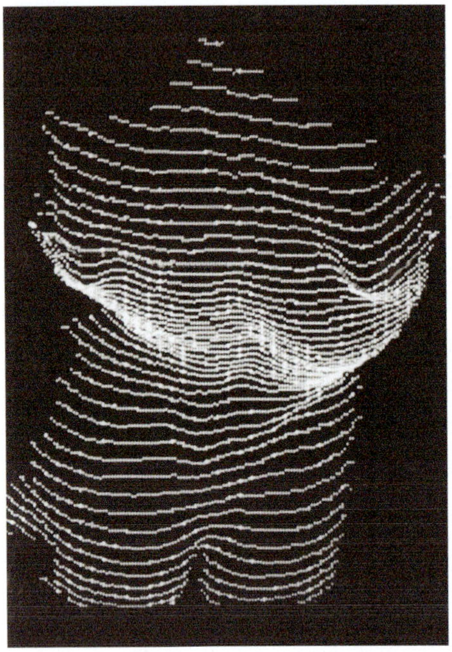

**Fig. 4.3** A patient with a right thoracic idiopathic scoliosis whose surface shape has been registered by the Quantec system.

humps, and lung volumes can be measured, it is not possible to obtain a single figure for overall surface shape.

Bunnell, with his great experience in the use of a scoliometer, originally suggested referral to a clinic for a child with a 5-degree angle, but then increased this to 7 degrees to reduce the number of false-positive results, with 12% of patients being referred for a 5-degree angle and only 3% for a 7-degree angle.[38] However, the number of false-negative results is the price for this. When 5 degrees of rotation is used, only 2% of 20-degree curves will be missed, and when this rises to seven degrees of rotation, 12% of 20-degree curves are missed.

Children referred for further assessment and in whom a clinically suspected scoliosis is confirmed then have a frontal radiograph of the spine. It is mandatory that this involve the lowest possible dose of radiation, and the Oxford Scoliosis Study Group devised a technique that reduces the radiation dosage in this procedure to less than 2% of that with a conventional film.[39] This is achievable by radiographing the patient in the posteroanterior (PA) direction, so that the full width of the torso will absorb X-rays before they meet the developing breast and thyroid, and by increasing the focus–film distance by a factor of 3 through the incorporation of an air gap (**Fig. 4.4**).

The Cobb angle is measured on the films obtained in this procedure, preferably by using Whittle's protractor with a free-hanging needle, which yields an error less than 1 degree,[40] rather than by drawing lines on the film with a pencil and dropping perpendiculars, the error of which can be as high as 10% (see **Figs. 2.6** and **2.7**).

## Prevalence Rates

Despite the aforementioned inconsistencies in the way in which screening programs have been described, the prevalence rates of different classes of scoliosis are remarkably similar, with just over 2% of patients shown to have a scoliosis of 11 degrees or more.[41,42] This decreases by an order of magnitude to 0.3% to 0.5% for curves in excess of 20 degrees, and falls to 0.1% to 0.3% for curves greater than 30 degrees (**Table 4.3**).[43] With increasing curve size, female-to-male dominance rises to more than 10:1 for curves in excess of 30 degrees. Thus, if the purpose of a screening program is early detection then eliminating boys from screening would improve the yield of the program at the expense of revealing less about the natural history of scoliosis in the screened population.

Thus, for instance, by examining the prevalence rates of curves of 5 degrees or more with age, the Oxford Study

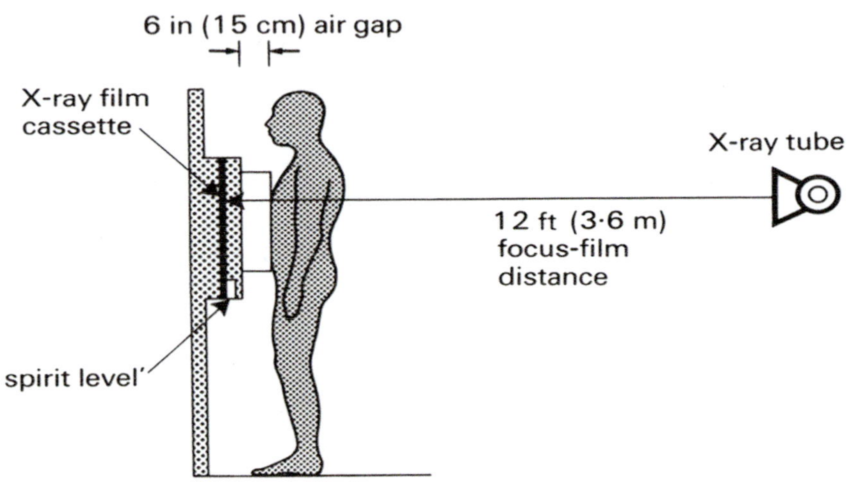


**Fig. 4.4** The Oxford low-dose radiographic technique. Taking the X-ray film in the PA direction, increasing the focus–film distance to 12 feet (3.6 m), and incorporating an air gap reduces the dosage received by the developing breast and thyroid to less than 2% of that with conventional radiography.

**Table 4.3 Prevalence of Adolescent Idiopathic Scoliosis**

| Cobb Angle (degrees) | Female-to- Male Ratio | Prevalence (%) |
|---|---|---|
| >10 | 1.4–2:1 | 2–3 |
| >20 | 5.4:1 | 0.3–0.5 |
| >30 | 10:1 | 0.1–0.3 |
| >40 | — | <0.1 |

*Source*: From Weinstein SL. Adolescent idiopathic scoliosis: Prevalence and natural history. In: Weinstein SL, ed. The Pediatric Spine. Principles and Practice, 1994. Copyright © by Lippincott-Raven. Reproduced with permission.

Group demonstrated that the prevalence rate of scoliosis in girls was seldom more than twice that in boys.[27]

The Oxford Study Group also found that 40% of children failing the screening test had a lumbar scoliosis in association with a hitherto undiagnosed leg-length inequality.[44] Fortunately this was spotted in the pilot-study phase of the investigation, before standardized reference grids were used, and as a result, the definitive study of more than 5000 Oxford schoolchildren incorporated a radio-opaque fluid level in the X-ray film as a horizontal reference point against which the inclination of the sacrum and position of the femoral heads could be measured. Pelvic-tilt scoliosis is defined as a lumbar scoliosis with the upper border of the sacrum as the lowest end-vertebra, with a pelvic tilt of S1 and a Cobb angle not bigger than twice the pelvic tilt (see **Fig. 2.3B**).

Most epidemiological surveys of idiopathic scoliosis have focused on the later years of adolescent growth, but the most recent study in the United Kingdom looked at 16,000 Leeds schoolchildren from the age of 6 to 14 so as to encompass all the years in which late-onset idiopathic scoliosis occurs (onset after 5 years of age).[42] When pelvic-tilt scoliosis was excluded, 1.1% of the children examined had a curve in excess of 5 degrees and 0.5% met the definition of idiopathic scoliosis (a curve of more than 10 degrees with concordant apical rotation) (**Table 4.4**). There were five times more girls than boys with scoliosis. The point-prevalence rate increased with age, being 0.1% for the age group from 6 to 8 years, 0.3% for the age group from 9 to 11 years, and 1.2% for the age group from 12 to 14 years. Idiopathic scoliosis was found in 2.2% of girls aged 12 to 14 years (**Table 4.5**).

When curve site was analyzed against curve size, thoracic curves became significantly more prevalent with increasing curve size, increasing from 40% of curves of 6 to 10 degrees to almost 70% of curves in excess of 15 degrees (**Table 4.6**).

The proportion of right-sided thoracic curves and left-sided lumbar curves increased with curve size to more than 10:1 for curves in excess of 20 degrees. However, for curves of less than 11 degrees, right- and left-sided curves were more equally distributed.

In comparing the prevalence data in the Leeds Study[42] with those in the Oxford Study, conducted almost 20 years earlier,[27] it would appear that late-onset idiopathic scoliosis is pursuing a more benign course with the passage of time (2.5% of teenage girls in Oxford versus 2.2% in Leeds).

What these epidemiological surveys have revealed is that some degree of scoliosis cannot be regarded as abnormal, as anatomists said centuries ago.[45] Rather like the situation with arthritis, it is not so much having the condition as the degree to which one has it. Fortunately, although 2% of teenage girls have idiopathic scoliosis, fewer than 1 in 1000 have a curve in excess of 40 degrees.[43] As will be entirely expected, the greater a curve the more likely it is to progress. This would accord with Euler's laws of flexible columns,[46] and would explain why the further the bell tower of the Cathedral of Pisa leans, the more likely it is to continue doing so (before it was stabilized). This is age dependent, and the probability of progression is very much associated with the adolescent growth spurt in females.

The epidemiology of idiopathic scoliosis of small magnitude is helpful with regard to the natural history of the condition. Right-sided thoracic curves and left-sided lumbar curves are more likely to progress, and we have already seen in-built transverse-plane asymmetry in both the thoracic and lumbar regions because of the effect of the descending thoracic and lumbar aorta (see **Figs. 3.22** and **3.23**).[46–48] Thoracic vertebrae are asymmetric to the right, and the transverse plane thus favors a right thoracic scoliosis, but there is also an in-built coronal-plane deformity in "normal

**Table 4.4 Overall Prevalence Rates of Idiopathic Scoliosis According to Curve Size in Children with Curves of 6 Degrees or More**

| Size of Curve (degrees) | No. of Patients | Prevalence | No. of Girls | No. of Boys | Prevalence Ratio: Girls to Boys |
|---|---|---|---|---|---|
| 6–10 | 93 | 0.6 | 63 | 30 | 2.3 |
| 11–15 | 47 | 0.3 | 37 | 10 | 4.0 |
| 16–20 | 18 | 0.1 | 26 | 3 | 9.3 |
| >20 | 11 | 0.07 | – | – | – |
| Total | 169 | 1.1 | 126 | 43 | 3.2 |

**Table 4.5 Overall Prevalence Rates of Idiopathic Scoliosis for Types of Curves According to Age Group**

| Age Group (yr) | No. of Patients | Prevalence | Prevalence in Girls (%) | Prevalence in Boys (%) |
|---|---|---|---|---|
| 6–8 | 4 | 0.1 | 0.1 | 0.1 |
| 9–11 | 16 | 0.3 | 0.4 | 0.1 |
| 12–14 | 56 | 1.2 | 2.2 | 0.3 |

children," with curvatures in the right and left directions being equally represented for small curves.[41] If therefore the pre-existing normal coronal-plane deformity is to the left, it will counter the adverse effect of right-sided transverse-plane asymmetry, with the two effectively canceling each other. If, however, there is a pre-existing right-sided coronal-plane deformity, the right-sided transverse-plane asymmetry may give momentum to a pre-existing thoracic lordosis (see **Table 3.1**).

With regard to the importance of the sagittal plane, the Leeds Group followed the cohort it had identified by screening, of just less then 1000 children, for 6 years, taking PA and lateral low-dose radiographs on an annual basis.[42] Because of the sensitivity of the screening test (a scoliometer reading of more than 4 degrees), screening programmes, the great majority of children in the Leeds cohort were indeed "normal," as is the case with all screening programs. The follow-up period of 6 years showed some of these normal children as developing idiopathic scoliosis during the study period. When the original radiographs were inspected and the PA film showed a straight spine, the lateral film showed the biomechanically dangerous flat back with a lordosis in the lower thoracic region (see **Fig. 3.20**).[46] This confirmed that this essential sagittal-plane lesion was primary and was the driving factor for subsequent buckling and deformation in the other two planes.

## Early-onset Idiopathic Scoliosis

Idiopathic scoliosis of early onset is a fascinating condition and is defined as an idiopathic scoliosis with an onset before the fifth year of life,[20] although for practical purposes the spinal curves in this condition develop in the first 2 years. This condition is common in Europe but much less so in the United States, for no obvious reason. Although there have been no epidemiological surveys of early-onset idiopathic scoliosis, there have been several retrospective studies that have provided crucial information about this very important condition. As noted previously, it is early-onset scoliosis and not late-onset scoliosis that gives rise to organic health problems.[23]

**Table 4.6 Distribution of Curve Sizes in Idiopathic Scoliosis According to Curve Site for Curves of 6 Degrees or More**

| | Size of Curve | | |
|---|---|---|---|
| Apex | 6–10 Degrees | 11–15 Degrees | >15 Degrees |
| Thoracic | 37(40) | 24(51) | 20(69) |
| Thoracolumbar | 28(30) | 17(36) | 8(28) |
| Lumbar | 28(30) | 6(13) | 1(3) |
| Total | 93 | 47 | 29 |

There are two distinct types of early-onset scoliosis: one that resolves in more than 90% of cases and one that has serious progression potential and accounts for just less than 10% of cases.[49] These are interesting proportions, showing the great majority of cases as resolving, and were not evident in early reports. The condition was first described in Holland in the 1930s by Harrenstein,[50] who did note that its spontaneous resolution could occur, but it was James in 1951 who first estimated the proportions of resolving to nonresolving cases.[51] Of his 33 cases, only 4 resolved and all involved small curves. James then went on to review a further 52 cases[52] and then another 212 cases, the latter being reported in 1959.[53] Of these 212 cases, 135 progressed and 77 resolved. They involved children referred to the London Scoliosis Clinic. Meanwhile, Scott and Morgan at the Nuffield Orthopaedic Centre in Oxford reported that four times as many of their cases progressed as resolved.[54]

Quite extraordinarily, the proportions resolving and progressing changed dramatically within 10 years, one group reporting in 1965 that 40 of 49 cases resolved, [55] whereas the same London Group that had reported many more cases progressing than resolving in 1959[53] reported in 1965 that 92 of a total 100 cases had resolved.[56] There has been no explanation for this dramatic spontaneous change in the natural history of the condition.

Notions that early-onset idiopathic scoliosis was caused by intrauterine molding were refuted by observations that the deformity resulted from postnatal pressure from a constant oblique supine position (**Fig. 4.5**).[57] Wynne-Davies confirmed in Edinburgh that all patients had plagiocephaly on the same side as the curve convexity, which was also on the same side as plagiopelvy, bat ear, and wry neck.[58] Wynne-Davies also recorded a high prevalence of mental retardation, but only in the group with progressive deformity, lending support to the notion that infantile idiopathic "malignant" progressive scoliosis might be a neurological problem rather than a real idiopathic one.

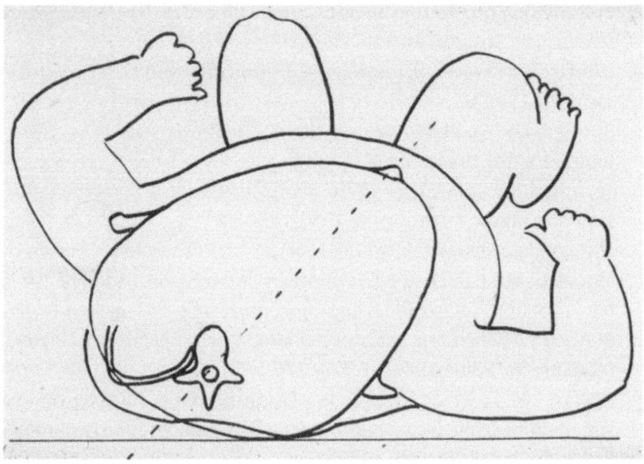

**Fig. 4.5** When babies lie in the oblique lateral decubitus position, body molding can occur.

Wynne-Davies also noted a much greater prevalence of congenital heart disease, inguinal hernia, congenital hip dislocation, older maternal age, and low birth weight among children with early-onset idiopathic scoliosis, recording congenital hip dislocation at five times the normal rate.

Early-onset idiopathic scoliosis affects males more often than females, in a ratio of three to two. Early reports tended to focus on thoracic scoliosis, but other curve patterns seen in late-onset scoliosis are also common.[53,56] However, three-quarters of thoracic curves in the early-onset condition are convex to the left, and girls with right-sided thoracic curves have the poorest prognosis. All double-structural curves have definite progression potential.[59]

Mehta, who has contributed much of what is known about infantile idiopathic scoliosis, analyzed several radiological parameters in an effort to identify on the first visit those infants that might have a poor prognosis.[60] Among other things, she measured the Cobb angle and the rib-vertebra angle difference (RVAD) at the apex of the curve (see **Fig. 2.11**). If a line is drawn along the neck of the ribs attached to the apical vertebra of the curve, and a vertical line is drawn down the longitudinal axis of that vertebra, the rib–vertebra angles are measured on each side. If the difference exceeds 20 degrees, the curve is likely to be progressive. Similarly, greater Cobb angles, above 30 degrees, are likely to indicate progressive deformity.

However, what both of these measures indicate is simply a bigger curve and, rather as in the case of the Leaning Tower of Pisa, the bigger the curve the more likely it is to progress. Mehta also described whether the rib heads overlapped the vertebral bodies, which is merely another measure of rotation and the magnitude of deformity.

Of considerable importance is the clinical status of the child with early-onset idiopathic scoliosis, and, as Wynne-Davies identified,[58] low-birth-weight children are at risk of having progressive deformity along with developmental delay, although curve flexibility is also crucial. If the infant is laid on his or her side over the examiner's knee, convex side of the infant's spinal curve facing downward, correction or reversal of the curve strongly indicates a resolving curve. A curve that is stiff and doesn't correct is perhaps the most important clinical feature of progressive infantile idiopathic scoliosis. With a double-curve pattern there isn't as much apical rotation as with a single curve and the RVAD may therefore not be more than a few degrees at the apex of the thoracic curve.

There is often a single curve with compensatory curves above and below it. With a single curve the ribs droop more vertically on the convex side than on the concave side, but if the 12th rib on the concave side droops more than that on the convex side, producing a negative RVAD, a progressive double-structural curve is likely to develop in due course.

In 1992 the Leeds Group reported its first 75 cases of early-onset idiopathic scoliosis, 70% had thoracic curves and 21 had an RVAD in excess of 20 degrees, for which casting was prescribed and controlled all curves.[59]

Recently, Mehta reported her total experience with 136 children with progressive infantile scoliosis, consisting of 72 boys and 64 girls, among whom twice as many children had left convex curves as right convex curves.[61] There were slightly more double and triple curve patterns than single. The mean age of detection of scoliosis was 9 months, and referral to a scoliosis center was made at a mean age of 1 year and 10 months. Mehta pointed out that children referred at an early age did very much better than those referred at a late age.

## References


1. Moe JH, Winter RB, Bradford DS, et al. Scoliosis and Other Spinal Deformities. Philadelphia: WB Saunders; 1978
2. Risser JC, Lauder CH, Norquist DM, et al. Three types of body casts. Instr Course Lect 1955;12:255–259
3. Harrington PR. Treatment of scoliosis. Correction and internal fixation by spine instrumentation. J Bone Joint Surg Am 1962;44A:591–610
4. Moe JH. Methods of correction and surgical techniques in scoliosis. Orthop Clin North Am 1972;3:17–48
5. Goldstein LA. The surgical treatment of idiopathic scoliosis. Clin Orthop Relat Res 1973;93:131–157
6. Moe JH. The Milwaukee brace in the treatment of scoliosis. Clin Orthop Relat Res 1971;77:18–31
7. Moe JH. Indications for Milwaukee brace non-operative treatment in idiopathic scoliosis. Clin Orthop Relat Res 1973;93:38–43
8. Blount WP. Use of the Milwaukee brace. Orthop Clin North Am 1972;3:3–16

9. Keiser RP, Shufflebarger HL. The Milwaukee brace in idiopathic scoliosis: Evaluation of 123 completed cases. Clin Orthop Relat Res 1976;118:19–24
10. Edmonsson AS, Morris JT. Follow-up study of Milwaukee brace treatment in patients with idiopathic scoliosis. Clin Orthop Relat Res 1977;126:58–61
11. Mellencamp DD, Blount WP, Anderson AJ. Milwaukee brace treatment of idiopathic scoliosis: Late results. Clin Orthop Relat Res 1977;126:47–57
12. Tolo VT, Gillespie R. The characteristics of juvenile idiopathic scoliosis and results of its treatment. J Bone Joint Surg Br 1978;60B: 181–188
13. Blount WP. The virtue of early treatment of idiopathic scoliosis. J Bone Joint Surg Am 1981;63:335–336
14. Winter RB, Carlson JM. Modern orthotics for spinal deformities. Clin Orthop Relat Res 1977;126:74–86
15. Reid L. Autopsy study of the lungs in kyphoscoliosis. In: Zorab PA, ed. Proceedings of a Symposium on Scoliosis. Action for the Crippled Child Monograph. London; 1965: 71–77
16. Nilsonne U, Lundgren KD. Long-term prognosis in idiopathic scoliosis. Acta Orthop Scand 1968;39:456–465
17. Nachemson A. A long-term follow-up study of non-treated scoliosis. Acta Orthop Scand 1968;39:466–476
18. Swank SM, Winter RB, Moe JH. Scoliosis and cor pulmonale. Spine 1982;7:343–354
19. Blount WP, Moe JH. The Milwaukee Brace. Baltimore: Williams & Wilkins; 1973.
20. Dickson RA. Conservative treatment for idiopathic scoliosis. J Bone Joint Surg Br 1985;67:176–181
21. Miller JA, Nachemson AL, Schultz AB. Effectiveness of braces in mild idiopathic scoliosis. Spine 1984;9:632–635
22. Davies G, Reid L. Effect of scoliosis on growth of alveoli and pulmonary arteries and on right ventricle. Arch Dis Child 1971;46: 623–632
23. Branthwaite MA. Cardiorespiratory consequences of unfused idiopathic scoliosis. Br J Dis Chest 1986;80:360–369
24. Rogala EJ, Drummond DS, Gurr J. Scoliosis: Incidence and natural history. A prospective epidemiological study. J Bone Joint Surg Am 1978;60:173–176
25. Lonstein JE, Winter RB, Moe JH, Bianco AJ, Campbell RG, Norval MA. School screening for the early detection of spine deformities. Progress and pitfalls. Minn Med 1976;59:51–57
26. Morais T, Bernier M, Turcotte F. Age- and sex-specific prevalence of scoliosis and the value of school screening programs. Am J Public Health 1985;75:1377–1380
27. Dickson RA, Stamper P, Sharp A-M, Harker P. School screening for scoliosis: Cohort study of clinical course. BMJ 1980;281:265–267
28. Span Y, Robin G, Makin M. The incidence of scoliosis in schoolchildren in Jerusalem. J Bone Joint Surg Br 1976;58B:379
29. Ascani E, Salsano V, Giglio G. The incidence and early detection of spinal deformities. A study based on the screening of 16,104 schoolchildren. Ital J Orthop Traumatol 1977;3:111–117
30. Smyrnis PN, Valavanis J, Alexopoulos A, Siderakis G, Giannestras NJ. School screening for scoliosis in Athens. J Bone Joint Surg Br 1979;61B:215–217
31. Golomb M, Taylor TK. Screening adolescent school children for scoliosis. Letter. Med J Aust 1975;1:761–762
32. Inoue S, Shinoto A, Ohti I. Moiré topography for the early detection of scoliosis and evaluation after surgery. Orthop Trans 1978;2:276
33. Commission on Chronic Illness. Chronic Illness in the United States. Cambridge, MA: Harvard University Press; 1957; vol 1
34. Whitby LG. Screening for disease. Definitions and criteria. Lancet 1974;2:819–821
35. Bunnell WP. An objective criterion for scoliosis screening. J Bone Joint Surg Am 1984;66:1381–1387
36. Terminology Committee of the Scoliosis Research Society. A glossary of scoliosis terms. Spine 1976;1:57–58
37. Dickson RA. Spinal deformities (Part 2). In: Benson MKD, Fixsen JA, Macnicol MF, Parsch K, eds. Children's Orthopaedics and Fractures, ed. 2, London: Churchill Livingstone; 2002: 512–547
38. Bunnell WP. The natural history of idiopathic scoliosis before skeletal maturity. Spine 1986;11:773–776
39. Ardran GM, Coates R, Dickson RA, Dixon-Brown A, Harding FM. Assessment of scoliosis in children: Low dose radiographic technique. Br J Radiol 1980;53:146–147
40. Whittle MW, Evans M. Instrument for measuring the Cobb angle in scoliosis. Lancet 1979;1:414
41. Dickson RA. Scoliosis in the community. Br Med J (Clin Res Ed) 1983;286:615–618
42. Stirling AJ, Howel D, Millner PA, Sadiq S, Sharples D, Dickson RA. Late-onset idiopathic scoliosis in children six to fourteen years old. A cross-sectional prevalence study. J Bone Joint Surg Am 1996;78: 1330–1336
43. Weinstein SL. Natural history. Spine 1999;24: 2592–2600
44. Walker AP, Dickson RA. School screening and pelvic tilt scoliosis. Lancet 1984;2:152–154
45. Farkas A. Physiological scoliosis. J Bone Joint Surg 1941;23: 607–627
46. Millner PA, Dickson RA. Idiopathic scoliosis: Biomechanics and biology. Eur Spine J 1996;5:362–373
47. Inkster RG. Osteology. In: Brash JC, ed. Cunningham's Textbook of Anatomy, ed. 9. London: Oxford Medical; 1953: 136
48. Kouwenhoven JWM, Vincken KL, Bartels LW, Castelein RM. Analysis of pre-existent vertebral rotation in the normal spine. Spine 2006; 31:E188–E191
49. Mehta M. The natural history of infantile idiopathic scoliosis. In: Zorab PA, ed. Scoliosis: Proceedings of a Fifth Symposium. London: Academic Press; 1977:103–122
50. Harrenstein RJ. Die Skoliose bei Saueglingen und ihre Behandlung. Z Orthop Chir 1930;52:1–40
51. James JIP. Two curve patterns in idiopathic structural scoliosis. J Bone Joint Surg Br 1951;33B:399–406
52. James JIP. Idiopathic scoliosis; the prognosis, diagnosis, and operative indications related to curve patterns and the age at onset. J Bone Joint Surg Br 1954;36B:36–49
53. James JIP, Lloyd-Roberts GC, Pilcher MF. Infantile structural scoliosis. J Bone Joint Surg Br 1959;41B:719–735
54. Scott JC, Morgan TH. The natural history and prognosis of infantile idiopathic scoliosis. J Bone Joint Surg Br 1955;37B:400–413
55. Walker GF. An evaluation of an external splint for idiopathic structural scoliosis in infancy. J Bone Joint Surg Br 1965;47: 524–525
56. Lloyd-Roberts GC, Pilcher MF. Structural idiopathic scoliosis in infancy: A study of the natural history of 100 patients. J Bone Joint Surg Br 1965;47:520–523
57. Watson GH. Relation between side of plagiocephaly, dislocation of hip, scoliosis, bat ears, and sternomastoid tumours. Arch Dis Child 1971;46:203–210

58. Wynne-Davies R. Infantile idiopathic scoliosis. Causative factors, particularly in the first six months of life. J Bone Joint Surg Br 1975;57:138–141
59. Millner PA, Helm R, Dickson RA. Early onset idiopathic scoliosis: Natural history and outcome. J Bone Joint Surg Br 1992;74(suppl III):303–304
60. Mehta MH. The rib-vertebra angle in the early diagnosis between resolving and progressive infantile scoliosis. J Bone Joint Surg Br 1972;54:230–243
61. Mehta MH. Growth as a corrective force in the early treatment of progressive infantile scoliosis. J Bone Joint Surg Br 2005;87:1237–1247

# 5 Clinical and Radiographic Evaluation of the Scoliotic Patient

*Alvin H. Crawford, Alan E. Oestreich, Linda P. D'Andrea, Joshua E. Heller, and Patrick Cahill*

The presentation of scoliosis is often the result of an incidental finding. Historically, a female patient came to attention because there was difficulty in hemming her garments or because her skirt was riding up on one side. Currently, the most frequent presenting history in patient's with scoliosis is a positive Adams bend test during school screenings or a physical examination for athletics. The Adams forward-bend test is performed by having the patient face away from the examiner, straighten the elbows, clasp hands, and bend over as though diving into a pool or touching the toes. The test is considered positive if there is rotation or a hump to one side of the spine. Occasionally, a child presents for evaluation after an outside observer notices some degree of truncal asymmetry, such as upon seeing the child in a bathing suit or attempting to adjust poorly fitting clothing. Questioning of the family often identifies a close relative who has been diagnosed with adolescent scoliosis. In most of these cases the family was unaware of the need for screening.

## History and Clinical Presentation

Typically the child with scoliosis will not have any complaints related to the condition. The most common presenting statement is, "I was told that I have scoliosis." However, up to 35% of patients may complain of some degree of back pain.[1] A study of more than 2400 patients with adolescent idiopathic scoliosis (AIS) revealed some degree of back pain on an original visit in 23% of the patients. An additional 9% developed pain later on during treatment. Of those with pain at presentation, ~58% were later symptom-free. Severe persistent back pain, or neurological symptoms including radicular pain, muscle weakness, sensory changes, and bowel or bladder incontinence or retention in a patient with AIS is extremely unusual. These symptoms should be evaluated fully and an alternative diagnosis considered.

In patients who present with pain, an evaluation of activities associated with spondylolysis, such as gymnastics, cheerleading, rowing, and weight lifting, is very important. Spondylolysis with subsequent progression to severe spondylolisthesis may initiate a reactive olisthetic scoliosis. Full details of the degree (pain score), location, radiation, and exacerbating and relieving factors for a patient's pain should be reviewed. Scoliosis may be the first sign of an intraspinal anomaly. Scheuermann's kyphosis, disc herniation, syringomyelia, tethered spinal cord, or an intraspinal tumor may all cause truncal malalignment in addition to pain. The presence of a left thoracic curve has been most predictive for discovering an underlying pathological condition. An abnormal neurological examination is even more suspect for intraspinal anomalies, especially in very young children. Thorough neurological and radiographic examination is mandatory. Early-onset spinal curves of >20 degrees in patients less than 10 years old should be suspected as indicating an underlying anomaly and should be thoroughly investigated (**Fig. 5.1**). On occasion, a patient with scoliosis will present with medial subscapular pain over the rib hump. This pain is often vague, occurs intermittently, and only rarely affects quality of life. Subscapular pain is often noted in these patients following surgery. Patients may also experience muscular flank pain from a truncal shift and asymmetric muscle contraction. The pain may resolve after surgery with correction of the truncal shift. On occasion a child may present with a painful scoliosis as the result of a benign osteoid osteoma. The pain characteristically occurs at night during rest, and is relieved by aspirin or non-steroidal anti-inflammatory drugs.

Other important aspects of the patient history include the date of initial observation of a truncal asymmetry, the perceived degree of progression, and the child's overall activity level. It is important to assess the menarchal status of female patients because this is related to their peak growth velocity and to curve progression. Girls are at greater risk for curve progression than are boys.[2] There is approximately a 7-to-1 ratio of female to male patients who will require surgery. Premenarchal girls are at risk of progression because they are still in the accelerated growth phase.

The patient's medical and surgical history may occasionally include conditions that put the patient at risk for developing spinal deformity, such as past intrathoracic procedures that may have led to distortion of the thoracic-cage anatomy. Prior irradiation of the chest wall may also occasionally result in a scoliotic deformity. A history of developmental hip dysplasia or a congenital foot condition giving rise to a limb-length discrepancy can also result in a compensatory scoliosis.

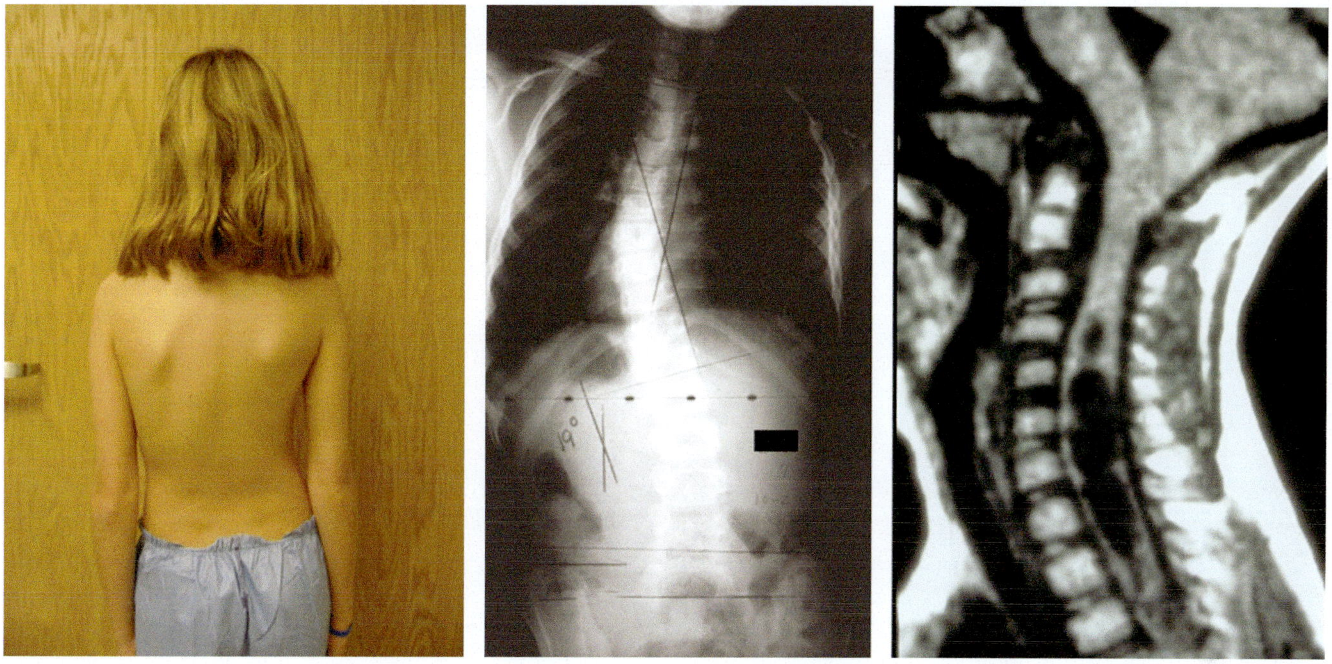

A–C

**Fig. 5.1** This 9-year-old girl presented with truncal imbalance and a 30-degree left thoracic curve. Her abdominal reflexes were questionable. An MRI scan showed thoracic "coin-on-end" syringomyelia. Curvatures of more than 20 degrees in children under 10 years of age justify an MRI scan. The yield of pathology is greater when the curve is to the left side and there is very little rotation in the curvature. Note that the pedicles show very little rotation in the apical portion of the curve. **(A)** Standing posterior view showing the truncal shift to the left. **(B)** PA X-ray film of the thoracolumbar sacral spine. **(C)** MRI scan illustrating cervical thoracic syrinx.

Several markers are helpful in assessing skeletal maturity. These include menarchal status, bone age (digital skeletal age [DSA]), the radiographic Risser grade, triradiate cartilage (TRC) status, parental height, and Tanner stage.[3–5] The adolescent peak height velocity is probably the most important factor to evaluate for the risk of curve progression. Patients in the earlier stages of Risser development (grades 0 or 1) are at greatest risk of curve progression. The Tanner staging correlates somewhat with skeletal maturity and indirectly reveals the risk of curve progression, but is not as accurate as other markers.

A family history of scoliosis may be elicited during a meeting with a patient, and although this may not affect a planned treatment, it may shed light on the family's familiarity with spinal deformity as well as on the family's expectations for the patient's outcome. The work-up of scoliosis can bring awareness to other undiagnosed musculoskeletal conditions that are associated with scoliosis and that may warrant additional testing and treatment. Such associated conditions include congenital muscular torticollis, Klippel–Feil syndrome, Scheuermann's kyphosis, Marfan disease, spondylolysis, spondylolisthesis, spondyloepiphyseal dysplasia, spinal cord or musculoskeletal tumors, and inflammatory conditions. All of these conditions may initiate primary or secondary deviations in a patient's standing balance, leading the healthcare provider to investigate for scoliosis. Idiopathic scoliosis is a diagnosis of exclusion, and can only be accepted after other pathologies have been ruled out.

## Physical Examination

With every effort made to protect the patient's modesty, it is extremely important to evaluate the patient in as little clothing as possible. Our preferred dress for the physical examination of female patients is a two-piece bathing suit (**Fig. 5.2**). Scoliosis is most frequently diagnosed by recognizing truncal asymmetry. The trunk may appear to sway toward one side, or there may be a greater gap between the rib cage and arm. A plumb bob is a useful tool in evaluating for scoliosis. In the normal spine, a plumb bob dropped from the occiput or cervical–thoracic junction will fall within 1 to 2 cm of the midline. In patients with scoliosis the bob will fall laterally. Spinal flexibility may be assessed by asking the patient to simulate a right and left "golf swing" while the patient's pelvis is stabilized by the examiner. Rib and flank prominences can be observed for reduction as the patient performs side-bending and rotation maneuvers.

The physical examination often reveals other musculoskeletal abnormalities associated with scoliotic deformity. There may be an elevation, or forward prominence, of the shoulder at the acromioclavicular joint, or elevation of the

A–D

E–H

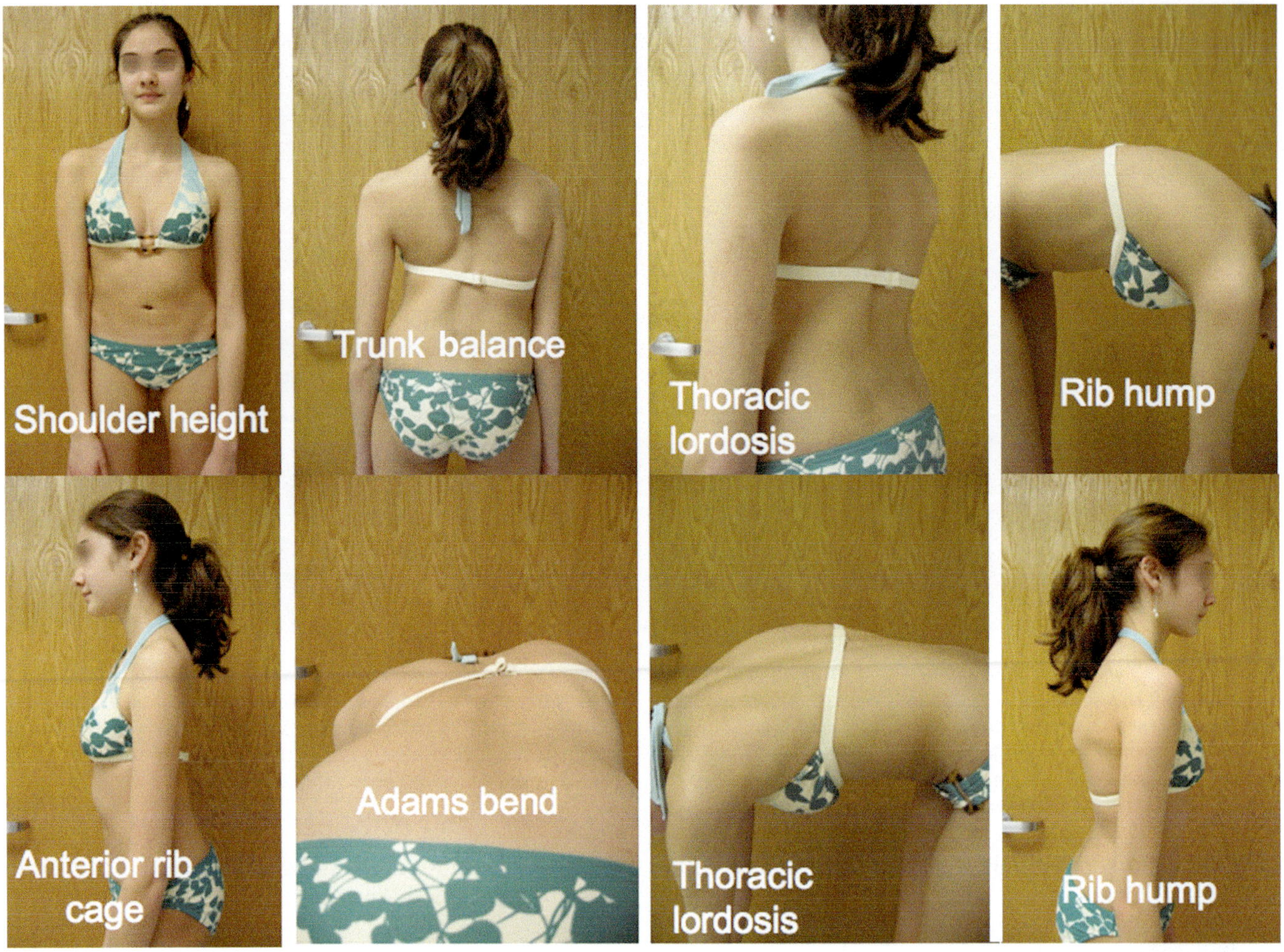


**Fig. 5.2** Physical examination. This 14-year-old girl has a 55-degree right thoracic curve. **(A)** Note the elevation of her right shoulder and a shift of her trunk to the right. **(B)** The right scapula is elevated from the rib cage and there is more space between the left arm and the trunk than between the right arm and trunk. **(C)** There is lordosis of the entire thoracic spine. **(D)** The Adams bend test, in a view from the right, shows a moderate rib hump. **(E)** There is prominence of the left rib cage. **(F)** The Adams forward-bend test shows the prominence and rotation of the right rib cage with very little deviation of the lumbar spine. **(G)** The Adams forward-bend test in a view from the left identifies the right rib hump and also confirms the lordosis of the thoracic spine. **(H)** An appreciation of the elevation and prominence of the right scapula.

scapula by the rib hump or other rotational prominence. The subscapular region should be palpated deeply to help rule out the presence of a subscapular osteochondroma, or, in patients with Sprengel deformity, in which an omovertebral bone forms a connection between the scapula and the lower cervical spine. The anterior chest cage must be assessed for flaring of the rib cage, pectus excavatum, or pectus carinatum. Although these abnormalities may be found in conjunction with scoliosis, it is important to recognize and inform the family that correction of scoliosis will not change the appearance of the anterior chest. A major concern for female patients is the presence of breast asymmetry. It is important for these patients to understand that this asymmetry may not change with spinal corrective surgery. It may help to educate such patients that some degree of breast asymmetry is normal and is a common finding in adolescent girls without scoliosis.

It is important to inspect the skin for cutaneous changes such as café au lait spots, freckling, or unusual hair-distribution patterns. The presence of more than five café au lait spots more than 1.5 cm in diameter are suggestive of neurofibromatosis type 1. Longer, linear café au lait spots with irregular borders may be a cutaneous sign of fibrous dysplasia. The lower back should be examined closely for abnormalities including vascular lesions, skin dimpling, dermal sinus tracts, or hairy patches (**Fig. 5.3**). These lesions when located above the gluteal cleft may be indicative of an intraspinal lesion.

The neurological evaluation of children with scoliosis is critical. The examiner should assess for muscle strength, bulk, and tone in all extremities. Any asymmetry found in

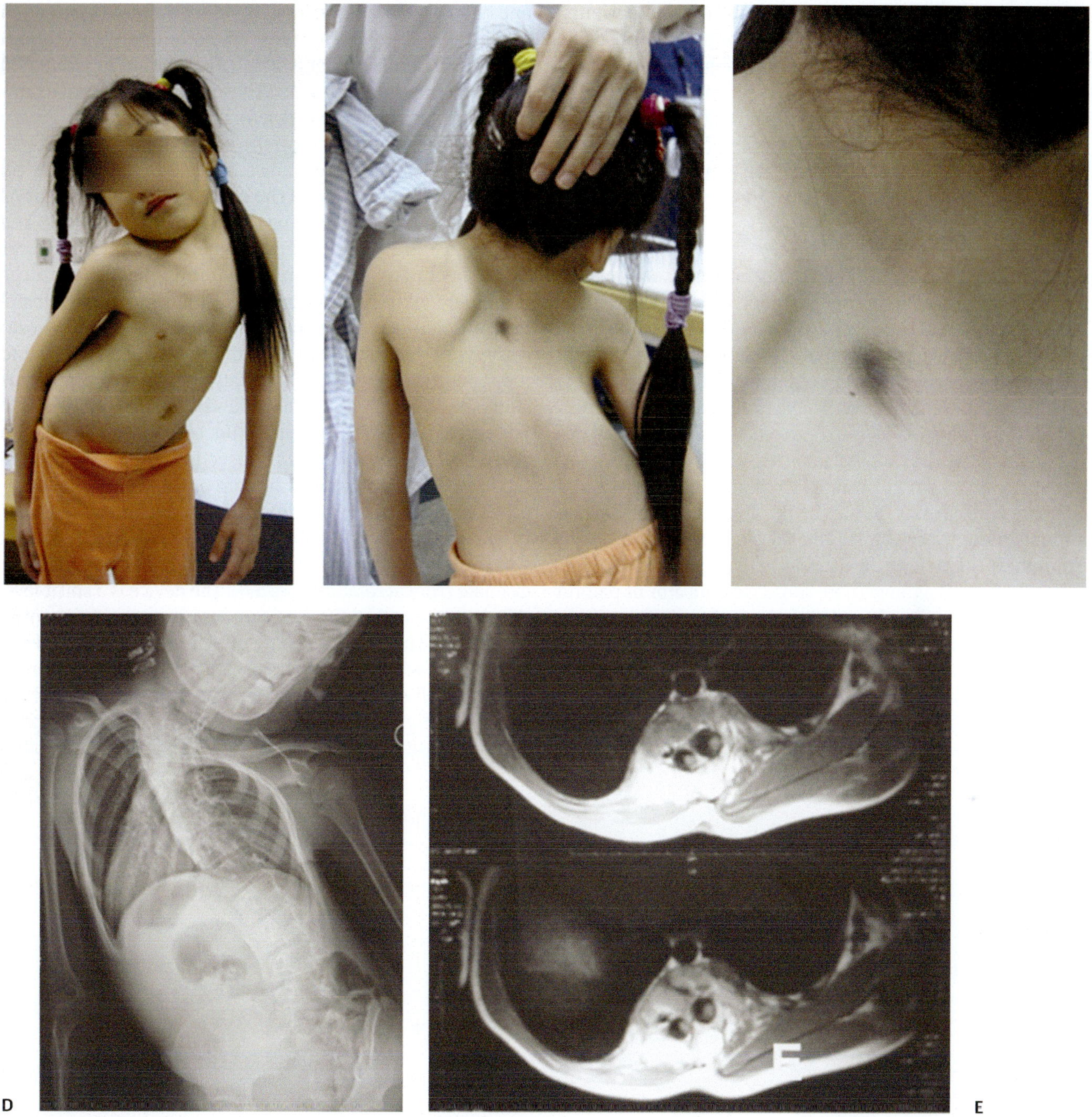


**Fig. 5.3** This 8-year-old child presented with a severely deformed rib cage and a hairy patch in the mid apical region. Her left leg was smaller than her right leg and she had a mild cavus deformity. The hairy patch was associated with a diastematomyelia. The radiographic triad is that of a widened interpedicular space on the apical vertebra, narrowed disc space, and presence of a bony spike. **(A)** Frontal view showing significant truncal imbalance. **(B)** A posterior view shows the hairy patch in the middle of the child's major spinal curve. **(C)** Close-up view of the hairy patch. **(D)** Plain X-ray film showing the triad mentioned above. **(E)** MRI scan showing spinal cord duplication at the midaxial cut.

the examination, such as weakness, atrophy, or limitation in range of motion, should raise the suspicion of an underlying neurological abnormality. Having a child walk, hop, or skip in the clinic hallway can bring subtle deficits to light. Sensation and reflexes should also be assessed. In addition to deep tendon reflexes (elbow/knee/ankle jerk), cutaneous reflexes, including the abdominal reflex, should be evaluated. The abdominal reflex is tested by gently scratching the skin of the abdomen and observing the reaction of the abdominal musculature. It should be tested in all four quadrants and any asymmetry in response should be noted. Absence of this reflex may be indicative of underlying neurologic problems.[6]

This response may be difficult to elicit in some patients, especially those that are ticklish. Although a fundoscopic examination is often unnecessary, the eyes should be observed for pupillary differences as well as abnormalities in movement, including nystagmus. A spinal magnetic resonance imaging (MRI) scan is indicated if any abnormal neurological findings are identified on the physical examination.

## Special Tests

As mentioned previously, the Adams forward-bending test, which is often used as a screening tool, is designed to identify the rotation of the chest wall that occurs in scoliosis. In addition to being used in school screenings, this test should be part of every well-child pediatric visit once a child is able to ambulate. Controversy exists about whether widespread screening leads to excessive specialist referrals for scoliosis.[7–9] In the Adams forward-bend test, the bend should exhibit a smooth "spinal rhythm." Any restriction or hesitancy of normal rhythm or motion, or lack of normal intersegmental motion (lumbosacral, midlumbar, thoracolumbar, thoracic), can usually be easily noted. Loss of spinal rhythm is a much more sensitive indicator of painful intersegmental disorders than is loss of range of motion (ROM), although both loss of rhythm and of ROM can clearly coexist. Abnormalities in spinal rhythm are not specific to any diagnosis, but will always occur when serious structural pathology exists.[10] Most children can bend sufficiently forward to extend their fingertips down to within one hand's length of touching the floor. Failure to extend to this level is abnormal. A child who upon repeat examination is still unable to bend adequately should be evaluated for hamstring contractures. A thorough neurological examination of such children is essential.

In having a child perform the Adams forward-bend test, the examiner should note any curvature of the spine or rib prominence on the side of the convexity of a spinal curve. This is best done by standing directly behind the child and looking in a straight line from the gluteal cleft of the buttocks to the neck. The procedure should be repeated with the examiner looking down from the head toward the buttocks. Previous surgical procedures such as a sternotomy, thoracotomy, or thoracoplasty may distort the chest wall and may cause the bend test to be "falsely" positive. The test is completed by evaluating the child's bend from both sides. A normal bend of the spine should be smooth, without a sharp peak or a hollow in its midsection when viewed from the side. If these abnormalities are present, they may indicate excessive kyphosis or lordosis.

The scoliometer is an excellent screening device that can be used in conjunction with the Adams forward-bend test to evaluate truncal rotation (**Fig. 5.4**). The device is a spirit level that when placed at different spinous processes can quantify rotation of the trunk. An angle of less than 7 degrees is considered within the limits of normal. When following a patient with scoliometer monitoring, the same vertebrae should ideally be used for each reading. The inter- and intrauser reliability of scoliometer testing has been evaluated

A–C

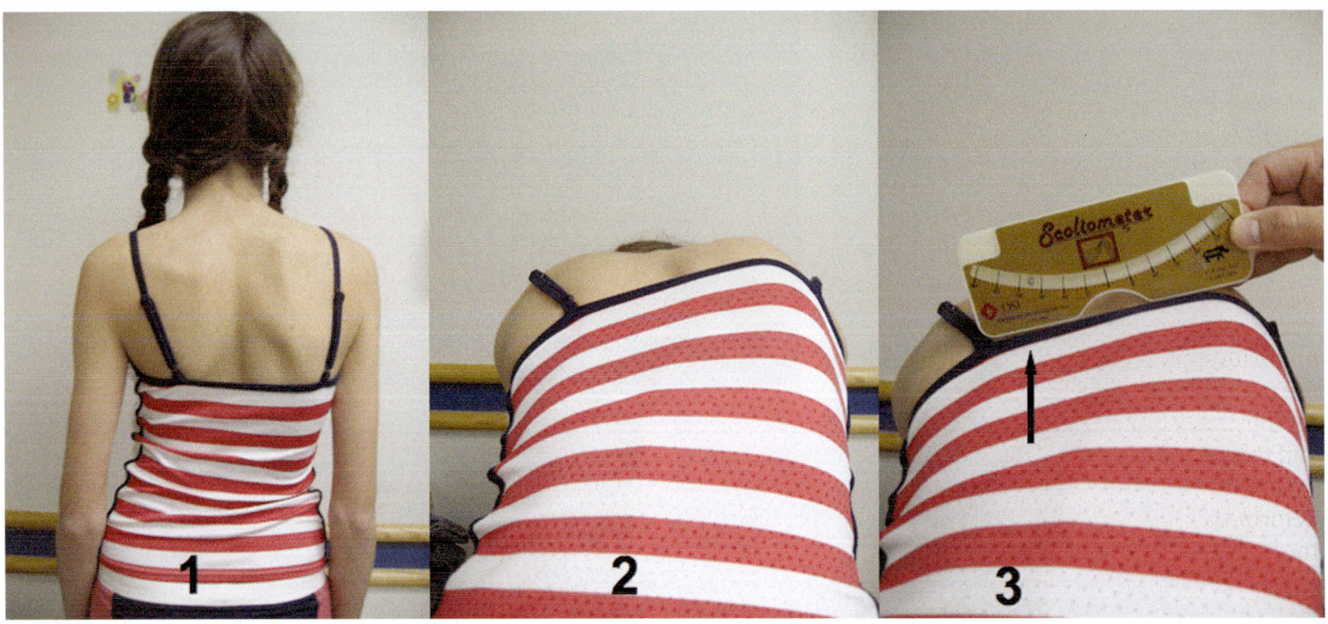


**Fig. 5.4** This 15-year-old girl has a 65-degree curve and is shown in the standing position and undergoing assessment of her rib rotation with a scoliometer while she performs the Adams forward-bend test. **(A)** Standing clinical photograph; note the rib prominence and scapular elevation. **(B)** Adams forward-bend test showing a prominent rib hump on the right. **(C)** Measurement with a scoliometer shows a 17-degree angle. The scoliometer measures the angle of trunk rotation (ATR), and is inexpensive and easy to use. It is a good screening tool and capable of reducing referrals. Referrals should be made only when a patient's spinal angulation is more than 7 degrees.

in the literature.[11,12] Although there is too much variation in inter-user reliability to permit substituting the Adams forward-bend test and scoliometer readings for routine radiography when a child is followed by multiple practitioners, the intra-user reliability of the test is sufficient to allow for extension of the time between radiographs as long as the patient is followed with frequent clinical examinations done by the same examiner.

### Limb-Length Evaluation

Limb-length discrepancy may result in pelvic tilt, which can induce a "compenstory scoliosis." A child with as much as a 3-cm leg-length discrepancy may have no functional difficulties, and these patients may go undetected until a positive Adams forward bending test prompts further investigation. Conventional teaching recommends absolute limb measurement from the anterior superior iliac spine (ASIS) to the medial malleolus, and relative limb measurement from the umbilicus to the medial malleolus. These measurements fail to include the foot, which in some cases may be up to an inch shorter than the other side due to anatomical differences or postsurgical changes. For this reason the authors recommend including the foot in clinical measurement of leg length. Measurements may be made from the ASIS to the lateral border of the sole of the foot just below the fibula. Conventional scanograms provide a radiographic means to assess limb length. Unfortunately, these studies often do not include the foot, and thus may not fully demonstrate a discrepancy. Standing blocks can also provide an effective means to evaluate limb length. They allow visual assessment of pelvic leveling. To use this technique, the ASIS is assessed from the front and the posterior superior iliac spine is assessed from the back. A difference of up to 2 cm in limb length is acceptable and should not be considered in the surgical correction equation if spinal fusion is considered.

In cases of limb-length discrepancy, X-ray films made with the patient in the standing position may show pelvic obliquity and a compensatory curve that is concave on the side of the longer limb. In addition to limb-length inequality, an unleveled pelvis may be caused by joint contractures in the lower extremity. It is extremely important to measure calf and thigh circumference for evidence of unilateral atrophy, which can be indicative of a neurological problem and thus possibly responsible for a compensatory scoliosis related to the limb-length discrepancy. A unilateral foot deformity, especially when associated with clawing of the toes or abnormal hair bearing, is highly associated with neurological disorders.

### Psychosocial Implications

Children with idiopathic scoliosis most often are completely asymptomatic. The effect of having a formal diagnosis of scoliosis is unpredictable in this age group. Most patients with a family history of scoliosis tend to take the diagnosis in stride. However, children who have heard frightening stories of intense pain, neurological deficit, and hardship of an affected relative or peer may confront the diagnosis and its treatment with much apprehension. Additionally, patients involved in competitive sports or intramural activities may be afraid that the condition and its treatment will prevent them from continuing or markedly limit their participation.

The method of intervention for scoliosis can have a profound effect on the psychological response of the child. There are essentially three options in the treatment of scoliosis (i.e., "the three O's"): observation, orthotic, or operation. Observation, although passive, may cause significant anxiety because of the lingering possibility that bracing or surgery may be required. In the case of children for whom an orthotic device has been prescribed, the physician needs to be aware that they may be threatened by the thought of having to wear a device that might make them look different. Even though modern braces can be nearly completely disguised by garment modification and loose clothing, these patients may be sufficiently disturbed about wearing a brace as to either refuse to wear it in school or request home schooling. A randomized controlled study of brace effectiveness (Bracing in Adolescent Scoliosis Trial [BrAIST]) sponsored by the National Institutes of Health is currently underway to determine whether bracing truly has the ability to alter the natural history of idiopathic scoliosis. As expected, patients for whom surgical treatment is recommended are typically concerned that it may harm them or that their scar will be unsightly. A multivariate assessment of patients and parents considering surgery revealed that despite their stated concerns about surgery, the most prevalent issue among them was the fear of paralysis.[13]

## ■ Radiographic Evaluation

Medical imaging for scoliosis allows quantification of the patient's spinal curvature and the diagnosis of underlying conditions that may have led to the deformity (e.g., sources of nonidiopathic scoliosis). Questions that radiographs may answer for the surgeon include the degree of deformity (in the coronal, sagittal, and axial planes), the flexibility of spinal curves, the levels of the spine requiring instrumentation, the quality of the pedicles, and the presence of associated spondylolisthesis.[14,15]

It is important to remember that patients with scoliosis will need multiple radiographic studies each year over a period of several years. Proper training of physicians in requesting radiographs and of technicians in obtaining radiographs can reduce the need for repeat studies and reduce overall radiation exposure for the patient. Proper radiation safety training is an essential part of a successful spinal-deformity practice.

## Plain Radiographs

The two most common radiographs used to evaluate patients with scoliosis are the standing posteroanterior (PA) and lateral views, utilizing full-length cassettes (14 × 36 in.) or digital equipment that allows accurate splicing of images (**Fig. 5.5**). The PA and lateral radiographs should include the lower cervical spine and shoulders, entire thoracolumbar spine, and pelvis. Properly made films allow assessment of the patient's overall skeletal balance as well as skeletal maturity. PA images are used rather than anteroposterior (AP) images in an attempt to reduce radiation exposure to the breast. An association between diagnostic imaging for scoliosis and an increased risk of breast cancer

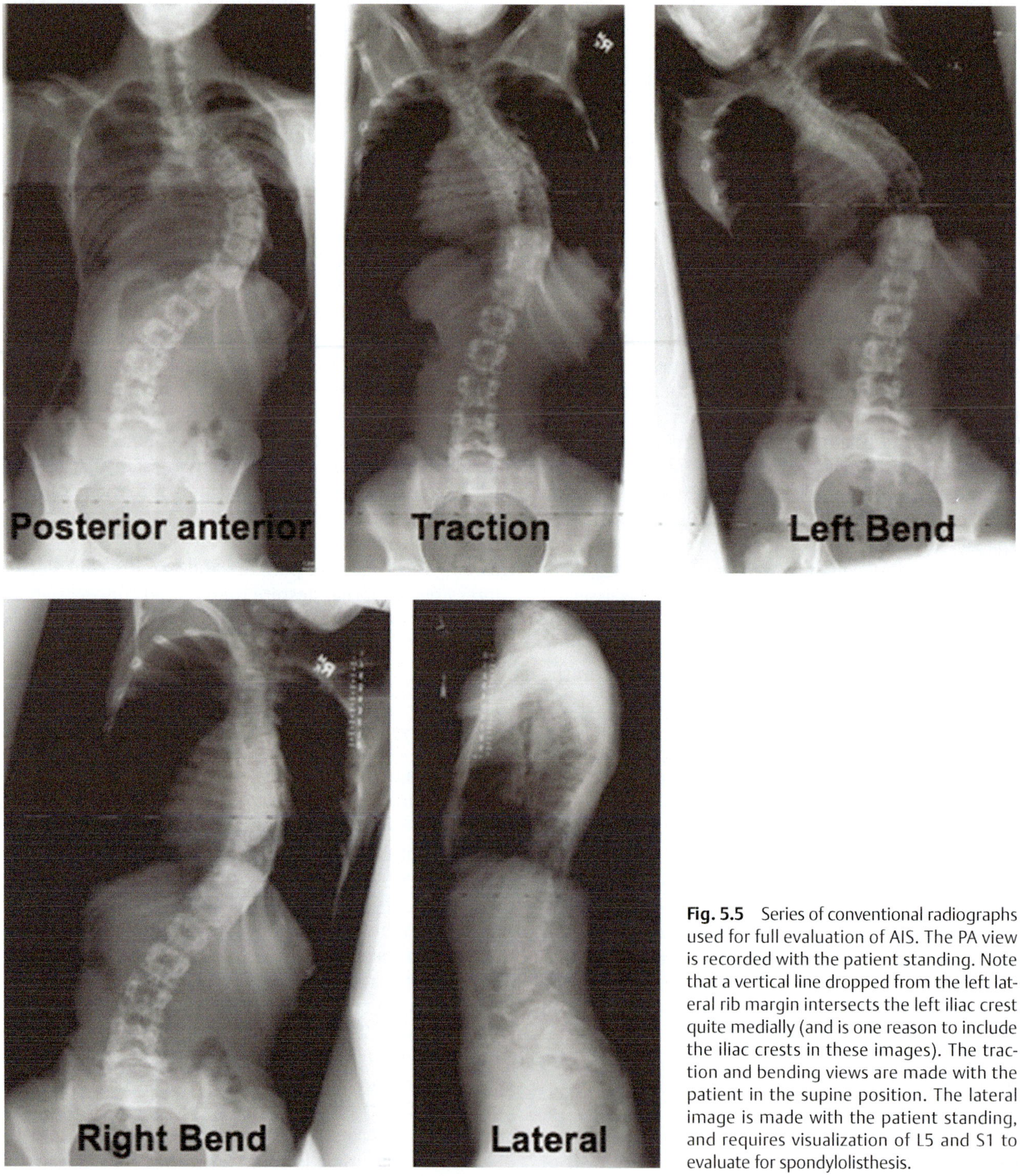


**Fig. 5.5** Series of conventional radiographs used for full evaluation of AIS. The PA view is recorded with the patient standing. Note that a vertical line dropped from the left lateral rib margin intersects the left iliac crest quite medially (and is one reason to include the iliac crests in these images). The traction and bending views are made with the patient in the supine position. The lateral image is made with the patient standing, and requires visualization of L5 and S1 to evaluate for spondylolisthesis.

in women has been established (see the section below on Radiation Hazards). PA radiographs of scoliosis, unlike most X-ray films, are displayed with the patient's right side on the right. This allows the films to be viewed as if the examiner were clinically examining the patient's spinal curve from a posterior position (e.g., with the patient standing in front). This is also the way in which the spine is viewed in the operating room when the patient is put in the prone position, which is the position used for a posterior spinal fusion.

An erect sitting position is an acceptable alternative to a standing view if the patient has a limb-length inequality or is only minimally ambulatory or wheelchair bound. It is well known that gravity can change the radiographic appearance of a spinal deformity, and a few minutes of sitting before the exposure allows a more accurate representation of the deformity. With supine radiographs there is an absence of the effect of gravity on the spine, and films made with the patient in this position can therefore show a very different curve magnitude and spinal balance as opposed to films made with the patient in a standing position. In the special case of oelisthetic scoliosis associated with high-grade spondylolisthesis, a remarkable decrease in the curve is often seen in the supine bending as compared with the standing position (**Fig. 5.6**).

It is important to obtain serial radiographs with a consistent method to demonstrate the true deformity in scoliosis and its progression. Radiographs should always be marked by the technician for technique, laterality, and patient position (i.e., supine, sitting, erect). If the patient has a limb-length inequality, an appropriate block may be placed under the shorter limb to level the pelvis before obtaining X-ray films. For more significant limb-length discrepancies, the film may be made with the patient in an erect sitting position or in the supine position, to negate the effects of pelvic obliquity and gravity. In either view, the iliac crests should be visible (**Fig. 5.5**). The offset of ribs with respect to the pelvic margins and to each other (including the double-rib contour sign) is important in the evaluation of scoliosis (**Fig. 5.7**).[16]

When PA and lateral views are obtained, the patient should be instructed to stand in a relaxed manner but not to slouch. In the PA radiograph, the arms are held out slightly from the sides to avoid overlap with the body's silhouette. Various studies have been done to evaluate the effect of arm positioning in acquisition of the lateral radiograph. The humeri need to be out of the way so that the spine can be visualized; however, holding the arms straight out from the body, as is done with a lateral chest radiograph, may influence the sagittal balance of the spine. When their arms are outstretched, patients tend to assume a "water skiing" position, with the spine leaning backward over the pelvis. One standard practice is to have the patient hold an intravenous infusion pole, or ski poles, to keep the arms at 45-degree angles from the trunk, with the poles supporting the weight of the arms.[17] Other described methods include having the

A

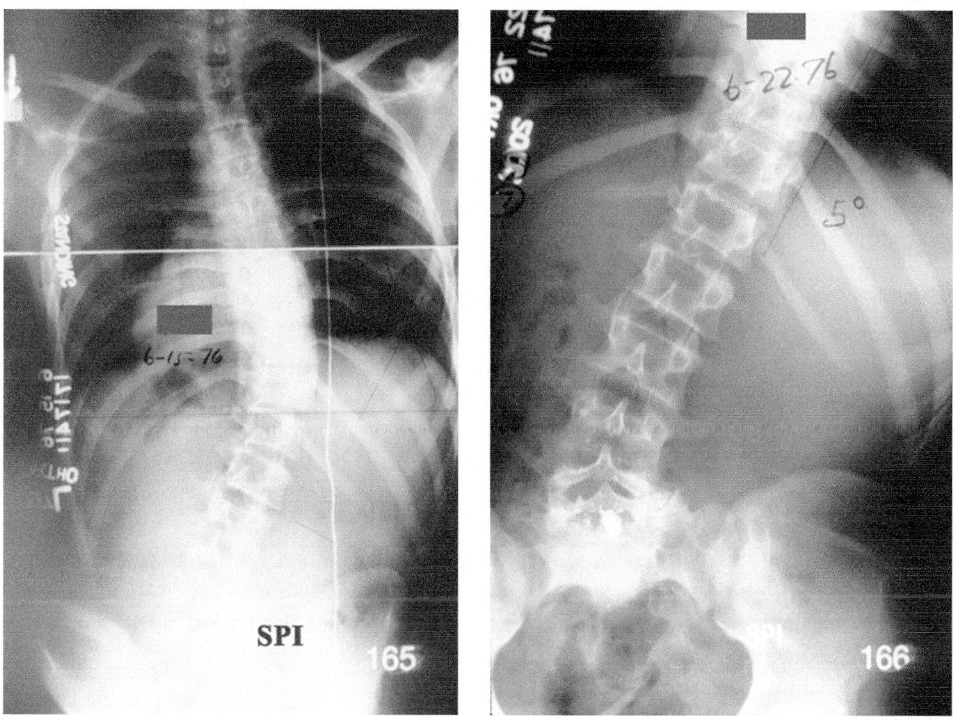


B

**Fig. 5.6** **(A)** Considerable scoliosis in an upright standing frontal image in a patient with severe L5/S1 spondylolisthesis. **(B)** The curve is almost entirely functional, as shown in this supine bending image.

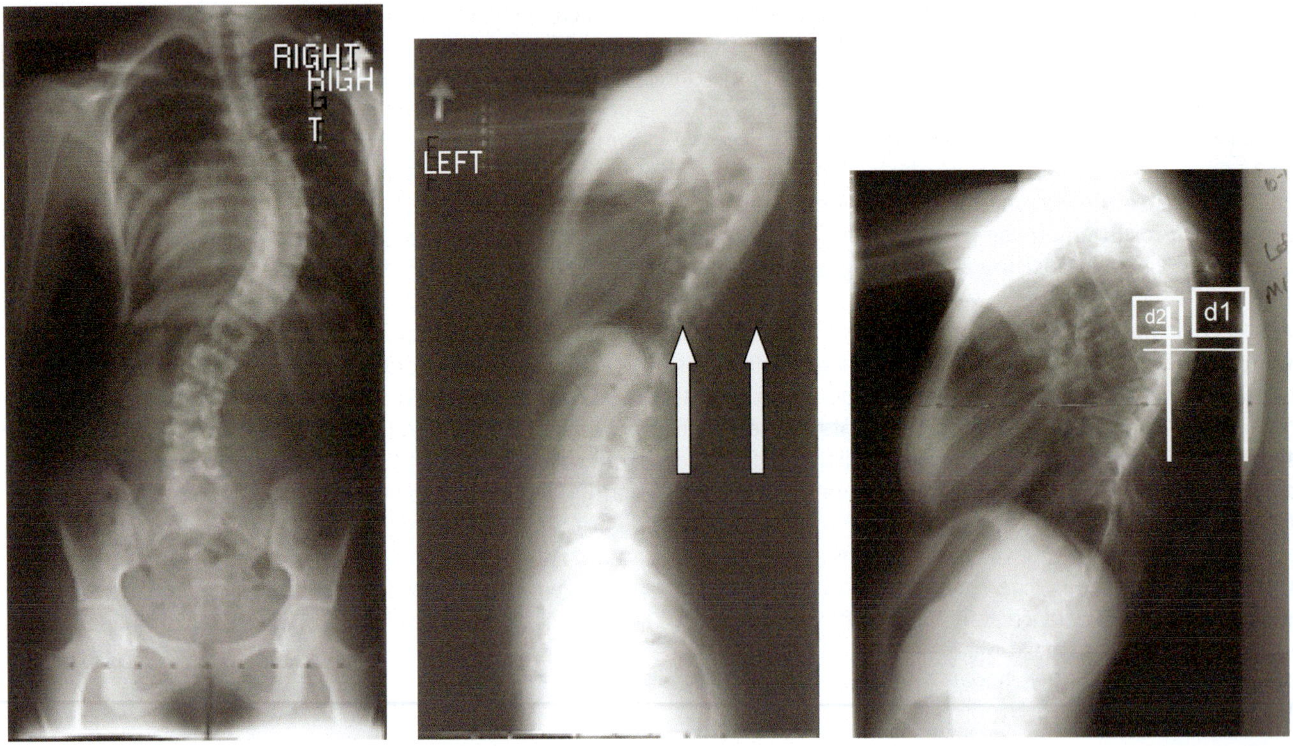


A–C

**Fig. 5.7** The double-rib contour sign is noted in these standing lateral x-ray films **(A)** Standing PA x-ray film of a 65-degree scoliosis. **(B)** Standing lateral x-ray of the same patient. The *arrows* point to the convex and concave ribs (hump) shadows. This identifies the rib hump, and can be compared with scoliometer findings. The length or height of the hump is measured from the posterior vertebral body to the tangent of the rib shadow. **(C)** The rib hump index is derived from vertical lines drawn tangential to the maximum concave/convex posterior rib shadows. The length of the convex (d1) over the concave (d2) shadows from the posterior body wall is the rib hump index. (RI) RI should equal one (1) for a symmetric thorax, with higher values indicating a greater (hump) deformity

patient stand with the arms folded or with the hands on the shoulders or midclavicles. Regardless of which method is chosen, it is important to standardize the method of image acquisition so that radiographs are comparable from one visit to another and from one patient to another.

Congenital anomalies and endplate changes associated with Scheuermann's kyphosis can sometimes be visualized only in a lateral view (**Fig. 5.8**). Generally, at least three anteriorly wedged vertebral bodies are seen at the apex of a true Scheuermann curve.

If the patient has complained of low back pain, then oblique views, and radiography of a spot lateral of the lumbosacral junction (if the long lateral does not suffice), may be ordered to look for a spondylolysis. If the patient has persistent back pain in another area, or if there is a history that raises suspicion of a tumor or infection, radiographs with a metallic marker placed over the area to be investigated can be helpful. A specialized oblique image, the Stagnara (Leeds) view, aims at lateral visualization of the apical vertebral bodies when there is severe scoliotic rotational deformity. The amount of obliquity (of the X-ray machine) required to achieve this view is related to the magnitude of the apical rotation of the spine. In the absence of a computed tomography (CT) image through the plane of the vertebral body, the patient is positioned for the Stagnara view so that the X-ray beam forms a tangent to the right and left posterior rib cage as positioned by the technologist. The Stagnara view is helpful because the anatomy and morphology of the pedicle, which is distorted in severe curves on routine PA films, can often be visualized through this technique, with less radiation exposure than is required in CT scanning.[18]

An AP Stagnara view can also be helpful because it often allows better visualization of the pedicle anatomy and morphology, which is often distorted in severe curves. The AP Ferguson view of the lumbosacral junction is very helpful for assessing sacral obliquity and hemivertebrae, as well as for the quality of a postoperative fusion. The Ferguson view is an upwardly oriented AP exposure of the sacrum so that it is seen *en face*, with the beam perpendicular to the estimated sacral inclination (**Fig. 5.9**). For the average sacrum this is about a 30-degree cephalad angulation of the beam.

Assessment of the flexibility of a scoliotic curve pattern is important for planning and predicting correction in a brace or Risser cast, determining fusion levels, and evaluating postoperative correction with growing rod instrumentation or instrumented fusion. The use of lateral or AP side-bending radiographs is a standard method of assessing the flexibility

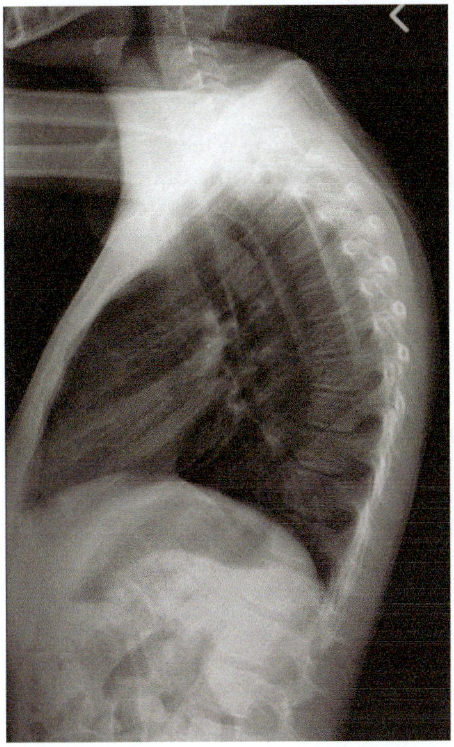

A

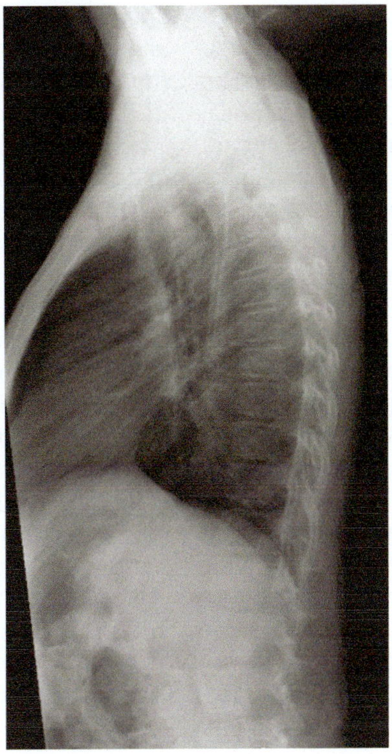

B

**Fig. 5.8** Evaluation of kyphosis. **(A)** Standing lateral view. Look for anteriorly wedged bodies at the apex of the curve in cases of Scheuermann's disease. This subject does not show this criterion for the disease. **(B)** Cross-table lateral supine view over a bolster demonstrates the flexibility of the kyphotic curve, as compared with the film in A made on the same day.

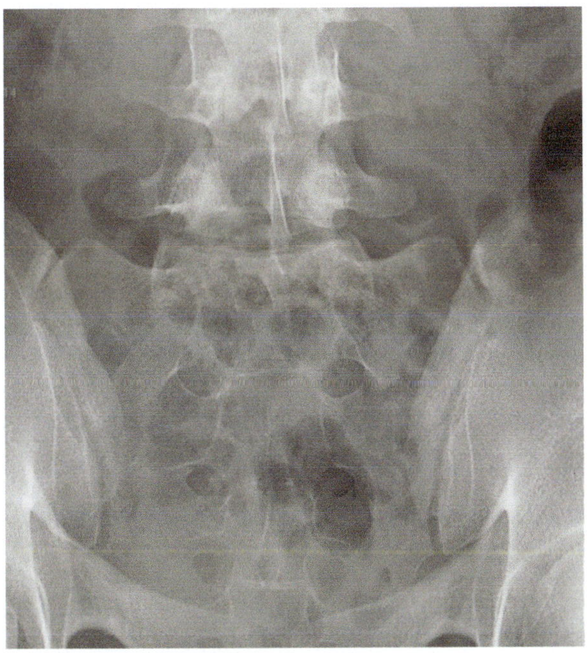

**Fig. 5.9** The angled frontal Ferguson view allows meticulous evaluation of the structure of the sacrum. Such findings, not evident in this patient, include sacral obliquity, facet trophism, interbody fusion, and fracture.

of a scoliosis. The patient is asked to make maximal effort when bending into and then away from the separate curves, and to hold those positions while the X-ray film is made (**Fig. 5.5**). These films are typically made with the patient in the supine position, but some authors have advocated prone positioning. In making supine bending radiographs for which the patient bends toward the concavity, the rib or flank prominence may increase in size and distort the view of the adjacent segments of the spine. This bias may be reduced by making these images with the patient in the prone position, in which the rib prominence will not be in contact with the X-ray plate. Images of the patient in supine traction (**Fig. 5.5**) have been proposed as an alternative to lateral bending views, but their usefulness is not yet fully established.

Luk et al have advocated fulcrum bending for evaluation of the flexibility of scoliotic curves, as this technique has been shown to be predictive of curve correction through posterior surgical techniques.[19] The test is performed by having the patient lie in the lateral position over a fulcrum (cylindrical bolster) placed beneath the apex of the curve. The fulcrum flexibility is the percentage correction of the Cobb angle of the patient's deformity as a result of this technique. This test, unlike erect side-bending films, does not require voluntary muscle activation by the patient.[19,20]

Push prone radiographs are also a good method for assessing curve flexibility, especially for patients who are unable to make a full bending effort.[21] In addition, these images can be obtained in the operating room after induction of anesthesia, to help predict the intraoperative correction of spinal curves. These radiographs require the assistance of additional persons to apply apical pressure and counterpressure above and below the specific curve for which surgery is being done. Radiographs made with supine traction show greater flexibility than side-bending films for patients with curves over 60 degrees.[22] These images are also useful for patients who have paralytic curves and are unable to move or bend in the ways needed for other methods. Radiographs of patients in Cotrel dynamic traction may be made with the use of a Risser traction table. This technique often requires anesthesia, because most young children cannot tolerate traction and lying on the bars of the Risser table while awake. Previously published studies using traction films to determine the end-instrumented vertebra have found frequent postoperative coronal decompensation.[23] Another study found that PA radiographs made during intraoperative traction showed better flexibility than radiographs made during supine bending, and this changed the operative plan for 11 of 13 patients, eliminating the need for anterior releases.[24]

Lateral radiographs made with backward bending over a bolster are appropriate for evaluating the flexibility of a kyphosis (**Fig. 5.8**). These images are obtained with the patient in a recumbent position. The technician must be able to judge where the bolster is to be placed (i.e., the apex of the kyphosis), on the basis of the physician's order and physical appearance of the patient. The technician must be experienced enough to ensure that the correct levels of the spine and ribs are captured on the image. If the initial lateral image does not reveal abnormality, lateral images on follow-up should be avoided unless needed for a full preoperative evaluation.

## Radiation Hazards

There is always some risk from exposure even to low doses of radiation, as is the case for routine X-ray films of the spine. However, the risk of tissue damage from medical imaging is low as compared with its potential benefits if it is clinically appropriate and performed with radiation protection. For perspective, the radiation exposure from a chest X-ray is about equal to the natural radiation exposure received during a round-trip airline flight from Boston to Los Angeles, or during 10 days of hiking in the Rocky Mountains. However, repeated exposure to low-level radiation for diagnostic imaging may carry an increased risk of neoplasia, such as breast cancer in women.[25]

Breast tissue and the thyroid gland are particularly sensitive to the cumulative effect of irradiation. Doody and colleagues examined a retrospective cohort of more than 5000 female patients with scoliosis treated between 1912 and 1965. They found that in this group there were 77 deaths from breast cancer, which represented a significant increase in the risk of death over that for the general population (standardized mortality ratio = 1.69). The expected number of deaths based on mortality data for the United States was 45.6. Doody and colleagues concluded that exposure to multiple radiographic studies during childhood and adolescence may increase the likelihood of breast cancer in women with scoliosis. Recognized confounding factors may relate to the degree of spinal deformity, amount of radiation exposure, and reproductive history.[26] The association between radiation exposure in adolescence and thyroid cancer has also been studied extensively. The evaluation of groups of patients exposed to thyroid irradiation in childhood (either as a result of medical treatment or as a consequence of exposure to a nuclear blast) makes it clear that the thyroid gland is highly sensitive to the carcinogenic effects of ionizing radiation.[27]

Currently, there is a far-reaching campaign in medical imaging, known by the acronym ALARA (as low as reasonably achievable), to minimize total body and local radiation dose, especially in children.[28] Techniques used to reduce excessive radiation exposure include collimation, shields, grids, and ultra-high-speed film. PA radiographs (versus AP films) allow the skin of the back to receive higher doses of radiation than the anterior breast and thyroid tissues.[29] However, when the AP versus PA view for chest radiography was studied clinically, the AP view was chosen because of concern for an increased risk of leukemia.[30] Gonadal shields are also important in reducing radiation exposure, and technicians should be educated in ensuring their proper placement. In obtaining films for evaluation of the TRC, which may be obscured by standard gonadal shields, a more tailored shield should be used to allow for its proper visualization. Posterior breast shields (blocking the posterior entrance site of the X-ray beam) can be used in an effort to reduce radiation exposure of the breast. These shields, however, can be counterproductive in cases of severe scoliosis, in that they may obscure visualization of the curved spine.

The best method for reducing total radiation exposure is to avoid radiographic testing unless it is truly necessary. Extending the interval between sessions of radiography when possible will also reduce the patient's lifetime radiation dose. The physician should avoid repeat radiography after an inadequate radiograph unless it is absolutely essential. Technicians also need to be educated about the proper placement of radiation shields and proper acquisition techniques for avoiding the need to repeat films.

## Other Techniques of Plain Radiography

The use of an antiscatter grid, an effective method of reducing scattered radiation, can greatly improve the quality of bone imaging. The grid is placed between the patient and the image intensifier, cassette, or digital detector, and absorbs a portion of the scattered radiation in its lead/aluminum plates. However, the use of this device may necessitate an increased dose of radiation to acquire an image. It is important to remember that the amount of radiation that reaches the image intensifier is not reduced until it has passed through the patient. The increased risk of additional radiation exposure must be weighed against the benefit of improved image quality.

The advent of digital radiography has led to better image quality, reduced radiation exposure, and improved transfer of information between physicians. In conventional radiography a great deal of signal degradation occurs before the image is displayed or printed. When a digital detector is used, less information is lost and thus more detail can be displayed, especially when an image is magnified at the viewing workstation. Other advantages to digital radiography are the easy storage and retrieval of images and the facility of transmission of images over Internet connections.

An issue with long digital images of scoliosis has been the imperfect stitching together of an upper and a lower image. Technical improvements in the machines used to perform this function have lessened this problem, but the possibility of error needs to be recognized.

Studies comparing Cobb-angle measurements of primary and secondary curves on digital radiographs with those made on traditional radiographs have shown no statistical difference in the intra- or inter-observer variance with the two techniques.[31] The radiation dose received by the patient is considerably reduced when digital imaging is used rather than conventional full-spine radiography (by two-thirds in the study cited here), and is further reduced with digital fluoroscopy.[32]

Close collaboration between physicists, biomechanical engineers, medical radiologists, and orthopedic surgeons has led to the development of a new low-dose radiation device named EOS™ (Biospace Med; Paris, France). The EOS system uses thin fan-beam collimation, which reduces most of the scattered radiation received by a patient during imaging and provides a high-quality image. Using a gaseous X-ray detector invented by Georges Charpak, who won the Nobel Prize in Physics in 1992, the system allows two-dimensional (2D) and three-dimensional (3D) image acquisition at much lower doses of radiation than with conventional methods. It is claimed that the dose used to obtain a 2D image of the skeletal system has been reduced by 8- to 10-fold. As compared with 3D reconstructions from axial CT slices, EOS can purportedly create 3D reconstructions with 800- to 1000-fold less radiation exposure of the patient.[33] The patient is examined in the standing (or seated) position, and can be scanned from head to feet, both frontally and laterally. This positioning represents a major advantage over conventional CT, which requires the patient to be horizontal. The 3D reconstructions of each element of the osteoarticular system imaged with the EOS technique are as precise as those obtained with conventional CT scanning. The EOS procedure is also relatively rapid, taking less than a minute to image the entire spine. In addition, Labele and colleagues in Montreal have shown value in the 3D imaging reconstruction techniques provided by the EOS system for operative planning and postoperative evaluation in scoliosis, including their use for direct vertebral derotation.[34]

## Computed Tomography

CT scanning has a limited role in diagnostic testing for idiopathic scoliosis, but may be useful in cases of severely rotated curves and congenital curves. The sagittal, coronal, reconstructed 3D images provided by modern CT scanning can be extremely helpful in appreciating the degree of a spinal deformity and in preoperative planning for its treatment. Preoperative assessment of a deformity, including the evaluation of pedicle diameter, can be helpful in selecting a surgical fixation technique and screw size for it. Such preoperative assessment is especially important for patients known to have neurofibromatosis 1, Marfan syndrome, and Larsen syndrome. Moreover, newer computer software can superimpose reconstructed images of blood vessels and other soft-tissue structures on CT scans if desired. CT scans can also help in evaluating other spinal pathologies such as spondylolysis (**Fig. 5.10**). Additionally, if the patient cannot undergo an MRI scan, a CT myelogram can provide considerable information about intraspinal pathology.

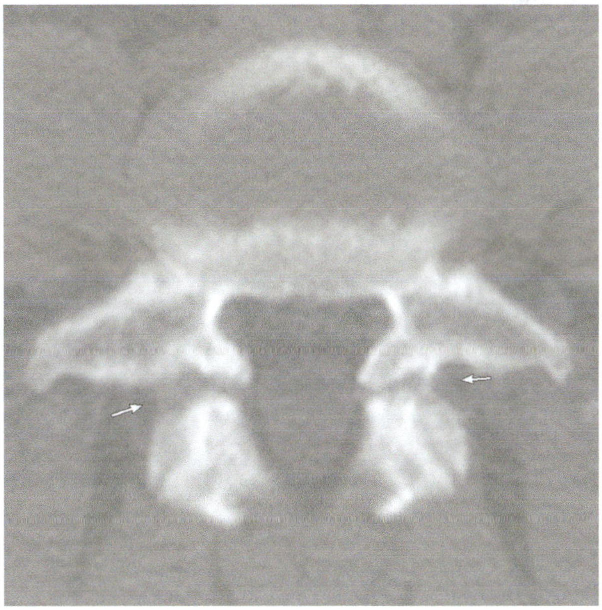

**Fig. 5.10** CT scan of bilateral spondylolysis (*arrows*) of vertebral body in a thin-section axial image with the gantry of the CT scanner appropriately tilted for optimal visualization.

The benefits of CT scanning must outweigh the risk of additional radiation exposure to justify its use. Newer multislice CT scanners can obtain images rapidly, and are designed to do so with less radiation (if proper protocols are utilized). However, CT scans still involve considerable radiation exposure. Additionally, younger children may need to be sedated if good CT images are to be obtained. The desired levels to be scanned and specific instructions regarding reconstructions should be clearly communicated to the CT technologist.

## Magnetic Resonance Imaging

MRI technology is invaluable in the diagnosis of soft tissue and bone pathology. In particular, MRI is very helpful in the diagnosis of neural axis pathology in children with scoliosis.[35–37] Assessment with MRI should be considered in all children under 11 years of age with scoliosis exceeding 20 degrees, and for patients with unusual curves, hyperkyphosis, back pain, or abnormal findings in a neurological examination.[38–40] A recent prospective study of 104 patients with Lenke type 1 idiopathic scoliosis found that 7 had abnormalities on MRI scans. In each of these cases, symptom onset was early (e.g., juvenile scoliosis), and the patients had complained of back pain. No patient who developed scoliosis after the age of 10 years had an intraspinal abnormality detected on MRI.[41]

An undisputed advantage of MRI over CT scanning is the absence of ionizing radiation delivered to the patient's tissues. However, there are concerns about magnets stronger than 1.5 Tesla producing a heating effect in the tissues of patients, especially those who have ferromagnetic metal implants. The specific absorption rate (SAR) measures this heating produced in tissues, and needs to be considered with the use of any magnet stronger than 1.5T. Another potential danger of MRI is nephrogenic systemic fibrosis, a devastating skin and muscle necrosis that can occur after a patient with impaired renal function receives intravenous gadolinium-containing contrast material.[42] It is thus necessary to ensure that the patient has normal renal function before considering the use of intravenous contrast material in an MRI study. Contrast material is rarely indicated in children with spinal deformity.

In addition to demonstrating intraspinal anatomy in great detail, spinal MRI has been shown to be effective for evaluating surrounding soft-tissue structures in children with scoliosis. Riccio et al, in a study of 153 patients with congenital scoliosis, found no instance of a renal abnormality that was noted on ultrasound examination but was absent on a spinal MRI scan (or vice versa).[43]

## Nuclear Imaging Studies

Bone scans provide information about the metabolic activity of bone and surrounding tissues, and for the evaluation of back pain. In the assessment of a scoliotic patient for a suspected nonidiopathic cause of the condition, a bone scan is used in conjunction with single-photon emission computed tomography (SPECT). This technique may also be helpful in the evaluation of acute back pain. A bone scan can demonstrate healing of a traumatic fracture, stress fracture activity, spondylolysis, tumor (such as osteoid osteoma), and altered growth-plate activity, such as after injury or infection (diskitis). A recent advance in nuclear medicine was the development of combination CT scanners. SPECT/CT and positron emission tomography/CT (PET/CT) allow the accurate overlay of metabolic information obtained in nuclear medicine on the anatomical detail provided by high-resolution CT scanning.

## Radiographic Measurements

### Cobb-Angle Method

In 1948 John Cobb described a technique to measure the frontal-plane magnitude of a scoliosis. In this technique, the angle of the spinal curve is subtended by lines drawn perpendicular to the endplates of the upper and lower vertebra of the curve, which are the vertebrae most tilted from the horizontal (**Fig. 5.11**). Because the Cobb angle measures those endplates (as does a line across the pedicle margins, if the endplates are not clearly imaged), it makes mathematical sense that the top of one spinal curve is automatically the bottom of the next curve and vice versa. Tools on picture archiving and communication system (PACS) workstations can allow angle measurements without the need to resort to the traditional use of a protractor to measure perpendiculars to endplate lines on films. There is ~3- to 5-degree measurement error inherent in the Cobb-angle technique. Therefore, the difference in a curve's measured magnitude would be considered a "real change" only if it was greater than 5 degrees. This method can be used in the sagittal plane to describe the amount of lordosis and kyphosis in different regions of the spine. When measured accurately and consistently, Cobb angles can provide information about curve progression, the effectiveness of bracing, the results of surgery, and the maintenance of curve correction over time. Any increase in an angle following fusion may signify a defect in the fusion mass and any associated instrumentation.

### Balance Assessment

In the coronal plane, overall balance can be assessed with a plumbline (easily produced by the tools on a PACS workstation). The C7 plumbline (C7PL) is a line dropped vertically from the center of the C7 vertebral body. This line should normally pass through the center of S1. Another technique is to erect a reference line from the center of S1. This line is called the center sacral vertical line (CSVL). The difference between the CSVL and the C7PL is the amount of coronal-

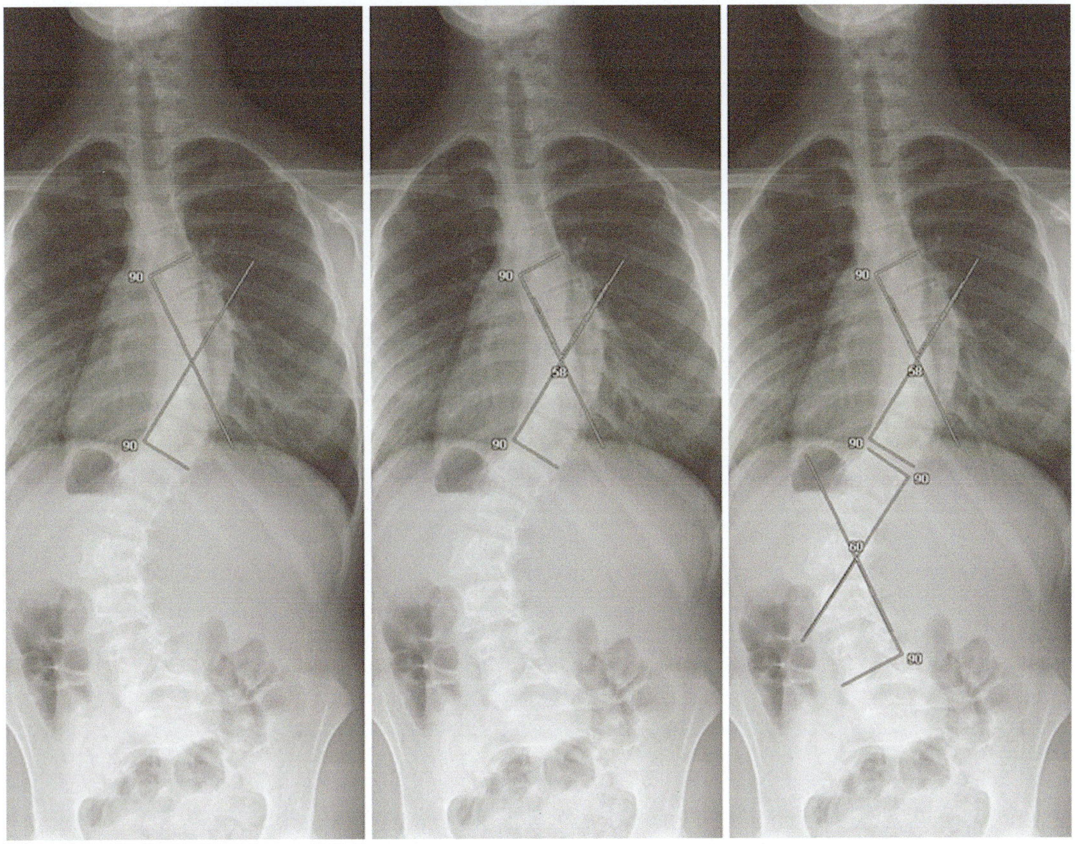


A–C

**Fig. 5.11** Cobb-angle measurement. **(A)** Select the top and bottom vertebra of the curve, shown by maximal tilting of the endplates from the horizontal. Draw the endplate lines and perpendiculars to those lines (the alternative to this manual method is to use PACS workstation toolbox functions). **(B)** The upper and lower angles at the point where the perpendiculars overlap give the measured Cobb angle. **(C)** The procedure is similar for the next curve, with an opposite convexity.

plane imbalance. A difference of less than 2 cm is considered acceptable (**Fig. 5.12**). Another method for assessing coronal trunk balance is to drop vertical lines tangential to the outermost perimeter of the rib cage on a frontal radiographic study. Both of these lines should fall within the bony pelvis.

Sagittal spinal balance is evaluated on the lateral radiograph by drawing the plumb line from the midpoint of the C7 vertebral body toward the sacrum. When normal, the line passes through the middle of the first sacral body (**Fig. 5.13**). Many authors have suggested other appropriate sacral reference points through which the plumbline reference can pass, such as the posterior-superior corner of S1. Others have suggested that patients are in acceptable sagittal balance if the C7PL falls through or behind the hip joints. Pre- and postoperative global sagittal balance is not typically a major concern in AIS. However, in adults, achieving and maintaining acceptable sagittal alignment may be the most important predictor of good long-term outcome, and is more important than correction in the coronal plane.

The most common sagittal-plane disturbance in AIS is thoracic lordosis (**Fig. 5.14**), or hypokyphosis. Although this sagittal plane malalignment is unlikely to cause significant global imbalance, it is often difficult to correct surgically and may leave the patient with a flat thoracic spine postoperatively. If the thoracic hypokyphosis is severe enough (i.e., lordotic), it may also affect the alignment of the cervical and lumbar spine.[44]

Over time, a junctional kyphosis may develop above or below the thoracic segment in AIS, eventually inducing kyphosis in either the cervical or lumbar spine. A thoracic hyperkyphosis in a curve considered otherwise idiopathic should be investigated for an underlying lesion such as syringomyelia.

## Vertebral Rotational Measurements

Although CT scanning permits the best evaluation of vertebral rotation, the Nash–Moe (**Fig. 5.15**) and Perdriolle methods can be used to evaluate rotation on plain radiographs. The Nash–Moe method categorizes vertebral rotation into

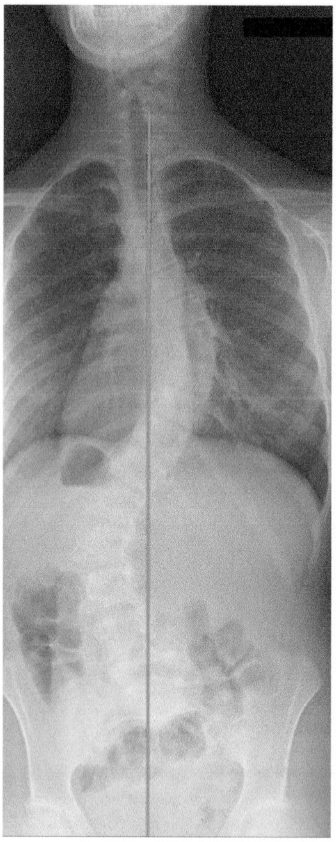

**Fig. 5.12** Use of plumbline for determining coronal balance. A vertical line constructed from the midpoint of C7 through the sacrum on upright PA image.

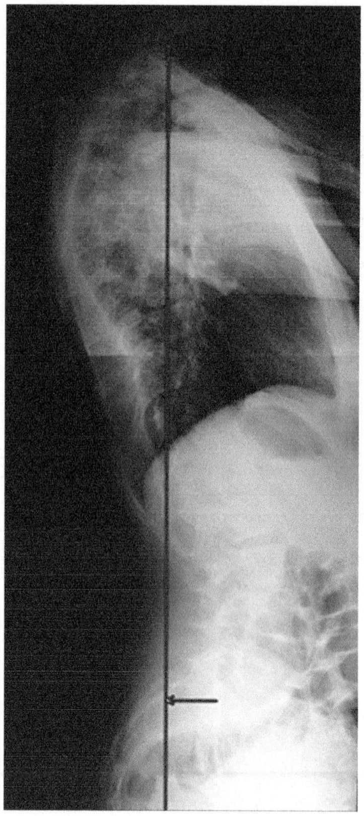

**Fig. 5.13** Plumbline for sagittal balance. A vertical line is constructed from the midpoint of the C7 vertebra through the pelvis on upright lateral image. Here it intersects S2. The relationship to the posterior border of S1 is to be evaluated.

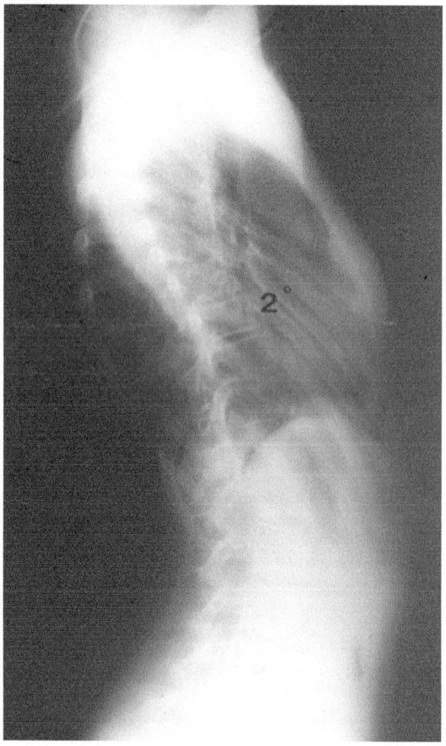


**Fig. 5.14** Thoracic lordosis of 2 degrees represents a severe form of hypokyphosis.

five grades. In this method the vertebra to be evaluated is divided into halves and then the convex half is divided into three equal segments. If the pedicles of these segments are equidistant from the lateral edges of the vertebral body, there is no significant rotation, and the rotation is classified as being of grade 0. In a rotation of grade 1, most of the convex pedicle is still within the first (lateral) one-third division of the vertebra, and the concave pedicle is beginning to disappear. With grade 2 the convex pedicle has rotated into the middle third segment of the vertebra and the concave pedicle may disappear. In grade 3 the convex pedicle has rotated into the medial third segment and the concave pedicle is not visible. In grade 4 rotation of the convex pedicle has gone past the midline of the vertebra and the concave pedicle is again not visible.[45] One recent study confirmed the accuracy of the Nash–Moe method despite any lateral tilting or forward–backward inclination of the spine.[46]

The Perdriolle method of measuring vertebral rotation is done with a device designed by Pedriolle and known as the torsiometer. In this technique the greatest diameter of the convex pedicle of the apical vertebra is marked as are the lateral edges of the waist of the vertebra. The transparent torsiometer is superimposed over the radiograph and

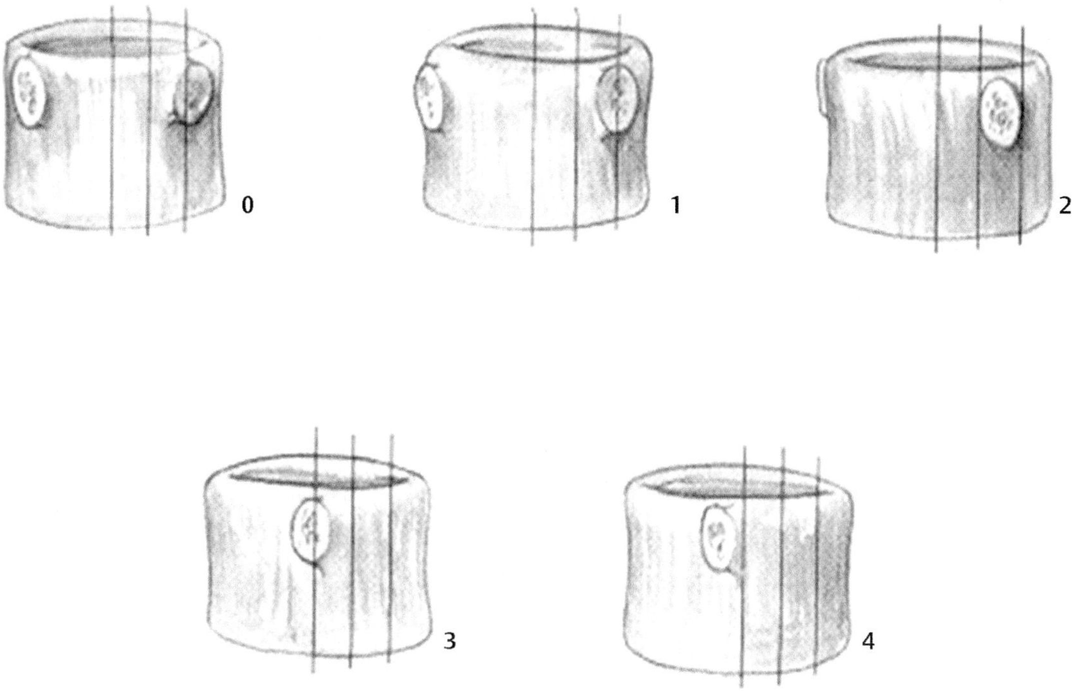


**Fig. 5.15** Nash–Moe method of measuring vertebral rotation.

the degree of rotation is determined from the line of the scale that intersects the midpoint of the pedicle (**Fig. 5.16**). This method has been shown to be both reliable and accurate by recent studies comparing the rotation measured on supine scanogram films with the rotation measured on CT scans. However, a difference was seen in measurements made on erect and those made on supine films.[47] This difference is a natural consequence of the effects of vertical loading as the result of gravity. Because most measurements of spinal curvature are made on erect radiographs, the evaluation of vertebral rotation should be done on erect radiographs as well as those made in other views.

In the recent report comparing the Nash–Moe, Perdriolle, and CT methods for determining rotation, the CT method demonstrated greater accuracy than the other methods when methodology was used to compensate for vertebral-body tilt. The gain in accuracy through CT scannning comes at the expense of greater radiation exposure, time taken by the procedure, and cost of the study.[48] Asghar et al and the Harms Study Group, in a recent study comparing all pedicle screw constructs versus hook-and-rod systems in AIS, used the axial CT method described by Aaro and Dahlborn to evaluate the degree of vertebral rotation. The angle of rotation of the vertebra is measured by using the angle between the junction of the laminae, the dorsal central aspect of the vertebral foramen and middle of the vertebral body, and the sagittal plane.[49,50] We found this technique to be reliable and easy to use with the measurement tools available in a modern PACS system.

## Scoring Systems

A 100-point radiographic scoring system was developed by the Harms Study Group to give an objective measurement of spinal deformity. A normal, straight and balanced spine would receive 100 points. The score is based on measurements made on standard PA and lateral radiographs of the spine, and accounts for the degree of coronal and sagittal (kyphotic and lordotic) deformity, spinal balance, shoulder and upper rib tilt, apical vertebra rotation and translation, end-instrumented vertebra (EIV) angulation, and disc below EIV angulation. Points are subtracted from a score of 100 on the basis of the degree of deviation from normal values. The weight or importance of each of the measurement components named above was determined by the consensus of opinions of surgeons experienced in treating spinal deformities. The system was developed to allow objective comparison of preoperative deformity and the postoperative results of correction. Multiple preoperative and postoperative radiographs can be grouped and compared by using this system. However, because numerous measurements are needed to produce a score, practical clinical implementation of the system may be difficult.

An awareness of the Lenke classification system[51] has also proven worthwhile, especially because it allows the comparison of outcomes at different centers. The six curve types in the system are: (1) main thoracic (the most common according to Lenke's data); (2) double thoracic;

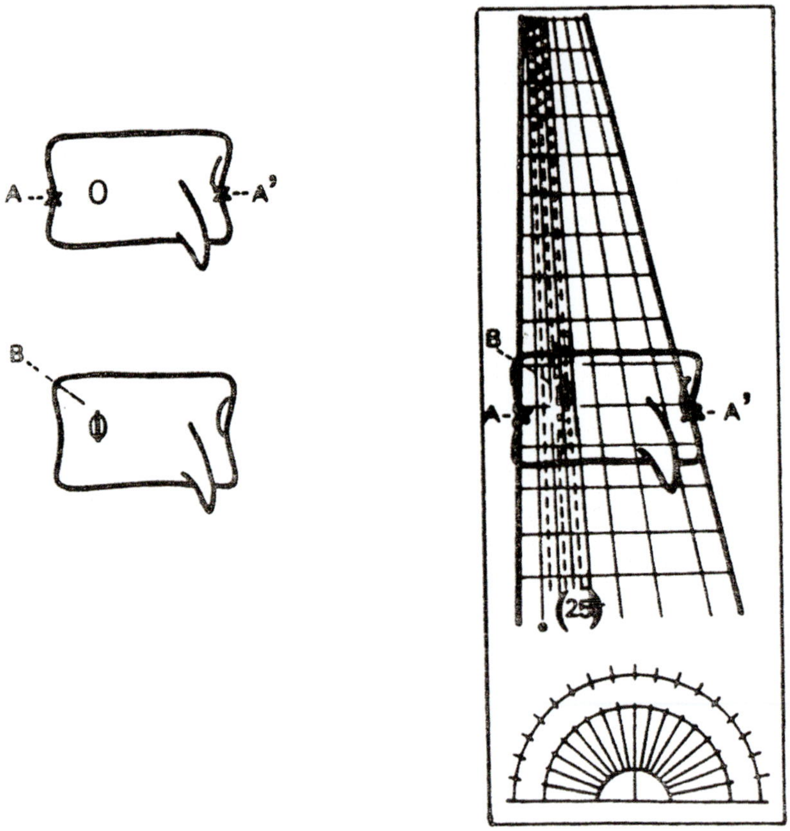


**Fig. 5.16** Perdriolle method of measuring vertebral rotation. The selected pedicles are highlighted on a radiograph and the torsiometer is then superimposed on the radiograph. The torsion angle is measured by constructing a vertical line through the pedicle on the convex side of the curve. (From Perdriolle R, Vidal J. Thoracic idiopathic scoliosis curve evolution and prognosis. Spine 10:785-791, 1985. Reprinted with permission.)

(3) double major; (4) triple major; (5) thoracolumbar/lumbar; and (6) thoracolumbar/lumbar–main thoracic. The other two components of the triadic Lenke classification system are a lumbar spine modifier (based on the association between the center sacral vertical line to the lumbar spine on an upright radiograph) and a sagittal thoracic modifier (hypokyphosis, normal, or hyperkyphosis) based on the upper-T5-to-lower-T12 angle, which is considered normal when between 10 and 40 degrees of kyphosis. The Lenke classification is intended to suggest the levels of the spine to be instrumented, fused, or both in a specific case of deformity.

## Assessment of Skeletal Maturity

The assessment of ossification centers and the subsequent timing of skeletal maturation and closure of growth centers are predictable and well described. The most common areas of bone growth used in determining a patient's level of skeletal maturity are the iliac apophysis, TRC, and hand and wrist. Other areas of potential value for estimating skeletal maturity are the olecranon apophysis at the elbow, the pelvis, and the spine. However, these centers are not always visible on routine radiographs, and are therefore not commonly used.

### Risser Sign

Risser described the gradual anterolateral-to-posteromedial ossification of the iliac crest apophysis and its eventual fusion with the ilium at skeletal maturity. His grading system (**Fig. 5.17**) divides the progression of skeletal maturity into five stages of ossification of the iliac apophysis: (1) Risser grade 0: no ossification; Risser grade 1: ossification of the lateral 25%; Risser grade 2: ossification of the lateral 50% of the apophysis; Risser grade 3: ossification of the lateral 75%; Risser grade 4: ossification of the entire apophysis without fusion to the ilium; and Risser grade 5: fusion of the ossified apophysis to the ilium.[5] The Risser staging system is convenient to use in evaluating radiographs of the spine for scoliosis, because the iliac apophyses are included in the long-standing film. There are, however, limitations in using spine films for this purpose, as a PA view results in poorer visualization of the apophyses than is possible with an AP view. It is noteworthy that the supine AP side-bending radiographs that are ordered to assess curve flexibility often permit excellent visualization of the iliac crests. Visualization of the iliac crest apophyses may be difficult in patients who have excessive pelvic tilt in the sagittal plane. The Risser sign may not be useful for predicting curve progression because

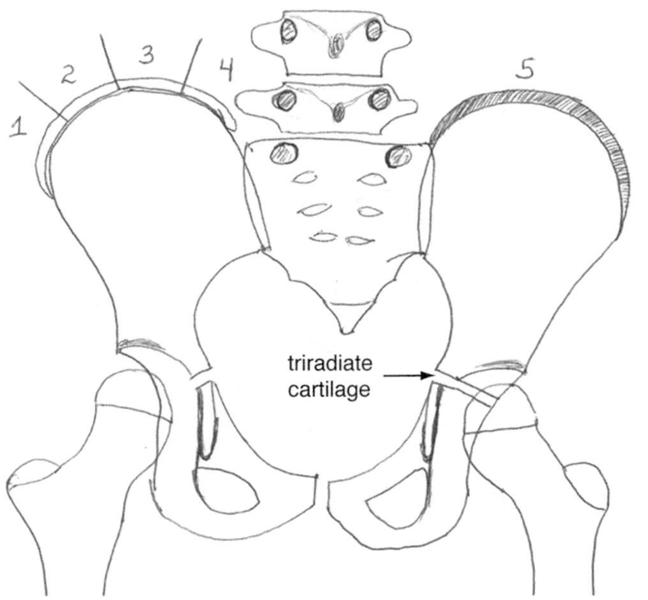


**Fig. 5.17** The Risser evaluation. The Risser stages are discussed in the text. The *arrow* points to the lucent zone (clear space) in the triradiate cartilage, between the pelvic bones.

grade 1 has been found to begin after the period of rapid adolescent growth or peak height velocity.[52] For girls, the mean period from the onset of ossification of the iliac apophysis to Risser grade 4 is 1 year. At Risser grade 4, only minimal skeletal growth potential remains. The Risser grading of boys with regard to skeletal maturity is not as reliable as that of girls. The changes in ossification of the iliac apophysis as a boy matures typically occur more slowly than in a girl, and boys can still grow by a significant amount when at Risser grade 4.[53]

## Triradiate Cartilage

The TRC of the acetabulum, which is visible throughout childhood and the prepubescent period, is also often conveniently visible on long-standing films of the spine. The TRC reliably begins to ossify in the early stages of puberty. In girls it is completely ossified by menarche, and in boys it is typically in the early stages of ossification when puberty begins. The cartilage is usually completely ossified by the time of the rapid growth phase. It is a reliable marker of skeletal immaturity when it is still cartilaginous or "open." However, the degree of ossification of the TRC is not useful in predicting the end of growth, and a proposed alternative has been the ossification of the olecranon process of the ulna.[54] The postoperative complication of crankshaft phenomenon, however, is unlikely to occur after the TRC has closed, presumably because the peak-height growth velocity has passed.[55]

## Hand and Wrist

Greulich and Pyle's *Radiographic Atlas of Skeletal Development of the Hand and Wrist* contains standardized tables and radiographic photographs with detailed descriptions of the bones and ossification centers that correlate with the degree of skeletal maturity.[56] Tables in the book also describe the range of variation for a particular skeletal age, and a range within a certain number of months that are included with that age. The Tanner–Whitehouse method for evaluation of individual bones of the fingers is currently far more tedious to use, but could eventually be useful for the computer-assisted calculation of maturity.[57] In 2008, Sanders and colleagues published a simplified method for evaluating skeletal maturity based on the key findings of the Tanner–Whitehouse method. Their method, which has been shown to be both rapid to use and reliable in predicting curve progression, depicts eight stages of skeletal maturity, ranging from stage 1: Juvenile slow to stage 8: Mature. The rapid phases of adolescent growth (stages 3 and 4 in their method) are differentiated by the closure of the distal phalangeal physes. The method has good intra- and inter-user reliability and is easy to use once the evaluator has become familiar with it. In our institution, a chart demonstrating the different stage descriptions and radiographic appearance of skeletal markers of growth is used at points of care to determine the approximate stage of a patient's growth and to counsel the patient and family (**Fig. 5.18**).

## Additional Imaging Findings

Many "incidental" findings on radiographs made to evaluate scoliosis, beyond routine measurements and the evaluation of predictive areas, may be of interest in the care of the patient. For example, careful documentation of the number of rib-bearing vertebral bodies (i.e., thoracic character plus any cervical ribs), as well as of the number of bodies of lumbar character, is important for accurate preoperative planning. This includes description of asymmetric vertebral levels (i.e., lumbar on one side and sacral on the other, or thoracic rib-bearing on one side and lumbar transverse process-bearing on the other). These Hox (homeobox)-gene variations may also eventually be important for forensic identification should the need arise in a disaster. Information seems to be accumulating that the presence of other than 12 rib pairs may imply a greater risk of malignancy of other systems,[59] although use of such information may currently be counterproductive. Other findings on imaging studies may move the diagnosis away from idiopathic scoliosis, such as the fusion of vertical laminae as a sign of diastematomyelia, ribbon ribs as a sign of neurofibromatosis, or repeated pneumonia in familial dysautonomia (Riley–Day syndrome). Indeed, an important part of the radiologist's role in imaging scoliosis is the elucidation of "other" findings beyond those made in standard evaluations, which additionally include renal, cardiothoracic, gastrointestinal,

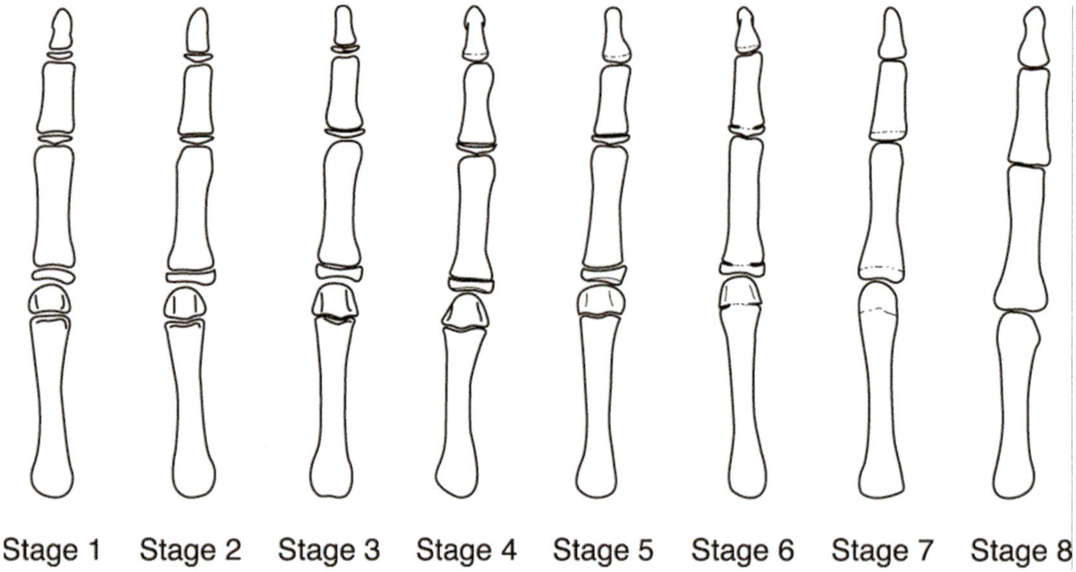


**Fig. 5.18** The Sanders classification system of skeletal maturity. Stage 1: Juvenile slow [G/P F 8–9 M 12.5]. Stage 2: Preadolescent slow (Tanner 2) [G/P F 10 M 13 ]. Stage 3: Adolescent rapid-early (Tanner 2–3, Risser grade 0, TRC open), Peak height velocity [G/P F 11–12 M 13.5–14 ]. Stage 4: Adolescent rapid-late (Tanner 3, Risser grade 0, TRC open) [G/P F 13 M 15 ]. Stage 5: Adolescent steady-early (Risser grade 0, TRC closed) [G/P F 13.5 M 15.5 ]. Stage 6: Adolescent steady-late (Risser grade >0) [G/P F 14 M 16 ]. Stage 7: Early mature [G/P F 15 M 17 ].

and even musculoskeletal abnormalities. The radiologist should also and in a most timely fashion recognize any potentially significant intraoperative or postoperative complications and inform the surgeon about them.[14,15]

## Conclusion

The complete diagnostic evaluation of the adolescent with scoliosis combines the patient's history and physical examinations with the psychosocial evaluation of the patient (including the patient's own perception of predicted progression of a spinal curve and the potential downside of treatment) and diagnostic imaging. Although giant strides in the understanding of scoliosis are anticipated in the near future through molecular genetic techniques, this information is not yet available. Continued utmost attention to the physical examination remains paramount for the proper care of patients with scoliosis. "It is important to remember that the pathology of a disease is always looking at you"; the ability to recognize it is what is important for the patient. It is our intent that a knowledge of the information presented in this chapter will equip the reader to better recognize obvious, as well as subtle, radiographic pathologies associated with adolescent idiopathic scoliosis

Through this chapter we have made an effort to identify obvious as well as subtle nuances presenting in children with scoliosis, to assist the reader in recognizing otherwise unknown causes of "idiopathic" spinal deformity. This information will aid in determining the appropriate management of a child's deformity. We wish to stress that any radiation involved in the diagnosis and follow-up of scoliosis must be balanced against the value to the patient of the information thus gained. Whenever possible, the ALARA concept should be used and unnecessary imaging should be avoided. Understanding the principles of the information that the spinal surgeon requires, and of how the surgeon can assist in the tailoring of imaging to those requirements, will help achieve this goal. Measurement methodology should be consistent and reproducible, and help convey standardized communication with other healthcare professionals.

### References

1. Ramirez N, Johnston CE, Browne RH. The prevalence of back pain in children who have idiopathic scoliosis. J Bone Joint Surg Am 1997; 79:364–368
2. Soucacos PN, Zacharis K, Gelalis J, et al. Assessment of curve progression in idiopathic scoliosis. Eur Spine J 1998;7:270–277
3. Sanders JO, Browne RH, McConnell SJ, Margraf SA, Cooney TE, Finegold DN. Maturity assessment and curve progression in girls with idiopathic scoliosis. J Bone Joint Surg Am 2007;89:64–73
4. Tanner JM. Growth and endocrinology of the adolescent. In: Gardner L, ed. Endocrine and Genetic Diseases in Childhood and Adolescence. Philadelphia: WB Saunders; 1975:14
5. Risser JC. The iliac apophysis: An invaluable sign in the management of scoliosis. Clin Orthop Relat Res 1958;11:111–119
6. Zadeh HG, Sakka SA, Powell MP, Mehta MH. Absent superficial abdominal reflexes in children with scoliosis. An early indicator of syringomyelia. J Bone Joint Surg Br 1995;77:762–767

7. Goldberg CJ, Dowling FE, Fogarty EE, Moore DP. School scoliosis screening and the United States Preventive Services Task Force. An examination of long-term results. Spine 1995; 20:1368–1374
8. Grivas TB, Samelis P, Polyzois BD, Giourelis B, Polyzois D. School screening in the heavily industrialized area: Is there any role of industrial environmental factors in idiopathic scoliosis prevalence? Stud Health Technol Inform 2002;91:76–80
9. Pruijs JE, van der Meer R, Hageman MA, Keessen W, van Wieringen JC. The benefits of school screening for scoliosis in the central part of The Netherlands. Eur Spine J 1996;5:374–379
10. Gaines RW. Clinical evaluation of the patient with a spinal deformity (scoliosis, kyphosis). In: DeWald RL, ed. Spinal Deformities: The Comprehensive Text. New York: Thieme; 2003
11. Harrop JS, Birknes J, Shaffrey CI. Noninvasive measurement and screening techniques for spinal deformities. Neurosurgery 2008; 63(3 suppl):46–53
12. Murrell GA, Coonrad RW, Moorman CT III, Fitch RD. An assessment of the reliability of the scoliometer. Spine 1993; 18:709–712
13. Bunch WH, Chapman RG. Patient preferences in surgery for scoliosis. J Bone Joint Surg Am 1985;67:794–799
14. Oestreich AE, Young LW, Young Poussaint T. Scoliosis circa 2000: Radiologic imaging perspective. I. Diagnosis and pretreatment evaluation. Skeletal Radiol 1998;27:591–605
15. Oestreich AE, Young LW, Poussaint TY. Scoliosis circa 2000: Radiologic imaging perspective. II. Treatment and follow-up. Skeletal Radiol 1998;27:651–656
16. Grivas TB, Dangas S, Polyzois BD, Samelis P. The double rib contour sign (DRCS) in lateral spinal radiographs: Aetiologic implications for scoliosis. Stud Health Technol Inform 2002;88:38–43
17. Marks M, Stanford C, Newton P. Which lateral radiographic positioning technique provides the most reliable and functional representation of a patient's sagittal balance? Spine 2009;34: 949–954
18. Letko L. The role of stagnara (true lateral, plan d'election) x-rays in the evaluation of the sagittal profile preoperatively in AIS. Abstract 317726, Poster 587. International Meeting on Advanced Spine Techniques, Paradise Island, Bahamas, 2007
19. Luk KD, Cheung KM, Lu DS, Leong JC. Assessment of scoliosis correction in relation to flexibility using the fulcrum bending correction index. Spine 1998;23:2303–2307
20. Little JP, Adam CJ. The effect of soft tissue properties on spinal flexibility in scoliosis: biomechanical simulation of fulcrum bending. Spine 2009;34:E76–E82
21. Vedantam R, Lenke LG, Bridwell KH, Linville DL. Comparison of push-prone and lateral-bending radiographs for predicting postoperative coronal alignment in thoracolumbar and lumbar scoliotic curves. Spine 2000;25:76–81
22. Polly DW Jr, Sturm PF. Traction versus supine side bending. Which technique best determines curve flexibility? Spine 1998;23:804–808
23. Vaughan JJ, Winter RB, Lonstein JE. Comparison of the use of supine bending and traction radiographs in the selection of the fusion area in adolescent idiopathic scoliosis. Spine 1996;21: 2469–2473
24. Davis BJ, Gadgil A, Trivedi J, Ahmed NB. Traction radiography performed under general anesthetic: a new technique for assessing idiopathic scoliosis curves. Spine 2004;29:2466–2470
25. Hoffman DA, Lonstein JE, Morin MM, Visscher W, Harris BS III, Boice JD Jr. Breast cancer in women with scoliosis exposed to multiple diagnostic X-rays. J Natl Cancer Inst 1989;81:1307–1312
26. Morin Doody M, Lonstein JE, Stovall M, Hacker DG, Luckyanov N, Land CE. Breast cancer mortality after diagnostic radiography: Findings from the U.S. Scoliosis Cohort Study. Spine 2000;25:2052–2063
27. Ron E, Lubin JH, Shore RE, et al. Thyroid cancer after exposure to external radiation: A pooled analysis of seven studies. Radiat Res 1995;141:259–277
28. Willis CE, Slovis TL. The ALARA concept in pediatric CR and DR: dose reduction in pediatric radiographic exams: A white paper conference. Am J Roentgenol 2005;184:373–374
29. De Smet AA, Fritz SL, Asher MA. A method for minimizing the radiation exposure from scoliosis radiographs. J Bone Joint Surg Am 1981;63:156–161
30. Boice JD Jr, Land CE, Shore RE, Norman JE, Tokunaga M. Risk of breast cancer following low-dose radiation exposure. Radiology 1979;131:589–597
31. Zmurko MG, Mooney JF III, Podeszwa DA, Minster GJ, Mendelow MJ, Guirgues A. Inter- and intraobserver variance of Cobb angle measurements with digital radiographs. J Surg Orthop Adv 2003; 12:208–213
32. Kluba T, Schäfer J, Hahnfeldt T, Niemeyer T. Prospective randomized comparison of radiation exposure from full spine radiographs obtained in three different techniques. Eur Spine J 2006; 15:752–756
33. Dubousset J, Charpak G, Skalli W, de Guise J, Kalifa G, Wicart P. [Skeletal and spinal imaging with EOS system]. Arch Pediatr 2008;15:665–666
34. Kadoury S, Cheriet F, Beauséjour M, Stokes IA, Parent S, Labelle H. A three-dimensional retrospective analysis of the evolution of spinal instrumentation for the correction of adolescent idiopathic scoliosis. Eur Spine J 2009;18:23–37
35. Cheng JC, Guo X, Sher AH, Chan YL, Metreweli C. Correlation between curve severity, somatosensory evoked potentials, and magnetic resonance imaging in adolescent idiopathic scoliosis. Spine 1999;24:1679–1684
36. Sun X, Qiu Y, Zhu Z, et al. Variations of the position of the cerebellar tonsil in idiopathic scoliotic adolescents with a Cobb angle >40 degrees: A magnetic resonance imaging study. Spine 2007; 32:1680–1686
37. Chu WC, Man GC, Lam WW, et al. A detailed morphologic and functional magnetic resonance imaging study of the craniocervical junction in adolescent idiopathic scoliosis. Spine 2007;32:1667–1674
38. Schwend RM, Hennrikus W, Hall JE, Emans JB. Childhood scoliosis: Clinical indications for magnetic resonance imaging. J Bone Joint Surg Am 1995;77:46–53
39. Ouellet JA, LaPlaza J, Erickson MA, Birch JG, Burke S, Browne R. Sagittal plane deformity in the thoracic spine: A clue to the presence of syringomyelia as a cause of scoliosis. Spine 2003;28:2147–2151
40. Inoue M, Minami S, Nakata Y, et al. Preoperative MRI analysis of patients with idiopathic scoliosis: A prospective study. Spine 2005;30:108–114
41. Benli IT, Uzümcügil O, Aydin E, Ateş B, Gürses L, Hekimoğlu B. Magnetic resonance imaging abnormalities of neural axis in Lenke type 1 idiopathic scoliosis. Spine 2006;31:1828–1833
42. Bhave G, Lewis JB, Chang SS. Association of gadolinium based magnetic resonance imaging contrast agents and nephrogenic systemic fibrosis. J Urol 2008;180:830–835, discussion 835
43. Riccio AI, Guille JT, Grissom L, Figueroa TE. Magnetic resonance imaging of renal abnormalities in patients with congenital osseous anomalies of the spine. J Bone Joint Surg Am 2007;89:2456–2459

44. Antonacci MD, Cahill P, Nydick J, et al. Cervical sagittal plane decompensation after pediatric AIS surgery. Paper presented at: North American Spine Society Annual Meeting. Toronto, Canada, 2008
45. Nash CL Jr, Moe JH. A study of vertebral rotation. J Bone Joint Surg Am 1969;51:223–229
46. Drerup B. Principles of measurement of vertebral rotation from frontal projections of the pedicles. J Biomech 1984;17:923–935
47. Kuklo TR, Potter BK, Lenke LG. Vertebral rotation and thoracic torsion in adolescent idiopathic scoliosis: What is the best radiographic correlate? J Spinal Disord Tech 2005;18:139–147
48. Lam GC, Hill DL, Le LH, Raso JV, Lou EH. Vertebral rotation measurement: A summary and comparison of common radiographic and CT methods. Scoliosis 2008;3:16
49. Aaro S, Dahlborn M. Estimation of vertebral rotation and the spinal and rib cage deformity in scoliosis by computer tomography. Spine 1981;6:460–467
50. Asghar J, Samdani AF, Pahys JM, et al; Harms Study Group. Computed tomography evaluation of rotation correction in adolescent idiopathic scoliosis: A comparison of an all pedicle screw construct versus a hook-rod system. Spine 2009;34:804–807
51. Lenke LG, Betz RR, Clements D, et al. Curve prevalence of a new classification of operative adolescent idiopathic scoliosis: Does classification correlate with treatment? Spine 2002;27:604–611
52. Little DG, Song KM, Katz D, Herring JA. Relationship of peak height velocity to other maturity indicators in idiopathic scoliosis in girls. J Bone Joint Surg Am 2000;82:685–693
53. Karol LA, Johnston CE II, Browne RH, Madison M. Progression of the curve in boys who have idiopathic scoliosis. J Bone Joint Surg Am 1993;75:1804–1810
54. Charles YP, Diméglio A, Canavese F, Daures JP. Skeletal age assessment from the olecranon for idiopathic scoliosis at Risser grade 0. J Bone Joint Surg Am 2007;89:2737–2744
55. Sanders JO, Little DG, Richards BS. Prediction of the crankshaft phenomenon by peak height velocity. Spine 1997;22:1352–1356, discussion 1356–1357
56. Greulich WW, Pyle SI. Radiographic Atlas of Skeletal Development of the Hand and Wrist, ed 2. Stanford, CA: Stanford University Press; 1959
57. Sanders JO. Maturity indicators in spinal deformity. J Bone Joint Surg Am 2007;89(suppl 1):14–20
58. Sanders JO, Khoury JG, Kishan S, et al. Predicting scoliosis progression from skeletal maturity: A simplified classification during adolescence. J Bone Joint Surg Am 2008;90:540–553
59. Loder RT, Huffman G, Toney E, Wurtz LD, Fallon R. Abnormal rib number in childhood malignancy: Implications for the scoliosis surgeon. Spine 2007;32:904–910

# 6 The Importance of the Sagittal Plane: Spinopelvic Considerations

*Frank Schwab, Virginie Lafage, Ashish Patel, and Michael F. O'Brien*

Analysis of the sagittal plane in the setting of spinal deformity is a rather modern concept. However, the last two decades have seen a substantial contribution to the understanding of the sagittal plane in terms of self-reported patient function, outcomes of treatment, and complications following surgery for spinal deformity.

A critical point of departure in discussing sagittal plane alignment relates to the need for including more than the spine in this topic. A study of spinal alignment during standing is not complete without understanding the importance of the pelvis, which has emerged as a key regulator of global balance, predominantly in the sagittal plane, between the spine proximally and the lower extremities distally. Whether in patients in good health or in the setting of spinal deformity, spinal balance and alignment are intimately intertwined with the pelvis. The importance of this concept has led Jean Dubousset[1] to coin the term *pelvic vertebra*. This chapter, related to spinal deformity, will expand the concept of sagittal-plane alignment to extend beyond the spine by using the term *spinopelvic* alignment.

To gain an understanding of the sagittal spinopelvic alignment and how it may relate to patients with spinal deformity, an appreciation for the normal spinopelvic axis must be pursued. Initial investigations have outlined the nature of the sagittal spinal alignment in the standing position and its interrelationship with the pelvis. Additionally, reports on the progressive modifications that occur in spinal alignment during growth have increased our knowledge of skeletal adaptation in the pediatric population. In the adult population the negative impact of spinal malalignment in the sagittal plane and spinopelvic mismatch offers critically important explanations of disabilities, poor outcomes, and failures in the treatment of spinal disorders.

## Sagittal Spinopelvic Parameters

Historically, scoliotic deformities were evaluated and treated primarily as coronal-plane entities, although appreciation of the three-dimensional nature of scoliosis is increasing, most specifically in the sagittal plane. Additionally, recognition that the spinal axis is only the proximal link in the entire global chain of mechanical alignment of the human standing posture has led to significant work directed toward understanding the role of the pelvis in this alignment and how it relates to global sagittal standing balance. Further research is needed to define the axial-plane component of standing alignment and optimal, patient specific, three-dimensional spinopelvic alignment, although this section of the present chapter is aimed at providing an outline of the important sagittal spinopelvic parameters appreciated to date and the observations made during investigations of the asymptomatic "normal" population.

### Sagittal Spinal Parameters

It can be understood without great intuition that the spine in the sagittal plane differs vastly from the "straight spine" in the coronal plane. The sagittal spine includes four curvatures, two "kyphotic" primary curves at the levels of the thoracic and sacral spine, respectively, and two secondary "lordotic" curvatures at the respective levels of the cervical and lumbar spine. Although specific regions of the spine may be labeled as kyphotic or lordotic, variability exists as to the nature of alignment at the individual vertebral levels, most notably at the junctional levels between regional curvatures.[2]

Radiographic analysis of the standing sagittal alignment in the asymptomatic population has demonstrated a broad range of normal values of thoracic kyphosis and lumbar lordosis. These values are listed in **Table 6.1** and provide a basic guideline of normal ranges and what would be considered abnormal. Additionally, reports suggest that sagittal spinal curvatures and alignment vary with age. Cil et al[3] conducted a radiographic analysis of the sagittal alignment of 151 asymptomatic children grouped by age (age range: 3 to 15 years). Significant differences in numerous parameters were identified among age groups. Older children stood with a more negative (backward) sagittal vertical axis (SVA). With an increased (positive) SVA in younger children, there is a greater L1 offset and more distal thoracic apex, resulting in a forward-leaning posture. With growth, the regional curvatures of both thoracic kyphosis (TK) and lumbar lordosis (LL) increase in angulation; the thoracic apex moves upward. As observed by Voutsinas and

**Table 6.1 Normative Distribution of Thoracic Kyphosis and Lumbar Lordosis among Children[3] and Adult[6] Populations**

| | Cil[3] Group I | Cil[3] Group II | Cil[3] Group III | Cil[3] Group IV | Jackson[29] |
|---|---|---|---|---|---|
| **No. of Subjects** | 51 | 37 | 32 | 31 | 100 |
| **Age (yr)** | 3–6 | 7–9 | 10–12 | 13–15 | 20 to 63 |
| **Kyphosis (degrees)** | 44.9 ± 11.4 | 47.8 ± 10.5 | 45.8 ± 10.6 | 53.3 ± 9.1 | 42.1 ± 8.9 |
| **Lordosis (degrees)** | − 11.0 | − 51.7 ± 11.5 | − 57.3 ± 10.0 | − 54.6 ± 9.8 | − 60.9 ± 12 |

colleagues,[4] and more recently by Mac-Thiong et al,[5] TK and LL tend to increase during childhood, although a longitudinal study of normal subjects is required to fully validate these observations (**Table 6.1**).

## Sacropelvic Parameters

Since the work published by Legaye and Duval–Beaupére and coworkers,[6] several studies[5,7–12] have emphasized the importance of pelvic morphology with regard to sagittal alignment during standing in both children and adults, particularly through its effect on LL. Three main parameters are utilized to define the morphology and positional characteristics of the pelvis.[6]

### Pelvic Incidence

Pelvic incidence (PI) is a morphological parameter described as the angulation joining the bicoxofemoral axis to the midsacral endplate and the perpendicular. PI has been suggested to remain set during adulthood, with a wide range of what are considered normal curves (40 to 65 degrees), although changes in PI during growth have been reported by several authors. Mangione and colleagues[13] demonstrated that PI tends to undergo a linear increase during childhood after the initiation of walking. Descamps et al[14] suggested that PI is relatively stable before the age of 10 years and then increases significantly until reaching its maximum at skeletal maturity. More recently Mac-Thiong et al[5] in a prospective radiographic study including 180 asymptomatic children, found a significant positive correlation between age and PI. They hypothesized that an increasing PI during childhood was a necessary mechanism for maintaining an adequate sagittal alignment during growth.

### Sacral Slope and Pelvic Tilt

Sacral slope (SS) and pelvic tilt (PT) are positional pelvic parameters that remain variable with changes in alignment, position, and posture. Significant variation has reported in the normative values of these parameters for adults (SS: 30 to 50 degrees, PT: 10 to 25 degrees). During adulthood, when PI remains stable, changes in one of these parameters negatively affects the other, such that $PI = SS + PT$. SS, the angulation of the sacral endplate with the horizontal, carries the strongest correlation with lumbar lordosis. A vertical SS is typically met with a large lordotic angulation, whereas the reverse holds true for lower values of SS. It has also been demonstrated that SS remains constant with growth, whereby SS through childhood does not differ significantly from that in childhood for a given individual.[5] Conversely, PT describes the position (rotation) of the pelvis centered on the hip joint. PT has been found to increase during childhood with increases in PI.[5] Positive changes in global spinal alignment typically lead to compensatory changes in PT; As the spine moves forward, increasing the SVA, PT increases (undergoes retroversion) to maintain ergonomic posture with spinal alignment over the pelvis.

Lafage et al[15] conducted a recent investigation of pelvic parameters and their impact on measures of health-related quality of life (HRQOL). This prospective study involved 125 adult patients (mean age: 57 years) who had spinal deformities. Full-length radiographs of patients in the free-standing position, and including the spine and pelvis, were available for all patients. Instruments for measuring HRQOL included Oswestry disability index (ODI), Health Outcome Short Form-12 (SF-12), and the Scoliosis Research Society (SRS-22) questionnaire. A correlation analysis of radiographic spinopelvic parameters with measures of HRQOL did not reveal any significant associations pertaining to coronal-plane parameters. However. significant sagittal-plane correlations were identified. Following SVA and truncal inclination, PT was the next most highly correlated parameter with patient-reported measures of HRQOL ($0.28 < r < 0.42$) (**Fig. 6.1**).

## Sagittal Spinopelvic Interaction during Standing Balance: An Introduction to Force-plate Technology and the Gravity Line

Ergonomical standing balance is the guiding principle explaining resilient compensatory mechanisms in the setting of spinal malalignment. Dubousset[1] outlined this principle in the term *cone of economy* (COE). As it was originally represented, the COE indicates that in the setting of standing balance, increased displacement of the upper body in relation to the feet requires increased effort until the displacement is so excessive that external support is necessary to prevent falling. This concept implies that any prolonged displacement of the center of gravity beyond an

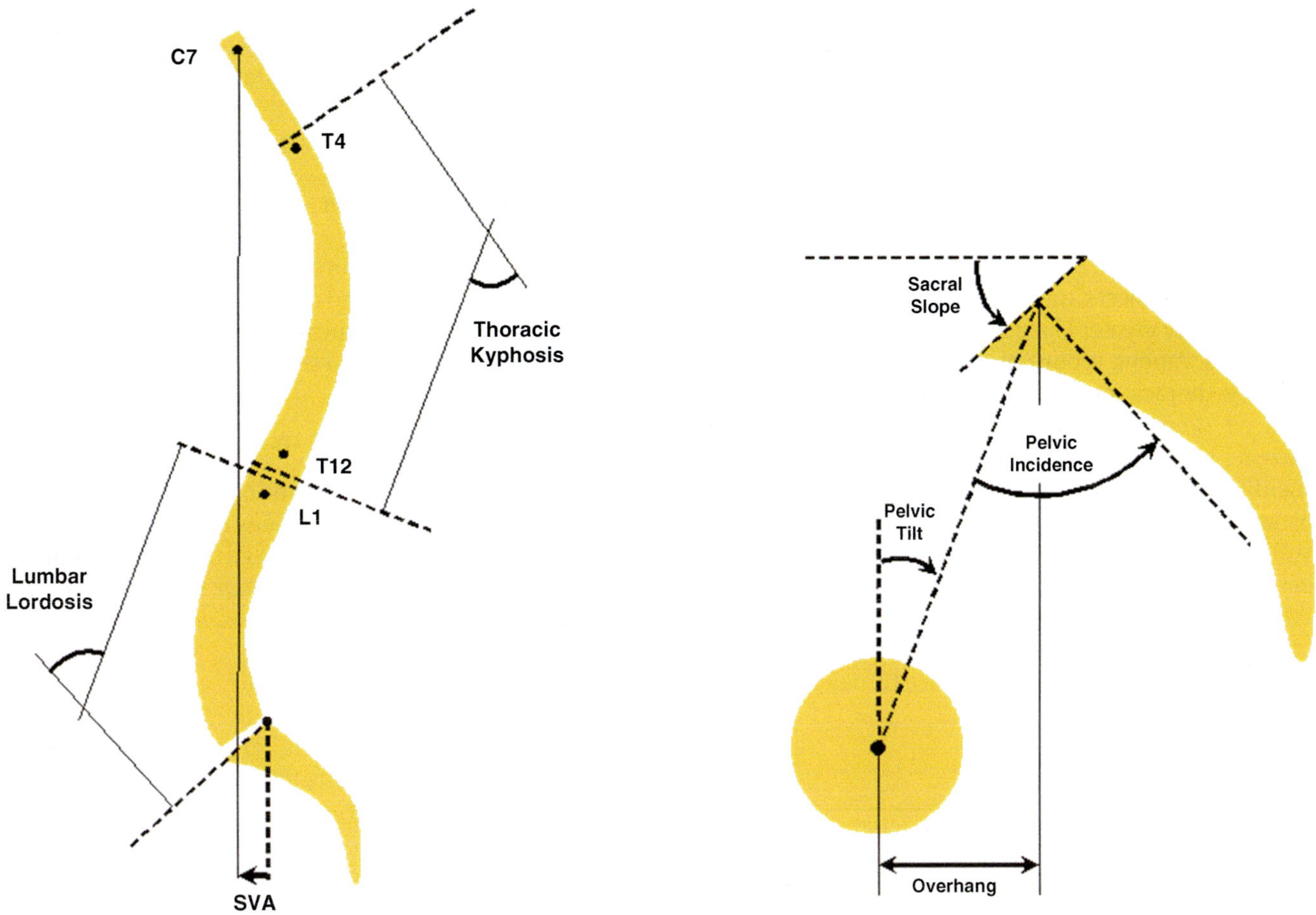


**Fig. 6.1** Key sagittal spinal, pelvic, and spinopelvic parameters in radiographic evaluation.

ideal point between the standing feet of an individual requires muscular effort, and therefore energy expenditure, and can eventually lead to fatigue and discomfort or pain. In the setting of spinal deformity, the concept of COE can explain observed disability when other obvious sources of pain (e.g., fracture, infection, focal instability, disc extrusion, etc.) have been excluded.

Several studies using force-plate technology have been conducted in an effort to quantify the concept of COE.[10,16,17] The force plate is a flat rectangular pad containing pressure sensors distributed evenly acros its surface, upon which a subject stands. From captured pressure measurements below both feet, the center of all pressures (COP) can be calculated. The COP represents the true gravity line (GL) of a given individual. Static force-plate analysis allows simultaneous determination of the GL and acquisition of radiographic data such that the offsets between the feet, pelvis, and spine can be precisely calculated.

An analysis of force-plate data in the asymptomatic population has shown that the GL travels in a very narrow ellipse centered between the feet of a standing individual.[10] Accordingly, it may be more precise to label optimal standing balance as occurring within an ellipse of economy (EOE). The dimensions of this ellipse are ~14 × 22 mm, and are generally located 11 cm anterior to the posterior border of the heels. Of significant interest is that the EOE is maintained within the same narrow range of offset from the heels in both asymptomatic subjects and those with a significant positive SVA. This is an essential concept because it demonstrates that dramatic shifts in spinopelvic alignment necessitate a driving effort (muscular) to maintain the GL within a narrow perimeter (the EOE).

## Sagittal Spinopelvic Alignment and Curve Type in Adolescent Idiopathic Scoliosis

Investigations directed at asymptomatic populations and the establishment of normal sagittal spinopelvic alignment permit interesting interpretations of the modifications observed among patients with adolescent idiopathic scoliosis (AIS). Mac-Thiong et al[18] investigated the possible relationship of

AIS curve types with sagittal spinopelvic parameters in a cohort of 160 patients. They found a significant reduction in TK in the primary thoracic curve of the spine as compared with the primary lumbar curves, and greater LL in patients with lumbar curves. No pelvic parameters were related to the type of deformity in this population. Similarly, Upasani and coworkers,[19] in a matched retrospective radiographic review, identified several sagittal spinopelvic differences between scoliotic groups and normal controls. In comparing normal and scoliotic subjects, they found that scoliotic patients have a significantly greater PI regardless of the type of their scoliotic curve. Among groups of scoliotic patients, those with primary thoracic curves (Lenke type 1a or 1b) exhibited reduced thoracic and thoracolumbar kyphoses, whereas patients with thoracolumbar curves (Lenke type 5) had a significantly larger thoracolumbar kyphosis. Sacropelvic parameters were not found to have a significant influence on scoliotic curve type, although interestingly, the relationship between sacropelvic parameters and degree of lordosis was maintained throughout the three groups, although, interestingly, the relationship between sacropelvic parameters (PI) and degree of lordosis was maintained throughout the three groups.

## Spinopelvic Considerations Drawn from Adult Patients

Much of the current understanding of the importance of pelvic parameters and compensatory mechanisms in the setting of spinal deformity is based on investigations conducted with adults. In the pediatric population, significant changes in spinal malalignment may be well tolerated because of a large compensatory reserve drawing from flexible spinal units and maintenance of muscle quality and quantity. However, it is evident that age-related changes have a marked effect on the ability to tolerate spinal deformity. Through the aging process, the ability to compensate for any malalignment becomes progressively reduced. The loss of ability to tolerate deformity is principally related to changes in soft tissues, comprising the intervertebral discs, ligaments, bone, and muscle. In the adult patient, degenerative changes with aging result in stiffening of spinal segments, loss of disc height, a global positive translation of the SVA, loss of hip hyperextension, and a general reduction of muscle mass and tone.

The effects of both spinal deformation and soft-tissue aging compound the problems of alignment related to scoliosis. This has the following profound effects on the ergonomical considerations of standing balance:

- Decreased capacity for compensatory spinal curvature in the setting of scoliosis
- Increasing recruitment of muscles that function less effectively with aging
- Pelvic retroversion and translation to offset sagittal imbalance
- Eventual exhaustion of hip extension to compensate for malalignment
- Need to enter knee flexion

Thus, an adolescent deformity in the spine may be well tolerated until stabilizing and compensatory mechanisms are overwhelmed. The full clinical impact of spinal deformity may become apparent only in adulthood.

### Sagittal Malalignment in the Adult

A wide variety of factors should be considered with disability in the setting of adult spinal deformity, although an important consideration is that of sagittal-plane alignment. This has been substantiated through work on the Adult Spinal Deformity Classification[20–22] as well as by Glassman and colleagues.[23,24]

Sagittal plane deformity in the adult, resulting in disability, is a global sagittal alignment issue. Although children can easily compensate for marked scoliosis and extensive spinal fusion, adults lose the reserve of compensatory mechanisms over time. This implies an increasing dependency on muscular endurance and strength. In return, such increased muscular effort to maintain standing balance and daily function translates into fatigue and disability. The problem of global sagittal alignment in the setting of adolescent idiopathic scoliosis in the adult (AISA) is most notably increased in the surgicaly treated patient in whom a sagittal alignment has been imposed through fusion. In some cases the problems of alignment become aggravated over time, particularly with the collapse of discs below a long fusion and loss of muscle tone and hip extension ability. Common names given to severe malalignment syndromes include flat back, flat buttock, kyphotic decompensation syndrome, and fixed sagittal imbalance.

The critical loss of compensatory mechanisms in AISA relate primarily to the lumbar spine and pelvis. Specifically, loss of LL and the increased stiffness seen with aging limit the ability to tolerate more proximal deformity in the sagittal plane. Pelvic retroversion occurs naturally with aging,[10] although its extent may be limited to permit rebalancing of the body in the setting of spinal deformity. In conjunction with this, hip motion must be able to accommodate pelvic position. The latter implies a progressive extension of the hip as the pelvis retroverts. This mechanism has limits and with aging the maximal extension possible becomes progressively reduced. When hip extension is no longer feasible, knee and ankle flexion become necessary to permit a balanced standing posture.

## Force-plate Investigations in the Adult Population

The observation of an EOE with a narrow relationship to the feet for both patients with deformity and volunteers makes it evident that spinal deformity requires recruitment of balancing (compensatory) mechanisms. This has been investigated through a follow-up force-plate study[25] of patients grouped by differences in radiographic sagittal alignment into the three groups of forward (SVA >5 cm), neutral (0 to 5 cm), and posterior (SVA <0 cm) alignment. As mentioned above, the GL offset from the heels did not differ among these groups, although significant differences were demonstrated in PI, PT, and pelvic position. PI was found to increase significantly with increasing SVA, from 48 degrees for the sagittal backward group to 52 degrees for the neutral group and to 56 degrees for the sagittal forward group. Similarly, PT was found to increase significantly with increasing SVA, from 10 degrees for the sagittal backward group to 16 degrees for the neutral group and to 21 degrees in the sagittal forward group (all $P < 0.001$). Analysis of the pelvic-location offset with regard to the projected heel line and GL demonstrated that when SVA increased, the pelvis translated posteriorly toward the heels. The combination of the pelvic shift and pelvic retroversion resulted in a decrease in the heel-to-S1 offset from 115 mm to 90 mm and to 56 mm for the sagittal backward, neutral, and sagittal forward groups, respectively (total translation = −58 mm). These important findings confirm the critical role of the pelvis in maintaining sagittal balance of the spinopelvic axis.

The implications of the findings stemming from studies of the spinopelvic axis are substantial. An optimal outcome of management of spinal deformity, whether in the pediatric or adult patient, must include an analysis of the pelvic parameters and the global spinopelvic alignment.

# Surgical Management in Adolescent Idiopathic Scoliosis

Scoliosis is a three-dimensional deformity of the spine,[1] which explains the limitations of its analysis in any one plane alone. With the advent of three-dimensional (3D) imaging techniques, more accurate evaluations of spinal deformity will be possible. Currently, it should be noted that even sagittal measurements on radiographs correspond to the lateral appearance of the spine but not to the true sagittal plane (which may be in an orientation not captured on a standing lateral radiograph).

Evaluation of the spinopelvic alignment should, at the minimum, begin with the review of full-length standing coronal and sagittal radiographs. Patients should be instructed to adopt a free-standing position with the hips and knees in a comfortable posture and the shoulders and elbows flexed, with the fingertips placed on the clavicles. This position minimizes changes in sagittal spinal contour and eliminates compensatory postures.[26] The spine should be visible proximally to C2, and the femoral heads must be visualized distally. It is of paramount importance that the pelvis (femoral heads) and proximal spine be visualized on the same film; the spinopelvic alignment, the spatial relationship between the head and the lower extremities, cues the physician about the global alignment adopted by the patient, including compensatory mechanisms for standing freely.

## Sagittal Considerations in the Treatment of Adolescent Idiopathic Scoliosis

In an investigation of the[27] long-term effects of Harrington rod fusion, Cochran et al, using full length radiographs and outcomes questionnaires, evaluated 95 AIS patients with a mean 9-year follow-up. Examination of the sagittal plane of patients with fusions extending to L4 and L5 revealed a mean 15.2 degrees of lordosis, showing that the distraction instrumentation resulted in a loss of physiological lordosis. More than 50% of the patients showed significant instability, radiographic changes below the level of fusion, and lower back pain.

Luk and colleagues[28] conducted an investigation into the effects of unfused lumbar mobile segments below a Harrington construct for scoliosis. They observed an increase in segmental lordosis at the unfused levels in an attempt to reachieve preoperative lumbar lordosis angulations (L1–S1) Similarly, arecent study published by Tanguay and co-workers[29] found that the relationship between pelvic parameters and lumbar curves was maintained after correction and fusion in AIS with modification of the alignment of the unfused lumbar segments. An increase in LL below the fusion site was noted, but no correlation was found between PI and fused lordosis. This study suggests that PI should be the basis of any surgical planning for AIS. An important goal of intervention for AIS should be to maintain the relationship between PI and LL so as to eliminate the need for compensatory modifications below a fusion.

The corrective surgical techniques in the setting of AIS have evolved over time with increasing understanding of the deformity in this condition, and of major important is that instrumentation systems with augmented anchorage have been developed for treating it. It is evident that the improved power of newer techniques will not only permit greater correction of certain parameters of deformity but will also have a more substantial effect on the nonfused segments of the spine. The secondary effects of arthrodesis include:

- Loss of mobility
- An imposed alignment through instrumentation
- Creation of stress risers at junctional levels

- Indirect correction of compensatory curves
- Increased demands on the muscular system as well as muscular denervation
- Modifications in pelvic position

Thus, given the considerations of optimal alignment and the power of current instrumentation systems for treating AIS, significant attention should be directed at establishing harmonious sagittal spinopelvic alignment. Failure to do so is likely to lead to long-term complications. However, ideal alignment in an adolescent is difficult to define given that spinopelvic parameters evolve during growth. It is thus uncertain whether the goal for alignment should be an age-matched one or one of a young adult (as opposed to an older adult). Finally, treating AIS so as to create sagittal alignment of an adult requires anticipation of a given patient's final spinopelvic alignment once growth is completed. The disproportionate consideration of the coronal plane (Cobb angle), and correcting malalignment in this plane for quantifiable proof of operative success, unfortunately minimizes the issues relating to the sagittal plane in AIS, which is the most important plane for long-term success in treating this condition.

## Conclusion

The spinal column performs several critical functions in the human body. As a structure, the spine is frequently defined by the vertebrae, discs, and surrounding soft tissues. It is evident, however, that when one considers the role of the spine in terms of balance and alignment, an isolated analysis of the spine is insufficient.

The goal of this chapter has been to introduce the important role of the sagittal spinopelvic axis in the setting of adolescent and adult idiopathic scoliosis, and to provide guidelines for sagittal treatment of the spine in the management of these conditions. Long-term success in the management of spinal deformity has been shown to depend primarily on effects in the sagittal plane, and most specifically on the spinopelvic relationship.

Early work on radiographic and force-plate analysis has increased the understanding of spinopelvic alignment in the setting of spinal deformity. Further research related to the effect of the axial-plane alignment in AIS, and the role of the lower extremities in alignment during standing, will improve the understanding of this complex three-dimensional disorder toward optimization of its treatment.

### References


1. Dubousset J. Three-dimensional analysis of the scoliotic deformity. In: Weinstein SL, ed. Pediatric Spine: Principles and Practice. New York: Raven Press; 1994
2. Roussouly P, Gollogly S, Berthonnaud E, Dimnet J. Classification of the normal variation in the sagittal alignment of the human lumbar spine and pelvis in the standing position. Spine 2005;30: 346–353
3. Cil A, Yazici M, Uzumcugil A, et al. The evolution of sagittal segmental alignment of the spine during childhood. Spine 2005;30: 93–100
4. Voutsinas SA, MacEwen GD. Sagittal profiles of the spine. Clin Orthop Relat Res 1986; (210):235–242
5. Mac-Thiong JM, Labelle H, Berthonnaud E, Betz RR, Roussouly P. Sagittal spinopelvic balance in normal children and adolescents. Eur Spine J 2007;16:227–234
6. Legaye J, Duval-Beaupére G, Hecquet J, Marty C. Pelvic incidence: A fundamental pelvic parameter for three-dimensional regulation of spinal sagittal curves. Eur Spine J 1998;7:99–103
7. Berthonnaud E, Dimnet J, Roussouly P, Labelle H. Analysis of the sagittal balance of the spine and pelvis using shape and orientation parameters. J Spinal Disord Tech 2005;18:40–47
8. Jackson RP, Hales C. Congruent spinopelvic alignment on standing lateral radiographs of adult volunteers. Spine 2000;25:2808–2815
9. Rajnics P, Templier A, Skalli W, Lavaste F, Illés T. The association of sagittal spinal and pelvic parameters in asymptomatic persons and patients with isthmic spondylolisthesis. J Spinal Disord Tech 2002;15:24–30
10. Schwab F, Lafage V, Boyce R, Skalli W, Farcy JP. Gravity line analysis in adult volunteers: Age-related correlation with spinal parameters, pelvic parameters, and foot position. Spine 2006;31:E959–E967
11. Vaz G, Roussouly P, Berthonnaud E, Dimnet J. Sagittal morphology and equilibrium of pelvis and spine. Eur Spine J 2002;11: 80–87
12. Mac-Thiong JM, Berthonnaud E, Dimar JR II, Betz RR, Labelle H. Sagittal alignment of the spine and pelvis during growth. Spine 2004;29:1642–1647
13. Mangione P, Gomez D, Senegas J. Study of the course of the incidence angle during growth. Eur Spine J 1997;6:163–167
14. Descamps H, Commare-Nordmann M, Marty C, et al. Modification of pelvic angle during the human growth. (in French) Biom Hum Anthropol 1999;17:59–63
15. Lafage V, Schwab F, Patel A, Hawkinson N, Farcy JP. Pelvic tilt and truncal inclination: Two key radiographic parameters in the setting of adults with spinal deformity. Spine 2009;34:E599–E606
16. El Fegoun AB, Schwab F, Gamez L, Champain N, Skalli W, Farcy JP. Center of gravity and radiographic posture analysis: A preliminary review of adult volunteers and adult patients affected by scoliosis. Spine 2005;30:1535–1540
17. Lafage V, Schwab F, Skalli W, et al. Standing balance and sagittal plane spinal deformity: Analysis of spinopelvic and gravity line parameters. Spine 2008;33:1572–1578
18. Mac-Thiong JM, Labelle H, Charlebois M, Huot MP, de Guise JA. Sagittal plane analysis of the spine and pelvis in adolescent idiopathic scoliosis according to the coronal curve type. Spine 2003;28:1404–1409

19. Upasani VV, Tis J, Bastrom T, et al. Analysis of sagittal alignment in thoracic and thoracolumbar curves in adolescent idiopathic scoliosis: How do these two curve types differ? Spine 2007;32:1355–1359
20. Schwab F, Farcy JP, Bridwell K, et al. A clinical impact classification of scoliosis in the adult. Spine 2006;31:2109–2114
21. Schwab F, Lafage V, Farcy JP, et al. Surgical rates and operative outcome analysis in thoracolumbar and lumbar major adult scoliosis: Application of the new adult deformity classification. Spine 2007;32(24):2723–2730
22. Schwab FJ, Lafage V, Farcy JP, Bridwell KH, Glassman S, Shainline MR. Predicting outcome and complications in the surgical treatment of adult scoliosis. Spine 2008;33:2243–2247
23. Glassman SD, Berven S, Bridwell K, Horton W, Dimar JR. Correlation of radiographic parameters and clinical symptoms in adult scoliosis. Spine 2005;30:682–688
24. Glassman SD, Bridwell K, Dimar JR, Horton W, Berven S, Schwab F. The impact of positive sagittal balance in adult spinal deformity. Spine 2005;30:2024–2029
25. Lafage V, Schwab F, Skalli W, et al. Standing balance and sagittal plane spinal deformity: Analysis of spinopelvic and gravity line parameters. Spine 2008;33:1572–1578
26. Horton WC, Brown CW, Bridwell KH, Glassman SD, Suk SI, Cha CW. Is there an optimal patient stance for obtaining a lateral 36″ radiograph? A critical comparison of three techniques. Spine 2005; 30:427–433
27. Cochran T, Irstam L, Nachemson A. Long-term anatomic and functional changes in patients with adolescent idiopathic scoliosis treated by Harrington rod fusion. Spine 2005;8:576–586
28. Luk KD, Lee FB, Leong JC, Hsu LC. The effect on the lumbosacral spine of long spinal fusion for idiopathic scoliosis. A minimum 10-year follow-up. Spine 1987;12:996–1000
29. Tanguay F, Mac-Thiong JM, de Guise JA, et al. Relation between the sagittal pelvic and lumbar spine geometries following surgical correction of adolescent idiopathic scoliosis. Eur Spine J 2007; April, 16(4):531–536

# 7 The Case for Bracing

*Suken A. Shah*

Perhaps no other issue in the management of scoliosis engenders as much debate and heated discussion as the topic of brace treatment. This chapter and the next present a dispassionate discourse on the two sides of this issue, based on the available scientific literature and the contributors' personal and institutional experience. The literature is confounded by the wide variety of brace designs, wearing schedules, and philosophies about the duration of treatment of scoliosis with braces. It seems that there are as many types of braces as there are ports-of-call in the world of sailing.

Another factor bound to add confusion and controversy to this subject is genetic testing. Indeed, nonoperative treatment of adolescent idiopathic scoliosis (AIS) may soon be guided by genetic analysis. Ogilvie et al[1] recently presented a paper demonstrating that the efficacy of brace treatment could be predicted by a genotype analysis of 30 genetic markers. Ninety-five percent of brace-compliant patients whose scoliosis progressed and required surgery had a calculated probability of progression of 0.35 or higher. Of those who had no progression, only 9% had a probability of progression of 0.35 or higher. The ability to predict brace failure increased to 100% when age and initial Cobb angle were included in the analysis.

The one thing about which the contributors to this chapter and Chapter 8 can agree is that there is a paucity of level-1 evidence to support or refute brace treatment for scoliosis. A large prospective, multicenter, randomized trial is required to resolve this issue. The trial should answer the fundamental question of whether the intent to treat with a brace is effective at decreasing curve progression and the need for surgery. Secondary outcome measures should answer questions about brace design, wearing schedules, and demographic factors predictive of successful treatment.

Fortunately, such a trial is underway. Led by Stuart Weinstein at the University of Iowa, a National Institutes of Health/National Institute of Arthritis and Musculoskeletal and Skin Disorders-funded multicenter trial is currently in the enrollment phase: 26 centers in the United States and Canada are participating. The study began enrolling patients in February 2007 and is expected to be completed in late 2010. The results of this trial should be the foundation of future recommendations for bracing in scoliosis.

## Introduction

The treatment of any condition should take into account the short- and long-term outcomes as well as the complications of that treatment modality. The three generally accepted treatment options for scoliosis are observation, use of a brace, and surgical stabilization. Others have proposed that treatment modalities such as electrical muscle stimulation, postural exercises, chiropractic manipulation, nutritional supplementation, and magnet therapy have a role in the care of scoliosis, but evidence to support these modalities is lacking. Valid scientific evidence does indicate that bracing and surgery alter the outcome of scoliosis as compared with observation alone; this chapter will focus on these nonoperative modalities of treatment for scoliosis.

## Screening

Early detection and school screening programs are widespread in North America. However, although these programs are mandated by many states and deeply rooted in tradition, recent studies have cast some controversy over their effectiveness. The objective of school screening is, ideally, to detect scoliosis in patients for whom brace treatment may alter the course of the disease at an early stage, rather than leave surgery as the only option.[2] A valid screening program must have a screening tool that is valid, cost-effective, ethical, and acceptable to the subjects, and which provides a diagnosis of a disease about which there exist knowledge and appropriate treatment interventions.[3]

Currently, knowledge about scoliosis seems to be well accepted. For example, curve progression is known to be most likely for skeletally immature girls (Risser grades 0 and 1) with curves measuring 30 degrees or more.[4] However, there is a paucity of data about small curves, including their progression potential and at what degree they constitute a serious health problem. The screening test used most widely for scoliosis is the Adams forward-bend test, which, when performed properly, is a sensitive method for identifying coronal-plane curvatures with concomitant axial-plane rotation. An inclinometer is frequently used in the forward-bend test to provide some objective measure of the rib prominence. A positive screen is applied to anyone with truncal asymmetry on this test, and such people are referred to a specialist. Viviani and colleagues tested the ability of trained nurses in the use of the Adams forward-bend test. They found the overall sensitivity of the test for curves >10 degrees to be 73.9%, the specificity 77.8%, and the positive predictive value 12.4%. The sensitivity for curves >20 degrees was 100%, with a specificity of 91%.[5] Beauséjour et al studied a population of patients referred to a Canadian scoliosis clinic in a community without school screening and found that of the 489 suspected cases of AIS, 206 (42%) had no significant deformity (Cobb angle <10 degrees) and could be considered as inappropriate referrals. Among subjects with confirmed AIS, 91 patients (32%) were classified as late referrals with regard to indications for brace treatment.[6]

Opponents of school screening cite concerns about the low predictive value of screening and the cost-effectiveness of referral. Additional factors are the possibility of unnecessary treatment, including the use of a brace and the effects of exposure to X-radiation during screening and examination. Costs involved in screening for scoliosis are relatively low on a societal level, and may be justified by the avoidance of surgery in some adolescents with scoliosis.[7] Patients without significant spinal deformity referred to specialists do not require X-radiography, and for those who do, it is important to note that current radiographic techniques involve significantly less radiation exposure than in the past.

Montgomery and coworkers, in 1993, supported school screening for scoliosis and demonstrated an 8-fold decrease in the relative risk of its progression into the surgical range. The authors concluded that screening decreased the demand for surgery, because smaller curves would be detected and braced at an earlier age, therefore having a better prognosis.[8] Conversely, Yawn et al[9] concluded that the positive predictive value of routine screening was low. Morais and colleagues[10] stated that the prevalence of scoliosis was too low to benefit from screening, and expressed concerns about radiation exposure following clinical screening.

To date, no studies based on level-1 evidence have been done on school screening for scoliosis, and unfortunately, such a study is unlikely to be performed in the future. In addition, there are no studies based on level-1 evidence studies that show effectiveness of bracing. Therefore, the U.S. Preventive Services Task Force has recommended eliminating school screening for scoliosis.[7] Definitive conclusions about the effectiveness of screening cannot be reached on the basis of the current body of literature. However, a study reported by Dolan et al in 2007 sought to examine professional opinion about the effectiveness of bracing relative to observation for AIS by polling experienced clinicians.[11] Although there was variability of opinion among experts, the overall panel stance was that bracing would decrease the risk of progression in premenarchal patients by 20 to 30%. Thus, it appears that many of those who most commonly treat scoliosis, in addition to the major subspecialty societies, perceive a potential positive effect of bracing.[7] Accordingly, it is important to identify patients with scoliosis at an early stage, either to begin bracing within a window of time when it is a viable option, or to allow surgical treatment at an earlier point in cases of severe deformity.

## The Use of Bracing

The goal of brace treatment of moderate scoliosis in growing children is to limit its further progression and, ideally, to avoid surgery. Spinal curves of 20 degrees or less before skeletal maturity are considered mild and are re-evaluated at 6-month intervals. Curves that progress by 5 to 10 degrees or curves of 30 degrees at presentation are moderate and are usually recommended for treatment with a brace because early, full-time bracing is considered to prevent curve progression and obviate the need for surgical intervention in most cases. Curves of less than 30 degrees rarely progress after maturity, but larger curves, especially in the thoracolumbar or lumbar region can increase during the life of the patient.[12] Fusion with instrumentation is indicated for curves >45 degrees in growing children, for curves >50 degrees at maturity, and for those curves that continue to progress after the cessation of brace treatment.

It is thought that brace correction of spinal curves occurs through molding of the spine, trunk, and rib cage during growth, specifically through the use of transverse forces to correct such curves with endpoint control. The application of transverse force and curve correction has an additive effect in improving critical load and stabilizing a curve.[13] Full-time bracing instituted early and with a well-fitting brace may reduce the size of a curve during the treatment period, but this correction rarely persists long after bracing is discontinued at skeletal maturity. The consensus among centers with a long track record of bracing is that the best outcome of bracing is the prevention of further deformity.

The Milwaukee brace was developed by Blount and Moe in the late 1940s as a substitute for postoperative casting in scoliosis and was then adapted for use in the nonoperative treatment of neuromuscular and idiopathic scoliosis. This CTLSO (cervical–thoracic–lumbar–sacral orthosis) consisted of a molded pelvic girdle that was attached to a metal superstructure, which supported lateral pads, trapezial pads, and axillary slings (for curves with an apex above T7). An occipital attachment and throat mold was used to stabilize the head and create traction forces; however, effectiveness of this component was later disproven.[14]

The Boston brace system was developed at Children's Hospital, Boston, in the 1970s and consisted of six standard prefabricated polypropylene pelvic and thoracolumbar modules, lined with polyethylene foam. The pelvic module is trimmed on the basis of X-ray findings and) pressure pads are added at the apex of the curve(s).[6] Lumbar lordosis is reduced by flexing the lumbar spine. For curves with a high apex, an axillary support can be added on the concave side with lateral pressure from a pad on the convex side. Today the Boston brace is the most commonly used brace for AIS worldwide, with more than 16 prefabricated modules available. Advantages of the Boston brace include its rapid fabrication time, curve correction of 50% in the brace, and better patient acceptance than the Milwaukee brace.[15]

The Wilmington brace was developed by Bunnell and colleagues at the Alfred I. duPont Hospital for Children in Wilmington, Delaware, also as an alternative to the Milwaukee brace.[16] Fashioned from Orthoplast, the total-contact custom jacket of this brace is made from a custom mold of the patient with the patient's scoliotic curve corrected on a Risser table with transverse, derotation, and traction forces. In the mold, transverse forces are applied at the apices of the curves, spinal balance is sought, and curve correction of 50% is attempted. Trim lines are cut high in the axilla and low over the pelvis, but still allow the patient to sit. An opening is cut in the front of the brace with an overlap that allows the patient to don and doff the brace over a cotton or synthetic-fiber undergarment with Velcro straps. Because of the intimate fit of the brace, convenience of its wear, and thinner material (3.2 mm) of which it is made, its acceptance by patients was superior to that of the Milwaukee brace. The breakdown of the Orthoplast material was, however, seen as a relative disadvantage of the Wilmington brace, although this deterioration of the brace documents compliance in its use. Patients who wear the brace full-time need an average of three fabrications.[17]

Other TLSO types of braces, constructed from more durable polypropylene include the Miami brace, Rosenberger brace, Providence brace, and Charleston bending brace. The Charleston brace was originally developed as an alternative to full-time brace wear for single thoracolumbar or lumbar curves. During production of this brace the orthotist maintains pressure over the apex of the patient's scoliotic curve while applying an unbending force above the curve, More than 75% curve correction is considered adequate. The Wilmington brace is intended for night-time wear only because of the awkward positioning of the patient in the brace.

## The Author's Preferred Bracing Method

Regardless of the type of brace, my own protocol, after the patient has received a brace and its proper fit is confirmed, involves an initial adjustment period as the straps are tightened and the patient increases brace-wearing to 22 to 23 hours per day. After one month of brace-wearing, a standing radiograph (a supine radiograph for the Charleston or Providence braces) of the patient should be obtained with the straps appropriately tightened to check pad placement, curve correction, and spinal balance. Curve correction of 50 to 60% can be expected from thoracic–lumbar–sacral orthoses (TLSOs) in younger patients with flexible spinal curves. Better initial correction seems to correlate with improved long-term outcome and decreased risk of progression.[18] At 4- to 6-month intervals, standing radiographs of the patient out of the brace are obtained to check for curve progression after a standard period of time (8 to 10 hours) without the brace at each session of radiography. Bracing is continued until skeletal maturity is reached in compliant patients after a weaning period of 6 to 12 months, during which the wearing time of the brace is gradually reduced to night-time wear. Skeletal maturity is considered to have occurred when there is lack of longitudinal growth in two successive office visits, or Risser grade 4 and 18 months postmenarche in girls, or fusion of the iliac apophyses, or a skeletal age of 16 years according to the criteria of the Gruelich and Pyle atlas in boys.[19] After skeletal maturity and the discontinuation of brace-wearing, patients should be followed for radiographic progression of their curves at increasing intervals for at least 2 years.

## Current Evidence in Support of Bracing

Conflicting evidence exists in the literature about the efficacy of bracing for AIS. Given differences in the type of orthosis used, wearing time, research methodologies, and statistical analyses, it is difficult to compare and contrast the studies discussed below of bracing outcomes.

A study by Lonstein and Winter of 1020 patients with AIS, all treated with a Milwaukee brace and compared with a natural-history group of 729 patients seen at the same hospitals, showed that bracing had a significant positive effect on the natural history of AIS ($P = 0.0001$). In the critical high-risk group of girls of Risser grade 0 to 1 with thoracic curves of 20 to 40 degrees, there was a failure rate of 43% with bracing as compared with a rate of 68% in the natural-history control group.[20]

In 1988, Durand published a doctoral thesis on the results of treatment with the Milwaukee brace of AIS in 477 patients.[21] In the highest-risk group, the "transpubertal" Risser grade 0 or 1 group, a 21% failure rate was found, compared with the 68% failure rate in the natural history group (at 5 years after skeletal maturity).

Fernandez-Filiberti and colleagues published the results for 54 compliant brace-treated patients compared with 47 untreated age-, gender-, and curve-matched patients. In resemblance to the findings by Durand, there was a 3-fold greater frequency of surgery or major curve increase in the control group than in the brace-treated group.[22]

Results with the Wilmington brace for the nonsurgical treatment of AIS are also favorable. The initial report by Bunnell and colleagues on 48 patients treated with this device showed that after initial correction of the curves of 74% in the brace, only the curves of 10% progressed by 5 degrees or more.[16] Bassett et al reported on 79 patients with curves of 20 to 39 degrees who were of Risser grade 1 or less, in whom initial correction of 50% occurred in the brace; 28% had curve progression of >5 degrees at a mean follow-up of 2.5 years.[23] In a subsequent report on these patients at 8 years of follow-up, only 12% had needed surgery.[24] These reports from Wilmington, along with the results of part-time versus full-time bracing, support the use of a TLSO in affecting the natural history of AIS in skeletally immature patients with moderate scoliotic curves.

Emans et al, in 1986, reported results with the Boston TLSO in 295 patients at an average follow-up of 1.4 years after the discontinuation of bracing.[25] Curve progression of 5 degrees or more was noted in 7% of the patients during treatment, and only 11% of the patients went on to surgery. Patients with low apex curves did best, whereas young age at brace initiation and large curves increased the risk of needing surgery. As did the Wilmington group, Emans and colleagues noted that initial brace correction of at least 50% correlated with better results.

A dynamic brace, using straps to provide transverse corrective forces, was developed in Montreal by Rivard and colleagues. Of the 170 patients followed to maturity after treatment in this SpineCor brace, 59% had no progression of spinal curvature during the treatment period. Forty-two patients (26%) required surgery because of curve progression or had curves >45 degrees at maturity.[26] Controlled studies and longer follow-up of this treatment are needed.

The only prospective controlled study of brace treatment for scoliosis was presented in 1993 and published in 1995 by Nachemson and Peterson.[27] In this long-term, multicenter study sponsored by the Scoliosis Research Society (SRS), 286 female patients were divided into three groups, consisting of: (1) a natural history group (no treatment of any kind); (2) brace treatment of at least 20 hours/day until the end of growth; and (3) electrical stimulation. Although the results with electrical stimulation were no different than those for the natural history group, the investigators were able to show that bracing significantly altered the natural history of AIS ($P < 0.0001$). Curve progression of 5 degrees or more was noted in 26% of the patients treated with braces, 67% of the electrical-stimulation group, and 66% of the natural-history group, demonstrating a clear advantage of bracing.

Because full-time brace-wearing (23 hours/day) is difficult, many centers have modified this to 16 hours/day[17,28] without finding any appreciable differences in the risk of progression with part-time versus full-time brace-wearing. A meta-analysis of the literature[29] found a relationship between the duration of brace-wearing per day and prevention of curve progression, suggesting that the more time a patient spends in a brace the less likely is the patient's curve to progress. This was corroborated in a study by Rahman and coworkers, which showed that more compliant patients had a favorable outcome with brace treatment in the Wilmington TLSO.[30]

## Conclusion and Future Directions

The studies described in this chapter show that bracing can be effective in the nonsurgical management of AIS, especially for mild and moderate curves (20 to 35 degrees), and does alter the natural history of curve progression in immature patients. However, skeptics continue to criticize the methodology of many of these studies as flawed science. Compliance can now be accurately assessed with temperature-sensitive monitors,[31] and criteria for consistent parameters of treatment evaluation, to allow valid and reliable comparisons of the findings in future bracing studies, have been outlined by the Bracing and Nonoperative Management Committee of the SRS. Richards and coworkers stated that assessment of brace effectiveness should include: (1) the percentage of patients who have curve progression of 5 degrees or less and the percentage of patients who have progression of 6 degrees or more at maturity; (2) the percentage of patients with curves >45 degrees at maturity or who have had surgery recommended or undertaken; and (3) a 2-year follow-up beyond maturity to determine the percentage of patients who subsequently undergo surgery. Additionally, information should be provided about all patients, regardless of compliance (intent to treat) and curves should be stratified by type and size.[32] As noted earlier in this chapter, a level-1 study incorporating all of these criteria is underway, consisting of a 5-year multicenter, randomized controlled trial of bracing sponsored by the NIH/NIAMS, which has been enrolling patients since 2007 and should provide the data needed to clearly answer the question of the role of bracing in AIS.

The decision to include bracing as part of the treatment algorithm in AIS can be difficult for the patient and family, but if the brace is to have any chance of success, a coordinated effort toward its use is necessary. The prescribing physician and orthotist must be knowledgeable and committed to fabricating an orthosis that is effective and comfortable for the patient. Continued maintenance and fitting to optimize curve correction and the application of transverse force are necessary to optimize results as well as maintain compliance. Periodic radiographic surveillance is required to detect the progression of scoliotic curves. The patient and family must be educated and counseled about brace-wearing and compliance, and must be honest in reporting their wearing schedule and appraisal of it. As Winter and Lonstein wrote, "Not all patients have a good response to a brace, but that should not deter us from giving the opportunity for a good result to all who are candidates. It is better to have tried and failed than never to have tried at all."[33]

Curves that show some correction at the end of treatment with a brace tend to regress toward their pretreatment magnitude at longer-term follow-up.[20,34] Gabos and colleagues examined 55 women who were treated with the Wilmington brace for curves caused by AIS that had an initial magnitude of 20 to 45 degrees at an average follow-up of 14.6 years after the completion of treatment, and found that most of these patients' curves remained stable at middle adulthood. Thirteen percent of the women studied demonstrated curve progression of 5 degrees or more as compared with the curvature present at the start of treatment; no curve progressed more than 17 degrees. The treatment group was compared with age-matched controls, and the two groups showed no significant overall difference in terms of back pain, physical activities, function, or self-care. Ninety-three percent of the treated women reported no subjective deterioration in their physical appearance, cosmesis, or self-image after the discontinuation of bracing.[35] Danielsson et al conducted a long-term follow-up of the original Swedish girls in the SRS study at a mean of 16 years, and found that girls in the brace-treatment group had an average of 6 degrees of correction during the bracing period, but that during the follow-up period, their curves returned to the curvature that had existed at the start of bracing. No girls in the brace-treated group needed surgery in adolescence or after maturity, whereas 10% of the observation group required surgery for curve deterioration.[36]

Ultimately, further knowledge of AIS will be critical in deciding which patients may benefit most from its nonoperative treatment. Accurate assessment of growth and an understanding of the genetics of AIS[1] will enable the clinician to determine which patients are the best candidates for an orthosis to prevent the progression of moderate scoliotic deformities.

## References


1. Ogilvie JW, Nelson LM, Chettier R, et al. Predicting brace resistant adolescent idiopathic scoliosis. Paper presented at: 43rd Annual Meeting of the Scoliosis Research Society, Salt Lake City, September 11, 2008
2. Parent S, Newton PO, Wenger DR. Adolescent idiopathic scoliosis: Etiology, anatomy, natural history and bracing. In: Birch J, ed. Instructional Course Lectures: Pediatrics. Rosemont, IL: American Academy of Orthopaedic Surgeons; 2006:159–166
3. Morrissy RT. School screening for scoliosis. Spine 1999;24:2584–2591
4. Nachemson A, Lonstein JE, Weinstein SL. Prevalence and natural history committee report. Paper presented at: 17th Annual Meeting of the Scoliosis Research Society, Denver, Colorado, September 25, 1982
5. Viviani GR, Budgell L, Dok C, Tugwell P. Assessment of accuracy of the scoliosis school screening examination. Am J Public Health 1984;74:497–498
6. Beauséjour M, Roy-Beaudry M, Goulet L, Labelle H. Patient characteristics at the initial visit to a scoliosis clinic: A cross-sectional study in a community without school screening. Spine 2007; 32:1349–1354
7. Richards BS, Vitale MG. Screening for idiopathic scoliosis in adolescents. An information statement. J Bone Joint Surg Am 2008;90: 195–198
8. Montgomery F, Willner S. Screening for idiopathic scoliosis. Comparison of 90 cases shows less surgery by early diagnosis. Acta Orthop Scand 1993;64:456–458
9. Yawn BP, Yawn RA, Hodge D, et al. A population-based study of school scoliosis screening. JAMA 1999;282:1427–1432
10. Morais T, Bernier M, Turcotte F. Age- and sex-specific prevalence of scoliosis and the value of school screening programs. Am J Public Health 1985;75:1377–1380
11. Dolan LA, Donnelly MJ, Spratt KF, Weinstein SL. Professional opinion concerning the effectiveness of bracing relative to observation in adolescent idiopathic scoliosis. J Pediatr Orthop 2007;27:270–276
12. Weinstein SL. Advances in the diagnosis and management of adolescent idiopathic scoliosis. J Pediatr Orthop 1994;14:561–563
13. Bunch WH, Patwardhan AG. Biomechanics of orthoses. In: Bunch WH, Patwardhan AG, eds. Scoliosis: Making Critical Decisions. St. Louis: CV Mosby; 1989:204–215
14. Galante J, Schultz A, Dewald RL, Ray RD. Forces acting in the Milwaukee brace on patients undergoing treatment for idiopathic scoliosis. J Bone Joint Surg Am 1970;52:498–506
15. Hall J, Miller ME, Schumann W, et al. A refined concept in the orthotic management of scoliosis: A preliminary report. Orthot Prosthet 1975;29:7–13
16. Bunnell WP, MacEwen GD, Jayakumar S. The use of plastic jackets in the non-operative treatment of idiopathic scoliosis. Preliminary report. J Bone Joint Surg Am 1980;62:31–38
17. Allington NJ, Bowen JR. Adolescent idiopathic scoliosis: Treatment with the Wilmington brace. A comparison of full-time and part-time use. J Bone Joint Surg Am 1996;78:1056–1062
18. Olafsson Y, Saraste H, Söderlund V, Hoffsten M. Boston brace in the treatment of idiopathic scoliosis. J Pediatr Orthop 1995;15: 524–527
19. Greulich WW, Pyle SI. Radiographic atlas of skeletal development of the hand and wrist. 2nd ed. Stanford: Stanford University Press, 1959
20. Lonstein JE, Winter RB. The Milwaukee brace for the treatment of adolescent idiopathic scoliosis. A review of one thousand and twenty patients. J Bone Joint Surg Am 1994;76:1207–1221
21. Durand MH. Faut-il abandoner le traitment orthopedique de la scoliosise. Doctoral thesis. University Paul Sabatier, Toulouse, France, 1988

22. Fernandez-Feliberti R, Flynn J, Ramirez N, Trautmann M, Alegria M. Effectiveness of TLSO bracing in the conservative treatment of idiopathic scoliosis. J Pediatr Orthop 1995;15:176–181
23. Bassett GS, Bunnell WP, MacEwen GD. Treatment of idiopathic scoliosis with the Wilmington brace. Results in patients with a twenty to thirty-nine-degree curve. J Bone Joint Surg Am 1986;68:602–605
24. Piazza MR, Bassett GS. Curve progression after treatment with the Wilmington brace for idiopathic scoliosis. J Pediatr Orthop 1990; 10:39–43
25. Emans JB, Kaelin A, Bancel P, Hall JE, Miller ME. The Boston bracing system for idiopathic scoliosis. Follow-up results in 295 patients. Spine 1986;11:792–801
26. Coillard C, Vachon V, Circo AB, Beauséjour M, Rivard CH. Effectiveness of the SpineCor brace based on the new standardized criteria proposed by the scoliosis research society for adolescent idiopathic scoliosis. J Pediatr Orthop 2007;27:375–379
27. Nachemson AL, Peterson LE. Effectiveness of treatment with a brace in girls who have adolescent idiopathic scoliosis. A prospective, controlled study based on data from the Brace Study of the Scoliosis Research Society. J Bone Joint Surg Am 1995;77: 815–822
28. Green NE. Part-time bracing of adolescent idiopathic scoliosis. J Bone Joint Surg Am 1986;68:738–742
29. Rowe DE, Bernstein SM, Riddick MF, Adler F, Emans JB, Gardner-Bonneau D. A meta-analysis of the efficacy of non-operative treatments for idiopathic scoliosis. J Bone Joint Surg Am 1997;79: 664–674
30. Rahman T, Bowen JR, Takemitsu M, Scott C. The association between brace compliance and outcome for patients with idiopathic scoliosis. J Pediatr Orthop 2005;25:420–422
31. Takemitsu M, Bowen JR, Rahman T, Glutting JJ, Scott CB. Compliance monitoring of brace treatment for patients with idiopathic scoliosis. Spine 2004;29:2070–2074, discussion 2074
32. Richards BS, Bernstein RM, D'Amato CR, Thompson GH. Standardization of criteria for adolescent idiopathic scoliosis brace studies: SRS Committee on Bracing and Nonoperative Management. Spine 2005;30:2068–2075, discussion 2076–2077
33. Winter RB, Lonstein JE. Use of the Milwaukee brace for progressive idiopathic scoliosis. J Bone Joint Surg Am 1997;79:954, author reply 954–955
34. Noonan KJ, Weinstein SL, Jacobson WC, Dolan LA. Use of the Milwaukee brace for progressive idiopathic scoliosis. J Bone Joint Surg Am 1996;78:557–567
35. Gabos PG, Bojescul JA, Bowen JR, Keeler K, Rich L. Long-term follow-up of female patients with idiopathic scoliosis treated with the Wilmington orthosis. J Bone Joint Surg Am 2004;86A:1891–1899
36. Danielsson AJ, Hasserius R, Ohlin A, Nachemson AL. A prospective study of brace treatment versus observation alone in adolescent idiopathic scoliosis: A follow-up mean of 16 years after maturity. Spine 2007;32:2198–2207

# 8 The Case Against Bracing

*Robert A. Dickson*

The previous chapter argued in favor of brace treatment; this chapter will make the case against it. To assess the role of bracing in the management of idiopathic scoliosis, it is crucial to understand this deformity and why it is treated.[1] We can then begin to understand why the results of bracing for idiopathic scoliosis have been so disappointing.

## What Deformity Are We Treating?

Chapter 3 of this book, on the pathogenesis of idiopathic scoliosis, describes in detail the geometry of idiopathic scoliosis and its development. The three-dimensional nature of structural scoliosis has been known for centuries,[2] and the essential features of the deformity are first a lordosis, second a rotation/torsion, and third a lateral deformity or scoliosis.[3–6] Scoliosis is fundamentally a front–back problem, not a right–left problem. Once the lordosis develops in the mid-lower thoracic region, it progressively gets closer to the axis of spinal-column rotation and tries to get out of the sagittal plane by buckling.[6] This is the basis of the Adams forward-bend test, developed in the early 1860s, which compresses the sagittal plane and enhances the rotational prominence in scoliosis (see **Fig. 3.5**).[2]

Going back to the geometry of the deformity in scoliosis, the posteroanterior (PA) view of the patient shows the lateral curvature with rotation such that the posterior elements turn into the curve concavity and it can be clearly seen that the back of the spine is shorter than the front (see **Figs. 3.6** and **3.7**).[7] However, above and below this central area of structural scoliosis are compensatory scolioses that act to bring the spine into straight alignment. The nature of these compensatory scolioses is that of asymmetric kyphoses balancing the central area of lordoscoliosis. This was precisely Roaf's concept of curve progression, holding that the central area of lordoscoliosis was compressed by the kyphoses above and below it.[4] His classic article should be compulsory reading for anyone trying to understand this three-dimensional deformity in scoliosis.

Unfortunately, the problem isn't so straightforward, because as soon as the lordosis buckles out of the sagittal plane, in comes the Hueter–Volkmann law to produce asymmetric epiphyseal loading and three-dimensional vertebral wedging that increases progressively toward the curve apex. As the Cobb angle increases progressively from 10 degrees, to 20 degrees, 30 degrees, 40 degrees, and beyond, so does the degree of asymmetric vertebral wedging (**Fig. 8.1**).[1,6,8] Supine, side-bending, or traction films of the patient now become progressively more like the erect film. The components of the jigsaw puzzle of the spinal column fit less well together and the resulting so-called stiffness or lack of flexibility does not come from an added component of soft-tissue stiffness, but simply from the progressive loss of stackability straightness of the spine the greater its curvature becomes. Therefore, if the word "unstackability" existed, it would very nicely describe the problems that occur with increasing curve size.

Even a 20-degree curve causes some loss of stackability, and it would challenge the most fertile mind to devise an orthosis that could not only stop the progression of curvature in scoliosis, but could actually produce some form of correction.

Meanwhile, looking at Scheuermann's disease, the adolescent idiopathic deformity opposite that of scoliosis, it is a thoracic hyperkyphosis with the sagittal plane of the spine moving progressively further behind the axis of spinal-column rotation (see **Fig. 3.11**).[6] Thus, Scheuermann's disease progresses in the sagittal plane without buckling potential. Because this is a uniplanar deformity, its correction requires extension, and indeed, 1 or 2 years in an extension cast or brace leads to a true physiological correction of the deformity.[9] If, therefore, hyperkyphosis needs extension for its correction, lordosis needs flexion, and it is flexion that renders it particularly rotationally unstable.[2] It therefore does not appear that the deformity of idiopathic lordoscoliosis is treatable without surgery.

## Why Are We Treating This Deformity?

James, in Edinburgh, divided idiopathic scoliosis according to its age of onset into the categories of infantile (birth to 4 years of age), juvenile (age 5 to 9 years), and adolescent (age 10 years to maturity).[10] There are, however, only two phases of increased growth velocity: during infancy and again during adolescence.[11] At birth, mean body length is 50 cm, and during the first year of life babies grow by half

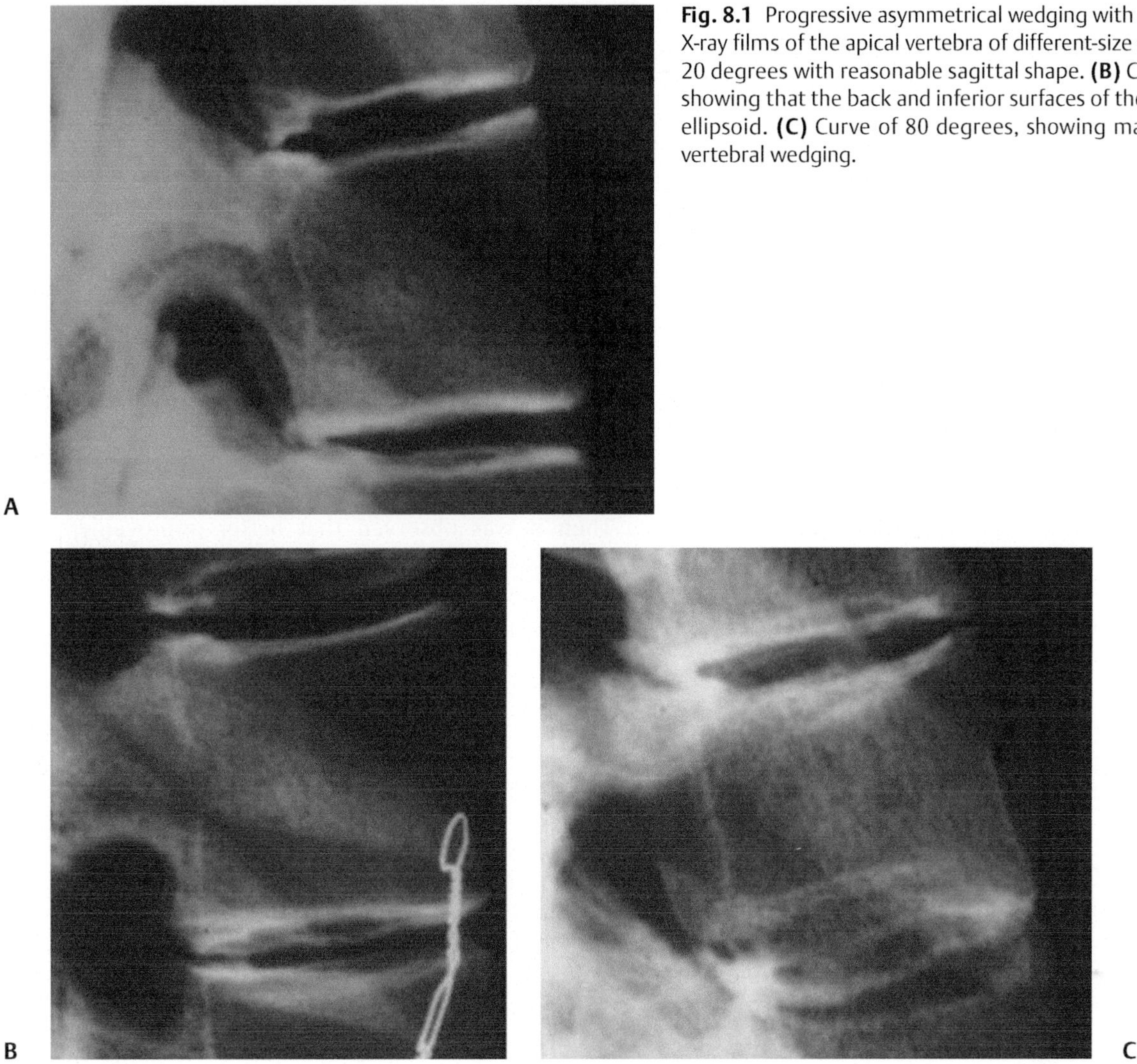


**Fig. 8.1** Progressive asymmetrical wedging with growth. True lateral X-ray films of the apical vertebra of different-size curves. **(A)** Curve of 20 degrees with reasonable sagittal shape. **(B)** Curve of 40 degrees, showing that the back and inferior surfaces of the vertebral body are ellipsoid. **(C)** Curve of 80 degrees, showing marked asymmetrical vertebral wedging.

of that (i.e., 25 cm). During the second year of life they grow by half of the latter figure (i.e., 12.5 cm), and in the third year of life they again grow by half of this (i.e., 6 cm).[12] The growth rate then remains steady until the adolescent growth spurt, when this trend reverses with increased growth velocity.

It is during the first year or two of life that a progressive thoracic scoliosis can impair the proper development of the heart and lungs,[13,14] and for this reason progressive infantile idiopathic scoliosis threatens health in adulthood. By contrast, there is no such risk if a deformity occurs after the age of 5 years.[15]

James had some difficulty in identifying true cases of idiopathic scoliosis of juvenile onset because if a deformity existed at, say, the age of 6 years, it was more likely to be a carryover from infancy than a disorder of true juvenile onset.[10] Consequently, there is much in favor of having two types of scoliosis according to age of onset: (1) early-onset idiopathic scoliosis beginning before the age of 5 years; and (2) late-onset idiopathic scoliosis beginning after the age of 5 years.[16]

Early-onset idiopathic scoliosis is therefore treated to prevent future cardiopulmonary problems, whereas treatment for late-onset idiopathic scoliosis is done to ease deformity and improve appearance, although not without the potential for producing significant psychosocial distress. Eating disorders are 10 times more common in girls with significant scoliosis than in their counterparts with straight backs, and at the worst end of the spectrum is frank osteoporosis just when peak bone mass occurs.[17] Once the deformity is corrected, such patients very quickly catch up with their straight-backed peers and become "normal" girls.

When bracing was first introduced for idiopathic scoliosis it was erroneously thought that preventing progression of the condition (particularly to beyond 60 degrees) would reduce the likelihood of the spine and chest providing a hostile environment for the internal organs.[18–20]

At the same time, surgery was a major undertaking, with the control of progression rather than correction being the main goal, and was accompanied by the possibility of serious neurological complications and pseudarthrosis requiring reoperation.[21] Indeed, James not only performed massive spinal fusions, but reinspected them at intervals of about 3 months to make sure that union was occurring, and if not, applied supplementary bone grafts.[10] Perhaps not unreasonably, children and families faced with the possibility of a hideous deformity with a shortened lifespan or a very major operation opted for any treatment offered, even to the point of spending 23 hours per day in a brace.

However, the deformity of late-onset idiopathic scoliosis is not and never has been a long-term organic health problem, and if the deformity does become unacceptable to the patient and family, a single modern surgical operation with only a few days spent in the hospital can easily restore body symmetry with minimal risks.

## Is the Deformity in Scoliosis Treated Successfully Without Surgery?

### Late-onset Idiopathic Scoliosis

All sorts of contraptions have been prescribed for scoliosis over the centuries. Most were in the form of racks or turnbuckles, from the design of which it would seem that pain was the chief objective.[22] Indeed, having a severe scoliosis was a serious stigma for which these sorts of horrific devices were deemed entirely appropriate. Unfortunately, patients with idiopathic scoliosis are, regrettably, still stigmatized, and endure continued bullying in schools. It is incomprehensible that idiopathic scoliosis can be regarded as a simple cosmetic condition when it can cause significant psychosocial distress at a very vulnerable age, weight loss, osteoporosis at the extreme, and social outcasting as the norm.[17] This is what drives scoliosis surgeons to ever-better goals for their patients.

The Milwaukee brace was introduced to support poliomyelitic scoliosis after surgical intervention, and was never designed to be a nonoperative treatment of any type of spinal deformity.[23] As the polio epidemics ended with successful vaccinations, the Milwaukee brace came to be prescribed for idiopathic scoliosis instead. Looking at the explanations and cases that Blount and Moe[23] reported in their textbook on treatment with the Milwaukee brace, it is clear that what was being treated was a straightforward right/left spinal asymmetry in the frontal plane, and indeed, that still seems to be the prevailing view. No adequate biomechanical explanation for the possible efficacy of brace treatment was put forward other than, to begin with, simple stretching of the spine with the upper part of the orthosis under the mandible and the lower part fitted to the pelvis. Serious problems with dentition then led to the orthosis having a cervical choker rather than an occipitomandibular piece.[24]

It was then conjectured that the Milwaukee brace might work by way of three-point fixation: at the top and bottom, and with a pad just below the middle on the convex side. X-ray films of patients in the brace were encouraging with, for example, a 30-degree standing curve when out of the brace and a 20-degree curve in the brace. The curve was not allowed to move from this semi-improved position for 23 hours a day, whereas a nonbraced child would move its spine through as full a range as possible thousands of times a day during normal activities of daily living.[16]

Then it was observed that better improvement was obtained when the pelvic component of upright posture flattened the lumbar lordosis of the scoliotic spine. No adequate biomechanical explanation was put forward for this, but clearly, with a flattened lumbar lordosis the upper torso was pitched forward, leading to spontaneous thoracic hyperextension, which in turn pushed the lordosis back towards the sagittal plane,[16] the opposite of the forward-bend test (see **Fig. 4.1**). Although this might reduce the magnitude of the scoliotic component of the deformity, it unquestionably increased the thoracic lordosis, with a reportedly detrimental effect on pulmonary function.[25]

"Evidence-based medicine" has now been an "in" phrase for several years, and means "the integration of individual clinical expertise with the best available external evidence from systematic research, particularly concerning the scientific principles governing treatment."[26] It is difficult to identify any criteria by which the nonoperative treatment of late-onset idiopathic scoliosis adheres to the principles of evidence-based medicine. Not only was the orthosis used for treating it devised for a completely different type of scoliosis under entirely different circumstances, but the early experience with this orthosis was reported at a time when it was not conventional to apply statistical methods or any other rigorous analytical approach to the problem. Yet this is what we have done, this is what has happened, and because we are the senior scoliologists of the day, we tell others that they had better do the same. None of us could possibly dissent. In the 1970s, the designer of the Milwaukee brace, Dr. Walter Blount, and his colleagues, reported retrospectively on only half of a total number of 94 patients treated with the brace.[27] Notwithstanding, they went on to state "there have been no published data with regard to long-term end results comparable to the available follow-up studies of untreated patients."

The Campbell Clinic reported on 52 patients, of an original cohort of 125, for whom treatment with the brace began at the age of 14 years and lasted until nearly the age of

17 years (despite spinal growth being effectively complete in girls by the age of 15 years).[27] Mean Cobb angles were initially >40 degrees, and improvement was between 0% and 20%. Then the Minneapolis Group reported their results with patients aged 8 to 16 years.[28] Of their original 133 patients, 30 were lost to follow-up and 29 were treated surgically "because of a poor response to the brace." Thus, 59 patients (44%) have to be regarded as having experienced treatment failure. The mean final curve in the 74 patients (56%) who were followed was only a few degrees smaller than the original curve. The authors stated quite rightly that "the role of the Milwaukee brace and the treatment of idiopathic scoliosis is still unclear." They then asked the important question: "What then is the proper role of the Milwaukee brace in scoliosis treatment?", and emphasized that "further follow-up must be obtained on these patients." Despite this important question, no scientific data were being gathered about the efficacy of the brace and no prospective studies were undertaken. Rather, it was stated by more senior scoliosis surgeons that the Milwaukee brace worked, and junior surgeons were obliged to agree.

Then, in 1984, Miller and his colleagues in Gothenburg pointed out that there were no controlled studies of brace treatment and reported retrospectively about 144 braced patients versus 111 untreated patients with both groups having a mean deformity of <30 degrees.[29] No evidence was provided in favor of bracing. Nonetheless, the Gothenburg investigators felt that a controlled, randomized prospective study was warranted. That was somewhat surprising, because this type of prospective investigation should be based on clear retrospective evidence of benefit, so as to determine, for example, how long treatment is required, for which group (boys or girls), and for what age range. Because the Swedish retrospective study demonstrated no benefit from brace treatment, the need for a prospective study is questionable.

In the next decade, Caroline Goldberg went from Dublin to Boston to determine the efficacy of the Boston underarm brace in late-onset idiopathic scoliosis. She and her coworkers compared 32 braced patients in Boston, for whom relevant data were adequate, with 32 nonbraced controls in Dublin, and their results were published in 1993.[30] There was again no difference between the braced and nonbraced patients, from which the authors concluded that "this raises very seriously the question of whether bracing can be considered an effective way of altering the natural history of late-onset idiopathic scoliosis."

Bracing has persisted despite the lack of new data in support of its efficacy. Its proponents state that "as high quality clinical research studies have been available in the 1980s and early 1990s the proper place of brace treatment for adolescent idiopathic scoliosis has become apparent,"[31] an extraordinary assertion in that precisely the opposite conclusion is contained in the literature.

In 1994 the Minneapolis Group published the results for more than 1000 patients who had been braced between 1954 and 1979.[32] The braced patients were compared with 727 patients who were not braced but were followed for evidence of curve progression. Overall, there was no curve progression in 77%, another 22% needed operative intervention, and the remaining 791 were managed with a brace only. Failure was defined as an increase in Cobb angle of at least 5 degrees or surgical intervention. The failure rate of curves of <30 degrees was 40% at the cessation of treatment and more than 50% at the latest follow-up. As compared with the previous study[29] it was suggested that failure rates were lower in the braced group. Noonan and Weinstein expressed concern about the large number of patients being excluded from the study and that only 28% of the study questionnaires had been completed.[33]

Then, in 1995, the Puerto Rico Group compared bracing in 54 patients with 47 controls.[34] There was a significantly greater number of patients in the control group who required surgery, but more than twice as many in the latter group (77%) had thoracic curves as did those in the treated group (46%). Thoracic curves have always been shown to be associated with a much greater progression potential than other spinal curves in scoliosis.[35] Furthermore, the Puerto Rico Group stated categorically that patients "fully complied with treatment," whereas the excellent study in Oxford by Houghton et al, using hidden compliance meters, showed that upper-middle-class Oxford schoolchildren didn't wear their braces much more than 10% of the prescribed time despite what they or their parents said.[36]

With so many stakeholders it was clear, despite the absence of any evidence-base from retrospective studies about bracing favorably altering the natural history of scoliosis, that a prospective controlled trial of bracing would be undertaken. The results of this trial were published in 1995,[37] and the authors quite rightly stated that as regards previous reports, "none of these studies met the stringent criteria for scientific evidence that must be used to prove the effectiveness of treatment."

They went on to state that "a well-designed study must include a large cohort of similar patients with similar patterns and sizes of deformity and that they should be randomized to different treatment methods and followed until at least skeletal maturity." Unfortunately, randomization was impossible because centers that used bracing would not stop using it and those that did not brace would not use a treatment that they did not believe worked. Furthermore, as will be seen, the patterns of deformity were significantly different.

They decided to use three arms in a study of 286 patients, consisting of: (1) 129 observed patients; (2) 111 braced patients; and (3) 46 electrically stimulated patients, although this last treatment had been discarded years earlier (**Table 8.1**). Perhaps they thought that the electrically stimulated patients would form another control group.

**Table 8.1 Results of Trial of Bracing, Observation, and Electrical Stimulation in Adolescent Idiopathic Scoliosis: I**

| | Brace | Observation | Electrical Stimulation |
|---|---|---|---|
| **No. of subjects** | 111 | 129 | 46 |
| **Failed*** | 40 | 56 | 29 |
| **Percent failure** | 36% | 52% | 63% |

*Failure = 6 degrees of progression.

Another problem was their selection of treatment failure as an increase of at least 6 degrees in the Cobb angle. That is close to the measurement error of the angle itself, but more importantly, a range of 20 degrees to 26 degrees is different from a range of 40 degrees to 46 degrees. As the lordosis in scoliosis buckles out of the sagittal plane, curve size diminishes with rotation. A curve of 40 degrees is therefore much more than twice the size of a curve of 20 degrees (see **Fig. 2.9**). Accordingly, mean values and percentage changes are difficult to interpret.

In any event, the braced patients did best, with a 36% failure rate, the observed patients had a 52% failure rate, and the electrical-stimulation group had a 63% failure rate. These differences in proportions were statistically significant, and from them it could be interpreted that bracing eases idiopathic scoliosis, observation does nothing, and electrical stimulation worsens the curves in scoliosisi!

On the face of it, therefore, the braced group in the study looked as if it had done better, but the following article, in the same edition of the *Journal of Bone and Joint Surgery* in which the study findings were published, reported on factors in the study that would be indicative of curve progression (**Table 8.2**).[38] The most dominant such factor was curve site, with thoracic curves being significantly more progressive than thoracolumbar curves. Meanwhile, when the trial investigators examined the proportions of the more progressive thoracic curves, they found that almost 90% in the stimulated group, 81% in the observed group, and a mere 68% in the braced group were thoracic curves. Similar proportions existed in the Puerto Rico Study. It would be difficult to better stack the odds in favor of bracing.

Then, in 1996, the Iowa Group reported on 102 of 111 patients treated with a Milwaukee brace, with a mean time from the cessation of bracing to follow-up of more than 6 years.[39] Although there were no controls, the authors did not favor bracing, and concluded that "it is currently impossible to state that bracing effectively alters the natural history in immature patients who are at high risk for curve progression."

**Table 8.2 Percentages of Thoracic and Thoracolumbar Curves in the Braced, Observed, and Electrical Stimulation Groups**

| | Brace | Observed | Electrical |
|---|---|---|---|
| Thoracic | 68 | 81 | 89 |
| Thoracolumbar | 32 | 19 | 11 |

When the available English-language literature was recently comprehensively reviewed, it showed no evidence in favor of bracing as altering the natural history of scoliosis.[40]

## Early-onset Idiopathic Scoliosis

Early-onset idiopathic scoliosis is the only type of scoliosis to definitely benefit from nonoperative treatment.[12,41–43] This condition is attributable to postnatal body molding among babies lying preferentially in the oblique lateral decubitus position (see **Fig. 4.5**). For the full-term, healthy, normotonic baby going through its milestones normally, any scoliosis resulting from postnatal molding will resolve. However, the floppy, low birth-weight hypotonic baby, developing slowly, often does not resist the positioning imposed on it, and thus may well develop progressive infantile idiopathic scoliosis. Progression is also associated with a big initial Cobb angle, a rib–vertebra angle difference (RVAD) in excess of 20 degrees, and a stiff spinal curve (see **Fig. 2.11**).[43]

Mehta and Morrell have shown that through the application of small plaster of Paris jackets under light general anesthesia (the application process takes about an hour), molding of the ribs on the convex side can straighten the spine and return the RVAD to normal.[41,43] The rationale for success with this technique is to capitalize on the infantile growth spurt, infants growing much faster during the first 3 years of life before they settle down to an average height gain of 6 cm a year until the adolescent growth spurt, when growth velocity again increases. Casting is repeated every 2 or 3 months until the end of the third year of life or earlier, should the curve be seen to resolve. Interestingly, it is the rotational component of the deformity that is the last to disappear, and although the spine may be straight in the frontal plane, radiography reveals that there is still a rib hump, which often persists until the age of ~10 years.

One of the biggest problems in treating infantile scoliosis is a lack of early referral. Conner in Glasgow analyzed this delay and found that the chief stumbling block was failure of the general orthopedic surgeon to refer such patients to the nearest scoliosis surgeon.[44] Mehta looked at this statistically in her first 67 children with progressive infantile scoliosis treated by extension–derotation–flexion (EDF) casting.[45] There were 49 patients in her group 1 whose referral was delayed for 12 months, as compared with 18 patients in group 2 whose referral was delayed for 20 months. The Cobb angle in the latter group was 52 degrees, and the curvature in this group took much longer to fully resolve.

Of the first 75 patients treated in Leeds, 47 were boys and 28 were girls.[42] Single thoracic curves were present in 70%, 20% had double thoracic and lumbar curves, and 10% had single thoracolumbar curves. Curves with an RVAD >20 degrees were significantly larger than those with an RVAD of <20 degrees. We treated 21 infants with EDF casting for a mean of 19 months, and in those with RVADs in excess of 20 degrees, casting significantly reduced curve size.

Recently, Mehta reviewed her prospective study of 136 children under the age of 4 years who had progressive infantile scoliosis treated with casting and who were followed for an average of 9 years.[12] She again stressed the importance of early referral. In children treated early and who had a mean Cobb angle of 32 degrees, scoliosis resolved by a mean age of 3 years and 6 months, without needing further treatment, and these children went on to lead normal lives. In the 42 children referred late, the Cobb angle was in excess of 50 degrees, and casting reduced but didn't reverse the deformity, with 15 of these children eventually requiring spinal fusion.

It is during the first 2 years of life, when a child grows by 25 cm and 12.5 cm, respectively, that serial EDF casting has its greatest beneficial effect. The Leeds experience with early-onset idiopathic scoliosis is now close to 300 cases, and our results with Mehta's EDF casting program are comparable to hers.

## References


1. Dickson RA. How to treat idiopathic scoliosis and why. Eur Instr Course Lect 2005;7:69–81
2. Adams W. Lectures on the Pathology and Teatment of Lateral and other Forms of Curvature of the Spine. London: Churchill and Sons; 1865.
3. Somerville EW. Rotational lordosis; the development of single curve. J Bone Joint Surg Br 1952;34B:421–427
4. Roaf R. The basic anatomy of scoliosis. J Bone Joint Surg Br 1966; 48:786–792
5. Dickson RA, Lawton JO, Archer IA, Butt WP. The pathogenesis of idiopathic scoliosis. Biplanar spinal asymmetry. J Bone Joint Surg Br 1984;66:8–15
6. Millner PA, Dickson RA. Idiopathic scoliosis: Biomechanics and biology. Eur Spine J 1996;5:362–373
7. Dickson RA. The aetiology of spinal deformities. Lancet 1988; 1331:1151–1155
8. Dickson RA. Spinal deformity: Adolescent idiopathic scoliosis. Nonoperative treatment. Spine 1999;24:2601–2606
9. Bradford DS. Juvenile kyphosis. Clin Orthop Relat Res 1977;128:45–55
10. James JIP. Idiopathic scoliosis; the prognosis, diagnosis, and operative indications related to curve patterns and the age at onset. J Bone Joint Surg Br 1954;36B:36–49
11. Tanner JM. Growth at Adolescence, ed. 2. Oxford: Blackwell Scientific; 1962
12. Mehta MH. Growth as a corrective force in the early treatment of progressive infantile scoliosis. J Bone Joint Surg Br 2005;87:1237–1247
13. Davies G, Reid L. Effect of scoliosis on growth of alveoli and pulmonary arteries and on right ventricle. Arch Dis Child 1971;46: 623–632
14. Pehrsson K, Bake B, Larsson S, Nachemson A. Lung function in adult idiopathic scoliosis: A 20 year follow up. Thorax 1991;46:474–478
15. Branthwaite MA. Cardiorespiratory consequences of unfused idiopathic scoliosis. Br J Dis Chest 1986;80:360–369
16. Dickson RA. Conservative treatment for idiopathic scoliosis. J Bone Joint Surg Br 1985;67:176–181
17. Smith FM, Latchford G, Hall RM, Millner PA, Dickson RA. Indications of disordered eating behaviour in adolescent patients with idiopathic scoliosis. J Bone Joint Surg Br 2002;84:392–394
18. Nachemson A. A long term follow-up study of non-treated scoliosis. Acta Orthop Scand 1968;39:466–476
19. Nilsonne U, Lundgren KD. Long-term prognosis in idiopathic scoliosis. Acta Orthop Scand 1968;39:456–465
20. Collis DK, Ponseti IV. Long-term follow-up of patients with idiopathic scoliosis not treated surgically. J Bone Joint Surg Am 1969; 51:425–445
21. American Orthopaedic Association Research Committee. End result study of the treatment of idiopathic scoliosis. J Bone Joint Surg 1941;23:963–977
22. Rang M. The Story of Orthopaedics. Philadelphia, PA: WB Saunders; 2000:157–162.
23. Blount WP, Moe JH. The Milwaukee Brace. Baltimore: Williams & Wilkins; 1973
24. Alexander RG. The effects on tooth position and maxillofacial vertical growth during treatment of scoliosis with the Milwaukee brace. Am J Orthod 1966;52:161–189
25. Winter RB, Lovell WW, Moe JH. Excessive thoracic lordosis and loss of pulmonary function in patients with idiopathic scoliosis. J Bone Joint Surg Am 1975;57:972–977
26. Sackett DL, Richardson WAS, Rosenberg W, Haynes RB. Evidence-Based Medicine: How to Practice and Teach EBM. London: Churchill Livingstone; 1997
27. Mellencamp DD, Blount WP, Anderson AJ. Milwaukee brace treatment of idiopathic scoliosis: Late results. Clin Orthop Relat Res 1977;126:47–57
28. Carr WA, Moe JH, Winter RB, Lonstein JE. Treatment of idiopathic scoliosis in the Milwaukee brace. J Bone Joint Surg Am 1980;62: 599–612
29. Miller JAA, Nachemson AL, Schultz AB. Effectiveness of braces in mild idiopathic scoliosis. Spine 1984;9:632–635
30. Goldberg CJ, Dowling FE, Hall JE, Emans JB. A statistical comparison between natural history of idiopathic scoliosis and brace treatment in skeletally immature adolescent girls. Spine 1993; 18: 902–908
31. Winter RB. The pendulum has swung too far. Bracing for adolescent idiopathic scoliosis in the 1990s. Orthop Clin North Am 1994; 25:195–204
32. Lonstein JE, Winter RB. The Milwaukee brace for the treatment of adolescent idiopathic scoliosis. A review of one thousand and twenty patients. J Bone Joint Surg Am 1994;76:1207–1221

33. Noonan KJ, Weinstein SL. Letter to Editor. J Bone Joint Surg Am 1997;76:954–955
34. Fernandez-Feliberti R, Flynn J, Ramirez N, Trautmann M, Alegria M. Effectiveness of TLSO bracing in the conservative treatment of idiopathic scoliosis. J Pediatr Orthop 1995;15:176–181
35. Weinstein SL, Ponseti IV. Curve progression in idiopathic scoliosis. J Bone Joint Surg Am 1983;65:447–455
36. Houghton GR, McInerny A, Tew A. Brace compliance in adolescent idiopathic scoliosis. Abstract. J Bone Joint Surg Br 1987;69:852
37. Nachemson AL, Peterson L-E. Effectiveness of treatment with a brace in girls who have adolescent idiopathic scoliosis. A prospective, controlled study based on data from the Brace Study of the Scoliosis Research Society. J Bone Joint Surg Am 1995;77: 815–822
38. Peterson L-E, Nachemson AL. Prediction of progression of the curve in girls who have adolescent idiopathic scoliosis of moderate severity. Logistic regression analysis based on data from The Brace Study of the Scoliosis Research Society. J Bone Joint Surg Am 1995;77: 823–827
39. Noonan KJ, Weinstein SL, Jacobson WC, Dolan LA. Use of the Milwaukee brace for progressive idiopathic scoliosis. J Bone Joint Surg Am 1996;78:557–567
40. Dickson RA, Weinstein SL. Bracing (and screening): Yes or no? J Bone Joint Surg Br 1999;81:193–198
41. Mehta MH, Morel G. The non-operative treatment of infantile idiopathic scoliosis. In: Zorab PA and Siegler D, eds. Scoliosis. Proceedings of the Sixth Symposium 1979. London: Academic Press; 71–84
42. Millner PA, Helm R, Dickson RA. Early onset idiopathic scoliosis: Natural history and outcome. J Bone Joint Surg Br 1992;74(suppl III): 303–304
43. Mehta MH. The rib-vertebra angle in the early diagnosis between resolving and progressive infantile scoliosis. J Bone Joint Surg Br 1972;54:230–243
44. Conner AN. Developmental anomalies and prognosis in infantile idiopathic scoliosis. J Bone Joint Surg Br 1969;51:711–713
45. Mehta M. The early treatment of infantile scoliosis: Early referral is crucial to the outcome. J Bone Joint Surg Br 1992;74(suppl I):97

# 9 Classification of Adolescent Idiopathic Scoliosis for Surgical Intervention

*David H. Clements, Joshua M. Pahys, and Patrick Cahill*

The first systematic classification of scoliosis was described by John R. Cobb in his classic article "Outline for the Study of Scoliosis," published in 1948. However, descriptions of scoliosis and its treatment may be traced back to Hippocrates and his "De Articulationes" in *Corpus Hippocraticum*. Understanding of the nature of the deformity by Hippocrates was based purely on the subjective appearance of the unfortunate patient; the treatment recommendation was primarily traction for all types of deformity, with results recognized to be poor. Galen later used Hippocrates' recommendations for treatment, and introduced the descriptive terms *kyphosis*, *lordosis*, and *scoliosis*. Despite the introduction of this appearance-based classification system, the treatment of scoliosis was largely unchanged until the late nineteenth century. After the discovery of roentgen rays in 1895, the description of scoliosis became more qualitative, as the deformed spine could now be visualized and more definitive treatment could be developed. With a better understanding of the geometry of the underlying spinal deformity, spinal fusion could then be attempted for certain types of scoliosis such as neuromuscular curves caused by polio, with some success.

When Cobb set forth to describe the classification and treatment of scoliosis, he was relying on only 30 years of experience in its surgical treatment, dating back to the first spinal fusion for scoliosis performed in 1914 by Hibbs. Cobb's descriptions of major and minor curves, structural curves, types of scoliosis, and etiological classification, as well as treatment recommendations based on these classification parameters, continue to influence the classification and treatment of scoliosis to this day. As more surgeons began to treat scoliosis, it became obvious that etiology, such as tuberculosis and neuromuscular disease, had an impact on the patterns of deformity, and also that identifying these patterns helped in predicting the response to the developing treatment modalities. It soon became apparent that sharing observations about deformity patterns and their response to treatment was an important next step in organizing the treatment of scoliosis. The founding of the Scoliosis Research Society in 1966, owing in large part to the ideas and enthusiasm of David B. Levine, MD, was the next important step in providing a platform for rationalizing and discussing treatments for scoliosis treatment and creating a body of literature about these.

## King Classification

In 1983, Howard A. King and colleagues published a review of the results of spinal fusion in thoracic idiopathic scoliosis. They reviewed and analyzed the cases of 405 patients treated by John Moe with Harrington rod instrumentation, attempting to define the criteria used by Moe to perform a selective thoracic fusion. Curves were defined and divided into five types (I to V). King's classification system was the first to specifically describe the most common type of idiopathic scoliosis, occurring in the thoracic spine, and recommend treatment based on the type of spinal curve in the disorder. More importantly, King et al presented recommendations for selectively fusing the thoracic spine and allowing the lumbar spine to undergo correction through compensation, thus preserving motion.[1]

### Description

The first concept that King et al described was that of the *stable vertebra*. This was defined as the vertebra most closely bisected by the center sacral vertical line (CSVL), a single line drawn through the center of the sacrum perpendicular to the iliac crests. Curve flexibility was an important concept in determining whether a curve was *structural* or *compensatory*. Flexibility was quantified by measuring the Cobb angle on films of the patient during bending, dividing it by the Cobb angle on the anteroposterior (AP) film of the spine in the erect position, and multiplying the result by 100%. The *flexibility index* was a concept defined as the percentage correction of the thoracic curve subtracted from the percentage correction of the lumbar curve on side-bending radiographs. King and Moe defined a type I curve as an S-shaped curve in which both the thoracic and lumbar curves cross the CSVL, with the lumbar curve larger than the thoracic curve, and with a negative flexibility index. A type II curve is also one in which both curves cross the CSVL, but the thoracic curve is greater than or of the same magnitude as the lumbar curve, with a positive flexibility index. A type III curve is a thoracic curve with a lumbar curve that does not cross the CSVL. Type IV curves are similar to type III, except that the fifth lumbar vertebra is centered over the sacrum and the fourth lumbar vertebra is tilted into the long thoracic curve. Type V curves are double thoracic curves, with the first thoracic vertebra tilted into the upper thoracic curve.

### Application

Guidelines for selecting levels of fusion were developed for each type of curve. It was recommended that type I curves be fused to L4. Type II curves could be treated with a selective thoracic fusion, with the fusion stopping at the stable vertebra and leaving the lumbar curve flexible and able to spontaneously correct. Type III and IV thoracic curves could also be fused to the stable vertebra. Type V curves were to be treated by fusion of both thoracic curves, with the fusion ending at the stable vertebra.

### Reliability

King and his coworkers noted that 4 of the 405 patients in their study had progression of the lumbar curve of their deformity, requiring a second operation to extend fusion into the lumbar spine. According to their treatment guidelines, these patients' spines were "inappropriately" fused either caudad or cephalad to the stable vertebra. From these findings, King et al concluded that for type II, III, IV, and V curves, selecting the stable vertebra rather than the neutral vertebra for the distal fusion level gave the most reliable results.

### Updates and Revisions

As segmental instrumentation systems began to gain favor over Harrington rods among surgeons, many patients with idiopathic scoliosis exhibited decompensation in the lumbar spine when King et al's recommendations for the distal level of instrumentation were followed. In 1992, Richards[2] examined 24 patients with type II idiopathic scoliosis and a flexible lumbar curve >40 degrees. All 24 patients underwent selective thoracic fusion with segmental spinal instrumentation (Cotrel–Dubousset or Texas Scottish Rite Hospital instrumentation). Despite the amount of preoperative lumbar-curve flexibility, these lumbar curves remained larger after surgery than did the instrumented thoracic curves, resulting in spinal imbalance. Richards concluded that lumbar-curve flexibility was not a reliable predictor of compensatory lumbar-curve correction with the selective fusion of King type II curves when the lumbar curve was >40 degrees.

Roye et al[3] published their results with treating scoliosis classified according to their King type with segmental instrumentation. They found significant decompensation in cases of King type II and III curves, whereas King type I, IV, and V curves had no decompensation. Also, in 1992, Knapp et al[4] published their results in which fusion levels in 253 patients were based on the classifications and recommendations of King and coworkers. They recommended including part of the lumbar curve in cases of King type II curves, and that King type IV curves could be safely fused at one level proximal to the stable vertebra.[4] Collectively, these studies suggest that the King system, developed during the era of Harrington-rod fixation, may not reliably predict the response of curves corrected with more powerful segmental instrumentation systems.

In addition to concerns about postoperative decompensation, concerns began to be raised about the reliability of the King classification system and its reproducibility among surgeons. In 1998, Cumming et al[5] published an article on both the inter- and intraobserver reliability of the King classification for idiopathic scoliosis. They found that the median kappa coefficient for interobserver reliability was 0.44 and that the kappa coefficient for intraobserver reproducibility was 0.64. They therefore concluded that the reproducibility of the system was fair and the reliability of the system was poor. Behensky et al,[6] assessing the reliability of the King classification in an article published in 2002, calculated a kappa coeficient of 0.45, indicating poor interobserver reliability. It was becoming more obvious that classifying curves according to the King classification system was somewhat unreliable. In combination with the instances of decompensation suggesting flaws in the King classification, concerns about lack of reproducibility of the King classification led to the development of a new classification system.

## ■ The Lenke Classification

The Lenke classification system was devised as a project by Lawrence Lenke and the Harms Study Group (HSG) to enhance the ability to accurately compare similar types of spinal curves among different treatment centers. The classification system was devised from the beginning to be descriptive, comprehensive, and reproducible with excellent inter- and intraobserver reliability. It sought to accomplish this goal by devising objective criteria for each type of curve, incorporating data on coronal deformity, flexibility, and sagittal alignment toward the goal of consistently classifying patterns of deformity and developing standardized treatment protocols for them, with reliable outcomes.

### Description

To fully define a curve by the Lenke system, one must identify its type, lumbar modifier, and thoracic sagittal profile. The types of curve defined by the system were based on the features of a major curve and the structural characteristics of the minor curves accompanying it. A few terms need to be defined to use the system. The major curve is the curve of greatest magnitude, and is always considered structural. Minor curves can be structural or nonstructural. A nonstructural curve is defined as one that bends to less than 25 degrees on a radiograph of the bending patient. With these terms, curves can be classified as being of one of six types. In a type 1 pattern (main thoracic [MT] curve), the major curve is in the thoracic spine and the proximal thoracic (PT) and thoracolumbar (TL) curves are minor and nonstructural. In a type 2 pattern (double thoracic curve) the MT curve is the major curve, with the PT curve being minor and structural and the TL curve being minor and nonstructural. The type 3 pattern (double major curve) has the MT curve as the major curve, the PT curve as nonstructural, and the lumbar curve as minor and structural. The type 5 pattern (triple major curve) describes the PT, MT, and TL curves as all being structural, with either the MT or the TL curve as the major curve. In the type 4 pattern (thoracolumbar/lumbar [TL/L] curves) the lumbar curve is the major and only structural curve, with the PT and MT curves being minor and nonstructural. In the type 6 pattern (TL/L and MT curves), the TL/L curve is the major curve, measuring at least 5 degrees more than the MT curve, which is minor but structural. A pattern in which the difference between the lumbar and thoracic curves is less than 5 degrees can be categorized as being of type 3, 4, or 5 on the basis of structural characteristics in the MT and TL/L regions.

Lumbar-spine modifiers in the Lenke classification system are defined by the location of the center sacral vertical line (CSVL) on the apical vertebra of the lumbar curve. The CSVL is defined as a vertical line bisecting the cephalad aspect of the sacrum and perpendicular to the true horizontal. An "A" is used as a modifier when the CSVL runs between the lumbar pedicles of the lumbar apical vertebra. The curve must have a thoracic apex at or cephalad to the level of the 12th thoracic disc. Therefore, the modifier A can be used only for MT curves of types 1 through 3. The modifier B is used when the CSVL touches the apex of the lumbar curve between the medial border of the lumbar concave pedicle and a concave lateral margin of the apical vertebral body or bodies. These curves were defined as having an apex in the main thoracic region. The modifier C is used when the CSVL falls completely medially to the margin of the vertebra at the apex of the lumbar curve. By their designation, curves with the modifier C would seem to be simply the next step in a progression of lateral deviations from curves designated by modifiers A and B; however, a curve with the modifier C may represent a distinct pathological entity and probably requires a treatment plan that deviates from those for curves with modifiers A and B. Lumbar curves designated by modifier C are more likely to have significant rotation at the apex and to deviate more from the midline than curves designated by the modifiers A or B. These features could result in a clinical deformity with a significant lumbar prominence. They may also contribute to the curve behaving more like a structural curve with continued deformity that does not improve in the same manner as that of a flexible, nonstructural curve designated by modifier A or B. Thus, curves with the modifier C, despite being considered strictly nonstructural, may occasionally be included at least partly in the levels of the spine that are instrumented and fused in treating a case of scoliosis.

For the first time in any classification system for scoliosis, the sagittal profile of the spine is included in the Lenke classification system. Sagittal thoracic modifiers are defined as normal (N) if sagittal thoracic alignment ranges from 10 to 40 degrees as measured from T5 to T12. Curves with less than 10 degrees of kyphosis from T5 to T12 are given a minus (−) modifier, and curves with more than 40 degrees of hyperkyphosis are given a plus (+) modifier.

In the original article describing the Lenke classification and its rationale, Lenke and colleagues presented their evaluation of the reliability of the system. The kappa value for the new system was noted to be 0.92, with interobserver reliability for determining a curve at 93%. When compared with the King classification, the intraobserver reliability of the Lenke classification system was calculated at 85%, with a kappa value of 0.83. The intraobserver reliability among five surgeons using the King classification was 69%, with a mean kappa value of 0.69. The interobserver reliability for the new classification system was 85%, with a mean kappa value of 0.83. From these data, Lenke and coworkers concluded that their new system was more reproducible and reliable than the King system.

A follow-up article published by Lenke et al and reporting a multi-surgeon assessment of the new system for surgical decision-making in idiopathic scoliosis showed a high level of agreement (84 to 90%) in curve classification, although choices for operative approaches and fusion levels still varied widely.[7] Subsequent reviews have focused on the intra- and interobserver reliability of the King and Lenke classifications. In an article published in 2006, Niemeyer et al[8] concluded that both classifications had good reliability. On nonmeasured radiographs, the higher the level of orthopedic training and experience of the measurers, the better the inter- and intraobserver reliability Likewise, Ogon et al[9] published a similar review of the reliability of the Lenke classification system, reporting that it was more reliable than the King classification, although proper classification of high thoracic and lumbar curves could be problematic. Most of these studies indicate that the Lenke classification provides a more reliable and reproducible way in which to communicate curve patterns than does the King classification, thus allowing surgeons to begin to speak the same language and compare results of different treatments in patients with similar curve patterns.

## Ability to Guide Treatment

Another key aspect of any useful classification system for spinal curvature in scoliosis is to guide its treatment. The Lenke classification system achieves this goal. Lenke types 1 and 5 curves are to be treated either anteriorly or posteriorly. The recommendation for Lenke types 2, 3, 4, and 6 curves is that they be treated completely posteriorly. The HSG reviewed its prospectively collected multicenter database to assess how often these recommendations were followed. Of the 1281 patients whose cases were reviewed, treatment recommendations based on the Lenke classification were not followed in 192 cases, indicating that the rules were broken 15% of the time. The greatest percentage (29%) of rule breaking occurred with Lenke type 3 curves and the least (6%) with Lenke type 1 curves. In addition, the Lenke classification recommends that only major structural curves be included in instrumentation and fusion, and that nonstructural curves be excluded. The development of the Lenke classification system within the HSG appears to have made the treatment of scoliosis more consistent. The incidence of "rule breaking" has decreased since publication of the classification system in 2001. The proportion of rule breakers was greater before the induction of the Lenke classification system, at 18%, than afterward, at 12%.

In 2003, Newton et al published a review of 203 patients with Lenke type 1B or 1C curves treated with surgical fusion.[10] Specifically, Newton et al's study examined whether the fusion done in these cases incorporated only the major structural thoracic curve (selective fusion) or included the nonstructural lumbar curve as well (nonselective). The Lenke classification dictates that only structural curves be fused, and therefore all fusions done on curves of Lenke type 1 and which include the lumbar curve are rule breakers. In Newton et al's review, the factors associated with rule breaking (fusion of the lumbar spine) included a lumbar curve of greater preoperative magnitude, greater displacement of the lumbar apical vertebrae from the CSVL, and a small ratio of thoracic-to-lumbar-curve magnitude. The rate of rule breaking was greater with type 1C curves than with type 1B curves, with the frequency of selective fusion being 92% for type 1B curves but only 68% for type 1C curves. These data indicate that the characteristics of the compensatory nonstructural lumbar curve play a role in surgical decision-making for treating spinal curves despite the designations made in the Lenke system. Newton et al's study further emphasized the continued disparity in the treatment algorithm for thoracic curves and the variability in application of selective fusion for thoracic curves. The study also showed that the most significant factor in whether Lenke's rules were broken was who performed the procedure, indicating a predilection among surgeons to fuse the lumbar curve rather than a rational application of the treatment algorithm. This raises the question of whether deviation from the recommendations of the Lenke classification system is secondary to surgeon education or to an unwillingness to fully adopt the suggested guidelines for lumbar C curves. Conversely, the data on rule breaking could also be an indication that the Lenke classification may not address all structural aspects of the lumbar curve in scoliosis, and specifically its rotation.

In summary, the Lenke classification, although comprehensive and potentially more reliable than the King classification in predicting treatment of the scoliotic spine, is still not perfect. It has helped guide the selection of scoliotic curves for fusion. However, surgeons still choose, rightly or wrongly, to deviate 15% of the time from the Lenke algorithm for treatment recommendations, despite its offering a more pragmatic protocol for selecting treatment than does the King classification. The Lenke classification does not help in selecting the end-vertebrae of the treatment construct, a matter that continues to be subjectively debated. Further studies with longer follow-up periods, and prospective randomized trials, are needed to more definitively resolve this dispute.

# The Classification of Multiplanar Deformity: The Next Generation

Increasing attention has been focused on the rotational component of the spinal deformity associated with scoliosis. The classification systems discussed previously are based only on the coronal and sagittal planes of this spinal deformity. The axial plane is intimately tied to the other two planes; altering the magnitude of the deformity in the coronal plane in one curve of a scoliosis is tied to the effect on the axial plane of another curve. Thus, the challenge in surgery for scoliosis lies in developing indices for properly characterizing the third dimension of scoliosis that can help direct the surgeon in predicting and guiding the response of uninstrumented curves.

Lee and colleagues[11] focused on the importance of addressing the axial rotation of spinal deformity and its implications for surgical curve correction. They devised a method of direct vertebral rotation (DVR) as an adjuvant intraoperative technique to improve overall curve correction in all three planes. The rotational angle of the apical vertebra relative to the sacrum (RAsac) was measured with computed tomography (CT) scans. In a group of 38 patients with adolescent idiopathic scoliosis (AIS), those treated with DVR as opposed to standard rod derotation (SRD) exhibited significantly better sagittal- and coronal-curve correction, as well as axial derotation. The average rotational correction of the apical vertebra was 42.5% in the DVR group as compared with only 2.4% in the SRD group. Lee and colleagues also noted that with DVR, distal fusion levels may be spared, because improved correction of thoracic axial rotation led the compensatory lumbar curve to "unwind" and often to "spontaneously correct." Patients in the DVR group exhibited significantly better three-dimensional (3D) correction of uninstrumented lumbar curves than did those in the SRD group. This was achieved by performing a DVR on the two lowermost instrumented vertebrae in cases of Lenke 1C curves, whereas this additional DVR was unnecessary for achieving a balanced lumbar curve in cases of Lenke types 1A and 1B curves.

Assessments of torsion and axial rotation have also been used in the research setting to evaluate spinal deformity.[12,13] However, these techniques required the use of additional measurement tools and complex interpretation methods, making them less likely to be applicable in a general spine clinic. A more desirable system would entail commonly used imaging modalities with computer-generated measurements to reduce inter- and intraobserver variability and assist with data interpretation. The Scoliosis Research Society (SRS) initiated the 3D Classification Working Group in 1994 in an effort to better characterize and classify all planes of spinal deformity in idiopathic scoliosis.

Cluster analysis has been used as a means for indentifying groupings of individuals according to a set of measurements. This allows the observer to use multiple measurement variables to analyze several patients collectively, and to search for "clusters" of patients having similar characteristics or patterns of spinal curvature. First presented by Duong et al,[14] cluster analysis was used to identify groupings of scoliosis patients on the basis of multiple measurements from calibrated biplanar radiographs, or through stereoradiography.[15] Duong and colleagues' study identified five classes of spinal curve patterns, which were similar to those in the King and Lenke classifications.

More recently, Stokes et al[16] and Sangole and co-workers[17] have built on the technique of using cluster analysis for stereoradiographic measurements of spinal deformity. They identified morphological parameters of each curve, using six anatomical landmarks for each vertebra.[18] The measurements utilized for the analysis were the Cobb angle, apical vertebra, axial rotation of the apical vertebra, and orientation of the plane of maximum curvature (PMC) with respect to the sagittal plane.[13,16,18–20] The PMC was defined as the plane passing through the vertebral-body centers of the two end-vertebrae of a curve and the apical vertebrae of each curve segment.[16] This measurement, combined with the parameters named above, allows assessment of a deformity in the coronal, sagittal, and axial planes.

In their most recent study, Stokes et al[16] examined 245 stereoradiographs of 110 patients with AIS. Four distinct groups were identified. Group 1 demonstrated a right "upper" (thoracic) kyphotic curve and left "lower" (lumbar) lordotic curve. The PMC in this group was rotated in a counterclockwise or "positive" direction when viewed from above for both curves. Group 2 was defined as having a right upper kyphotic curve with a "negative" (clockwise) PMC and a left lower kyphotic curve with a positive rotation of the PMC. Group 3 was characterized as having a left upper kyphotic curve and a right lower lordotic curve, with the PMC rotated in the negative direction for both curves. Patients in group 4 had a left upper kyphotic curve with a negative rotation of the PMC and a right lower kyphotic curve with a positive rotation of the PMC. These generated groupings were found to be significantly distinct, having minimal overlap of patient data from one group to another. This is in contrast to other measurements of spinal deformity (Cobb angle, apex level, and axial rotation of the apical vertebrae), in which distinct groupings could not be created because of substantial overlap of patient data if the rotation of the PMC was not included.

The currently described 3D model may provide a better description of overall spinal shape in scoliosis. However, the 3D classifications described above currently provide little direct guidance with regard to treatment decisions for spinal curvatures. More long-term studies are warranted to further delineate the validity and applicability of these new 3D assessments to common clinical practice.

## Genetic Classification

Extensive laboratory and clinical research has been conducted in an effort to determine the etiology of idiopathic scoliosis. A multitude of genetic factors have been identified that may play a role in the development of spinal deformity.[21] Wynne-Davis,[22] and later Robin and Cohen,[23] postulated a multiple gene inheritance pattern on the basis of examining multiple patients with idiopathic scoliosis and their families. More recently, Miller et al,[24] Alden et al,[25] and Chan et al[26] identified possible candidate regions for a genetic origin of idiopathic scoliosis on chromosomes 6, 9, 16, 17, and 19. The eventual goal of this research is to develop a test to help predict which patients will eventually require surgery and which patients have curves that will not progress and can potentially be spared multiple follow-up radiographs, long courses of bracing treatment, or both. Medical treatment of scoliosis may some day even supplant surgery and bracing.

Melatonin was discovered as playing a potential role in the development of spinal deformity when it was found that animals developed scoliosis after undergoing pinealectomy with subsequent melatonin dysfunction.[27,28] Further study in humans revealed a possible defect in the melatonin signal-transduction pathway of patients with AIS. Moreau et al[29] discovered a melatonin signaling defect in 100% of the osteoblasts isolated from a small group of AIS patients undergoing surgery. Their study identified three distinct groups of AIS patients who were identified on the basis of the extent of deficiency of melatonin signal transduction. This information led to the first scoliosis screening assay in the hope of helping to identify children at high risk of developing AIS. Continued study of this signaling pathway and the screening assays is currently underway.

Further research has produced a 30-marker genetic panel in an effort to predict the likelihood of progression to severe AIS.[30,31] Ward and colleagues[30] conducted a genome-wide association study comparing 1200 patients with severe AIS (defined as a curve >40 degrees in a skeletally immature patient or a curve >50 degrees in a skeletally mature patient) with 1500 control patients. A total of 30 genetic markers were identified as the "most useful prognostic markers" for progression to severe AIS. This panel has since been expanded to include more than 50 markers and is now marketed to clinicians as the ScoliScore™ AIS Prognostic Test (Axial Biotech; Salt Lake City, UT). Peer-reviewed reports of the results with this genetic panel concluded that it could be used as early as in the initial clinical evaluation to predict which patients' deformities would or would not progress to severe AIS.

Ogilvie et al[31] expanded the research for this genetic panel to potentially identify those patients presenting with AIS curves of 25 to 40 degrees who would be resistant to brace-wearing and whose curves would progress to require surgery.[31] This is significant, as it has been shown that one-third of patients of Risser grade 0/1 with curves of 20 to 29 degrees will not have scoliosis that progresses to the point of requiring surgery if left untreated, and that conversely, 20% will fail brace-wearing and progress to have severe AIS.[31–33] Ogilvie and coworkers' study examined 57 AIS patients whose curves were "brace-resistant." This was defined as a 25- to 40-degree initial AIS curve, treated with standard bracing, that progressed to require surgical intervention. Utilizing the 30-marker genetic panel described above, these researchers were able to calculate the probability of a "brace-resistant" curve in 95% (54 of 57) of the patients in the study, based solely on their genetic profile. Conversely, the same study identified only a 9% false-positive rate in 500 patients with initial curves <25 degrees. These patients' curves were predicted by genetic analysis to progress to within the range requiring surgery, but remained at <25 degrees at the time of final evaluation.

The genetic tests described above may prove invaluable to the clinician. Potentially, a patient presenting with a mild curve and a low probability of curve progression based on genetic testing may be spared from multiple follow-up radiographs to monitor curve progression, or from a long course of brace-wearing treatment, or both. On the other hand, a patient with a similar presenting curve pattern but a high genetic probability of curve progression may be more closely monitored and counseled at an earlier stage of disease on the basis of a greater likelihood of eventually needing surgical intervention.

## ■ Conclusion

The goals of a classification system for any disease process must be that it distinguish between clinically significant groups of persons with the disease, be easy to apply in clinical settings, be reproducible over time and among observers, guide treatment, and predict outcomes. The ideal classification system for AIS continues to elude researchers. However, the system devised by Lenke and the HSG has proven invaluable for advancing care and research in the field of idiopathic scoliosis. Many groups continue to devise classification systems as both surgical techniques and the understanding of scoliosis are refined.

### References


1. King HA, Moe JH, Bradford DS, Winter RB. The selection of fusion levels in thoracic idiopathic scoliosis. J Bone Joint Surg Am 1983; 65:1302–1313
2. Richards BS. Lumbar curve response in type II idiopathic scoliosis after posterior instrumentation of the thoracic curve. Spine 1992; 17(8, suppl):S282–S286
3. Roye DP Jr, Farcy JP, Rickert JB, Godfried D. Spine 1992;17(8 suppl): S270–3
4. Knapp DR Jr, Price CT, Jones ET, Coonrad RW, Flynn JC. Choosing fusion levels in progressive thoracic idiopathic scoliosis. Spine 1992;17:1159–1165
5. Cummings RJ, Loveless EA, Campbell J, Samelson S, Mazur JM. Interobserver reliability and intraobserver reproducibility of the system of King et al. for the classification of adolescent idiopathic scoliosis. J Bone Joint Surg Am 1998;80:1107–1111
6. Behensky H, Giesinger K, Ogon M, et al. Multisurgeon assessment of coronal pattern classification systems for adolescent idiopathic scoliosis: Reliability and error analysis. Spine 2002;27: 762–767
7. Lenke LG, Betz RR, Haher TR, et al. Multisurgeon assessment of surgical decision-making in adolescent idiopathic scoliosis: Curve classification, operative approach, and fusion levels. Spine 2001; 26:2347–2353
8. Niemeyer T, Wolf A, Kluba S, Halm HF, Dietz K, Kluba T. Interobserver and intraobserver agreement of Lenke and King classifications for idiopathic scoliosis and the influence of level of professional training. Spine 2006;31:2103–2107; discussion 2108
9. Ogon M, Giesinger K, Behensky H, et al. Interobserver and intraobserver reliability of Lenke's new scoliosis classification system. Spine 2002;27:858–862

10. Newton PO, Faro FD, Lenke LG, et al. Factors involved in the decision to perform a selective versus nonselective fusion of Lenke 1B and 1C (King-Moe II) curves in adolescent idiopathic scoliosis. Spine 2003;28:S217–S223
11. Lee SM, Suk SI, Chung ER. Direct vertebral rotation: A new technique of three-dimensional deformity correction with segmental pedicle screw fixation in adolescent idiopathic scoliosis. Spine 2004;29:343–349
12. Poncet P, Dansereau J, Labelle H. Geometric torsion in idiopathic scoliosis: three-dimensional analysis and proposal for a new classification. Spine 2001;26:2235–2243
13. Stokes IA. Axial rotation component of thoracic scoliosis. J Orthop Res 1989;7:702–708
14. Duong L, Cheriet F, Labelle H. Three-dimensional classification of spinal deformities using fuzzy clustering. Spine 2006;31:923–930
15. Delorme S, Petit Y, de Guise JA, Labelle H, Aubin CE, Dansereau J. Assessment of the 3-d reconstruction and high-resolution geometrical modeling of the human skeletal trunk from 2-D radiographic images. IEEE Trans Biomed Eng 2003;50:989–998
16. Stokes IA, Sangole AP, Aubin CE. Classification of scoliosis deformity three-dimensional spinal shape by cluster analysis. Spine 2009;34:584–590
17. Sangole AP, Aubin CE, Labelle H, et al. Three-dimensional classification of thoracic scoliotic curves. Spine 2009;34:91–99
18. Stokes IA, Bigalow LC, Moreland MS. Three-dimensional spinal curvature in idiopathic scoliosis. J Orthop Res 1987;5:102–113
19. Villemure I, Aubin CE, Grimard G, Dansereau J, Labelle H. Progression of vertebral and spinal three-dimensional deformities in adolescent idiopathic scoliosis: A longitudinal study. Spine 2001;26:2244–2250
20. Stokes IA. Three-dimensional terminology of spinal deformity. A report presented to the Scoliosis Research Society by the Scoliosis Research Society Working Group on 3-D terminology of spinal deformity. Spine 1994;19:236–248
21. Kouwenhoven JWM, Castelein RM. The pathogenesis of adolescent idiopathic scoliosis: Review of the literature. Spine 2008;33: 2898–2908
22. Wynne-Davies R. Familial (idiopathic) scoliosis. A family survey. J Bone Joint Surg Br 1968;50:24–30
23. Robin GC, Cohen T. Familial scoliosis. A clinical report. J Bone Joint Surg Br 1975;57:146–148
24. Miller NH, Justice CM, Marosy B, et al. Identification of candidate regions for familial idiopathic scoliosis. Spine 2005;30:1181–1187
25. Alden KJ, Marosy B, Nzegwu N, Justice CM, Wilson AF, Miller NH. Idiopathic scoliosis: identification of candidate regions on chromosome 19p13. Spine 2006;31:1815–1819
26. Chan V, Fong GC, Luk KD, et al. A genetic locus for adolescent idiopathic scoliosis linked to chromosome 19p13.3. Am J Hum Genet 2002;71:401–406
27. Thillard MJ. Deformation de la colonne vertebrale consecutives a l'epiphysectomie ches le poussin. C R Assoc Anat 1959;46:22–26
28. Machida M, Dubousset J, Imamura Y, Iwaya T, Yamada T, Kimura J. An experimental study in chickens for the pathogenesis of idiopathic scoliosis. Spine 1993;18:1609–1615
29. Moreau A, Wang DS, Forget S, et al. Melatonin signaling dysfunction in adolescent idiopathic scoliosis. Spine 2004;29: 1772–1781
30. Ward K, Nelson LM, Chettier R. Genetic profile predicts curve progression in adolescent idiopathic scoliosis. Paper presented at: Scoliosis Research Society Annual Meeting. Salt Lake City, UT, 2008
31. Ogilvie JW, Nelson LM, Chettier R. Predicting brace-resistant adolescent idiopathic scoliosis. Paper presented at: Scoliosis Research Society Annual Meeting. Salt Lake City, UT, 2008
32. Danielsson AJ, Hasserius R, Ohlin A, Nachemson AL. A prospective study of brace treatment versus observation alone in adolescent idiopathic scoliosis: A follow-up mean of 16 years after maturity. Spine 2007;32(20):2198–2207
33. Dolan LA, Weinstein SL. Surgical rates after observation and bracing for adolescent idiopathic scoliosis: An evidence-based review. Spine 2007; 32(19, suppl):S91–S100

# 10 Biomechanics and Reduction of Scoliosis

*Thomas R. Haher, Jahangir Asghar, Loren Latta, and Patrick Cahill*

The spinal-deformity surgeon applies forces to favorably affect the spine's geometry and morphology. To accomplish this, patients are placed in a thoraco–lumbo–sacral orthosis (TLSO) or force anchors are inserted into the vertebrae. Forces are also applied to the spine when physical therapy is prescribed. The force may be applied by the adjacent muscles of the spine, passively through the surrounding soft tissues, or directly to the vertebrae by instrumentation. In each instance, the forces applied are directed to counteract an abnormal group of forces that are producing spinal imbalance. The spine surgeon must be able to identify, locate, and correct those abnormal forces so as to achieve correction of a deformity and subsequent spinal balance. The forces should be applied harmoniously, to prevent stress risers; safely, to preserve the integrity of the surrounding anatomy; and efficiently, to achieve the desired spinal profile.

This chapter describes the mechanisms of failure of a long slender column such as the spinal column and describes the forces that cause that failure. These forces and others that contribute to the progression of a spinal deformity will be defined as critical forces (Fcr) or abnormal forces (Fab). Corrective forces (F+) are applied by the surgeon. The mode of application of these forces is important to understand, and the effect of these forces will be described and identified. F+ are applied to the spine via longitudinal members through force anchors, which are any devices used to transmit applied forces to the spine. They include hooks, screws, and wires. Techniques for enhancing the efficiency of force transmission by instrumentation, as well as failure of the implants used to transmit forces, will be presented together with pertinent metallurgical and biomechanical concepts.

It is the authors' belief that a firm knowledge of the mechanical behavior of soft tissue, the effect of deforming and F+ applied to the spine, and techniques for applying corrective forces will improve the surgeon's ability to correct spinal deformities.

## The Biomechanics of the Spine: A Biological Column

Leonhard Euler in the 1700s discovered a relationship between the dimensions of a long slender column and the force needed to cause the failure of that column by buckling. The beam theory was developed from this and from the work of Bernoulli. The beam theory allows the prediction of load-carrying characteristics and deflection of a simple beam. The relationship is valid for an ideal column that is perfectly straight, homogenous in composition, and free of all and any initial stresses. The relationship of forces and failure of a beam derived by Euler and Bernoulli is:

$$\text{Critical force} = \text{K}\pi\text{EI}/L^2$$

where E = the modulus of elasticity of the beam (slope of the stress–strain curve)

I = moment of inertia (resistance of the beam to bending)

$L$ = length of the beam

K = a constant depending on the conditions of end support of the beam

The failure of columns may vary according to their geometry. Short, wide columns may fail by yielding (**Figs. 10.1, 10.2**). Long, slender columns fail by buckling (**Figs. 10.3, 10.4**).

The Fcr needed for buckling is proportional to the moment of inertia, I, and the modulus of elasticity, E, and not to the strength of the column, as one might expect.

Boundary conditions have an effect on the critical load capacity of a slender column. The critical boundary conditions for column stability are the type of mechanical supports provided at the ends of the column. The greater the resistance to bending at the ends, the more stable the column will be. However, boundary conditions also reflect other physical conditions or properties of the surrounding environment. Boundary conditions usually model supports, but may also model load points and moments. In the case of a spinal column, the surrounding bone and soft tissue would affect its mechanical behavior. Boundaries may determine the mode of bending and the number of inflection points of a column. An inflection point occurs when the curvature of a column changes from concave to convex. The closer the inflection points are to one another, the greater the load capacity of the column.

In Euler's formula, the modulus of elasticity, E, the moment of inertia, I, for the structure, and $\pi$ are constants.

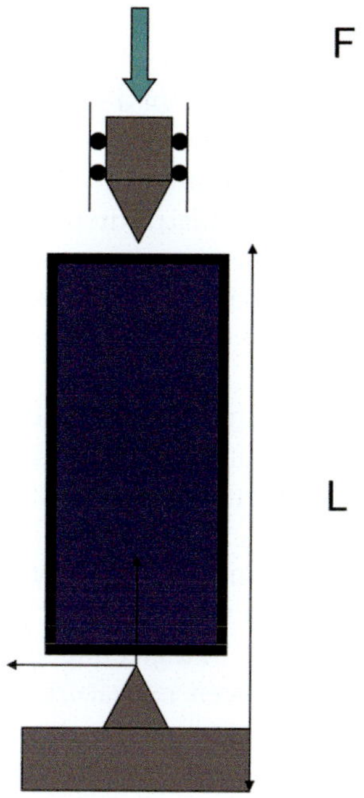


**Fig. 10.1** A short column with an axial load applied.

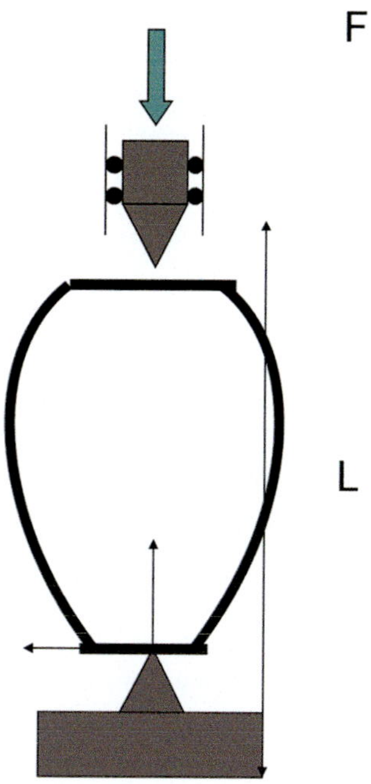


**Fig. 10.2** A short column failing under a critical load by yielding.

The modulus of elasticity is defined as the slope of the stress–strain curve for the beam material in the elastic region (**Fig. 10.5**). Additionally, the beam in Euler's formula must be made of a single material that is homogeneous and isotropic. The spine is neither. Therefore, Euler's formula cannot be applied directly to the spine. However, the "effective" stiffness of the materials of which it is composed, and their interactions with surrounding structures, are directly proportional to the Fcr for the spinal column. The moment of inertia, I, is the resistance to bending of the cross-section of a structure, and is a function of the structure's geometry. In Euler's formula, I must be uniform along the length of the beam to which the formula applies. This is not true for the spine, and the formula

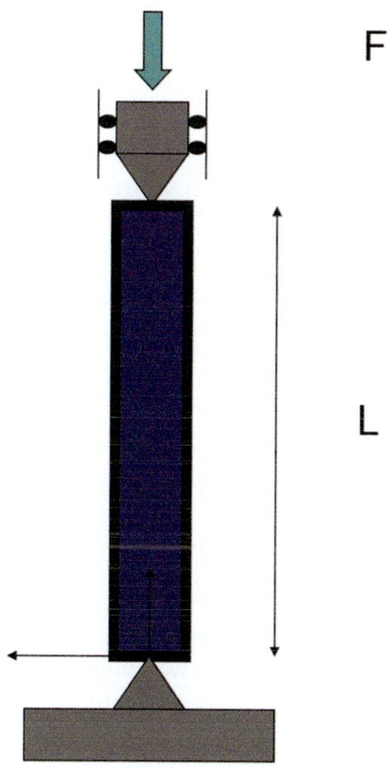


**Fig. 10.3** A long slender column with an axial load applied.

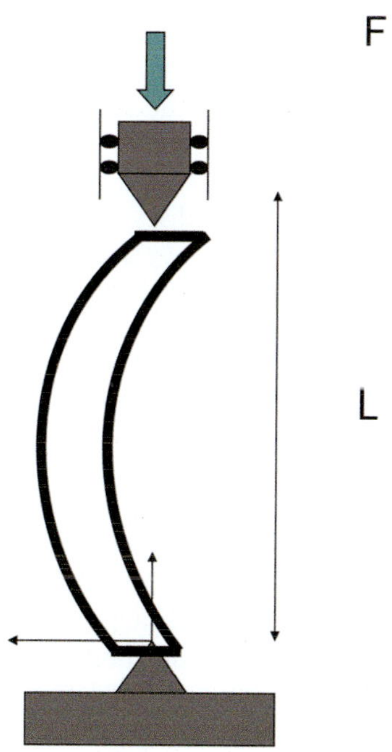


**Fig. 10.4** A long slender column failing under a critical load by buckling.

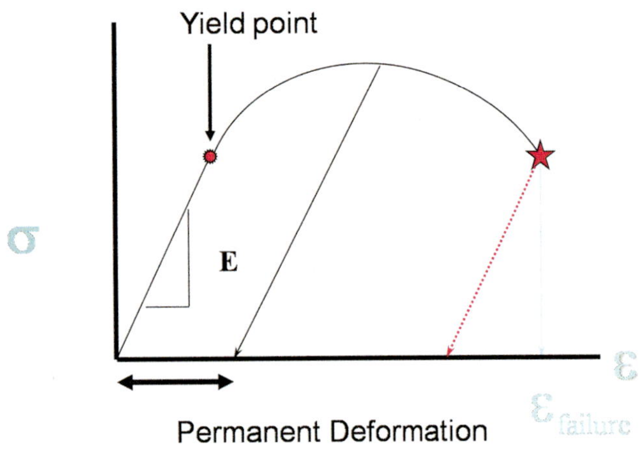


**Fig. 10.5** A stress–strain curve showing the elastic portion of the curve up to the yield point. There is no permanent deformation in this region. The plastic portion of the curve from the yield point to the ultimate tensile strength. Failure of the material at the ultimate tensile strength (*star*).

therefore cannot be applied directly to the spine. The diameter or breadth of the cross-section of the beam is the critical dimension for I. The resistance to bending of the beam is roughly proportional to the fourth power of its diameter. Therefore, if one spine is 20% smaller in diameter than another, its I would be only 41% that of the wider spine, and its Fcr would be ~41% less.

The Fcr needed for buckling of the beam in Euler's formula is inversely proportional to the length of the beam squared. Increasing the length of the beam significantly reduces the force needed to produce buckling of the beam. This relationship is appealing in that adolescent idiopathic scoliosis (AIS) occurs during a rapid growth spurt when the length of the spine is rapidly changing. It may also reflect variations in the mechanical properties of the spine that predispose to its buckling. More specifically, changes in E for that individual spine may reduce the Fcr needed for its buckling. The changes may affect ligaments, discs, and bone itself during the period of rapid growth, thereby predisposing the spine to buckling. Also of interest is Dickson's concept of thoracic lordosis (bending) as the driving force in the development of thoracic scoliosis.

Euler's equation does not specifically reflect the mechanical behavior for a spine, for the following reasons:

1. The structure must consist of an isotropic material, and must have equal physical properties along all of its axes. It must therefore be made of a homogenous material. The axial skeleton does not meet these criteria. It is composed of bone (compact and cancellous), ligaments, and discs. All of which have nonhomogeneous and anisotropic properties.
2. The spine in its normal state is prebuckled. The spine has normal sagittal contours, cervical lordosis, thoracic kyphosis, and lumbar lordosis. This condition is not included in Euler's equation.
3. Scoliosis develops slowly over time; it is not a sudden, catastrophic event as is the buckling of a beam.
4. To satisfy Euler's equation, a column must be a one-dimensional object, be straight, have a distributed load that is contained in one plane, and must be without torsion. Once again the geometry and mechanics of the axial skeleton do not meet these criteria.

The conditions in Euler's formula do predict the failure of a long slender column resembling what is seen in scoliosis. Variations in the E of the spine will predispose to buckling and allow buckling to occur.

Euler, however, gives further insight into the etiology of scoliosis. The terms in his equation are constants except for the length of a given column. Yet spines of a given length do not often progress to develop a given curvature or geometry (moment of inertia, I). The remaining variable is E, the modulus of elasticity. This modulus is a function of the mechanical behavior of the material of which Euler's beam is made. The value of E may vary among spines of a given length if the biological substrate should change. Variations in supporting spinal muscle composition, strength, or both may also result in a global change in the E of the spine. The Fcr needed to produce buckling should not be the focus of attention, but rather factors that alter the composition of the biological substrate. These changes may affect the overall strength of the spine more substantially and allow buckling. Decreasing the value of E would result in reducing Fcr, perhaps resulting in a deformity. A genetic predisposition that resulted in a change in the mechanical properties of the soft tissue of the back, uncoupled neuro-osseous growth, or an anterior–posterior growth mismatch could all affect the value of E of the spinal column. The Fcr needed to precipitate changes in the value of E for the spine could be such that a smaller Fcr would produce a deformity, thereby increasing the risk for curve development in an individual.

## Vertebral Rotation and Coupled Motion

The preceding formulae describing beam deflection and buckling assume that the bending or buckling of the beam or both will occur about the neutral axis. The neutral axis is in the cross-section of a beam or shaft along which there are no longitudinal stresses or strains. If the section is symmetric (in both geometry and materials), the neutral axis is at the geometric centroid. Bending of the beam or shaft about the geometric centroid will not produce rotation. If, however, the axis of rotation is not the neutral axis then rotation will occur with bending. This relationship is called

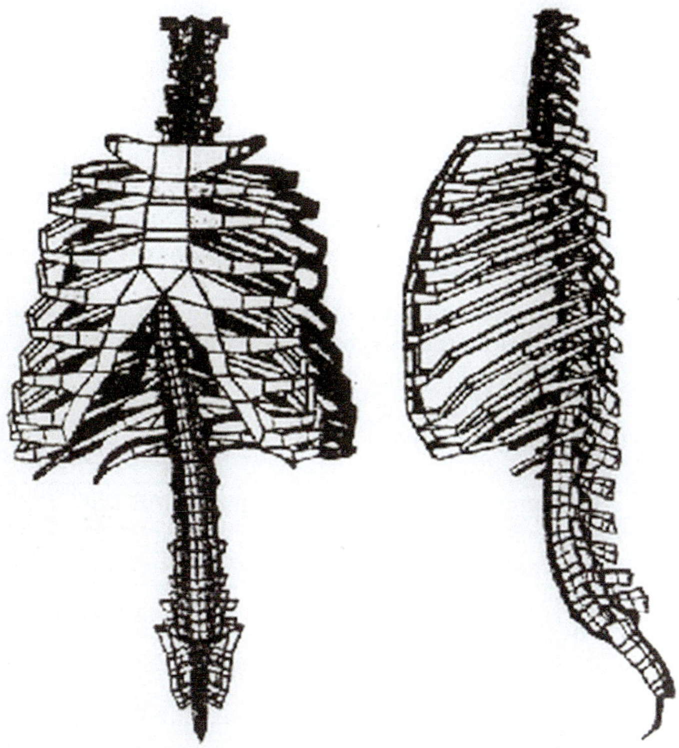

**Fig. 10.6** A finite element model of the spine with the thoracic cage included. Bending and rotation of the spine can be appreciated as described by Azegami.

*coupled motion*. Rotation will result in lateral bending and lateral bending will result in rotation. Coupled motion is the basis for correction of a spinal curve using the derotation maneuver. Derotation of the spine will result in decreasing the lateral bend of a spinal curve. The correction can be achieved without elongation, and a distraction force is therefore not required.

# Anterior Overgrowth Theory

## Uncoupling of Anterior and Posterior Spinal Growth

The spine grows or elongates by anterior and posterior column growth. A balance between these two directions of growth will result in the normal coronal and sagittal planes of the spine. Uncoupled growth, as seen with anterior overgrowth, will result in a deformity. Anterior overgrowth with posterior tethering causes rotation and bending of the spine.[1] This has been called *rotational lordosis*, and results in lordosis, rotation, and lateral deviation.[2]

Scoliosis is an axial rotational deformity. Although it has been postulated as a cause of scoliosis, no empirical evidence exists for rotation as a causative factor in initiating the deformity in scoliosis. Anterior vertebral overgrowth has also been postulated as a causative factor, yet this is difficult to prove in a human or animal model. By using a finite-element model of the human spine including the rib cage, Azegami has attempted to create a deformity by rapid apical vertebral growth.[3] Azegami was able to achieve a 23-degree curve with 7 degrees of rotation by producing rapid growth of the vertebral bodies from T4 to T10. This model provided the proof that uncoupled vertebral growth can precipitate a three dimensional (3D) vertebral deformity similar to scoliosis (**Fig. 10.6**).

## Force Application in the Creation of a Deformity

A 3D spinal deformity may be simulated by the application of force.[4] A model of the thoracolumbar spine was made with vertebrae composed of a synthetic resin and silicon discs. The model was fixed to a metal frame, and the spinal deformation caused by loading was determined relative to 3D coordinates set in the frame. The application of forces to the spine may result in scoliosis. However, these forces must be applied in a distinct order. The most severe scoliosis occurs when the order of loading is rotation, followed by lordosis, followed by lateral flexion (**Fig. 10.7**).

Therefore, factors that promote buckling of the spinal column and the development of scoliosis include:

1. Uncoupled anterior–posterior vertebral growth (vertebral growth modulation)
2. Application of an Fcr to the column (Euler's equation)

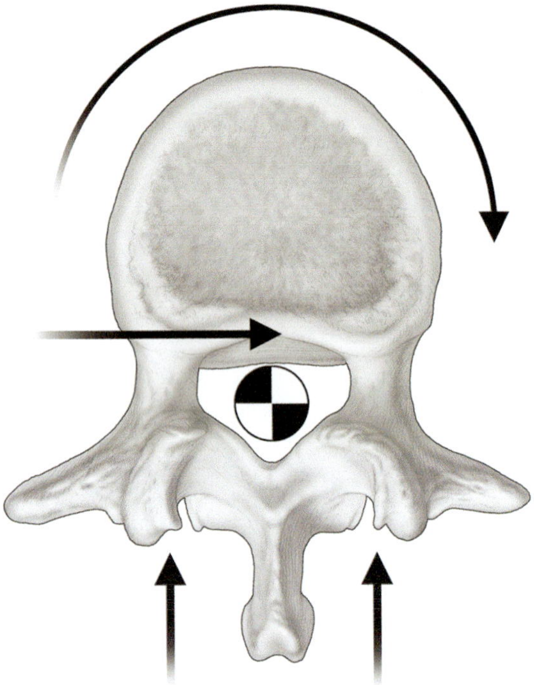

**Fig. 10.7** The application of forces to the spine may result in scoliosis. However, these forces must be applied in a distinct order. The most severe scoliosis occurs when the order of loading is rotation followed by lordosis followed by lateral flexion, as described by Takemura.

3. Application of force to the spine to produce rotation of the vertebral column followed by lordosis and lateral bending (asymmetrical loading)

## Biomechanics of Surgical Correction of Scoliosis

F+ required to overcome or reverse the Fcr causing an abnormal spinal curvature must reverse the lateral bending and the rotation of the spine. Because lateral bending and rotation are coupled, a reversal of one will affect the other. How should the F+ be applied in such a situation? The location of the axis of rotation of the spine will explain the forces required to achieve correction of a deformity.

### The Instantaneous Axis of Rotation

The instantaneous axis of rotation (IAR) is a point about which all other parts of a structure will rotate. It constitutes the center about which the muscles and instrumentation applied to a spinal curve exert their moment during flexion, extension, and torsion. The axis of rotation always migrates to the stiffest part of the structure. This is the mechanical premise for all osteotomies including pedicle subtraction osteotomy (PSO), the Smith–Peterson osteotomy (SPO), and Ponte's innovative osteotomy for kyphosis. As the posterior column of the spine is compromised and shortened, the IAR migrates to the anterior column. The spine rotates about the anterior column. This allows the restoration of sagittal alignment without destroying the anterior column.

### Positive Mechanical Advantage

Increasing the moment arm (the distance over which a force is applied from the IAR) has a positive mechanical advantage. Less force is required to achieve the same moment.

$$\text{Moment} = \text{Force} \times \text{Distance}$$

F+ applied at a distance from the IAR will have a mechanical advantage in controlling and correcting a deformity. Where is the IAR of the spine? Where is the IAR of a scoliotic spine (**Fig. 10.8**)?

The IAR of the spine in rotation is located in the region of the spinal canal. Structures located at a distance from the axis of rotation will have an advantage in controlling motion. This is called a positive mechanical advantage and is the result of a force applied at a distance from the IAR.

The greater the distance from the IAR for a given force the larger the moment observed. If the IAR is located in the anterior column of the spine, the facet joints will have a positive mechanical advantage in resisting rotation, owing to their distance from the IAR and the consequently larger

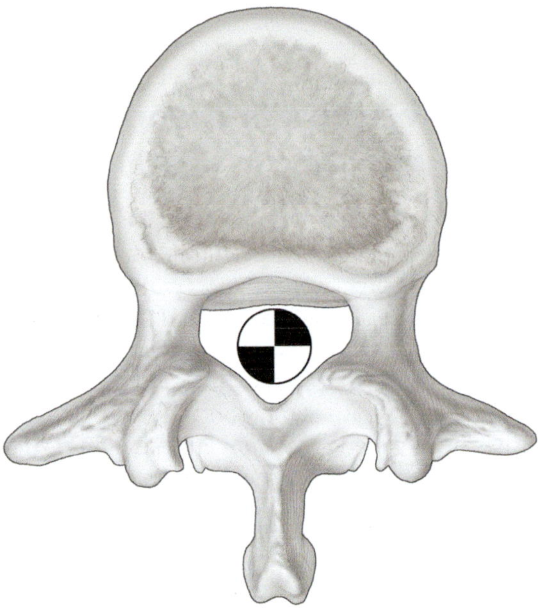

**Fig. 10.8** The IAR of the spine in rotation is located in the region of the spinal canal. Structures at a distance from the axis of rotation will have an advantage in controlling motion.

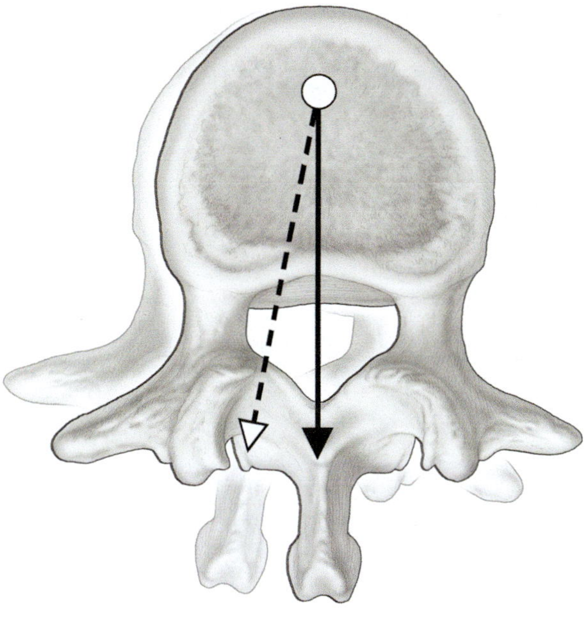

**Fig. 10.9** If the IAR is located in the anterior column of the spine, the facet joints will have a positive mechanical advantage in resisting rotation owing to the distance from the IAR and the larger moment arm.

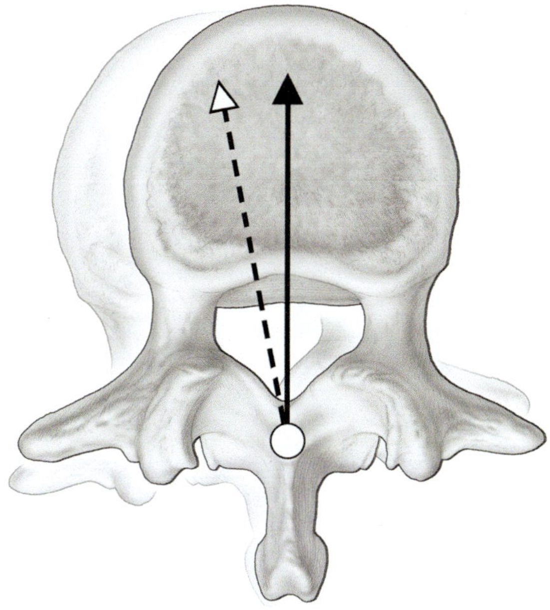

**Fig. 10.10** If the IAR is located in the middle or posterior column the disc has a mechanical advantage due to the larger moment arm. The IAR for the human spine in rotation is located in the vicinity of the middle column. Structures at a distance from the IAR have a mechanical advantage in resisting rotation and force applied further from the IAR have a mechanical advantage in promoting rotation.

moment arm (**Fig. 10.9**). If the IAR is located in the middle or posterior column, the disc has a mechanical advantage owing to the resultingly larger moment arm (**Fig. 10.10**). The IAR for the human spine in rotation is located in the vicinity of the middle column. Structures at a distance from the IAR have a mechanical advantage in resisting rotation, and forces applied further from the IAR have a mechanical advantage in promoting rotation. The clinical application for this is multifold. First, the use of pedicle screws in a construct for correcting a thoracic deformity, and the three-column purchase achieved, significantly improves the ability to predictably treat the entire deformity. Traditionally, the problem of inadequate fixation of the spine and the inability of the construct being used to achieve fixation to withstand the magnitude and vector of the corrective forces applied has often led to minimal correction of an axial deformity. Put simply, posterior instrumentation with a hook (a form of single-column fixation)-and-rod system could not generate sufficient torque for the needed vertebral rotation because the axis of hook fixation was posterior to that of vertebral rotation. This has been validated by studies showing the limited rotational correction achieved with a hook-and-rod construct.[5] The use of pedicle-screw instrumentation and the ability to provide a biomechanically superior construct has advanced the approach to treating spinal deformities posteriorly. With the resulting improved purchase and the freedom to develop corrective tools that increase the distance from the IAR, a rapid evolution of surgical techniques has dramatically improved the coronal and rotational correction of spinal deformities. The most poignant example of this is the technique for direct vertebral body derotation (DVR). Lee and colleagues showed significant coronal-, axial-, and sagittal-plane correction with this technique.[6] The authors' (JA and PC) evaluated CT scans confirmed and quantitated the significantly better axial-plane correction achieved with an all-pedicle-screw (60%) construct than with a hook-and-rod construct (22%).

Furthermore, Suk et al concluded that the pedicle-screw fixation technique effectively spares fusion levels at the distal end of a construct by improving the 3D correction of a deformity and proposed a strategy for determining distal fusion levels based on the neutral vertebrae and potentially shortening curves in single-curve constructs.

## The Anterior Column and its Effect on the Rigidity of a Curve

Destruction of the anterior column has a significant effect on reducing the rotational stiffness of the spine.[7] With removal of the anterior two-thirds of a disc, the spine loses 90% of its rotational stiffness. The middle column has no significant effect on rotational stiffness. Destruction of the

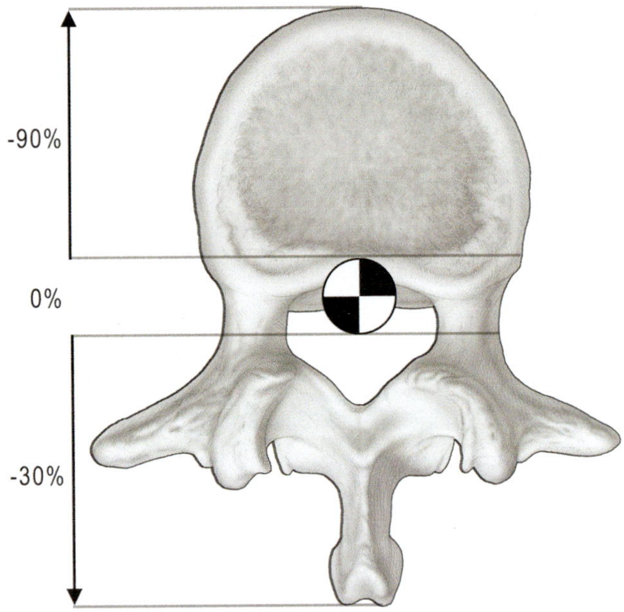


**Fig. 10.11** Destruction of the anterior column has a significant effect on reducing the rotational stiffness of the spine. Removal of the anterior two-thirds of the disc leads to the loss of 90% of rotational stiffness of the spine. The middle column has no significant effect on rotational stiffness. Destruction of the posterior column results in a 30% reduction in spinal stiffness.

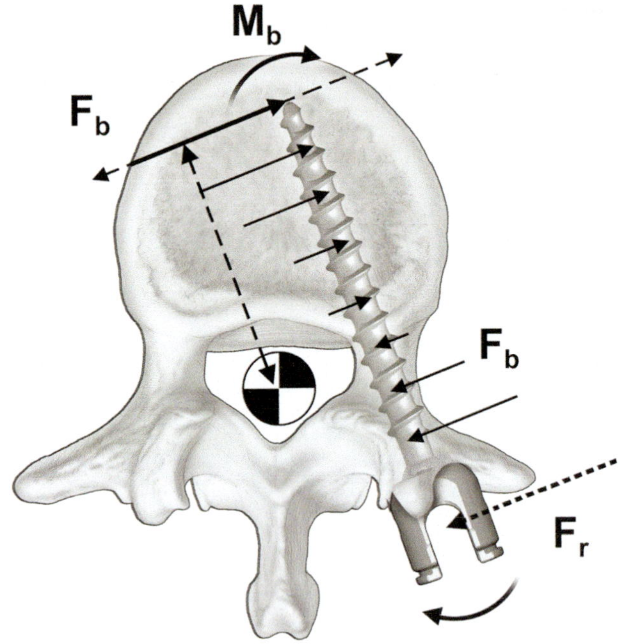


**Fig. 10.12** The mechanical advantage of pedicle screws is apparent because they will transmit forces to all three columns of the spine.

posterior column results in a 30% reduction in spinal stiffness (**Fig. 10.11**).

## Application of Corrective Forces to Restore Coronal- and Sagittal-Plane Curvature

Because the anterior column of the spine is responsible for rotational stiffness, removal of the anterior column (discectomy), application of anterior forces at a distance from the IAR, or both will result in the most efficient application of forces for correcting a deformity. Forces may be applied to the anterior column of the spine while maintaining distance from the IAR through the use of pedicle screws or anterior instrumentation.[6,8–13] The mechanical advantage of pedicle screws is apparent, in that they will transmit forces to all three columns of the spine (**Fig. 10.12**). Lamina hooks have a mechanical disadvantage owing to their proximity to the IAR and their inability to transmit forces to all three columns (**Fig. 10.13**).

The concept that pedicle screws affect all three columns of the spine is supported by force analysis in spinal models.[14] Sawbones® spine models instrumented with posterior screw constructs without transverse connectors were, on average, 482% more rigid than spine models with simulated anterior fusion instrumented with hook constructs and lacking transverse connectors.

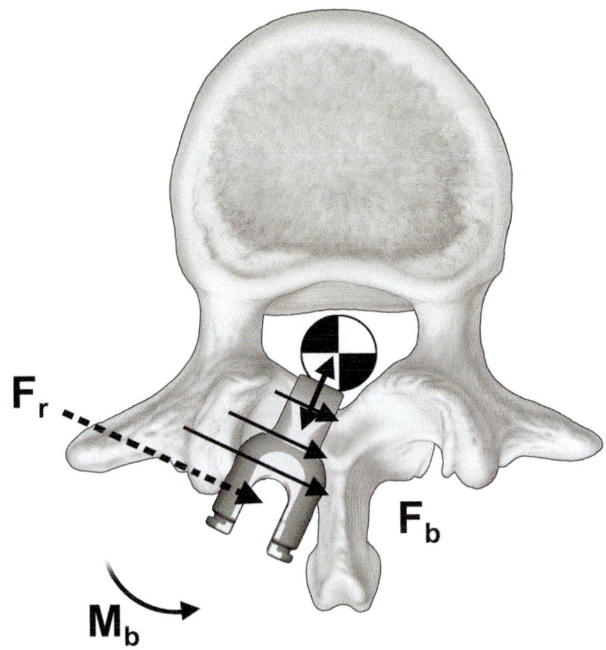


**Fig. 10.13** Lamina hooks have a mechanical disadvantage because of their proximity to the IAR and their inability to transmit forces to all three columns of the spine.

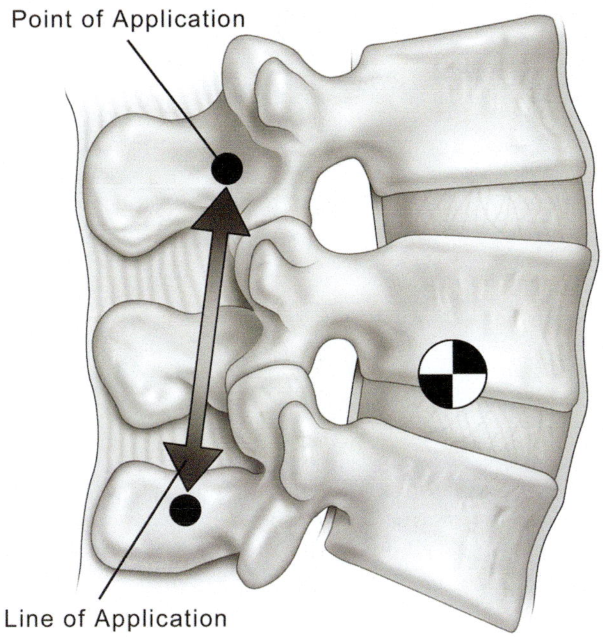


**Fig. 10.14** Knowledge of the magnitude of an applied force, the point and line of application of the force, and the location of the IAR may be used to predict the spine's response to the force as well as the implants ability to resist the applied force.

## Control of the Sagittal Plane as a Function of the IAR

Knowing the magnitude of a force, the point and line of application of the force, and the location of the IAR, the response of the spine to the force may be predicted, as may also the ability of an implant to resist the applied force (**Fig. 10.14**).

The IAR for flexion and extension is located in the vicinity of the disc space of the inferior vertebrae (**Fig. 10.15**).[15]

A distraction force applied posterior to the IAR in the sagittal plane will decrease lumbar lordosis (**Fig. 10.16**). A compressive force applied anteriorly will have the same effect (**Fig. 10.17**).

The response of the spine to the force will also be a function of the distance of the force from the IAR. Posterior constructs should therefore always first compress the convexity of a spinal curve, followed by distraction of the concavity of the curve (**Fig. 10.18**).

## The Kyphogenic Aspects of Anterior Instrumentation

Compression forces anterior to the spine in the sagittal plane are also anterior to the IAR. Therefore, anterior instrumentation in compression produces kyphosis in the thoracic and lumbar spine (**Fig. 10.17**). Such instrumentation is indicated for thoracic curves with hypokyphosis or thoracic lordosis. It is contraindicated with thoracic kyphosis

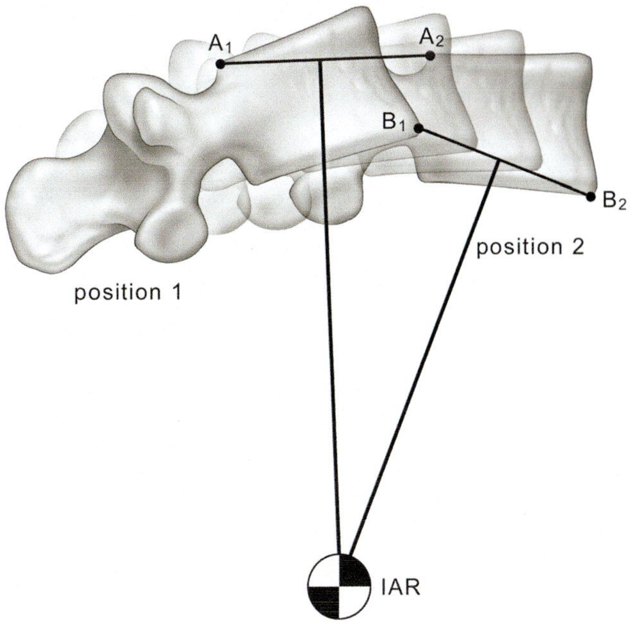


**Fig. 10.15** In the spine, the IAR for flexion and extension is located in the vicinity of the disc space of the inferior vertebrae.

of >40 degrees unless the sagittal profile is recreated with structural interbody grafts.

## Shortening of the Posterior Column in the Treatment of Thoracic Kyphosis

Shortening of the posterior column over each vertebral level in a kyphosis will effectively reduce the kyphosis, sparing the middle and anterior columns. With this, the

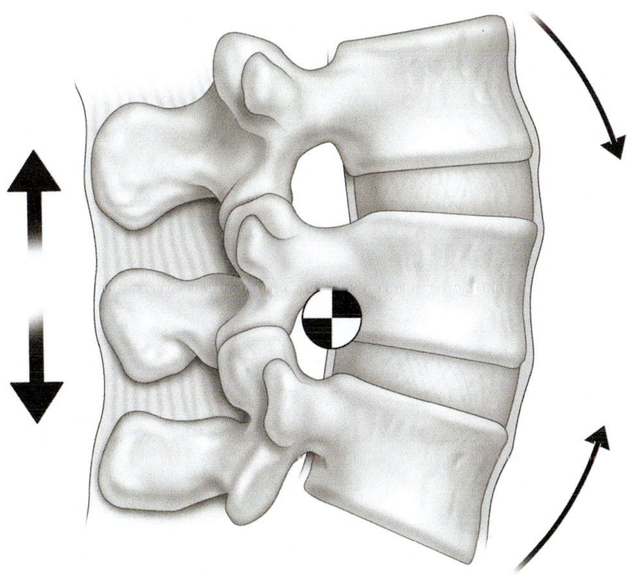

**Fig. 10.16** A distraction force applied posterior to the IAR in the sagittal plane will decrease lumbar lordosis.

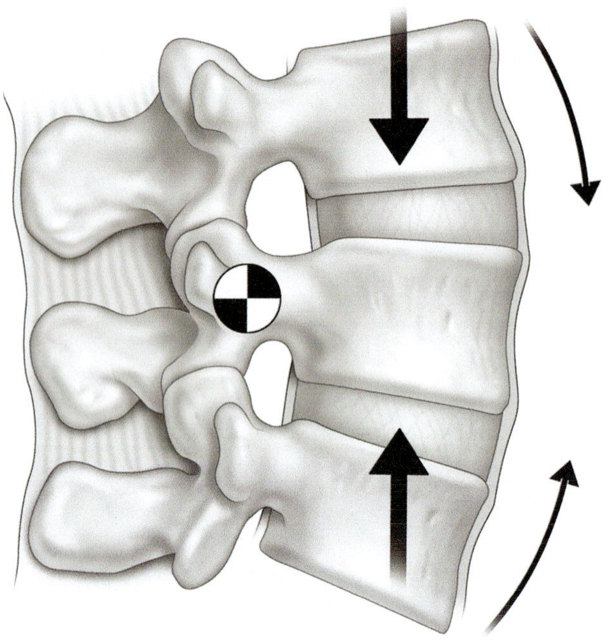

Fig. 10.17 A compressive force applied anteriorly to the IAR in the sagittal plane will decrease lumbar lordosis. Anterior instrumentation in compression will also produce kyphosis in the thoracic and lumbar spine.

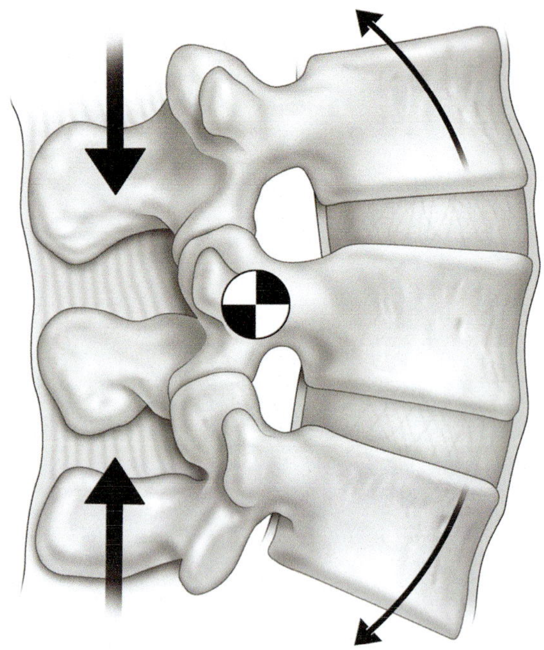

Fig. 10.18 The response of the spine to an applied force will also be a function of the distance of the force from the IAR. Posterior constructs should therefore always compress the convexity of a curve first, followed by distraction of the concavity of the curve.

IAR migrates anteriorly to the anterior aspect of the disc (now the stiffest aspect of the spine). The correction should be harmonious, with an equal distribution of force at each anchor site. This reduces the concentration of stress at the distal hook or screw sites, thereby eliminating distal junctional kyphosis,[16,17] and the same is true for the proximal fixation points.

If a harmonious distribution of forces is not practical, augmentation of the anterior column may be considered. Stiffness in spinal flexion may be significantly increased and rod strains may be significantly reduced when anterior cages are added to each construct in both models and cadaveric spines.[18] Pedicle screws were found to provide more rigid constructs than hooks, but also increased rod strain.[19] Anterior support with titanium cages provides an immediate increase in stiffness of spinal flexion and reduces hardware loading at the distal end of a construct at the price of increasing strains on the superior, adjacent segment.[20]

### The Effect of Cross-links in a Short-Construct Mechanics: The 4R Four-Bar Linkage

Without load-sharing in a single-level experimental model, instability of a four-bar mechanism was clearly demonstrated when all four pedicle screws were parallel.[21] The use of cross-links significantly reduced the rate of failure of this mechanism. The addition of transverse connectors to hook constructs led to an average increase of 380% in rigidity over that of posterior screw constructs without transverse connectors. The addition of transverse connectors to posterior screw constructs increased rigidity by 567% over models that were anteriorly fused and instrumented with hook constructs without transverse connectors. The addition of transverse connectors to posterior-only screw constructs increased the rigidity by 450%.[22]

## The Effect of Implant Geometry on Spinal Stability: Is Bigger Always Better?

### Moment of Inertia

The moment of inertia, I, of a structure is a geometric property of the cross-sectional area of the structure. It describes the spatial distribution of the material in a section of the structure in relation to the neutral axis of the structure. The moment of inertia is a sectional property and is not related to the type of material of which the structure is made. It reflects the ability of this material to resist bending. Essentially, the ability of a rod to support the spine is very sensitive to the diameter of the rod. A small change in the rod diameter has a dramatic effect on the resistance of

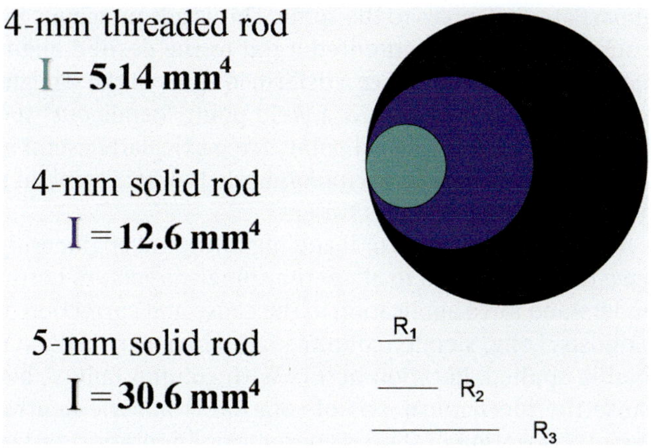


**Fig. 10.19** The moment of inertia, I, of a rod is proportional to the fourth power of the rod radius (*r*). A very small increase in the radius has a large effect on the resistance of the rod to bending.

the rod to bending. For a spinal rod, the area moment of inertia is defined as:

$$I = (\pi/4)r^4$$

where I is proportional to the fourth power of the rod radius, *r*. Thus, a very small increase in rod radius has a large effect on the resistance of the rod to bending, as noted earlier. This effect is shown graphically in **Fig. 10.19**.

The I of a 4-mm threaded rod is 12.56 $mm^4$, whereas the I of a 7-mm rod is 118.0 $mm^4$. The I of a 7-mm rod is therefore 10 times that of a 4-mm rod. The value of I may be calculated for a rod by simply knowing the radius of the rod. When a rod is implanted in the spine, however, the effect of the diameter of the rod on the overall mechanical behavior of the construct of which it is a part becomes more complex. A construct for the treatment of scoliosis is composed of more than one material, with each material having a different stiffness. The equations dealing with the resistance to bending of a construct member composed of multiple materials is complicated.

## Rod Diameter versus Outcome – Linear or Nonlinear

Instruments for measuring outcomes are efficient and effective means of assessing patient satisfaction with a specific treatment. The Harms Study Group database was utilized to correlate the effect of rod diameter in the correction of scoliosis with patient satisfaction. Linear and nonlinear analyses using rod diameter were done and the results compared with outcomes based on the Scoliosis Research Society (SRS-24) health-related quality of life (HRQOL) instrument. All records were sorted according to rod diameter. Entries with non-numerical or missing data were excluded from the analysis. The linear analysis did not show significant correlations between rod diameter and the database parameters. Variations in rod diameters resulted in a fitted $R^2$ of 0.96, calculated with a quadratic equation, in the examination of both functional level of activity and lordosis. Patients with small-diameter rods had higher functional levels of activity at 1- and 2-year follow-up. Despite greater resistance to bending with the use of a bigger rod, clinical outcomes seem to be inversely related to rod diameter. Bigger may not be better!

## The Effect of Yield-point Magnitude on Rod Insertion

In the treatment of scoliosis, corrective forces are applied to the spine through devices such as rods, plates, cables, and even springs. These devices or members of a construct must be orders of magnitude stiffer and stronger than the structure they are supporting. If a device such as a rod is too stiff, it may prove difficult to engage a force anchor (hook, screw, etc.) to the rod, or the anchor may disengage from the bone into which it has been inserted when the rod is engaged. Is it possible to maintain the stiffness and strength of a rod while decreasing its resistance to bending? The answer lies in the concept of yielding or the location of the yield point on the stress–strain curve for the rod (**Fig. 10.20**).

The yield point or yield strength is defined as the stress needed to achieve permanent deformation of a structure. It is the point at which the elastic (nonpermanent) deformation

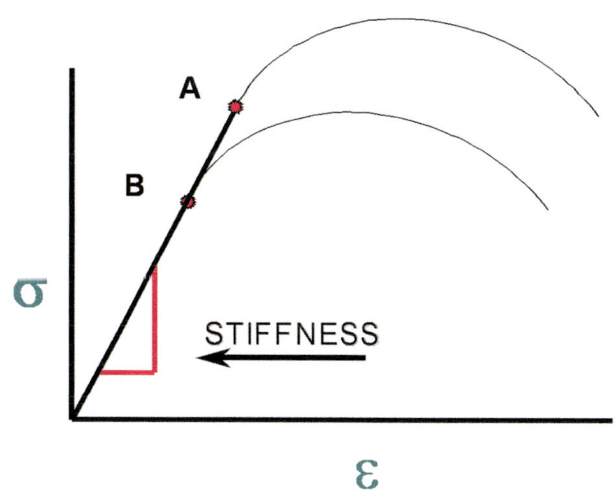


**Fig. 10.20** The yield point or yield strength is defined as the stress needed to achieve permanent deformation of a structure. It is the point where elastic (nonpermanent) deformation ends and plastic (permanent) deformation begins. It is independent of the stiffness (modulus) and strength of the rod.

of the structure ends and plastic (permanent) deformation begins. The yield point is independent of the stiffness (modulus) and strength of a structure such as a rod; stiffness refers to the point on the stress–strain curve at which the rod fractures. The yield point may be reduced while the stiffness and strength of the rod remain constant. Materials with this property are currently available for use; they constitute the family of commercially pure titanium (CP Ti) metal. Rods with a lower yield point are ideal for in situ bending, which facilitates their engagement to the anchor in complex curves. One should therefore consider the manufacturer's disclosed yield point of a rod as well as its strength and stiffness in evaluating its suitability for inclusion in a construct.

## Construct Stiffness as a Function of the Number of Anchors

Orchowski et al[19] investigated the relationship between rod size and hook numbers in construct stiffness. In three-point bending tests, the expected stiffness values for rods of varying diameters were as predicted; increasing rod diameter in the model construct produced an increase in stiffness. Interestingly, increasing hook number also had a significant effect on construct stiffness (**Fig. 10.21**).[23] A smaller-diameter rod with a low yield point, used in conjunction with multiple anchors, could be affixed to the anchors with relatively low stress to the anchors and the anchor–bone interface, but still have high overall rigidity owing to the high implant density.

Surgeons often require rods with high yield points. These rods maintain their shape when stressed and in turn impart applied forces to the spine. This is advantageous for a surgeon who has contoured a rod to the desired alignment and wishes to reduce a deformed spine to the straight rod. A rod that has too low a yield point "bends out" too easily. Rods with high yield points are particularly useful in imparting kyphosis to a hypokyphotic thoracic spine in a typical idiopathic scoliosis patient.

Concepts from structural and metallurgical engineering have been presented to allow the spinal surgeon to better understand force application in the cause and correction of scoliosis. Long, slender columns fail when a critical axial load is applied. Rotation occurs with column failure, because the mechanical axis of rotation is not the neutral axis. The location of the axis of rotation in rotation and in flexion has been defined so that the surgeon may better understand the effects of an applied force to the spine. A rod with a lower yield point requires the application of less force to achieve a permanent deformation, and the stiffness of a construct may be increased by increasing the number of anchor points. The understanding of these simple concepts will enhance the surgeon's ability to achieve 3D correction of a deformity. Clinically, however, an increase in the density of anchor points has a detrimental effect on the sagittal plane, apical rotational thoracic lordosis. Clements et al found a loss of preoperative kyphosis with increasing implant density.[22] Similarly, a statistically significant loss of preoperative kyphosis was noted to depend on implant type, in terms of whether an implant was anchored with hooks alone, or used hybrid anchoring, or was an all-pedicle-screw construct.[5] All pedicle screw constructs decreased the thoracic kyphosis more than the other two anchor constructs.

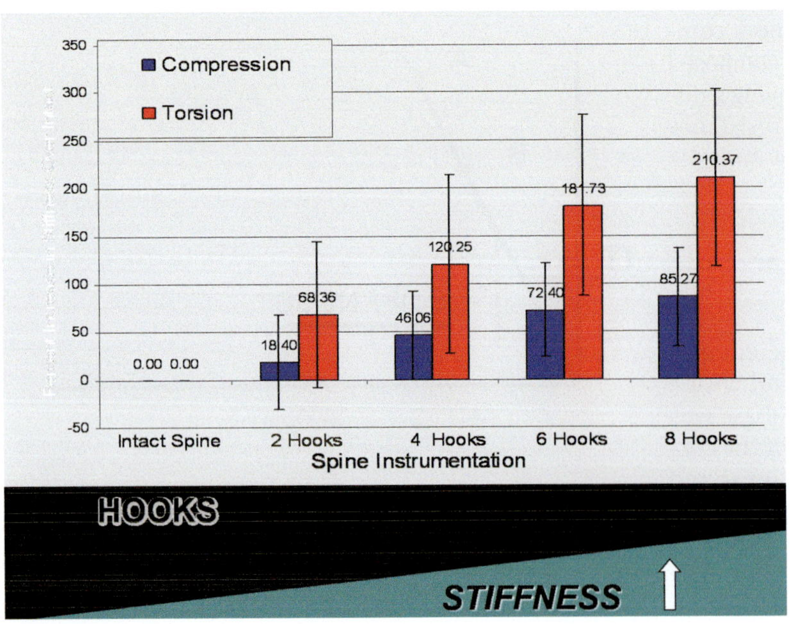


**Fig. 10.21** Increasing the number of anchors has a significant effect on the stiffness of a construct for treating scoliosis.

# Appendix: Glossary

## Euler–Bernoulli Beam Theory

For a long, slender, one-dimensional (1D) beam made of isotropic material, it can be shown that the elastic curve of the beam must satisfy:

$$\frac{\partial^2}{\partial x^2}\left(EI\,\frac{\partial^2 u}{\partial x^2}\right) = w$$

This is the Euler–Bernoulli equation. The curve u(x) describes the deflection u of a beam at some position $x$ (recall that the beam is modeled as a 1D object). The result, $w$, is a distributed load, or in other words a force per unit length (analogous to pressure); it may be a function of $x$, $u$, or other variables.

Note that E is the elastic modulus and that I is the second moment of area. I must be calculated with respect to the centroidal axis perpendicular to the applied loading; for a beam to which the Euler–Bernoulli equation applies, this axis is called the neutral axis.

Often, $u = u(x)$, $w = w(x)$, and EI is a constant, so that:

$$EI\,\frac{d^4u}{dx^4} = w(x)$$

This equation is very common in engineering practice: it describes the deflection of a uniform, static beam.

Successive derivatives of u have important meaning:

- $u$ is the deflection of the beam.
- $\frac{\partial u}{\partial x}$ is the slope of the beam.
- $EI\frac{\partial^2 u}{\partial x^2}$ is the bending moment in the beam.
- $-\frac{\partial}{\partial x}\left(EI\frac{\partial^2 u}{\partial x^2}\right)$ is the shear force in the beam.

## Engineering Terms and Definitions

A. Terms related to loading on or within objects

1. Load: A general term describing the application of a force, a moment (torque), or both to an object. The unit of measure for the force is the newton (N), or pound force (lbs), and the unit of measure for the moment is the newtonmeter (Nm) or foot-pound (ft-lb).
2. Compression: The normal force that tends to push together material fibers or finite material units. The unit of measure is the newton (N; pound force).
3. Tension: A normal force that tends to elongate the fibers or finite material units of a material oriented in the direction of load. The unit of measure is the newton (N; pound force).
4. Shear: A force parallel to the surface upon which it acts, which tends to angulate the material fibers or finite material units oriented perpendicularly to the surface.
5. Moment: (Couple) A pair of equal and opposite parallel forces acting on a body and separated by a distance. The moment or torque of a couple is defined as a quantity equal to the product of one of the forces and the perpendicular distance between the forces. The unit of measure for the torque is the newton·meter ((N · m)foot-pound force).
6. Torsion: A type of load that is applied by a force couple (two forces parallel and directed opposite to each other) about the long axis of a structure. The load is called torque. It produces relative rotation of different axial sections of the structure with respect to each other. For a straight structure, all the sections are subjected to the same torque on the ends of the structure. The magnitude of bending with torsion depends on the orientation of the particular cross-section at which bending occurs with respect to the torque axis.
7. Force: Any action that tends to change the state of rest or motion of a body to which it is applied. The unit of measure for the magnitude of force is N or lbs.
8. Stress: The force per unit area acting on an object, and a measure of the intensity of the force or distribution of the force throughout the object. There are two kinds of stress: normal and shear. The normal stress on an object is perpendicular to the plane of a cross-section of the object. The normal stress can be tensile or compressive. Shear stress is parallel to a cross-section of the object. The unit of measure of stress is newtons per square millimeter ($N/mm^2$) or megapascals (MPa), or pound force per square inch (psi).
9. Pressure: The contact stress between two surfaces, or the stress generated in a fluid under load. The unit of measure of pressure is MPa or psi.
10. Static load: A load applied to a specimen is called static if it remains constant with respect to time.
11. Dynamic load: A load applied to an object is called dynamic if it varies with time.
12. Steady state: A condition in which regular, dynamic loads are applied to a structure in cycles and the response of the structure is the same for each cycle.

B. Terms related to distortion within or movement of an object

1. Deflection: The relative movement of any two points on an object as the result of distortion of that object under load.
2. Displacement: The relative movement of any point on an object in relation to a fixed reference frame. Such movement may or may not involve distortion of the object.
3. Strain: The change in length or angle of a material subjected to a load. There are two types of strain: normal

and shear. The former is defined as the change in length of a material divided by its original length. Normal strain can be tensile or compressive. The latter is defined as the change in angle of a material under the influence of a load. The units of measure of strain are dimensionless (i.e., mm/mm, inches/inch, or % change).

4. Angulation: An angular change in the shape or position of an object as the result of an applied loads.
5. Rotation: An angular change in the position of an object.
6. Bending: A distortion that occurs when a load is applied to a long structure that is not directly supported at the point of application of the load. The structure deforms by moving with the direction of the load, with the supported portion remaining in place.
7. Twisting: A deformation of a long structure that is not directly supported at the point of application of a load when a moment is applied to the structure. The structure deforms by rotating in the direction of the moment, but the supported portion remains in place.

C. Terms related to the graphical representation of loading and distortion or movements

1. Stress–strain curve: A graphical representation of the relationship between the stress and strain in the material of an object at a fixed position in the object under a load. Terms associated with the stress–strain curve include:
2. Load–deflection curve: A graphical representation of the relationship between the load on an object and the deflection of a given point on the object.
3. S/N curve: A graphical representation of fatigue-test plotting stress (or load) versus the number of cycles to failure for a cyclic (dynamic) loading of an object. The number of cycles is usually represented in a logarithmic scale.
4. Creep curve: A plot of the strain or deformation versus time for an object under a static load.
5. Relaxation curve: A plot of the stress or load versus time for an object under a static deformation, deflection, or strain.

D. Terms related to the stiffness or rigidity of objects

1. Modulus of elasticity: The ratio of normal stress to normal strain (slope of the elastic portion of the stress–strain curve) in a material. The unit of measure for the modulus of elasticity is MPa, or gigapascals (GPa), or pounds per square inch (psi) (also known as Young's modulus, elastic modulus).
2. Stiffness: A measure of resistance offered to external loads by a specimen or structure as it deforms. This phenomenon is characterized by the stiffness coefficient.
3. Structural rigidity or structural stiffness: The resistance of a structure to compression, tension, bending, or rotational loading. The slope of the load–deflection curve for a given structural test of an object. Structural rigidity is a function of the modulus of elasticity and size and shape (length, cross-sectional area, area and polar moments of inertia) of an object, and for structures with joints, of the neutral zone(s). Structural rigidity is expressed in load/deformation (i.e., N of force/mm of deformation, N · m of moment or torque/degree of deformation, etc.)
4. For structures of uniform cross-section and consisting of a single material, the structural stiffness of the member can be expressed as the modulus of elasticity, E, times the appropriate moment of inertia, I, which quantifies the distribution of material in the cross-section. In bending, the area moment of inertia, Ixx, is calculated relative to the X-axis perpendicular to the plane of bending. In torque, the polar moment of inertia, Ip, is calculated in polar coordinates relative to the axis of rotation of the torque load.

E. Terms related to the strength characteristics of an object

1. Yield stress is the maximum stress that the material of an object can bear in the elastic range of behavior; all stress above this level will cause plastic deformation of the object (also known as yield strength, proportional limit, elastic limit).
2. Ultimate stress is the maximum stress that the material of an object can bear (ultimate strength, ultimate limit).
3. Column stability: The resistance of a column-like structure to buckling. Column stability is related to the width-to-length ratio of the column, the degrees of freedom and resistance to rotation of the ends of the column, and the curvature of the column, in addition to the location and type of loading applied to the column.
4. Energy to yield, ultimate, or other failure: The area under the stress–strain curve for a structure to the point at which the desired event occurs.
5. Fatigue limit (low cycle): The load or stress level that an object can withstand without failure for a given number of cycles.
6. Endurance limit: The load or stress level that an object can withstand without failure for an infinite number of cycles.

F. General terms relating to mechanical behavior or material characteristics that influence mechanical behavior

1. Material behavior: Any description of the mechanical properties of a material (without regard to the size or shape of any objects made of that material).
2. Structural behavior: Any description of the mechanical characteristics of an object taking into account its size, shape, materials, orientation to loads, etc.
3. Isotropic material: A material whose mechanical properties are the same in all directions.
4. Anisotropic material: A material whose mechanical properties vary as a function of direction within a structure or object made of the material.

5. Homogeneous: A term referring to a structure or object whose mechanical properties are the same in all locations.
6. Nonhomegeneous: A term referring to a structure or object whose mechanical properties vary as a function of position within the structure or object.
7. Elasticity: Property of a material or structure to return to its original form following the removal of a deforming load.
8. Plasticity: Property of a material or structure to remain permanently deformed after the removal of a deforming load.
9. Viscoelastic: A term describing materials that exhibit time-dependent mechanical behavior (both viscous and elastic behavior).
10. Creep: Increasing strain or distortion with time of a material under constant load.
11. Stress relaxation: Under constant deforming stress, decreasing resistance to a load or stress with time.
12. Strain-rate/load-rate dependence: Variable resistance to a load related to the rate at which the load is applied.
13. Moment of inertia of an area: A measure of the distribution of material around a central axis or plane. This distribution influences the strength and stiffness of a material under bending or torsional loads. The unit of measure of the moment of inertia of an area is millimeters to the fourth power (inches to the fourth power).
14. Degrees of freedom: The number on independent coordinates, in a coordinate system, needed to completely specify the position or movement of an object in space.
15. Rigid-body analysis: A method of simplifying the behavior of moving objects or structures made up of components that have very significant differences in stiffness so that the distortions or strains in the relatively rigid components may be ignored.
16. Vector: A representation of a force or load with an arrow that has the properties of sense, direction, and magnitude.
17. Equilibrium: A condition in which the loads on an object are balanced between the actions and reactions of the object so that no movement of the object takes place.
18. Ductile: Capable of sustaining large plastic deformations without fracture (e.g., in metals, the ability to be drawn into a wire).
19. Brittle: Having little tendency to deform (or strain) before fracture.
20. Notch sensitivity: A measure of the reduction in strength of a metal caused by the presence of stress concentration. Values of notch sensitivity can be obtained from static, impact, or fatigue tests.
21. Wear: A process in which interaction of the surface(s) or bounding face(s) of a solid with the working environment results in dimensional loss of the solid, with or without loss of material.
22. Micromotion: Minute, relative movement ($<1$ mm in magnitude) of two surfaces or interfaces relative to one another.

## References


1. Azegami H, Murachi S, Kitoh J, Ishida Y, Kawakami N, Makino M. Etiology of idiopathic scoliosis. Computational study. Clin Orthop Relat Res 1998;357:229–236
2. Takemura Y, Yamamoto H, Tani T. Biomechanical study of the development of scoliosis, using a thoracolumbar spine model. J Orthop Sci 1999;4:439–445
3. Haher TR, O'Brien M, Felmly WT, et al. Instantaneous axis of rotation as a function of the three columns of the spine. Spine 1992; 17(6, suppl):S149–S154
4. Haher TR, Felmy W, Baruch H, et al. The contribution of the three columns of the spine to rotational stability. A biomechanical model. Spine 1989;14:663–669
5. Clements D, Betz R, Newton P, et al. Correlation of scoliosis curve correction with the number and type of fixation anchors. Spine 2009.
6. Lee SH, Shufflebarger HL, Milne EL, et al. Mechanical effect of anterior column support in the distal lumbar spine in a long fusion model. Paper presented at: 45th Annual Meeting of the Orthopedic Research Society, 1999
7. Hall JE. The anterior approach to spinal deformities. Orthop Clin North Am 1972;3(1):81–98
8. Harms J, Jeszenszky D, Beele B. Ventral correction of thoracic scoliosis. In: Bridwell K, DeWald R, eds. The Textbook of Spinal Surgery, ed. 2. Philadelphia, PA: Lippincott-Raven; 1997:616.
9. Betz RR, Lenke LG, Harms J. Anterior instrumentation. Spine 2000;14:115
10. Betz RR, Harms J, Clements DH III, et al. Comparison of anterior and posterior instrumentation for correction of adolescent thoracic idiopathic scoliosis. Spine 1999;24:225–239
11. Haher T, Merola A, Gorup J, et al. The treatment of AIS using VDS: A clinical study in 50 patients. Orthop Trans 1997;21:357–358
12. Kaneda Y, Shono Y, Satoh S, et al. Anterior correction of thoracic scoliosis with Kaneda anterior spinal system. Orthop Trans 1997;21:25
13. Haher TR, Bergman M, O'Brien M, et al. The effect of the three columns of the spine on the instantaneous axis of rotation in flexion and extension. Spine 1991; 16(8, suppl):S312–S318
14. Ponte A, Siccardi GL. Scheuermann's kyphosis: posterior shortening procedure by segmental closing wedge resections. Orthop Trans 1995;19:603
15. Ponte A. Posterior column shortening for Scheuermann's kyphosis: an innovative one state technique. In: Haher TR, Merola AA, eds. Surgical Techniques for the Spine. New York: Thieme, 2003:304

16. Lee JY, Shufflebarger HL, Milne EL, et al. Anterior column support in long segment kyphosis constructs. J Spinal Disord 2000
17. Carson WL, Duffield RC, Arendt M, Ridgely BJ, Gaines RW Jr. Internal forces and moments in transpedicular spine instrumentation. The effect of pedicle screw angle and transfixation: The 4R-4bar linkage concept. Spine 1990;15:893–901
18. 32nd Annual Meeting of the Scoliosis Research Society. St. Louis, MO, Sept. 1997
19. Lonner B, Muller E, Betz R, Crawford A, Lowe T, Newton P. The effect of rod diameter on scoliosis correction. E-poster at 13th IMAST Athens, Greece. July 12–15, 2006. Shah S, Newton P, Lonner B, Shufflebarger H, Bastrom T, Marks M. Harms Study Group. Rod strength: Is it an important factor in coronal and sagittal realignment after surgery for adolescent idiopathic scoliosis? Podium presentation at the 44th Annual Meeting of the Scoliosis Research Society. San Antonio, TX, Sept. 23–26, 2009
20. Malik A, Gonzales A, Milne EL, et al. Torsional rigidity of long scoliotic constructs: Hooks versus screws. Biomed Eng. Miami: Miami, School of Engr, 2004
21. Orchowski J, Polly DW Jr, Klemme WR, Oda I, Cunningham B. The effect of kyphosis on the mechanical strength of a long-segment posterior construct using a synthetic model. Spine 2000;25: 1644–1648
22. Clements D, Betz R, Newton P, et al. Are we improving postoperative sagittal contour with new posterior instrumentation compared to "old school" instrumentation. Paper presented at: 44th Annual Meeting of the Scoliosis Research Society. San Antonio, TX, Sept. 23–26, 2009
23. Helgeson MD, Shah S, Newton P, et al. Evaluation of proximal junctional kyphosis in adolescent idiopathic scoliosis following pedicle screw, hook, or hybrid instrumentation. Manuscript in preparation 2009

# 11 Anesthesia for Scoliosis Surgery

*Elizabeth Demers Lavelle, Mohamed Mahmoud, See Wan Tham, Mark Vadney, and Sara Lozano*

Although surgery on pediatric patients was attempted before the introduction of anesthesia into clinical medicine in 1846, the lengths and types of procedures that children could endure significantly limited surgical practice.[1] Pediatric spine surgery, particularly the correction of scoliosis, has now become a routine element of pediatric anesthesia practice. Patients undergoing scoliosis surgery present unique physiological and pharmacological challenges for the anesthesiologist. Pediatric anesthesia is rapidly advancing as new anesthetic techniques, pharmacological options, blood-replacement modalities, neurophysiological monitoring, and surgical techniques become available.

## Preoperative Evaluation and Preparation

A multidisciplinary approach is needed in the preoperative preparation of a patient for spinal deformity surgery. Both the surgeon and anesthesiologist must evaluate and explain the risks and benefits of all components of the surgical procedure to the patient and patient's family. Scoliosis carries several risks that need significant consideration before the induction of anesthesia. The primary physiological concern is the patient's cardiopulmonary function. Patients must also have hematological, nutritional, and neurological preoperative evaluation.

### Pulmonary Considerations

The pulmonary system is the most obvious preoperative concern, and can be significantly affected by the structural changes brought about by a scoliotic spine. In cases of extreme scoliosis, exercise tolerance testing is the best screening tool for pulmonary performance. Patients should undergo preoperative pulmonary function tests if they have:

- A history of poor exercise tolerance
- A curve >60 degrees associated with a history of reactive airway disease,
- A curve >80 degrees
- Neuromuscular scoliosis

Patients for whom an anterior approach is planned should receive additional consideration for pulmonary evaluation. The most common respiratory defect in scoliosis is restrictive, with a decrease in vital capacity (VC) and forced expiratory volume in 1 second (FEV1) as the scoliotic angle increases. The respiratory compromise may take the form of chronic alveolar hypoventilation, atrial hypoxia, ventilation–perfusion (V-Q) mismatch, and pulmonary hypertension with progression to cor pulmonale.[2] Patients with preoperative Cobb angles >100 degrees can have a significantly diminished VC, nearing 45% of normal. A VC of 45% or less or a forced vital capacity (FVC) of 30% less than predicted is an indicator of the possible need for postoperative ventilation.[3] Patients with severe Cobb angles can have difficulty with clearing their airways through coughing, particularly with the coupling of postoperative pain. This can result postoperatively in atelectasis, pneumonia, and possible aspiration.

### Cardiac Considerations

Depending on the magnitude of a patient's scoliosis and the patient's coexisting disease state, preoperative cardiac testing may be required. This includes an electrocardiogram (ECG), echocardiogram, or stress testing. The cardiac system can be secondarily affected by severe deformities, possibly leading to cor pulmonale. Patients with scoliosis associated with genetic deformities have a significantly higher rate of cardiac deformities and merit preoperative investigation. Mitral valve prolapse, coarctation, and cyanotic heart disease are the most commonly found pathologies in patients with scoliosis.[2] Duchene muscular dystrophy can present as septal hypertrophy, which can lead to cardiomyopathy and manifest as arrhythmias or heart blocks.[4]

### Hemotological and Nutritional Considerations

Patients with scoliosis should have blood work done to evaluate their initial hematocrit and platelet count. Because major blood loss (>50% blood volume) may occur during scoliosis surgery, a blood type and crossmatch analysis should be obtained preoperatively. Nutritional status, particularly in patients with neuromuscular scoliosis, should be evaluated with blood testing, including assays for albumin and vitamin K, and a basic metabolic panel. Clotting abnormalities are associated with patients with poor nutrition and vitamin K deficiency.[5] These concerns need to be corrected before surgery to optimize the patient's status for surgery. Discussions should be initiated about blood replacement during surgery and the possibility of autologous donation. Murray et al reported that 90% of adolescent patients with scoliosis who had autologous predonation of blood avoided allogenic red-cell transfusions.[6] Postoperative facial swelling should be discussed with the patient's family because it may result from necessary fluid replacement as well as from placement of the patient in the prone position for an extended period.

### Neurological Considerations

A neurological evaluation should be done before surgery to monitor for deficits and identify whether any changes have occurred in the patient's neurological status. To this end, a basic discussion of neurophysiological monitoring and the possibility of a wake-up test should be discussed with the patient and the patient's family.

### Fasting Guidelines

Guidelines for adolescents and adults undergoing scoliosis surgery require that nothing be taken by mouth after midnight of the night before surgery, with the exception of a sip of water with morning medications. Younger patients may be given clear liquids until 2 hours before surgery, breast milk until 4 hours before surgery, and a light meal or cow's milk until 6 hours before surgery.[7]

## Preoperative Medication

Adolescent patients preparing for scoliosis surgery may decide to proceed with preoperative intravenous catheter placement or with oral benzodiazepines followed by an inhalational induction of anesthesia. If a patient elects to have an intravenous catheter inserted, traditional intravenous premedication with anxiolytic agents is warranted for appropriate candidates. Further medication may be warranted for this specific surgery. Use of gabapentin has been discussed as a means for addressing neuropathic postoperative pain if it is started preoperatively. Albuterol may be helpful for patients who have a bronchial restrictive pattern to their disease process. Narcotics or medications that would depress respiration should be avoided preoperatively, including anticholinergic drugs.

## Induction and Maintenance of Anesthesia

The mechanisms of anesthesia can be described as the presence of three linked conditions: (1) amnesia and hypnosis; (2) analgesia; and (3) muscle relaxation. In providing care for the surgical correction of scoliosis, these three conditions must be carefully managed and balanced. Profound analgesia is necessary to provide optimal conditions for neurophysiological monitoring, wake-up testing, or both. General anesthesia including intubation and mechanical ventilation constitutes standard care for all patients having spinal surgery.[8]

### Induction

Anesthesia in pediatric patients can be induced either through an inhalational or intravenous technique. Patients with airways that are difficult to intubate should have an intravenous catheter placed before the induction of anesthesia whenever possible. Sevoflurane is currently the most commonly used volatile agent for induction of anesthesia via a face mask. Its advantages include a nonpungent odor, low incidence of respiratory irritation, and little myocardial depression and arrhythmia in normal clinical use. Sevoflurane may be combined with nitrous oxide to hasten the onset of induction. Although the choice of intravenous induction for IV induction may vary depending on the patient's comorbidities, propofol is the most commonly used intravenous induction agent.

Intubation of the trachea may be facilitated by use of a muscle relaxant. The choice of muscle relaxant is based on the required onset and duration of paralysis, with consideration also given to the side effects and comorbidities of the individual patient. Muscle relaxation with a nondepolarizing neuromuscular blocking agent such as rocuronium, vecuronium, cisatracurium, or atracurium produce paralysis for ~20 to 30 minutes, which typically coincides with the period needed to obtain vascular access, place monitors, and position the patient. Succinylcholine is the only depolarizing neuromuscular blocking agent available, and can have adverse side effects including malignant hyperthermia in susceptible patients, severe hyperkalemia leading to cardiac arrest, myalgias, bradycardia, and flushing. Typically, succinylcholine is held in reserve by pediatric anesthesiologists as an emergency drug.

### Airway Management

After the induction of anesthesia, maintaining and managing the patient's airway is of utmost importance to the anesthesiologist. Typically, the patient is mask ventilated until adequate muscle relaxation is obtained. This is accomplished with a face mask and bag technique with the patient's head tilted and jaw lifted anteriorly. An oral or

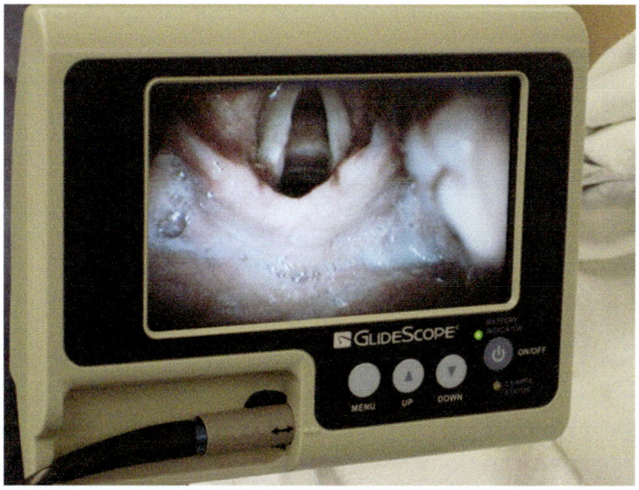


**Fig. 11.1** View of the vocal cords through the GlideScope.

nasal airway device can be inserted as necessary to maintain a patent upper airway.

Children with adolescent idiopathic scoliosis (AIS) rarely present difficulty in airway management and intubation. However, patients with coexisting syndromes may present a more difficult situation, and the anesthesiologist should make preoperative airway management plans for them. Klippel–Feil syndrome, spondyloepithelial dysplasia, any of the mucopolysaccharidoses, arthrogryposis multiplex, mandibulofacial dystosis, or Goldenhar syndrome can be associated with particularly difficult airway anatomy. These patients may require a fiberoptically guided intubation under sedation and use of additional airway equipment, such as a laryngeal mask airway or the GlideScope (**Fig. 11.1**).

A wire-reinforced endotracheal tube may be considered for avoiding tube kinking and occlusion when turning the patient from the supine to the prone position. After the airway is secured, particular attention must be given to securing the endotracheal tube, because the patient will remain in the prone position and may have secretions that pool around the mouth.

### Maintenance

The maintenance of anesthesia for patients undergoing surgical correction of scoliosis largely depends on the necessity of monitoring the spinal cord and on surgical preference. Monitoring of somatosensory evoked potentials (SSEPs) and motor evoked potentials (MEPs) is accepted as the standard of care for neurophysiological monitoring during scoliosis surgery.[9] The impact of anesthetic agents on spinal cord monitoring increases as more synapses in the neurological pathways are monitored.[10] Because inhalational anesthetic agents considerably depress the amplitude of transcranial electrical MEPs (TceMEPs) in a dose-dependent manner, total intravenous anesthesia (TIVA) has been increasingly used during spine surgery to provide adequate anesthesia with minimal interference of monitored neurophysiological signals. TIVA techniques with propofol and narcotic infusion as a central component have been advocated for optimizing the monitoring of TceMEPs. Because of its sedative, analgesic, and neuroprotective properties, dexmedetomidine has recently been added to TIVA regimens to reduce infusion rates of propofol and to facilitate emergence from anesthesia for the intraoperative wake-up test and at the completion of surgery.[11] The other consideration of the anesthesiologist in determining the maintenance of anesthesia is minimizing blood loss through specific fluid management, drug therapy, and careful positioning of the patient to minimize venous congestion and abdominal compression.[12]

## Monitoring During Surgery

### Cardiovascular Monitoring

Surgical correction of scoliosis and kyphosis may involve extensive fusion of the spine accompanied by notable fluid shifts. Hemodynamic monitoring should routinely include ECG, pulse oximetry, capnography, and monitoring of blood pressure and anesthetic agent dosing and of temperature. Prolonged anesthesia in the prone or lateral decubitus positions, combined with significant blood loss, and where appropriate, controlled hypotension, necessitates detailed monitoring of the cardiovascular system, and frequent evaluation of acid–base balance, hematocrit, and the coagulation profile. Invasive arterial pressure monitoring is mandatory in these procedures. Monitoring of central venous pressure (CVP) should be done for patients with associated cardiac disease and when major blood loss is anticipated. Recently, esophageal Doppler ultrasonography has been validated as a noninvasive alternative to pulmonary artery catheterization for the continuous assessment of cardiac output, stroke volume, preload, and systemic vascular resistance.[13]

### Respiratory Monitoring

Monitoring of the respiratory system should always include the measurement of end-tidal carbon dioxide concentration and peak airway pressure. Patients with severe respiratory dysfunction as a result of scoliosis may have an increased alveolar-arterial oxygen gradient, which may be further increased during prolonged anesthesia because of regional hypoventilation.[14]

### Temperature Monitoring

Body temperature may be difficult to maintain because of the duration of surgery and environmental factors. Because hypothermia has been shown to increase infection rates and blood loss, the use of temperature monitoring, warming of all intravenous fluids, and a warm air mattress device is recommended for the duration of the procedure.[15] Kurz et al found a 3-fold increase in wound infection when patients' temperatures were decreased by 1.9°C, with a 20% longer duration in hospitalization.[15] Room temperature should be maintained at 29°C from the time of a patient's entry into the operating room until the patient is draped.

## Intraoperative Neurophysiological Monitoring

Knowledge of the influence of anesthesia on neuromonitoring is essential. A close working relationship among the members of the neuromonitoring team, the anesthesiologist, and the surgeon is mandatory for the successful conduct and interpretation of neuromonitoring. The effect of anesthetic agents on neurophysiological monitoring increases with the number of synapses in the pathway being monitored, because all anesthetic agents produce their effects by altering neuroexcitability through changes in synaptic function or axonal conduction.[16]

## Somatosensory Evoked Potentials

The subcortical SSEP can be very useful intraoperatively because it is not very susceptible to anesthetic effects (**Table 11.1**).[17] Most studies consider a decrease in amplitude of 50% or more, an increase in latency of 10% or more, or both to be significant changes in SSEP reflecting loss of integrity of a neural pathway, provided these changes are not caused by anesthetic agents or temperature.[18–20] All volatile anesthetic agents produce a dose-dependent increase in SSEP latency and a decrease in SSEP amplitude.[21–23] Sevoflurane and desflurane are associated with less amplitude reduction than isoflurane in the range of minimum alveolar anesthetic concentration (MAC) of 0.7 to 1.3%.[24] In contrast to their effects on the cortical SSEP, all volatile anesthetic agents, even at concentrations above 1.0 MAC, only minimally affect the subcortical waveform, resulting in a high recordability and reliability of the SSEP.[25] Nitrous oxide (60 to 70%) generally diminishes cortical SSEP amplitude by ~50% while leaving cortical SSEP latency and subcortical waves unaffected.[26,27] Intravenous anesthetic agents generally affect SSEPs less than do inhaled anesthetic agents. Human SSEPs are preserved even at high doses of narcotics and barbiturates, but are abolished at high concentrations of volatile anesthetic agents. Neuromuscular blocking drugs do not directly influence SSEPs. However, they may improve the waveform quality of SSEPs by favorably reducing myogenic noise, allowing quicker and more reliable SSEP information.[28]

## Motor Evoked Potentials

Despite reports of improved outcomes obtained with SSEP monitoring, there have been case reports of isolated motor injury with normal sensory function during anesthesia, making it clear that monitoring of motor-function is needed. All currently used inhalational anesthetic agents have been found to markedly attenuate transcranial motor-induced compound muscle action potentials (CAMPs).[29–32] This includes sevoflurane, isoflurane, desflurane, and nitrous oxide in concentrations >50%.[33] Therefore, numerous studies have determined that TIVA techniques optimize the monitoring of TceMEP.[33–35]

**Table 11.1 Effects of Anesthetic Agents on Evoked Potentials**

| Monitoring | Type of Anesthesia | |
|---|---|---|
| | **Anesthetic** | **Dose** |
| Somatosensory evoked potential (SSEP) | • Volatile agent | • 0.5–1 MAC acceptable |
| | • $N_2O$ | • 50–70% acceptable if baseline SSEP is not compromised |
| | • IV anesthetics | • No limitations |
| | • Muscle relaxant | • No limitations |
| Electromyography | • Volatile agent | • No limitations |
| | • $N_2O$ | • No limitations |
| | • IV anesthetics | • No limitations |
| | • Muscle relaxant | • Try to avoid |
| Transcortical and cortical muscle evoked potentials | • Volatile agent | • Limited use; 0.3 MAC maximum |
| | • $N_2O$ | • 50–70% acceptable |
| (Bispectral index monitoring recommended especially in long cases) | • IV anesthetics | • No limitations |
| | • Muscle relaxant | • Try to avoid |

*Abbreviations:* IV: intravenous; MAC: monitored anesthesia care; SSEP: somatosensory evoked potential.

The newer synthetic opioids sufentanil, alfentanil, and remifentanil moderately decrease the amplitude (peak to trough) of motor-evoked potential waveforms.[36] Fentanyl and morphine have shown a strong effect after bolus administration as compared with continuous infusion.[37] Propofol seems to be the most popular agent used in TIVA because of its easy titratability, although it has also been shown to depress motor evoked potentials (MEPs).[38] Use of dexmedetomidine as an anesthetic adjunct at target plasma concentrations up to 0.6 ng/mL does not change somatosensory or motor evoked potential responses during complex spine surgery by any clinically significant amount.[39]

### Wake-Up Test

Before the mid-1970s, the only method for detecting spinal cord injury during corrective scoliosis surgery was the Stagnara wake-up test, which consisted of waking the patient intraoperatively and observing voluntary lower-extremity movement. It is occasionally done to verify the clinical alarm triggered by changes in SSEP and MEP. The performance of a wake-up test requires use of anesthetic technique that allows rapid awakening of the patient to a level of consciousness at which a response to commands can be effected. Ultrarapid-acting opioids such as remifentanil can have an important role in rapid recovery to the point of the ability to follow commands. Short-acting hypnotics (such as propofol) are also of great value. In a recent study, however, the new volatile anesthetic desflurane had a shorter wake-up time than did propofol.[40]

## Fluid Management

The prolonged duration of surgery for scoliosis, extensive surgical manipulation, and likelihood of significant blood loss necessitate judicious fluid administration for the patient. Inadequate fluid replacement can lead to hypotension, hemodynamic instability, and renal failure. Overhydration can lead to fluid overload, congestive cardiac failure, pulmonary edema, dilutional anemia, and coagulopathy, and may preclude early extubation. For optimal management of the fluid status of patients undergoing scoliosis surgery, all components of their fluid loss must be addressed. This includes replacement of the fluid deficit from patients' preoperative fasting (NPO) status, maintaining hourly fluid requirements, and compensating for third-space losses and blood loss. The deficit is calculated as the hourly fluid requirement multiplied by the duration of the patient's NPO status in hours. Deficits are usually corrected by 50% replacement in the first hour of surgery and replacement of the remainder over the next 2 hours (**Table 11.2**). The patient's blood loss is estimated, and the general practice is to replace each milliliter of lost blood with 3 mL of crystalloid or 1 mL of colloid or blood.

**Table 11.2 Calculation of Maintenance Fluid Requirement**

| | Maintenance Fluid Requirements | |
|---|---|---|
| **Weight (kg)** | **Hour** | **Day** |
| <10 | 4 mL/kg | 1000 mL |
| 10–20 | 40 mL +2 mL/kg for every kg >10 kg | 1000 mL + 50 mL/kg for every kg >10 kg |
| >20 | 60 mL + 1mL/kg for every kg >20 kg | 1500 mL + 20 mL/kg for every kg >20 |

Fluid replacement through crystalloid administration has been the traditional practice in surgery in general. However, it has been recognized that this may result in a patient's receiving an enormous amount of fluid, which may lead to the complications of overhydration. This has led to a trend to restrict the volume of fluid administered during surgery.[41] In addition, the choice of fluid replacement with crystalloids versus colloids is a matter of ongoing debate. There is evidence that the use of colloids yields a better recovery profile than the sole use of crystalloids. Patients receiving colloids were found to have less tissue edema, nausea, and vomiting, and a lower incidence of severe pain.[42] Alternatively, systematic reviews of colloid versus crystalloid use suggest an unchanged mortality associated with colloid use. Currently, many centers use crystalloid for fluid maintenance and colloid for managing acute blood loss during surgery, as directed by vital signs and urine output.[43] Lactated Ringer's solution is the choice as a maintenance crystalloid, because 0.9% normal saline is slightly hypertonic and in larger quantities may result in hyperchloremic metabolic acidosis.

## Minimizing Blood Loss and Blood Conservation Techniques

Substantial blood loss during surgery can lead to serious adverse events and it is therefore highly desirable to minimize the risk of blood loss and need for transfusion. It is useful to determine the maximal allowable blood loss (MABL) before surgery because this provides an estimate of the need for transfusion based on the volume of blood lost (**Table 11.3**).

**Table 11.3 Maximum Allowable Blood Loss Calculation**

MABL = Patient's weight (kg) × EBV × (patient's Hct − minimally accepted Hct)

Patient's Hct

- MABL = Maximal allowable blood loss
- EBV = Estimated blood volume (in an adolescent, it is estimated to be 70 mL/kg)
- Hct = Hematocrit

The minimum accepted hematocrit is generally 25% in an otherwise healthy child; however, the decision to transfuse should be based on a clinical evaluation of the patient and the progress of the surgery.

In spine surgery, blood loss has been shown to be progressively greater the greater with increased numbers of vertebral levels incorporated into the fusion and the longer the procedure.[10,44] Intraoperative blood loss typically ranges from 600 to 1500 mL for posterior spinal fusion procedures and 350 to 650 mL in anterior spinal fusion procedures. Blood loss may further increase with more complex procedures, such as osteotomies and vertebral column resections. On average, the blood loss per vertebral level involved in a fusion procedure is 60 to 160 mL. Posterior spinal fusions have been accompanied by a greater volume of blood loss when from 9 to 12 vertebral levels are fused, whereas for anterior spinal fusions this number is usually between 4 and 7 vertebral levels.[44] The literature reports blood transfusion as being required in from 37 to 85% of spine-surgery procedures.[45]

Many strategies have been described for limiting perioperative blood loss and the need for transfusion of allogeneic blood products. These include blood conservation techniques such as acute normovolemic hemodilution (ANHD), preoperative autologous blood donation (PABD), hypotensive anesthesia (HA), intraoperative blood-salvage methods (cell saver–closed drainage systems), and the use of antifibrinolytic agents. Each of these techniques has been shown to be efficacious, and the techniques have successfully been used in combination.

## Acute Normovolemic Hemodilution

Acute normovolemic hemodilution refers to the controlled removal of a volume of the patient's whole blood at the beginning of surgery. The quantity removed depends on the preoperative hematocrit, typically reducing the hematocrit to 28%, and varies from 1 to 3 units. Each milliliter of whole blood removed is then replaced with 3 to 4 mL of colloid or crystalloid to maintain normovolemia.[46] The blood can then be reinfused intraoperatively or postoperatively as needed. This technique has been shown to reduce the requirement for perioperative allogeneic blood transfusion.[47–50]

## Preoperative Autologous Blood Donation

PABD has been proposed to reduce the risks from allogenic blood transfusions. These include disease transmission, infusion of microbial components introduced during blood processing, allergic reactions, volume overload, and immunosuppression.[51] Although blood products are currently safe from infectious hazards, the U.S. Food and Drug Administration (FDA) continues to report deaths from hemolytic transfusion reactions.[52] Thus, autologous transfusion has been advocated and widely used. PABD reduces allogeneic transfusion requirements after lumbar or scoliosis surgery.[53] However, one retrospective case–control study concluded that 51% of patients had at least one autologous unit wasted or were transfused unnecessarily at a high hematocrit (>30%).[54] Risks inherent in blood banking apply to PABD, including risks in blood processing, storage, and misidentification.

## Hypotensive Anesthesia

HA, also known as deliberate hypotensive anesthesia, has been advocated for decreasing the amount of blood loss during surgery. The generally accepted mean arterial pressure (MAP) in this procedure is 50 to 60 mm Hg.[55] Recently, more conservative recommendations are to limit the MAP to 70 mm Hg because of the risk of spinal cord ischemia during spinal instrumentation.[56,57] HA can be used in a patient who is otherwise healthy, but is contraindicated in the setting of end organ injury or ischemia. There is some evidence of reduction in blood loss with HA. Sum and colleagues concluded that HA decreased estimated blood loss by nearly 55%, with a matched reduction in transfusion rates.[58] However, Brodsky et al found that operative technique rather than HA plays a greater role in reducing blood loss.[59] HA can be achieved with direct venous and arterial vasodilators. Numerous medications including nitroprusside, nitroglycerin, inhalation agents, $\beta-$ and $\alpha$-receptor antagonists, $\alpha 2$ adrenergic agonists, and dopamine agonists have been investigated.

## Cell Salvage

Red blood cell recycling or intraoperative cell saving refers to the autotransfusion of shed blood. This is accomplished by using blood processing devices that aspirate, anticoagulate, wash, and reinfuse into the patient the cell suspension from the blood or directly reinfuse the unwashed filtered blood. Although this technique is commonly used, its "added value," when balanced against its cost, is controversial.[47,60]

## Antifibrinolytic Agents

Antifibrinolytic agents such as epsilon aminocaproic acid ($\varepsilon$-ACA), tranexamic acid (TXA), and aprotinin are used to decrease perioperative blood loss. The mechanism of action of these agents is the inhibition of fibrin degradation, which results in improved clot formation. Systematic reviews of randomized controlled trials support the use of antifibrinolytic drugs to reduce perioperative blood loss and the amount of blood transfused in children undergoing scoliosis surgery.[61]

$\varepsilon$-ACA binds to the lysine site on plasminogen and plasmin and prevents plasmin from binding to fibrin. It has been shown to be safe and effective for reducing perioperative blood loss in patients undergoing spinal fusion for scoliosis.[62,63] Complications with its use were of low frequency, with no reported thromboembolic or other reported adverse events. Contraindications to using ε-ACA include active intravascular clotting disorders, disseminated intravascular coagulation, bradycardia, an increase in creatinine phosphokinase levels, muscle weakness, pulmonary embolism, and thrombosis.

TXA is a synthetic antifibrinolytic agent that competitively blocks lysine binding sites on plasminogen, plasmin, and tissue plasminogen activator. It is similar to ε-ACA, but has 10 times the potency of the latter. TXA was shown in one study to be effective in reducing intraoperative blood loss during spinal surgery in children with scoliosis.[64] Neilipovitz et al found that the patients who received TXA had significantly lower blood transfusion requirements in the perioperative period than those who did not despite the lack of a difference in intraoperative blood losses.[65] The majority of evidence suggests that TXA can be safely used. However, the patient sample sizes in which it has been studied have so far been small, and future studies are needed to determine its effectiveness and safety.

Aprotinin is a serine protease inhibitor with antifibrinolytic properties through its effects on fibrinolytic and clotting pathways, the inflammatory response, and platelet function. Aprotinin had been the most widely studied antifibrinolytic agent in spinal surgery and is well documented as an effective blood-conserving agent,[66,67] but the FDA removed it from the market in November 2007 because of concerns about its safety. Its use was accompanied by greater mortality from associated perioperative renal dysfunction, cardiovascular events, and pulmonary embolism. The status of aprotinin awaits a comprehensive review that proves its safety.

### Other Agents

Other agents that have been investigated for decreasing perioperative blood loss include erythropoietin, desmopressin acetate (DDAVP), and Factor VII. Erythropoietin is used in a blood conservation strategy that increases the ability to donate autogenous blood, contributes to higher preoperative hematocrits, and reduces the need for postoperative allogenic transfusions.[68] Despite initial successes, there is no current evidence that DDAVP reduces blood loss in patients undergoing scoliosis surgery.[69–71] Preliminary reports indicated that recombinant Factor VIIa had efficacy in decreasing red cell transfusion, but there is insufficient evidence that this is better than or even as good as conventional therapy.[72]

Studies have shown that a combined approach to blood conservation makes it possible to avoid allogenic blood transfusions.[45,53,73,74] However, until their efficacy and adverse effects are resolved through further trials, clinicians must weigh the cost and consequences of hemostatic medications and blood conservation techniques against the risk of substantial perioperative blood loss and of allogenic blood transfusions.[75]

## ■ Postoperative Pain Management

Posterior scoliosis surgery remains one of the most common orthopedic surgeries for children and adolescents, and also one of the most painful. Analgesia decreases respiratory complications postoperatively by promoting deep breathing, early mobilization, and rehabilitation. Deep somatic pain and muscular reflex spasms follow spine surgery as results of the massive nociceptive inputs of periarticular tissues. In animal models, significant nociceptive input to the spinal cord produces hyperexcitability of the dorsal horn. The occurrence of pain after scoliosis surgery is not unanticipated because of the extensive surgical incision involved, the high degree of bone and soft-tissue dissection, and C-fiber stimulation from periosteal stripping.

The large incision and extensive tissue trauma in major spinal surgery result in severe postoperative pain, particularly during the first 24 to 48 hours,[76–78] with moderate pain lasting through postoperative days 4 to 7. Debate persists about the optimal postoperative method of pain control for children and adolescents undergoing surgical correction of pediatric scoliosis.[78] Opioids, either systemic or spinal; local anesthetic techniques; and nonsteroidal anti-inflamatory drugs (NSAIDs) are the most commonly used means for controlling pain. Gabapentin has become a recent addition to the available means for pain control.

### Intravenous Patient-controlled Analgesia with Narcotics

The most common technique for pain management remains intravenous patient-controlled analgesia (IV PCA) with opioids. Intravenous opioids carry the risks of excessive sedation, pruritus, nausea and vomiting, urinary retention, constipation, and ileus. The PCA mode of delivering medication has potential advantages because of its more rapid ability to meet patient needs, greater patient satisfaction, and lower overall requirement for analgesic use.[79,80]

### Single-Dose Intrathecal Narcotic

Several studies have shown the efficacy of preoperative single-dose intrathecal morphine for controlling pain.[81–84] Intrathecal morphine decreases postoperative pain scores, intraoperative narcotic requirements, and intraoperative bleeding. Because it is a hydrophilic drug, it remains in the cerebrospinal fluid (CSF) for an extended period, allowing it to migrate in a cephalad direction after a lumbar injection.[85]

After injection, morphine works directly on the opioid receptors in the dorsal horn of the spinal cord.[86] Dosing ranges of 2 to 25 mcg/kg of intrathecal morphine have been studied, with the most recent retrospective review supporting doses of 9 to 19 mcg/kg as safe and effective, with minimal complications.[87] As with intravenous opioids, intrathecal opioids carry the risk of pruritus, nausea and vomiting, urinary retention, ileus, and respiratory depression. Monitoring of SSEPs and MEPs has not been affected by intrathecal narcotic dosing.

## Epidural Analgesia

Postoperative continuous epidural analgesia using local anesthetic agents, opioids, or both has been described as having good success after the posterior correction of scoliosis (**Fig. 11.2**); however, the use of epidural analgesia for pediatric patients after spinal-deformity surgery is still limited to an institution-related basis.[88–91] A study reported in 2001 by the Scoliosis Research Society found that only 33% of surveyed scoliosis surgeons used epidural analgesia for postoperative pain control.[92] Sanders et al reported similar numbers in a survey published in 2006.[93] Epidural analgesia has been explored in both continuous and patient-controlled analgesia. Single- and double-catheter methods have been used, with double catheters used to enhance the control of pain in the upper and lower limits of the surgical field. Epidural analgesia is recognized as offering the possibility for significant analgesia with a decreased side-effect profile, in that it involves the delivery of medication regionally and not systemically. Numerous studies have demonstrated decreased pain scores at rest and with motion, a decreased need for rescue narcotic use, and a decreased incidence of side effects (pruritus, nausea/vomiting, constipation, and ileus) with epidural analgesia.[88–90,94–97]

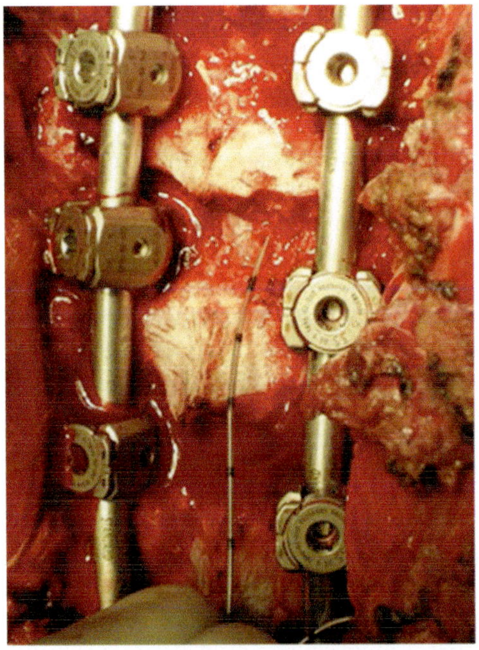

**Fig. 11.2** Placement of epidural catheter for postoperative control of pain.

Our group has recently completed a trial that found efficacy for epidural analgesia even in the setting of a violated epidural space, such as in Smith–Peterson osteotomies. The use of regional anesthesia had been limited by its potential for having adverse effects, including the delayed diagnosis of surgical causes of lower-extremity paralysis, as reported by Purnell in 1982.[98] With the use of neurophysiological monitoring and delaying the infusion of epidural medication until a reliable postoperative neurological assessment has been made, epidural analgesia may become increasingly popular for the postoperative control of pain.

## Nonsteroidal Anti-inflammatory Drugs

NSAIDs are widely used as adjuvant agents for decreasing narcotic consumption in the postoperative period. Studies have demonstrated enhanced analgesia when NSAIDs, most popularly ketorolac, are added to the regimen of postoperative analgesia for spine surgery.[99,100] Ketorolac has been found to decrease rescue narcotic use and shorten hospital stays.[101] However, controversy about bone healing and inhibition of spinal fusion with ketorolac and NSAIDs has limited their use.[102] NSAIDs, not including acetaminophen, are known in animal models to inhibit bone metabolism through the disruption of prostaglandin synthesis, reduction in immune responses, and inhibition of osteoblast production at bone surfaces. A higher incidence of pseudarthrosis was found when ketorolac was given in adult spinal surgery.[103] However, studies of adolescent patients have not found this greater incidence of inhibition of spinal fusion.[101,104] Because failed fusions are rare in AIS, the frequency of effects of NSAIDs on fusion rates would need to be exceedingly high to demonstrate causation.

## Ketamine

Ketamine, an N-methyl-D-aspartate (NMDA) receptor antagonist, has been shown to have an opioid sparing effect in the pharmacological management of postoperative pain, and to be useful in preventing morphine-induced hyperalgesia.[105,106] Both intraoperative infusions and postoperative continuous infusions of ketamine have been studied. Limitations and side effects of ketamine infusion must also be considered. As reported by Tsui et al, ketamine may interfere with the results and interpretation of SSEPs during surgery.[104] It was also found to delay the postoperative voluntary motor response as compared with an opioid regimen. A further issue with ketamine infusion is the need to assess the patient for adverse psychogenic effects such as hallucinations.

### Gabapentin

Studies currently are being conducted on the use of gabapentin begun preoperatively and continued postoperatively for the management of postoperative pain following scoliosis surgery. Gabapentin is a safe and well-tolerated γ-aminobutyric acid (γ-GABA) analogue, with few side effects and few drug interactions. The investigators conducting its clinical trials in scoliosis surgery hypothesize that gabapentin may improve analgesia and decrease opioid requirements. Gabapentin may also decrease persistent neuropathic pain.

Because pain after scoliosis surgery involves multiple mechanisms and neural pathways, a multimodal approach to analgesia may be most effective. This may also decrease the side effects of each class of drug used. Adequate pain control is important not only for short-term patient comfort, but also to prevent more significant and long-term pain.[95,96] Our group recently completed a study that found lower long-term pain scores in patients who had good pain control within the first 24 hours after spinal surgery.

## Special Considerations

Several special considerations in scoliosis surgery warrant additional attention from an anesthetic standpoint.

### Congenital Heart Disease

The incidence of scoliosis is higher in patients with congenital heart disease (CHD) than in the general population, ranging from 4 to 12%.[106–109] Perioperative complications are more common in patients with complex CHD, reaching 42.4% in a retrospective analysis.[110] The majority of patients with CHD requiring surgical correction of scoliosis will present with corrected or palliated congenital heart defects. Patients with residual abnormalities or palliated CHD can have long-term sequelae including valvular dysfunction, arrhythmias, hypoxia, cardiac failure, thromboembolic disorders, and paradoxical air embolism. The preoperative evaluation of such patients should address these concerns, and their cardiac function should be documented.

After complete repair, patients with normal cardiovascular function may not require modifications in anesthetic management other than prophylaxis against endocarditis. However, in patients with complex cardiac physiology or those with abnormal cardiac function, additional monitoring may be necessary. A retrospective review of seven patients who had a Fontan repair of a single-ventricle pathology showed no intraoperative complications during scoliosis surgery. In this study, all of the patients had Swan–Ganz monitoring catheters placed before the surgery and a cardiac anesthesiologist providing anesthesia.[111] Intraoperative transesophageal echocardiography (TEE) has also been found useful as a monitoring tool. It provides real-time information about preload, ventricular filling, contractility, and cardiac output, and may be an alternative to the use of a Swan–Ganz catheter.[112]

### Down Syndrome

Down syndrome (DS) or trisomy 21 is the most common genetic disorder in humans, occurring in 1 in 600 to 1 in 800 live births. Reports have shown an incidence of scoliosis ranging from 9 to 52% in patients with DS.[113–115] Craniofacial and cardiac anomalies seen in DS increase these patients' risk of complications during anesthesia.[116] Craniofacial features that have adverse implications during anesthesia include a short neck, macroglossia, and midfacial and mandibular hypoplasia. Generalized hypotonia, a narrowed nasopharynx, obesity, and tonsil and adenoid hypertrophy are also characteristic of these patients. Abnormalities of the cervical spine seen in DS include atlantoaxial instability (AAI) and atlanto-occipital instability. Cardiac defects are present in 40 to 50% of patients with DS.[117]

Combinations of the foregoing abnormalities predispose patients undergoing spine surgery to upper-airway obstruction, making their airway management difficult. Normal films of the cervical spine in patients with DS are reassuring, particularly during intubation and positioning for scoliosis-related procedures. The incidence of bradycardia on induction of anesthesia in patients with DS is greater than average, and premedication with an anticholinergic agent should be considered.[116]

### Neuromuscular Scoliosis

The most common causes of neuromuscular scoliosis (NMS) are cerebral palsy, myelomeningocele, muscular dystrophy, and spinal muscular atrophy. Concerns about NMS patients include increased blood loss, poor respiratory and muscular function, and possible cardiac pathology.

Blood loss is a major issue in patients with NMS. A literature review of intraoperative blood loss in pediatric spinal fusion surgery concluded that patients with NMS had the highest mean blood loss.[118–120] Many patients with cerebral palsy are taking antiepileptic medications such as valproic acid, which is known to be hepatotoxic and affects the platelet count and platelet function. Preoperative use of valproic acid has been shown to be associated with increased blood loss and increased use of blood products.[121] Patients with neuromuscular disorders are often malnourished and underweight, impairing their production of vitamin K-dependent clotting factors. Postoperative respiratory complications are common in children with NMS. Frequently, these children have muscle weakness and abnormal hypopharyngeal tone leading to chronic aspiration, recurrent pneumonias, and hypoxia. Respiratory status must be evaluated and optimized before the surgery and the need for postoperative ventilatory support must be anticipated. Because right-ventricular dysfunction can develop in patients with cor pulmonale, echocardiography should be part of their preoperative evaluation.

### Malignant Hyperthermia

Malignant hyperthermia (MH) is a disorder of calcium regulation in skeletal muscle that presents as a hypermetabolic response to volatile anesthetic agents and succinylcholine. The incidence of MH ranges from 1 in 20,000 to 1 in 40,000 anesthetic procedures. A known or suspected myopathy should alert the clinician of the possibility of MH. Central core disease (CCD), a myopathy with a genetic link to MH, is associated with progressive kyphoscoliosis.[122] Other disorders associated with MH are Multi–Minicore disease and King–Denborough syndrome.

The earliest signs of MH are muscle rigidity, tachycardia, hypercapnia, and hypertension. Hyperthermia is usually a late sign. Other clinical manifestations of MH include acidosis, rhabdomyolysis, hyperkalemia, ventricular arrhythmias, an increased creatine kinase concentration, myoglobinuria, and coagulopathy. MH-susceptible children should have a formal anesthesia consultation and their anesthetic management should consist of a nontriggering technique, including the use of intravenous anesthetic agents. Dantrolene, a specific antagonist of the pathophysiological changes in MH, should be readily available for use in these patients.

## ■ Conclusion

With advances in pharmacology and physiology, the surgical and anesthetic considerations for children undergoing surgical correction of scoliosis continue to evolve. Progress has been made in continuous intraoperative neurophysiological monitoring, blood-conservation techniques and blood-loss minimization, and postoperative pain management. The surgical treatment of scoliosis requires a team approach to the patient for a safe and successful outcome.

### References

1. Keys TE. The History of Anesthesia. New York, Schumans; 1945.
2. Smyth RJ, Chapman KR, Wright TA, Crawford JS, Rebuck AS. Pulmonary function in adolescents with mild idiopathic scoliosis. Thorax 1984;39(12):901–904
3. Salem MR, Klowden AJ. Anesthesia for Orthopedic Surgery. In: Gregory GA, ed. Pediatric Anesthesia. Churchill Livingstone, New York; 2002:617–661
4. Raw DA, Beattie JK, Hunter JM. Anaesthesia for spinal surgery in adults. Br J Anaesth 2003;91:886–904
5. Jevsevar DS, Karlin LI. The relationship between preoperative nutritional status and complications after an operation for scoliosis in patients who have cerebral palsy. J Bone Joint Surg Am 1993;75:880–884
6. Murray DJ, Forbes RB, Titone MB, Weinstein SL. Transfusion management in pediatric and adolescent scoliosis surgery. Efficacy of autologous blood. Spine 1997;22:2735–2740
7. Practice guidelines for preoperative fasting and the use of pharmacologic agents to reduce the risk of pulmonary aspiration: Application to healthy patients undergoing elective procedures: A report by the American Society of Anesthesiologists Task Force on Preoperative Fasting. Anesthesiology 1999;90(3): 896–905
8. Soundararajan N, Cunliffe M. Anaesthesia for spinal surgery in children. Br J Anaesth 2007;99:86–94
9. Padberg AM, Wilson-Holden TJ, Lenke LG, Bridwell KH. Somatosensory- and motor-evoked potential monitoring without a wake-up test during idiopathic scoliosis surgery. An accepted standard of care. Spine 1998;23(12):1392–1400
10. Gibson PRJ. Anaesthesia for correction of scoliosis in children. Anaesth Intensive Care 2004;32:548–559
11. Mahmoud M, Sadhasivam S, Sestokas AK, Samuels P, McAuliffe J. Loss of transcranial electric motor evoked potentials during pediatric spine surgery with dexmedetomidine. Anesthesiology 2007;106:393–396
12. Eyres R. Update on TIVA. Paediatr Anaesth 2004;14:374–379
13. Almenrader N, Patel D. Spinal fusion surgery in children with non-idiopathic scoliosis: Is there a need for routine postoperative ventilation? Br J Anaesth 2006;97:851–857
14. Kafer ER. Idiopathic scoliosis. Gas exchange and the age dependence of arterial blood gases. J Clin Invest 1976;58:825–833
15. Kurz A, Sessler DI, Lenhardt R. Study of Wound Infection and Temperature Group. Perioperative normothermia to reduce the incidence of surgical-wound infection and shorten hospitalization. N Engl J Med 1996;334:1209–1215
16. Sloan TB. Anesthetics and the brain. Anesthesiol Clin North America 2002;20:265–292
17. Sebel PS, Erwin CW, Neville WK. Effects of halothane and enflurane on far and near field somatosensory evoked potentials. Br J Anaesth 1987;59:1492–1496
18. Brown RH, Nash CL Jr, Berilla JA, Amaddio MD. Cortical evoked potential monitoring. A system for intraoperative monitoring of spinal cord function. Spine 1984;9:256–261
19. Nuwer MR, Dawson E. Intraoperative evoked potential monitoring of the spinal cord: Enhanced stability of cortical recordings. Electroencephalogr Clin Neurophysiol 1984;59:318–327
20. Faberowski LW, Black S, Trankina MF, Pollard RJ, Clark RK, Mahla ME. Somatosensory-evoked potentials during aortic coarctation repair. J Cardiothorac Vasc Anesth 1999;13:538–543
21. Samra SK, Vanderzant CW, Domer PA, Sackellares JC. Differential effects of isoflurane on human median nerve somatosensory evoked potentials. Anesthesiology 1987;66:29–35

22. Peterson DO, Drummond JC, Todd MM. Effects of halothane, enflurane, isoflurane, and nitrous oxide on somatosensory evoked potentials in humans. Anesthesiology 1986;65:35–40
23. McPherson RW, Mahla M, Johnson R, Traystman RJ. Effects of enflurane, isoflurane, and nitrous oxide on somatosensory evoked potentials during fentanyl anesthesia. Anesthesiology 1985;62: 626–633
24. Rehberg B, Rüschner R, Fischer M, Ebeling BJ, Hoeft A. [Concentration-dependent changes in the latency and amplitude of somatosensory-evoked potentials by desflurane, isoflurane and sevoflurane]. Anasthesiol Intensivmed Notfallmed Schmerzther 1998;33: 425–429
25. Porkkala T, Jäntti V, Kaukinen S, Häkkinen V. Nitrous oxide has different effects on the EEG and somatosensory evoked potentials during isoflurane anaesthesia in patients. Acta Anaesthesiol Scand 1997;41:497–501
26. Schindler E, Müller M, Zickmann B, Osmer C, Wozniak G, Hempelmann G. Modulation of somatosensory evoked potentials under various concentrations of desflurane with and without nitrous oxide. J Neurosurg Anesthesiol 1998;10:218–223
27. Wolfe DE, Drummond JC. Differential effects of isoflurane/nitrous oxide on posterior tibial somatosensory evoked responses of cortical and subcortical origin. Anesth Analg 1988;67:852–859
28. Sloan TB. Nondepolarizing neuromuscular blockade does not alter sensory evoked potentials. J Clin Monit 1994;10:4–10
29. Zentner J. Influence of anesthetics on the electromyographic response evoked by transcranial electrical cortex stimulation. Funct Neurol 1989;4:299–300
30. Kawaguchi M, Sakamoto T, Ohnishi H, Shimizu K, Karasawa J, Furuya H. Intraoperative myogenic motor evoked potentials induced by direct electrical stimulation of the exposed motor cortex under isoflurane and sevoflurane. Anesth Analg 1996;82:593–599
31. Kawaguchi M, Shimizu K, Furuya H, Sakamoto T, Ohnishi H, Karasawa J. Effect of isoflurane on motor-evoked potentials induced by direct electrical stimulation of the exposed motor cortex with single, double, and triple stimuli in rats. Anesthesiology 1996;85:1176–1183
32. Ku AS, Hu Y, Irwin MG, et al. Effect of sevoflurane/nitrous oxide versus propofol anaesthesia on somatosensory evoked potential monitoring of the spinal cord during surgery to correct scoliosis. Br J Anaesth 2002;88:502–507
33. Thees C, Scheufler KM, Nadstawek J, et al. Influence of fentanyl, alfentanil, and sufentanil on motor evoked potentials. J Neurosurg Anesthesiol 1999;11:112–118
34. Ubags LH, Kalkman CJ, Been HD, Drummond JC. Differential effects of nitrous oxide and propofol on myogenic transcranial motor evoked responses during sufentanil anaesthesia. Br J Anaesth 1997;79:590–594
35. Lo YL, Dan YF, Tan YE, et al. Intraoperative motor-evoked potential monitoring in scoliosis surgery: Comparison of desflurane/nitrous oxide with propofol total intravenous anesthetic regimens. J Neurosurg Anesthesiol 2006;18:211–214
36. Lotto ML, Banoub M, Schubert A. Effects of anesthetic agents and physiologic changes on intraoperative motor evoked potentials. J Neurosurg Anesthesiol 2004;16:32–42
37. Pathak KS, Brown RH, Cascorbi HF, Nash CL Jr. Effects of fentanyl and morphine on intraoperative somatosensory cortical-evoked potentials. Anesth Analg 1984;63:833–837
38. Nathan N, Tabaraud F, Lacroix F, et al. Influence of propofol concentrations on multipulse transcranial motor evoked potentials. Br J Anaesth 2003;91:493–497
39. Bala E, Sessler DI, Nair DR, McLain R, Dalton JE, Farag E. Motor and somatosensory evoked potentials are well maintained in patients given dexmedetomidine during spine surgery. Anesthesiology 2008;109:417–425
40. Grottke O, Dietrich PJ, Wiegels S, Wappler F. Intraoperative wake-up test and postoperative emergence in patients undergoing spinal surgery: A comparison of intravenous and inhaled anesthetic techniques using short-acting anesthetics. Anesth Analg 2004;99:1521–1527
41. Nisanevich V, Felsenstein I, Almogy G, Weissman C, Einav S, Matot I. Effect of intraoperative fluid management on outcome after intraabdominal surgery. Anesthesiology 2005;103:25–32
42. Drummond JC, Petrovitch CT. Intraoperative blood salvage: Fluid replacement calculations. Anesth Analg 2005;100:645–649
43. Ornstein E, Berko R. Anesthesia techniques in complex spine surgery. Neurosurg Clin N Am 2006;17(3):191–203, v
44. Shapiro F, Sethna N. Blood loss in pediatric spine surgery. Eur Spine J 2004;13(suppl 1):S6–S17
45. Joseph SA Jr, Berekashvili K, Mariller MM, et al. Blood conservation techniques in spinal deformity surgery: A retrospective review of patients refusing blood transfusion. Spine 2008;33(21): 2310–2315
46. Epstein NE. Bloodless spinal surgery: A review of the normovolemic hemodilution technique. Surg Neurol 2008;70:614–618
47. Epstein NE, Peller A, Korsh J, et al. Impact of intraoperative normovolemic hemodilution on transfusion requirements for 68 patients undergoing lumbar laminectomies with instrumented posterolateral fusion. Spine 2006;31:2227–2230, discussion 2231
48. Epstein NE, Peller A, Korsh J, et al. Normovolemic hemodilution: an effective method for limiting postoperative transfusion following complex lumbar spinal decompression with instrumented fusion. Spinal Surgery 2004;18:179–188
49. Hur SR, Huizenga BA, Major M. Acute normovolemic hemodilution combined with hypotensive anesthesia and other techniques to avoid homologous transfusion in spinal fusion surgery. Spine 1992;17:867–873
50. Guay J, de Moerloose P, Lasne D. Minimizing perioperative blood loss and transfusions in children. Can J Anaesth 2006; 53(6, Suppl):S59–S67
51. Roback JD, Su L, Zimring JC, Hillyer CD. Transfusion-transmitted cytomegalovirus: Lessons from a murine model. Transfus Med Rev 2007;21:26–36
52. Linden JV, Wagner K, Voytovich AE, Sheehan J. Transfusion errors in New York State: An analysis of 10 years' experience. Transfusion 2000;40:1207–1213
53. Anand N, Idio FG Jr, Remer S, Hoppenfeld S. The effects of perioperative blood salvage and autologous blood donation on transfusion requirements in scoliosis surgery. J Spinal Disord 1998;11: 532–534
54. Bess RS, Lenke LG, Bridwell KH, Steger-May K, Hensley M. Wasting of preoperatively donated autologous blood in the surgical treatment of adolescent idiopathic scoliosis. Spine 2006;31:2375–2380
55. Zuckerberg A. Myron Yaster Anesthesia for Pediatric orthopedic surgery. In: Motoyama EK, Davis PJ, eds. Smith's Anesthesia for Infants and Children, ed. 7. St. Louis: CV Mosby;2006:737–769

56. Mooney JF III, Bernstein R, Hennrikus WL Jr, MacEwen GD. Neurologic risk management in scoliosis surgery. J Pediatr Orthop 2002;22:683–689
57. Barcelona SL, Thompson AA, Coté CJ. Intraoperative pediatric blood transfusion therapy: a review of common issues. Part II: Transfusion therapy, special considerations, and reduction of allogenic blood transfusions. Paediatr Anaesth 2005;15:814–830
58. Sum DC, Chung PC, Chen WC. Deliberate hypotensive anesthesia with labetalol in reconstructive surgery for scoliosis. Acta Anaesthesiol Sin 1996;34:203–207 Erratum in: Acta Anaesthesiol Sin 1997;35:59
59. Brodsky JW, Dickson JH, Erwin WD, Rossi CD. Hypotensive anesthesia for scoliosis surgery in Jehovah's Witnesses. Spine 1991; 16:304–306
60. Cha CW, Deible C, Muzzonigro T, Lopez-Plaza I, Vogt M, Kang JD. Allogeneic transfusion requirements after autologous donations in posterior lumbar surgeries. Spine 2002;27:99–104
61. Florentino-Pineda I, Thompson GH, Poe-Kochert C, Huang RP, Haber LL, Blakemore LC. The effect of amicar on perioperative blood loss in idiopathic scoliosis: The results of a prospective, randomized double-blind study. Spine 2004;29:233–238
62. Thompson GH, Florentino-Pineda I, Poe-Kochert C, Armstrong DG, Son-Hing JP. The role of Amicar in same-day anterior and posterior spinal fusion for idiopathic scoliosis. Spine 2008;33: 2237–2242
63. Thompson GH, Florentino-Pineda I, Poe-Kochert C. The role of amicar in decreasing perioperative blood loss in idiopathic scoliosis. Spine 2005; 30(17, suppl):S94–S99
64. Neilipovitz DT, Zurakowski D, Brustowicz RM, Bacsik J, Sullivan LJ, Shapiro F. Tranexamic acid for major spinal surgery. Eur Spine J 2004;13(suppl 1):S62–S65
65. Neilipovitz DT, Murto K, Hall L, Barrowman NJ, Splinter WM. A randomized trial of tranexamic acid to reduce blood transfusion for scoliosis surgery. Anesth Analg 2001;93:82–87
66. Cole JW, Murray DJ, Snider RJ, Bassett GS, Bridwell KH, Lenke LG. Aprotinin reduces blood loss during spinal surgery in children. Spine 2003;28:2482–2485
67. Tryba M. Epoetin alfa plus autologous blood donation and normovolemic hemodilution in patients scheduled for orthopedic or vascular surgery. Semin Hematol 1996; 33(2, suppl 2):34–36, discussion: 37–38
68. Guay J, Reinberg C, Poitras B, et al. A trial of desmopressin to reduce blood loss in patients undergoing spinal fusion for idiopathic scoliosis. Anesth Analg 1992;75:405–410
69. Alanay A, Acaroglu E, Ozdemir O, Erçelen O, Bulutçu E, Surat A. Effects of deamino-8-D-arginin vasopressin on blood loss and coagulation factors in scoliosis surgery. A double-blind randomized clinical trial. Spine 1999;24:877–882
70. Henry DA, Moxey AJ, Carless PA, et al. Desmopressin for minimising perioperative allogeneic blood transfusion. Cochrane Database Syst Rev 2001;2:CD001884
71. Kolban M, Balachowska-Kosciolek I, Chmielnicki M. Recombinant coagulation factor VIIa: A novel haemostatic agent in scoliosis surgery? Eur Spine J 2006;15:944–952
72. Weiskopf RB. The use of recombinant activated coagulation factor VII for spine surgery. Eur Spine J 2004;13(suppl 1):S83–S88
73. Verma RR, Williamson JB, Dashti H, Patel D, Oxborrow NJ. Homologous blood transfusion is not required in surgery for adolescent idiopathic scoliosis. J Bone Joint Surg Br 2006;88:1187–1191
74. Lisander B, Jonsson R, Nordwall A. Combination of blood-saving methods decreases homologous blood requirements in scoliosis surgery. Anaesth Intensive Care 1996;24:555–558
75. Erstad BL. What is the evidence for using hemostatic agents in surgery? Eur Spine J 2004;13(Suppl 1):S28–S33
76. Amaranath L, Andrish JT, Gurd AR, Weiker GG, Yoon H. Efficacy of intermittent epidural morphine following posterior spinal fusion in children and adolescents. Clin Orthop Relat Res 1989;249(249): 223–226
77. Joshi GP, McCarroll SM, O'Rourke K. Postoperative analgesia after lumbar laminectomy: Epidural fentanyl infusion versus patient-controlled intravenous morphine. Anesth Analg 1995;80:511–514
78. Borgeat A, Blumenthal S. Postoperative pain management following scoliosis surgery. Curr Opin Anaesthesiol 2008;21:313–316 Review
79. Walson PD, Graves PS, Mortensen ME, Kern RA, Torch MA. Patient-controlled versus conventional analgesia for postsurgical pain relief in adolescents. Dev Pharmacol Ther 1992;19:32–39
80. Saudan S, Habre W, Ceroni D, et al. Safety and efficacy of patient controlled epidural analgesia following pediatric spinal surgery. Paediatr Anaesth 2008;18:132–139
81. Dalens B, Tanguy A. Intrathecal morphine for spinal fusion in children. Spine 1988;13:494–498
82. Blackman RG, Reynolds J, Shively J. Intrathecal morphine: dosage and efficacy in younger patients for control of postoperative pain following spinal fusion. Orthopedics 1991;14:555–557
83. Gall O, Aubineau JV, Bernière J, Desjeux L, Murat I. Analgesic effect of low-dose intrathecal morphine after spinal fusion in children. Anesthesiology 2001;94:447–452
84. Urban MK, Jules-Elysee K, Urquhart B, Cammisa FP, Boachie-Adjei O. Reduction in postoperative pain after spinal fusion with instrumentation using intrathecal morphine. Spine 2002;27:535–537
85. Chaney MA. Side effects of intrathecal and epidural opioids. Can J Anaesth 1995;42:891–903
86. Cousins MJ, Mather LE. Intrathecal and epidural administration of opioids. Anesthesiology 1984;61:276–310
87. Tripi PA, Poe-Kochert C, Potzman J, Son-Hing JP, Thompson GH. Intrathecal morphine for postoperative analgesia in patients with idiopathic scoliosis undergoing posterior spinal fusion. Spine 2008;33:2248–2251
88. Arms DM, Smith JT, Osteyee J, Gartrell A. Postoperative epidural analgesia for pediatric spine surgery. Orthopedics 1998;21:539–544
89. Shaw BA, Watson TC, Merzel DI, Gerardi JA, Birek A. The safety of continuous epidural infusion for postoperative analgesia in pediatric spine surgery. J Pediatr Orthop 1996;16:374–377
90. Cassady JF Jr, Lederhaas G, Cancel DD, Cummings RJ, Loveless EA. A randomized comparison of the effects of continuous thoracic epidural analgesia and intravenous patient-controlled analgesia after posterior spinal fusion in adolescents. Reg Anesth Pain Med 2000;25:246–253
91. Turner A, Lee J, Mitchell R, Berman J, Edge G, Fennelly M. The efficacy of surgically placed epidural catheters for analgesia after posterior spinal surgery. Anaesthesia 2000;55:370–373
92. Winkelpleck M, Auffant R, Ferguson R. Post-Operative Epidural Analgesia for Spine Fusion in Adolescent Idiopathic Scoliosis, Current Utilization at Spine Centers. Abstract. 36th Annual Meeting, Scoliosis Research Society
93. Sanders JO, Haynes R, Lighter D, et al. Variation in care among spinal deformity surgeons: Results of a survey of the Shriner's hospitals for children. Spine 2007;32:1444–1449

94. Van Boerum DH, Smith JT, Curtin MJ. A comparison of the effects of patient-controlled analgesia with intravenous opioids versus epidural analgesia on recovery after surgery for idiopathic scoliosis. Spine 2000;25:2355–2357
95. Tobias JD, Gaines RW, Lowry KJ, Kittle D, Bildner C. A dual epidural catheter technique to provide analgesia following posterior spinal fusion for scoliosis in children and adolescents. Paediatr Anaesth 2001;11:199–203
96. Ekatodramis G, Min K, Cathrein P, Borgeat A. Use of a double epidural catheter provides effective postoperative analgesia after spine deformity surgery. Can J Anaesth 2002;49:173–177
97. Blumenthal S, Min K, Nadig M, Borgeat A. Double epidural catheter with ropivacaine versus intravenous morphine: A comparison for postoperative analgesia after scoliosis correction surgery. Anesthesiology 2005;102:175–180
98. Purnell RJ. Scoliosis correction and epidural analgesia. Prolonged block following Harrington rod insertion. Anaesthesia 1982;37: 1115–1117
99. Reuben SS, Connelly NR, Steinberg R. Ketorolac as an adjunct to patient-controlled morphine in postoperative spine surgery patients. Reg Anesth 1997;22:343–346
100. Turner DM, Warson JS, Wirt TC, Scalley RD, Cochran RS, Miller KJ. The use of ketorolac in lumbar spine surgery: A cost-benefit analysis. J Spinal Disord 1995;8:206–212
101. Sucato DJ, Lovejoy JF, Agrawal S, Elerson E, Nelson T, McClung A. Postoperative ketorolac does not predispose to pseudarthrosis following posterior spinal fusion and instrumentation for adolescent idiopathic scoliosis. Spine 2008;33:1119–1124
102. Glassman SD, Rose SM, Dimar JR, Puno RM, Campbell MJ, Johnson JR. The effect of postoperative nonsteroidal anti-inflammatory drug administration on spinal fusion. Spine 1998;23: 834–838
103. Vitale MG, Choe JC, Hwang MW, et al. Use of ketorolac tromethamine in children undergoing scoliosis surgery. An analysis of complications. Spine J 2003;3:55–62
104. Tsui BC, Wagner A, Mahood J, Moreau M. Adjunct continuous intravenous ketamine infusion for postoperative pain relief following posterior spinal instrumentation for correction of scoliosis: A case report. Paediatr Anaesth 2007;17:383–386
105. Sveticic G, Eichenberger U, Curatolo M. Safety of mixture of morphine with ketamine for postoperative patient-controlled analgesia: an audit with 1026 patients. Acta Anaesthesiol Scand 2005;49:870–875
106. Jordan CE, White RI Jr, Fischer KC, Neill C, Dorst JP. The scoliosis of congenital heart disease. Am Heart J 1972;84:463–469
107. Luke MJ, McDonnell EJ. Congenital heart disease and scoliosis. J Pediatr 1968;73:725–733
108. Roth A, Rosenthal A, Hall JE, Mizel M. Scoliosis and congenital heart disease. Clin Orthop Relat Res 1973;93:95–102
109. Kawakami N, Mimatsu K, Deguchi M, Kato F, Maki S. Scoliosis and congenital heart disease. Spine 1995;20:1252–1255, discussion 1256
110. Coran DL, Rodgers WB, Keane JF, Hall JE, Emans JB. Spinal fusion in patients with congenital heart disease. Predictors of outcome. Clin Orthop Relat Res 1999;364:99–107
111. Hedequist DJ, Emans JB, Hall JE. Operative treatment of scoliosis in patients with a Fontan circulation. Spine 2006; 31:202–205
112. Vischoff D, Fortier LP, Villeneuve E, Boutin C, Labelle H. Anaesthetic management of an adolescent for scoliosis surgery with a Fontan circulation. Paediatr Anaesth 2001;11:607–610
113. Diamond LS, Lynne D, Sigman B. Orthopedic disorders in patients with Down's syndrome. Orthop Clin North Am 1981;12:57–71
114. Krompinger WJ, Renshaw TS. Scoliosis in Down syndrome. Orthop Transplant 1984;8:157
115. Milbrandt TA, Johnston CE II. Down syndrome and scoliosis: A review of a 50-year experience at one institution. Spine 2005;30: 2051–2055
116. Borland LM, Colligan J, Brandom BW. Frequency of anesthesia-related complications in children with Down syndrome under general anesthesia for noncardiac procedures. Paediatr Anaesth 2004;14:733–738
117. Kobel M, Creighton RE, Steward DJ. Anaesthetic considerations in Down's syndrome: Experience with 100 patients and a review of the literature. Can Anaesth Soc J 1982;29:593–599
118. Shapiro F, Sethna N. Blood loss in pediatric spine surgery. Eur Spine J 2004;13(suppl 1):S6–S17
119. Edler A, Murray DJ, Forbes RB. Blood loss during posterior spinal fusion surgery in patients with neuromuscular disease: Is there an increased risk? Paediatr Anaesth 2003;13:818–822
120. Meert KL, Kannan S, Mooney JF. Predictors of red cell transfusion in children and adolescents undergoing spinal fusion surgery. Spine 2002;27:2137–2142
121. Winter SL, Kriel RL, Novacheck TF, Luxenberg MG, Leutgeb VJ, Erickson PA. Perioperative blood loss: The effect of valproate. Pediatr Neurol 1996;15:19–22
122. Gamble JG, Rinsky LA, Lee JH. Orthopaedic aspects of central core disease. J Bone Joint Surg Am 1988;70:1061–1066

# 12 Selective versus Nonselective Surgery for Adolescent Idiopathic Scoliosis

*Daniel J. Sucato*

The goals of surgical treatment in adolescent idiopathic scoliosis (AIS) are to prevent progression of the curve and to correct the spinal deformity while maintaining overall coronal and sagittal balance of the patient. These two goals should be achieved with fusion of as few spine motion segments as possible. The most common curve pattern in AIS is a single thoracic curve with an associated lumbar curve. This lumbar curve may be compensatory and not require inclusion in the fusion, or may be structural, necessitating its inclusion in the fusion levels. When the lumbar curve is not included into the fusion levels, the fusion is known as a *selective thoracic fusion*, a concept first introduced by Winter and Moe as a method to satisfy the two goals of surgery for scoliosis while leaving the patient with a mobile lumbar spine.

The ability to determine whether the lumbar curve in scoliosis is compensatory or structural has been challenging. With the passage of time, several definitions have been developed to determine this. In addition to defining those lumbar curves that do not require instrumentation and fusion, several factors play a role in accomplishing good correction of a spine deformity while maintaining the patient's overall coronal and sagittal balance.

The purpose of selective fusion of the thoracic spine in scoliosis is to obtain correction of the thoracic deformity while preserving the mobility of the lumbar segments of the spine.[1,2] The premise is that a flexible lumbar compensatory curve will respond to any coronal-plane correction in the thoracic spine, leaving the patient balanced in the coronal plane. In 1983, King and colleagues described a classification for AIS to assist surgeons in identifying those curve patterns that were amenable to selective thoracic fusion.[3] They recommended that patients with a King II pattern, defined as a major thoracic curve with a compensatory lumbar curve, undergo a selective fusion (**Fig. 12.1**). The King classification system was derived with the use of the Harrington distraction system, and generally worked well with the corrective forces imparted to the spine in this way.[4–6] The concept of selective fusion, although promising, led to some complications, including the "adding on" of adjacent spinal segments to the scoliotic curve, and truncal decompensation with a shift to the left (**Fig. 12.2**). These became more evident with the use of Cotrel–Dubousset (CD) instrumentation, which provided greater coronal-plane correction than the previously used Harrington instrumentation. The improved thoracic coronal-plane correction would often lead to decompensation to the left because of the inability of the lumbar curve to respond to thoracic-curve correction, and strategies to improve these outcomes have since been discussed and

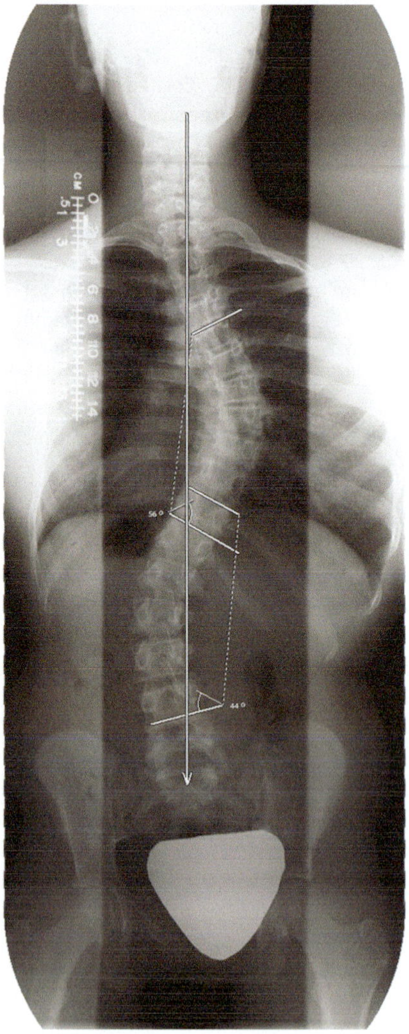

**Fig. 12.1** King II curve pattern. The thoracic curve has a larger measured coronal Cobb angle (56 degrees) and is structural, whereas the coronal angle measured for the lumbar curve (44 degrees) is smaller and the curve is considered a compensatory curve.

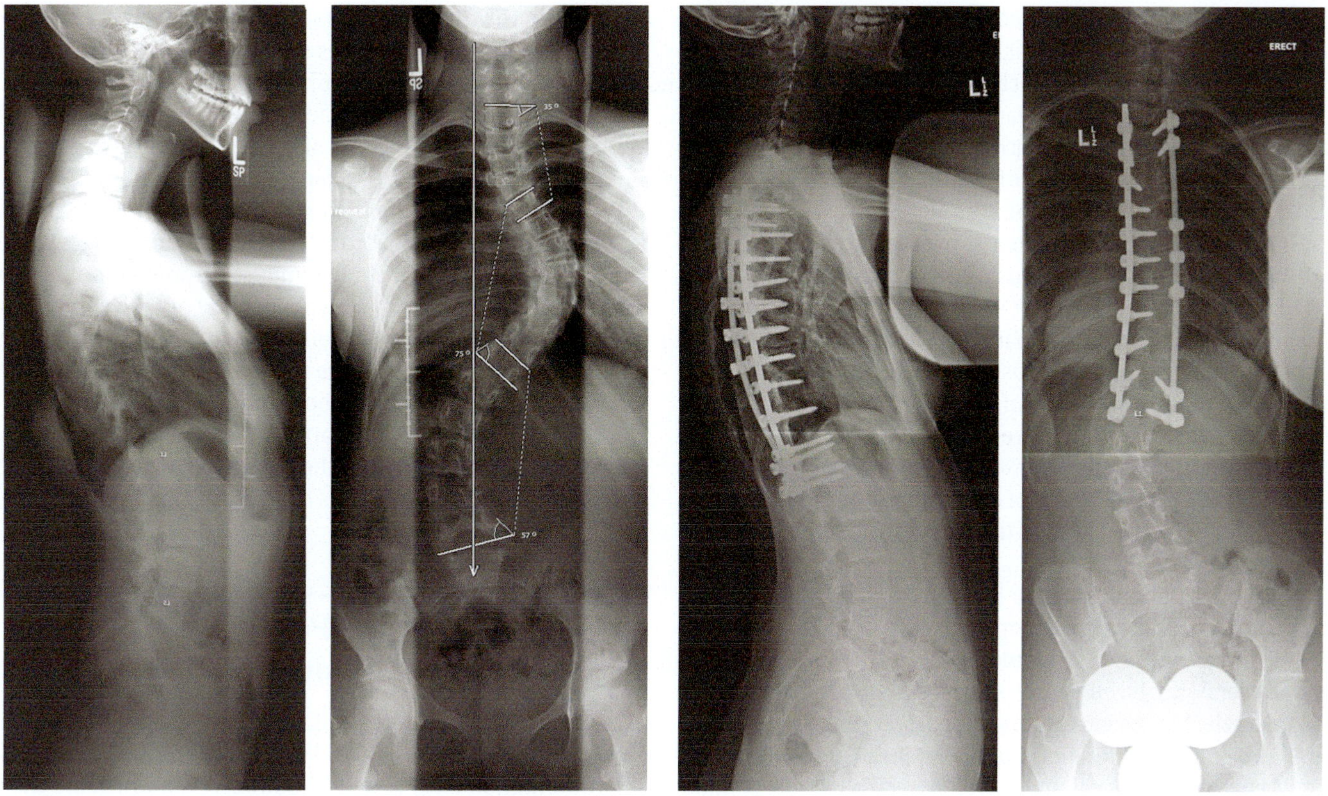


**Fig. 12.2** Trunk decompensation following selective thoracic fusion with modern implant systems. **(A,B)** Preoperative radiographs demonstrating a 75-degree thoracic curve and a 57-degree lumbar curve. **(C,D)** Two-year postoperative radiographs demonstrating good overall correction of the thoracic curve; however, the lumbar curve has not responded to the thoracic correction, and the patient demonstrates a significant truncal shift to the left.

studied.[7–10] The Lenke classification system for AIS is a more comprehensive system and improves upon the definitions used to define a compensatory lumbar curve.[11] Greater attention to defining a lumbar compensatory curve, which has improved the planned selection of fusion levels and the planning of thoracic-curve correction, has been a benefit of the Lenke classification system. In addition, the introduction of thoracic pedicle screws and anterior fusion in specific situations appears to have improved the results of surgery, with less coronal imbalance.[12–15]

## Advantages and Disadvantages of Selective Thoracic Fusion

The advantages of selective fusion are maintenance of lumbar motion segments of the spine and correction of the primary deformity in scoliosis, the main thoracic curve. Motion of the spine occurs predominantly at the thoracolumbar junction and in the lumbar segments. It is logical to assume that preservation of these motion segments will provide better long-term health of the spine. Studies have determined that a more proximal fusion level in AIS results in greater motion of the spine.[16,17] Wilk et al compared 34 patients who had fusion for AIS, 32 patients who did not have fusion, and 25 control patients, and demonstrated less motion in those patients who had fusion into the lumbar spine than in those who had thoracic fusion only.[16] Greater mobility of the lumbar spine appears to be important in the long-term health of the spine and is the primary reason for performing selective thoracic fusion when possible. Clinical studies have substantiated some of the perceived problems with fusion into the lumbar spine. Paonessa and Angler[18] reported greater back pain scores, difficulties with normal daily activities, increased need for pain medications, and more episodes of back pain with fusion to L3 or caudally than with fusion to more proximal levels.[18] Cochran and coworkers analyzed the long-term functional changes in patients with AIS and demonstrated more low back pain, degenerative facet-joint changes, and disc space narrowing in patients with fusion to L4 or L5.[19,20] However, it should be noted that the patients in this study were treated with Harrington implants that flatten the lumbar spine and lead to a flatback deformity and resultant pain and disability. With current segmental fixation and attention to maintaining lumbar lordosis, the long-term results, although yet to be determined, should be improved. Besides permitting greater mobility, a selective thoracic fusion is a shorter and less complicated surgical procedure than is fusion into the lumbar spine.

The disadvantages of selective thoracic fusion include less correction of the coronal-plane deformity in scoliosis, with greater risk of decompensation. For patients who wish to have significant correction of a thoracic deformity, a selective fusion will not allow the complete correction of deformity in the thoracic or lumbar spine. The greatest potential disadvantage of selective fusion is that it may lead to left decompensation, requiring an additional procedure to achieve fusion into the lumbar spine so as to provide coronal balance. This extension of fusion into the lumbar spine may require a more distal level of fusion than would have been needed if the fusion had been done in the primary procedure. It should be remembered that extension of fusion into the lumbar spine because of decompensation following an attempted selective thoracic fusion is a relatively uncommon occurrence.[6,7,13,21]

Although selective fusion is often the goal in surgery for scoliosis, a variety of opinions exist for when it should be performed and how it should be performed. Newton and coworkers[22] analyzed factors involved in the decision to perform a selective fusion for King type II and Lenke type 1B and 1C curves at five different centers. Despite all of the curves being Lenke type 1 curves and therefore requiring side-bending lumbar curve correction of <25 degrees, there was wide variation in the frequency of selective fusion, ranging from 67 to 94%. Newton and colleagues demonstrated that the rate of selective fusion was higher for Lenke 1B than for Lenke 1C curves, at 92% versus 68%. Radiographic factors associated with the fusion of both types of curve included a larger preoperative lumbar curve (42 degrees vs. 37 degrees), greater displacement of the lumbar apical vertebra (3.1 vs. 2.2 mm), and a smaller ratio of thoracic-to-lumbar curve magnitude (1.3 vs. 1.4). However, the most important predictor of fusion into the lumbar spine was the philosophy of each surgeon at each site, with those who felt strongly about preserving motion segments being more likely to perform a selective fusion. If there is a question about the appropriateness of selective thoracic fusion, the matter should be thoroughly discussed with the patient and the patient's parents, including details of the risks and benefits of selective thoracic fusion.

## Anterior versus Posterior Approach for Selective Fusion

Two main approaches are available for fusion of the thoracic spine: anterior and posterior. The anterior approach utilizes instrumentation with vertebral-body screws, which are then connected by single or dual rods to gain correction (**Fig. 12.3**).

A–D

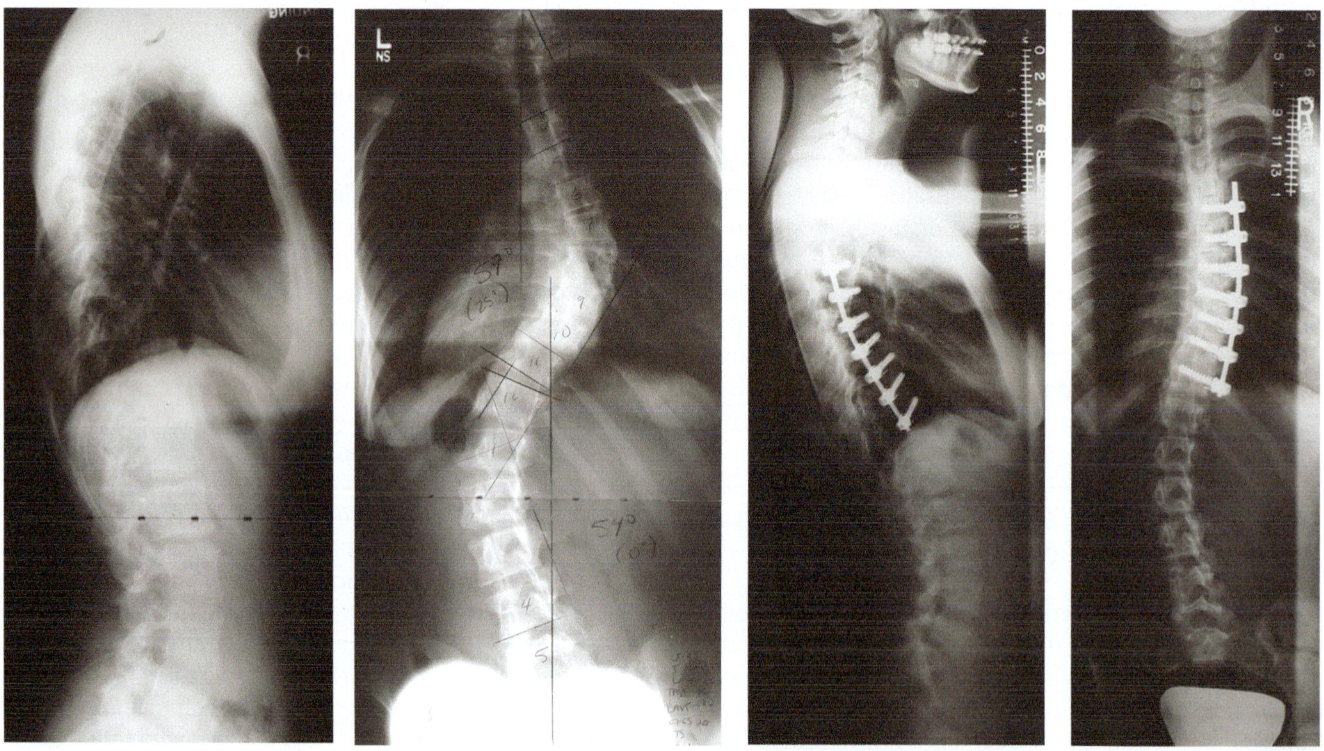

**Fig. 12.3** Selective thoracic fusion using anterior instrumentation and fusion for a Lenke 1C lumbar-curve pattern. **(A,B)** The preoperative PA radiograph demonstrates a 55-degree thoracic curve and a lumbar curve of 53 degrees that is very flexible, bending to zero degrees on supine-bend radiographs. **(C,D)** Two-year radiographs following a thoracoscopic anterior spinal fusion and instrumentation from T6 to T11, with excellent overall coronal and sagittal balance.

The correction maneuvers are typically cantilevering and compression, although rod rotation has also been utilized. The advantage of anterior surgery for a selective thoracic fusion is that, in general, fewer motion segments are fused because this technique allows instrumentation and fusion of the measured Cobb angle, which may not be possible with posterior fusion. Selective thoracic fusion utilizing anterior instrumentation may influence the lumbar curve to a lesser degree than posterior instrumentation if fewer motion segments are included. In addition, the correction mechanics of anterior surgery may not impart a significant rotational force to the lumbar spine, with a correspondingly reduced risk of creating coronal imbalance and decompensation. However, anterior surgery does require entry into the chest, which may injure vital organs and structures and will affect pulmonary function. Yet the use of thoracoscopic techniques limits the negative effect of an anterior approach on pulmonary function.[22]

The posterior approach to instrumentation and fusion of the thoracic spine is more familiar to most surgeons. It is a straightforward approach that can be performed quickly and most commonly produces outstanding results. Posterior instrumentation and fusion, however, does disrupt the paraspinal musculature, and may therefore have long-term health benefits with respect to back pain. The posterior approach often requires fusion to a more caudal extent than anterior surgery, although the use of thoracic pedicle screws may allow greater ability to preserve motion segments. The use of thoracic pedicle screws readily permits segmental manipulation of the spine to a desired correction through multiple correction strategies including cantilevering, segmental in situ bending, translation, direct vertebral rotation, and incomplete rod rotation (**Fig. 12.4**). Early reports of posterior techniques with Cotrell–Dubousset and Texas Scottish Rite Hospital instrumentation to accomplish selective fusion included some concern about creating coronal decompensation.[7,8,10,23,24] These techniques used all-hook constructs, which may not be comparable to the all-pedicle-screw constructs in use today. Several factors were thought to cause coronal decompensation with these all-hook constructs, including instrumenting into the lumbar curve, overcorrection of the thoracic curve, and continued obliquity of the L4 vertebra relative to the pelvis.

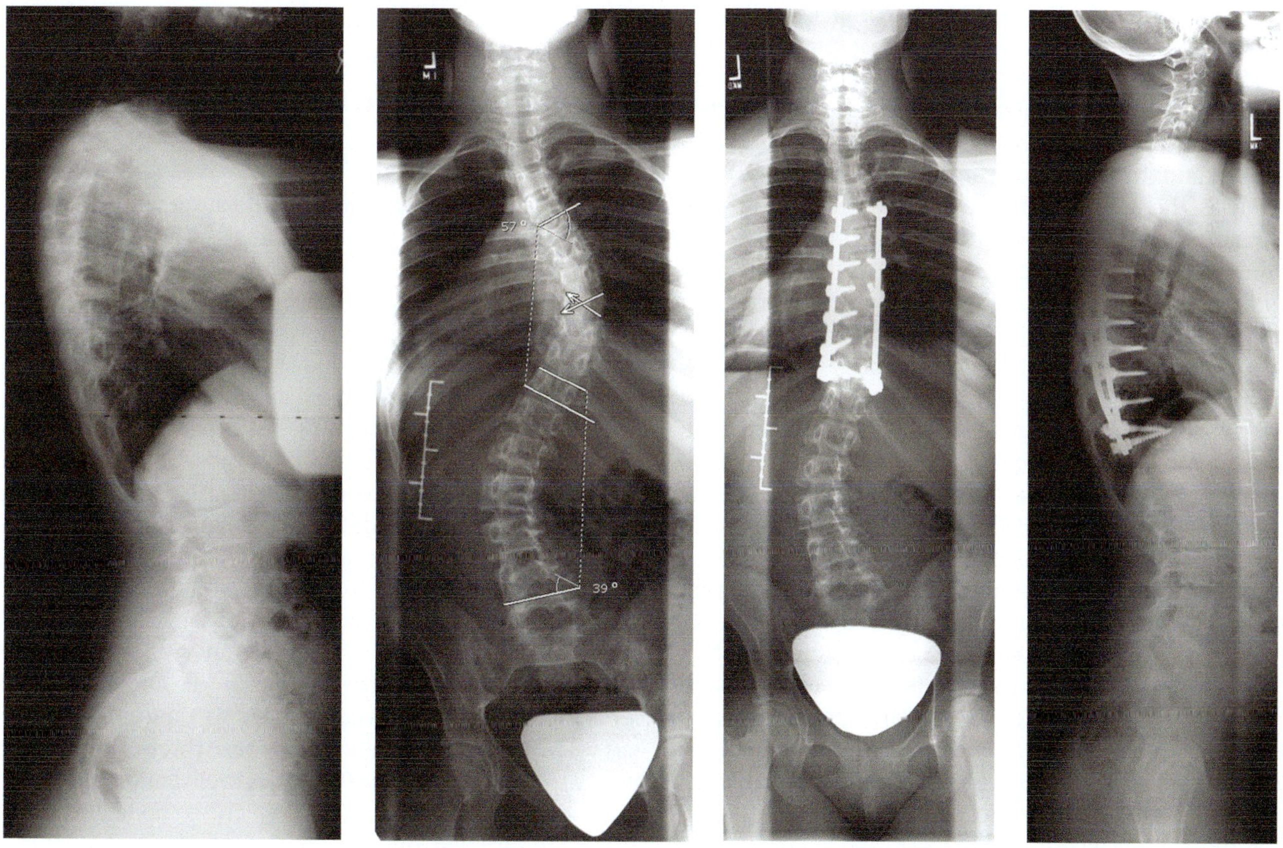


**Fig. 12.4** Selective thoracic spinal fusion done with a posterior approach and instrumentation with pedicle-screw fixation. **(A,B)** Preoperative radiographs demonstrating a 62-degree thoracic curve and a 45-degree lumbar curve. **(C,D)** Two-year postoperative radiographs demonstrating good coronal correction of the thoracic curve, with a good response of the lumbar curve and overall coronal balance.

Early comparisons of the anterior and posterior approaches to selective fusion demonstrated superior results with the anterior approach.[21,25] Betz and colleagues reviewed their experience with 78 patients who underwent anterior spinal fusion with flexible threaded rods in comparison with 100 patients who underwent posterior spinal fusion with multisegmental hook systems. The anterior approach saved 2.5 motion segments (mean) in that many of these patients did not have fusion into the lumbar spine. Surgeons treating these patients felt that anterior surgery could more often be used to perform a selective thoracic fusion, because posterior instrumentation often led to decompensation.[21] To specifically compare the anterior and posterior techniques in a selective-fusion setting, Lenke and colleagues analyzed the cases of 123 patients with selective fusions done either anteriorly or posteriorly. The thoracic-curve correction was superior for the anteriorly treated group (58% vs. 38%) and resulted in greater spontaneous correction of lumbar curves (56% vs. 37%).[25] Lenke and colleagues distinguished lumbar curves on the basis of the position of the apical lumbar vertebra relative to the center sacral vertical line (CSVL), as in their subsequent classification of lumbar curves into those with an "A" modifier (CSVL between pedicles), "B" modifier (CSVL touching the vertebra), and "C" modifier (apical vertebra not touching CSVL). The anterior approach produced greater compensatory lumbar correction in all three of these types of lumbar curves, which was most dramatic for type C lumbar curves. These early comparisons of the anterior and posterior approaches were made with posterior techniques in which only hooks were used and the lowest instrumented vertebra (LIV) was selected as the stable vertebra. A more recent study, in which hybrid and all-screw posterior constructs were used, demonstrated no difference between the anterior and posterior approaches for spontaneous lumbar-curve correction in a series of patients matched for LIV, lumbar-curve flexibility, and percent thoracic-curve correction.[26]

Suk et al were the first to describe thoracic pedicle-screw fixation, demonstrating outstanding overall results with good safety with this technique.[27] They reviewed their experience with selective thoracic fusion with segmental pedicle fixation in 203 patients, and showed 69% correction of thoracic curves with a compensatory lumbar-curve correction of 66%. There were no instances of junctional kyphosis; however, coronal decompensation occurred in 10 patients (5%). Also, 17 patients experienced "adding on" to their spinal curves, most likely because of fusion levels that were too short.[15] Dobbs and colleagues compared posterior hooks with posterior pedicle screws for the selective fusion of thoracic curves in a series of 66 patients, all of whom had lumbar C modifiers. The thoracic pedicle-screw group had greater thoracic correction (53% vs. 34%) and a greater lumbar-curve response (38% vs. 30%) with fewer instances of decompensation than did the posterior-hook group at 2-year follow-up. There were no complications or reoperations in either group. Pedicle-screw instrumentation allows surgeons to keep the lowest instrumented vertebra appropriately tilted, and provides greater ability to "dial-in" the amount of thoracic correction desired on the basis of preoperative thoracic- and lumbar-curve flexibility.[28] These studies support the concept that pedicle screws offer the ability to improve the thoracic curve in scoliosis without decompensation.

In analyzing only patients with a lumbar type C curve, and who were treated with mixed instrumentation consisting of all-hook, all-screw, and hybrid constructs, Edwards and coworkers, at an average 5-year follow-up, demonstrated a 36% overall correction in the patients' thoracic curvature, accompanied by a 34% lumbar-curve correction, which occurred primarily in the more cephalad segments of the lumbar curve.[29] The majority of patients did well with respect to spontaneous correction of their lumbar curvature, although preoperative coronal imbalance was a predictive factor for postoperative coronal balance. Those patients who had a coronal imbalance postoperatively had poorer functional outcome scores, as measured with the Scoliosis Research Society (SRS)-24 instrument. This series had mixed instrumentation, all hooks, all screws, and hybrids.

## Surgical Decision-Making Before Selective Fusion

### Radiographic Evaluation

King and Moe developed their classification of AIS to determine fusion levels for thoracic scoliosis.[3] This classification distinguishes a single thoracic curve with a compensatory lumbar curve (King–Moe type II) from a double major curve in which the lumbar curve is usually larger than the thoracic curve (King–Moe type I). Lenke et al attempted to further define King–Moe type II curves on the basis of several parameters on the standing posteroanterior (PA) radiograph, and side-bending radiographs.[8] They analyzed 50 consecutive patients who were classified as having King type II or III curves, and defined distinguishing features of these curves based on overall radiographic outcome. A successful selective thoracic fusion was more likely if the preoperative ratio of the thoracic-to-lumbar-curve magnitude was $>1.2$, the apical vertebral rotation (AVR) ratio of the thoracic to the lumbar curve was $>1.0$, and the apical vertebral translation of the thoracic to the lumbar curve was $>1.2$ (**Fig. 12.5**). When two of these three criteria were met, 21 of 21 patients (100%) had well-balanced spines postoperatively, however, but when one or none of the criteria were satisfied, only 50% of the patients had balanced spines. Lenke and colleagues defined an exception to their criteria as occurring when the lumbar curve was large in

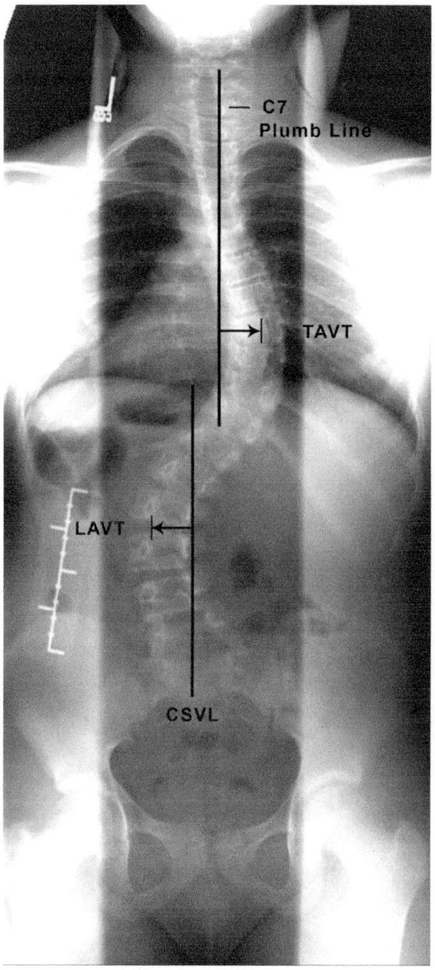


**Fig. 12.5** Method for measuring apical vertebral translation and apical vertebral rotation of both the thoracic and the lumbar curves in scoliosis. The AVT of the thoracic curve is always measured with the C7 plumbline. whereas the AVT of the lumbar curve is measured from the CSVL.

magnitude (>60 degrees) or had significant rotation (>grade 2.5 and deviation of >4 cm from the plumbline used to assess verticality). Richards retrospectively reviewed 24 patients with King type II scoliosis after they underwent selective thoracic fusion.[24] The review focused on the lumbar curve, which in all cases was >40 degrees preoperatively. The patients' overall preoperative thoracic curve was 61 degrees, which improved to 24 degrees postoperatively (a 61% improvement), and at a minimum follow-up of 2-years averaged 32 degrees (47.5%). The lumbar curve responded from a preoperative average of 49 degrees with postoperative improvement to 29 degrees (a 41% improvement) and at a follow-up of at least 2-years was 36 degrees (a 26.5% improvement). Preoperative lumbar rotation was not predictive of lumbar-curve response, spinal balance, or overall truncal balance. Lenke and colleagues compared those patients whose lumbar curves were ≤50 degrees with those whose curves were >50 degrees and found that the larger lumbar curves had truncal imbalance, although this was not significant. They then determined that the lumbar obliquity measured between L4 and the pelvis remained unchanged, averaging 14 degrees, and was accompanied by a truncal shift of 1.5 cm, and strongly recommended careful evaluation of this lumbar obliquity preoperatively in the planning of a selective fusion (**Fig. 12.6**). More recently Jansen et al made similar findings, in which the response of the lumbar curve was found to occur in the proximal aspect of the curve rather than its distal aspect.[30] McCall and Bronson found that lumbar curves >45 degrees and in which the flexibility index was low were more likely to decompensate if a selective thoracic fusion was performed.[31] In addition to the assessment of the coronal-plane deformity and spinal flexibility in scoliosis, some have recommended careful evaluation of the axial-plane deformity with the Perdriolle method. Behensky et al determined that less than 40% derotation of the lumbar apical rotation accurately predicted coronal spinal decompensation postoperatively.

The Lenke classification has improved the definitions of scoliosis in describing whether the lumbar curve is structural or compensatory to the thoracic curve.[32] Two parameters are specifically analyzed to assist in determining whether the lumbar curve is considered a compensatory curve, which allows treatment of the patient with a selective thoracic fusion. The first parameter is the flexibility of the lumbar curve on a radiograph of a supine best-bend to the opposite side of the curve. If the coronal-plane measurement is <25 degrees on this radiograph, the curve is considered to be a compensatory curve and not to require inclusion in the fusion. The second parameter is the lumbar modifier, which denotes the degree of apical vertebral translation (AVT) by the position of the apical vertebral body relative to the CSVL. The greater the translation of the apical vertebra from the CSVL, the more likely it is that a curve is structural and requires inclusion in the fusion levels. When the CSVL is between the pedicles, the lumbar curve falls into the group with an A modifier in the Lenke classification; when the CSVL is between the pedicle and the lateral vertebral body, the lumbar curve is designated as being of class B. A C modifier is applied when the CSVL does not touch the apical vertebra in the lumbar curve.

The term *selective fusion* assumes that there are structural characteristics to a lumbar curve, including complete translation of the apical vertebra, and this term is used for lumbar C modifiers, predominantly. An A modifier should automatically exclude discussions of selective versus nonselective fusion for a lumbar curve, and indicates that a lumbar curve should go unfused. With a B or C modifier. the decision about whether to include the

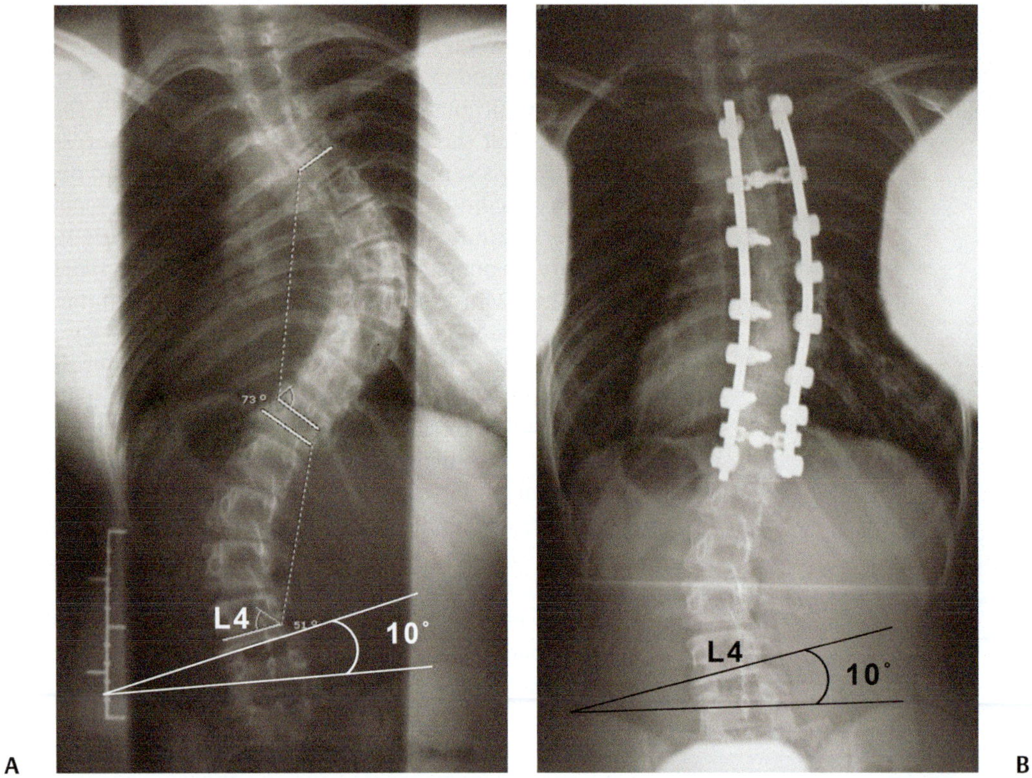


**Fig. 12.6** Measurement of the L4 obliquity relative to the pelvis partly predicts the response of the lumbar curve to selective thoracic fusion. **(A)** Preoperative measurement of the obliquity of L4 demonstrates a final angle of 10 degrees. **(B)** Coronal radiograph at 2 years after a selective thoracic fusion, demonstrating a similar obliquity of L4 relative to the pelvis as that seen preoperatively.

lumbar curve in a thoracolumbar fusion or to perform a selective thoracic fusion is challenging, and several parameters need to be examined before this decision is made. In general, because a B modifier indicates that the apical vertebra is not as far from the midline as in the case of a C modifier, curves with a B modifier are less likely to need fusion, and selective fusion is more often considered in such cases. Many would suggest, in fact, that no lumbar curve with a B modifier requires inclusion in the fusion and instrumentation. However, studies do suggest that lumbar curves with C modifiers do not necessarily have to be included in the fusion mass, and that consideration of a selective fusion is warranted.[29] An additional characteristic for determining whether a lumbar curve is structural is the measured kyphosis between T10 and L2, which, if >20 degrees, defines junctional kyphosis and the presence of two structural curves. The ratio of the thoracic-to-lumbar-curve magnitude, AVT, and AVR help to determine whether selective thoracic fusion is appropriate.[8] If the ratio of the magnitude of the thoracic to that of the lumbar curve is >1.2, the AVT is >1.2, and the AVR is >1.0, it is more likely that a well-balanced correction will be achieved with a selective thoracic fusion. However, if one or more of these criteria are not met, it is more likely that decompensation will occur, because the lumbar curve has a more structural character.

## Clinical Examination

The most important parameter in selecting surgical treatment for a spinal deformity is the clinical appearance of the patient. This certainly holds true when deciding whether to perform a selective fusion for patients with Lenke type 1B and type 1C curve patterns. The overall preoperative coronal balance should be to the right or neutral when planning a selective thoracic fusion. Patients who have a truncal shift to the left most likely have a structural lumbar curve, and selective fusion is contraindicated (**Fig. 12.7**). Evaluation of the rotational deformity of a patient's spine with the scoliometer, or clinical assessment with the Adams forward-bend test, is important for determining whether the patient's lumbar curve appears to be structural relative to the thoracic curve. A minor lumbar-rotational deformity in the presence of a large thoracic rotational deformity usually indicates that selective fusion can be performed.

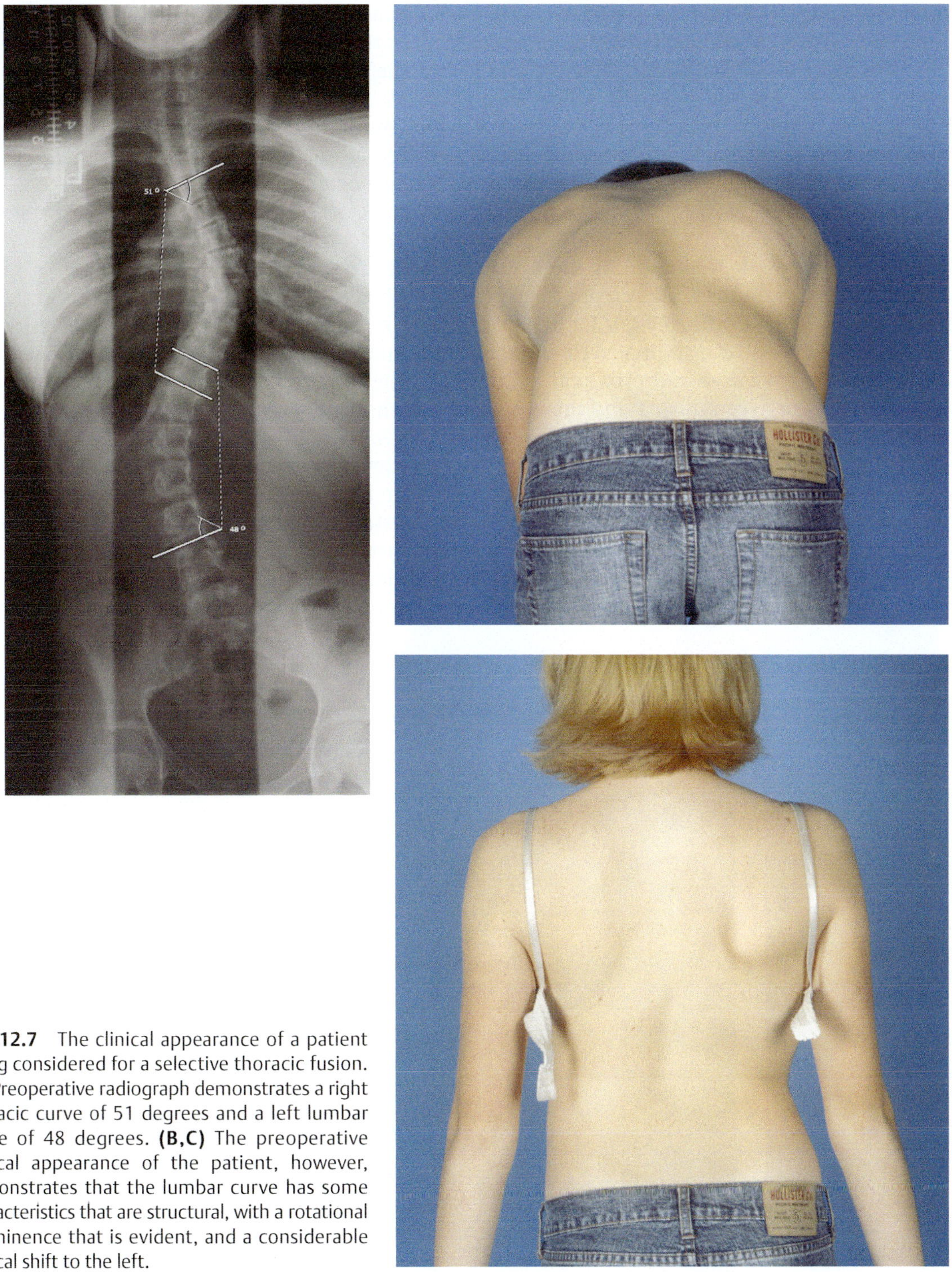


A B C

**Fig. 12.7** The clinical appearance of a patient being considered for a selective thoracic fusion. **(A)** Preoperative radiograph demonstrates a right thoracic curve of 51 degrees and a left lumbar curve of 48 degrees. **(B,C)** The preoperative clinical appearance of the patient, however, demonstrates that the lumbar curve has some characteristics that are structural, with a rotational prominence that is evident, and a considerable truncal shift to the left.

## Surgical Planning for Selective Fusion

The options in performing a selective thoracic fusion are an anterior approach or a posterior approach. Much has recently changed in the making of this decision, as posterior constructs have become more rigid and segmental fixation is more often utilized.[14] However, with good preoperative planning and careful surgical technique, anterior instrumentation and fusion has traditionally produced outstanding results.[21,25,33-35]

When choosing the upper instrumented vertebra (UIV) in a selective thoracic fusion, it is most common to choose the proximal end-vertebra of the main thoracic

(MT) curve. The proximal thoracic (PT) curve should be evaluated radiographically as well as clinically to determine whether it requires inclusion in the fusion. Selection of the LIV depends on several factors, including the surgical approach to be taken (anterior vs. posterior), the type of thoracic anchors to be used (hooks vs. screws), and the relationship of the distal end-vertebra to the CSVL. The goal in choosing the LIV is to allow for adequate control and correction of the MT curve while avoiding any influence of the proximal portion of the thoracolumbar/lumbar (TL/L) curve that would create a risk for decompensation. As a general rule, the LIV for a selective thoracic fusion should be the transitional vertebra (distal end-vertebra of the MT curve and proximal end-vertebra of the TL/L curve) between the MT and the TL/L curves. The translation of the transitional vertebra should be assessed relative to the CSVL and should be touched by this line, especially when the posterior approach is utilized (**Fig. 12.8**). In general, the distal level of fusion for the anterior approach should be at the distal end-vertebra (**Fig. 12.9**), whereas the posterior approach uses the most proximal vertebra touched by the CSVL. A variety of approaches to choosing the LIV have been reported. For the posterior approach, Suk et al[15] relates the LIV to the neutral vertebra. The "gap" or distance from the LIV to the neutral vertebra should not be greater than one vertebra, or decompensation may occur. Others utilize the stable vertebra as a reference to choose the LIV as being one or two levels proximal to it.[28]

The author (D.J.S.) generally analyzes the following three parameters to determine the LIV of the thoracic curve: (1) the distal end-vertebra of the thoracic curve; (2) the last vertebra touched by the LIV; and (3) the status of the disc space below the end-vertebra. The LIV for a posterior construct is the end-vertebra if it is the most proximal vertebra touched by the CSVL and the disc below this vertebra is opened into the lumbar curve. If the disc below the end-vertebra is parallel, then LIV becomes the next most distal vertebra, to allow inclusion of the parallel disc. Anterior instrumentation and fusion are generally considered when one or two distal fusion levels can be saved. This most often occurs when the end-vertebra does not touch the CSVL on the preoperative curve, and a posterior fusion will require fusion one or two levels below the end-vertebra. In

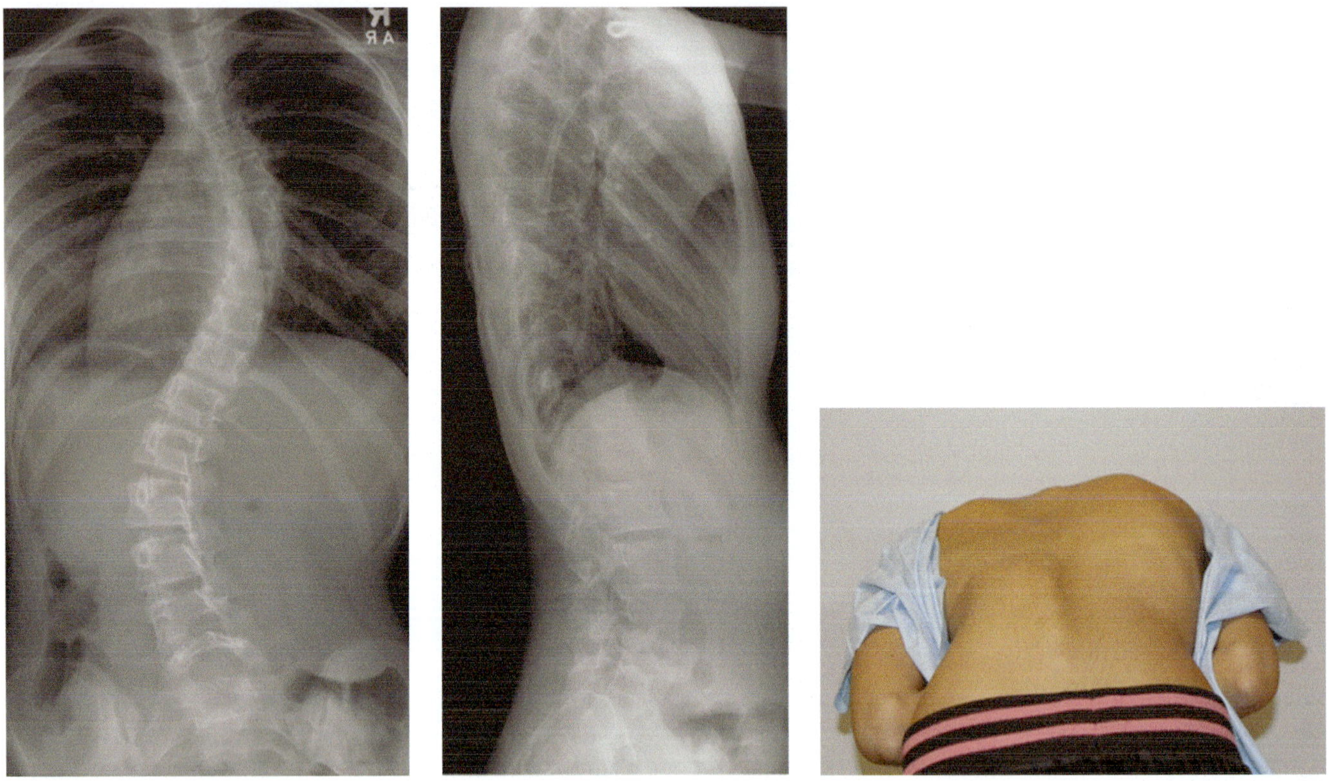

A–C

**Fig. 12.8** The selection of fusion levels when performing posterior instrumentation and fusion in a patient treated with selective fusion. **(A)** In this Lenke 1C curve pattern, the patient's thoracic curve measures 55 degrees and her lumbar curve measures 48 degrees. The apical vertebral translation (AVT), not the thoracic curve, is larger than the lumbar curve **(B)** The sagittal plane is unremarkable. **(C)** The lumbar rotation is <2 degrees. The thoracic prominence is much larger than the lumbar prominence. The patient is a good candidate for a selective thoracic fusion.

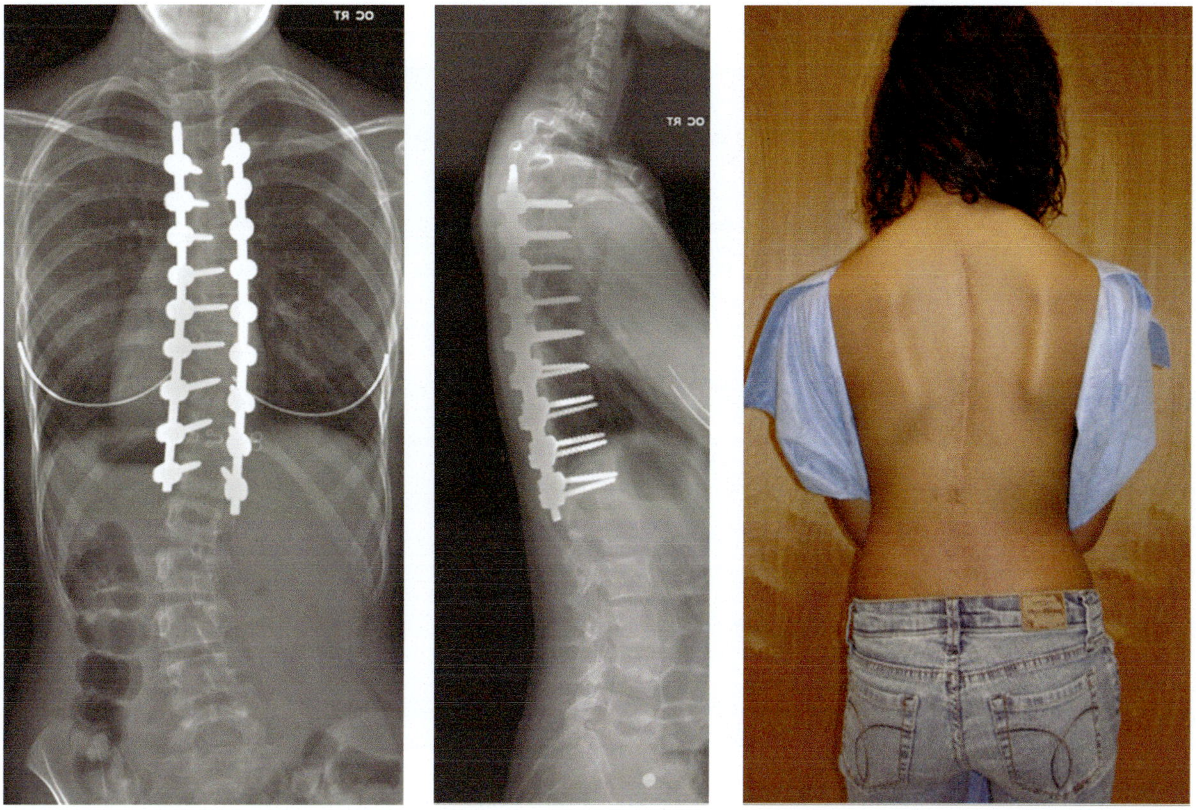

D–F

**Fig. 12.8** (*Continued*) **(D,E)** Selective thoracic fusion with an all- screw construct has produced xcellent balance. Note the tilt remaining in T12, blending with the lumbar curve. **(F)** The patient's clinical appearance is excellent.

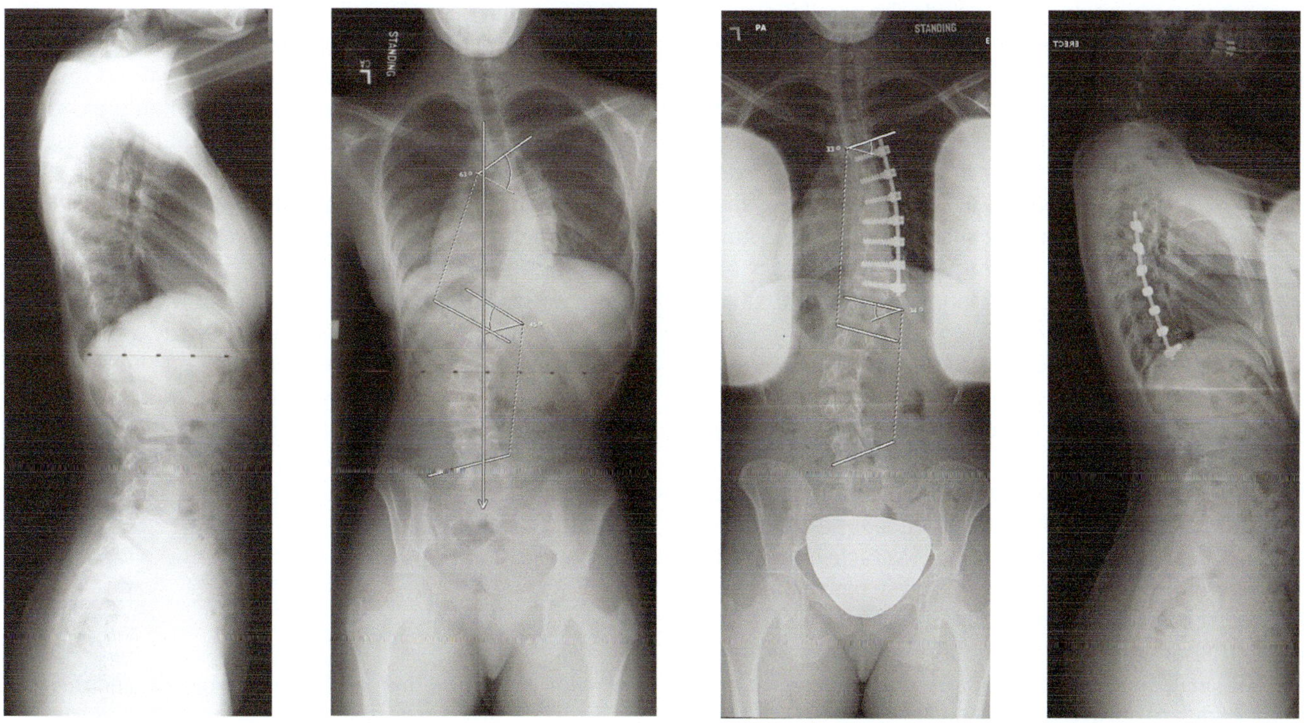


**Fig. 12.9** The selection of fusion levels when performing anterior instrumentation and fusion in a patient treated with selective fusion. **(A,B)** Preoperative AP and lateral radiographs demonstrating a 63-degree right thoracic curve measured from T5 to T11 and a lumbar curve measured from T11 to L4. Because T11 is the transitional vertebra (distal end-vertebra of the thoracic curve and proximal end-vertebra of the lumbar curve), one can consider performing an anterior selective fusion to this level. **(C,D)** Five-year postoperative radiographs demonstrate balanced 33-degree curves.

(*Continued on page 146*)

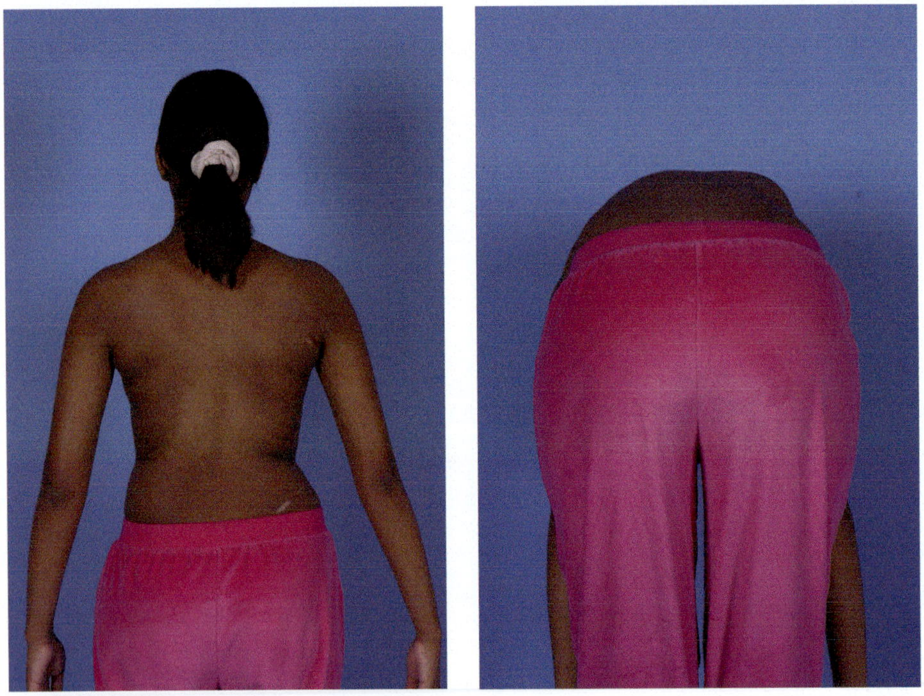

E,F

**Fig. 12.9** (*Continued*) The selection of fusion levels while performing anterior instrumentation and fusion in a patient treated with selective fusion. **(E,F)** Clinical photographs at 5 years demonstrate excellent overall balance in the coronal plane. Preservation of motion in the lumbar spine allows outstanding flexibility.

the author's view, the distal end-vertebra can always be the LIV for a selective thoracic fusion when the anterior approach is used and does not include the parallel disc.

A balance exists between obtaining thoracic-curve correction and creating decompensation through overcorrection of the thoracic curve that influences the lumbar curve. The first step in attaining this balance is to predetermine the magnitude of correction of the thoracic curve to be achieved at surgery, which is based on a variety of factors. First among these factors are the magnitude and flexibility of the lumbar curve, because this seems to influence the amount of response to thoracic-curve correction. A smaller lumbar curve (<45 degrees) that is very flexible is more likely to respond to greater thoracic-curve correction. A very flexible lumbar curve, which bends to less than 10 degrees, is more likely to respond to thoracic-curve correction, whereas a stiff lumbar curve will not. The second factor in predetermining the thoracic-curve correction in surgery is the flexibility of the thoracic curve, which can be assessed on a supine best-bend film or a push–prone radiograph. A thoracic curve with a flexibility index of >50% on a supine best-bend film may be easily corrected at the time of surgery, with little influence on the lumbar curve. Just as important as measurement of the Cobb angle in the coronal plane is the residual tilt of the LIV following surgical correction, which is based on the parameters named above, with a general residual tilt of 10 to 20 degrees being desirable. Intraoperative radiographs are important for assessing the amount of coronal-plane correction achieved, as well as for assessing the extent of tilt, so as to allow the surgeon to change these parameters to the desired correction (**Fig. 12.10**).

Correction strategies for selective fusion vary with the approach, type of posterior anchors to be used, and philosophy of the surgeon. Some suggest partial rod rotation to avoid a full 90-degree rod rotation, which will impart forces to the lumbar curve, whereas others suggest the use of more distraction and translational forces.[36] Recently, Chang et al recommended using a cantilever bending technique (CBT) of the convex rod, and reported achieving 83% coronal-plane correction of the thoracic curve, with a similar response of the lumbar curve.[12] Anterior correction strategies include cantilevering of the rod with sequential compression, using a thoracoscopic approach, and rod rotation with an open thoracotomy approach. The most important point with all approaches and techniques is to have incomplete correction of the thoracic curve, and a curve apex with residual tilt of the thoracic end-vertebra at the completion of surgery.

## Postoperative Course

Following a selective thoracic fusion, the patient and the family should understand that the patient will have truncal imbalance with a shift to the left in the early postoperative period. In addition, splinting by the patient after anterior surgery may accentuate this coronal imbalance as the patient tries to remain comfortable. Families may be alarmed at the

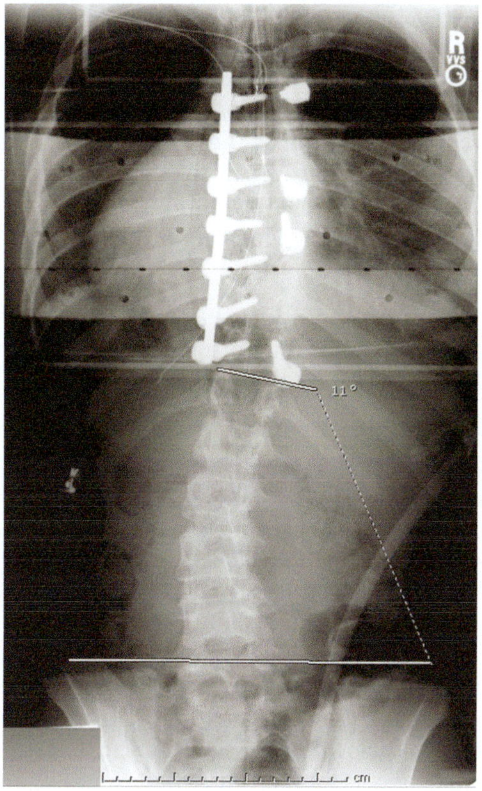


**Fig. 12.10** This intraoperative radiograph of the patient in Figure 12.4 demonstrates some intended residual tilt of the LIV to prevent decompensation.

initial appearance of the patient's radiographs and clinical appearance of the patient, and this should be explained before surgery as an expected occurrence. The patient's coronal balance should improve over time, and usually stabilizes within 6 to 12 months. The ability to reduce this decompensation generally comes at the expense of a lumbar curve that increases so as to bring the patient back into coronal balance. In the skeletally immature patient (Risser grade 0 and open triradiate cartilage), a brace can be used to prevent further lumbar curve progression, although this is often unnecessary.

## Recent Data from the Harms Study Group

The Harms Study Group (HSG) analyzed 230 patients who had Lenke 1 or 2 curves and compared those patients who had a selective fusion with those who had a fusion of both the thoracic and lumbar curves. There were 184 patients in the selective-fusion group and 46 in the nonselective-fusion group. There were no differences in the selective- and nonselective-fusion groups with respect to age (14.4 ± 1.9 vs. 14.6 ± 2.3 years) or gender (89.1% female vs. 82.6% female). Preoperatively, the magnitude of the thoracic curve was the same in the two groups (52.6 ± 8.4 degrees vs. 56.1 ± 12.9 degrees), as was the spine flexibility index (48.0 ± 15.6% vs. 43.0 ± 18.5%). There were some differences in the characteristics of the lumbar curve in the two groups, in that the magnitude of the curve was smaller (37.6 ± 7.5 degrees vs. 41.4 ± 9.5 degrees), the flexibility was greater (74.2 ± 17.1% vs. 70.0 ± 13.9%), and the apical translation of the TL/L curve was less (20.9 ± 8.3 mm vs. 25.3 ± 11.9 mm) in the selective-fusion group than in the nonselective-fusion group. The preoperative end-vertebral translation was also smaller in the selective-fusion group (11.0 ± 7.8 mm vs. 17.8 ± 8.8 mm). Sagittal-plane parameters showed that junctional kyphosis distally was less marked in the selective-fusion group (3.5 ± 4.0 degrees vs. 15.4 ± 11.5 degrees). The greatest difference between the two groups was in the distribution of Lenke curve types, with a greater percentage of C lumbar modifiers in the group of patients that had fusion into the lumbar spine. Among patients who had a selective fusion, 35.8% had a type C lumbar curve as compared with 54% who had fusion into the lumbar spine.

Postoperatively, there was intentionally less correction of the thoracic curve in the selective fusion group (20.3 ± 8.5 degrees vs. 17.7 ± 8.9 degrees), with a smaller percent correction (61.7 ± 14.2 vs. 68.2 ± 14.6%) but no postoperative difference in the thoracic apical translation (11.7 ± 9.8 mm vs. 11.2 ± 10.2 mm). There was a nice response of the lumbar curve to selective thoracic fusion, with a postoperative thoracic curve of 22.0 ± 8.1 degrees. As one would expect, the lumbar curve correction was greater in patients who had fusion of the lumbar curve, with a postoperative curve of 15 ± 7.8 degrees. Greater residual apical translation of the TL/L curve was seen in the selective fusion group (21.3 ± 11.5 mm vs.15.6 ± 8.9 mm). The overall postoperative coronal balance as measured by the distance between the C7 plumbline and the sacrum was no different in the the groups (14.9 ± 11.3 mm vs. 14.6 ± 9.3 mm).

At a minimum follow-up of 2 years, the magnitude of the thoracic curve was greater in the selective- than in the nonselective-fusion group (24.6 ± 10.1 degrees vs. 20.4 ± 9.9 degrees), and the overall thoracic curve correction was smaller (53.4 ± 17.1% vs. 62.8 ± 17.5%); however, thoracic apical translation was similar in the two groups (15.1 ± 11.8 mm vs. 13.5 ± 10.1 mm). Similarly, the magnitude of the lumbar curve was greater in the selective-fusion group (21.0 ± 8.4 degrees vs. 17.9 ± 10.2 degrees), but the TL/L apical translation in the two groups was similar at 2 years (15.5 ± 9.2 mm vs. 16.0 ± 10.5 mm). The sagittal-plane parameters in the two groups were fairly similar, although at 2 years the thoracic kyphosis as measured from T5 to 12 was greater in the selective-fusion group (27.3 ± 10.5 degrees vs. 23.2 ± 9.6 degrees). The overall balance as measured with the C7 plumbline showed greater coronal imbalance in the selective-fusion group (22.0 ± 1.3 mm vs. 17.7 ± 10.4 mm) ($P = 0.008$).

The functional scores at a minimum of 2 years showed greater SRS total scores on the SRS-24 instrument in the selective- than in the nonselective-fusion group (82.5 ± 37.4 vs. 59.2 ± 46.5) ($P = 0.01$). When the specific domains in the SRS-24 instrument were analyzed, the selective-fusion group had greater scores with respect to function after surgery (5.1 ± 2.9 vs. 3.1 ± 3.1), functional level of activity (11.6 ± 5.5 vs. 8.1 ± 6.5), general self-image (10.9 ± 5.1 vs. 8.2 ± 6.4), pain (25.0 ± 11.6 vs. 17.9 ± 14.5), and patient satisfaction (10.9 ± 5.4 vs. 8.1 ± 6.4). The total score on section 1 of the SRS-24 instrument was also greater (55.5 ± 24.9 vs. 39.6 ± 31.0), as was the total score for section 2 of the instrument (27.1 ± 13.4 vs. 19.6 ± 16.1).

Because of the retrospective nature of the study, there may have been some selection bias in favor of including the lumbar spine in the fusion levels for those patients who had larger lumbar curves, which crossed the midline. To limit this bias, a subanalysis was done to compare matched groups of patients with similar curve characteristics, specifically matching curve magnitude and flexibility of both the thoracic and lumbar curves. The two groups in the subanalysis contained of 46 patients each, and because of the matching process, the magnitudes and flexibilities of the thoracic and lumbar curves of patients in the selective- and nonselective-fusion groups were the same (thoracic curve: 54.6 degrees vs. 56.1 degrees, and 48.5% vs. 43.5%; lumbar curve: 41.8 vs. 41.4 degrees and 72.2% vs. 70.0%). At 2-year follow-up, the selective-fusion group had a greater thoracic curve magnitude (25.6 degrees vs. 20.4 degrees), less thoracic-curve correction (53.3% vs. 62.8%), a lumbar curve of greater magnitude (23.4 degrees vs.17.9 degrees), and less lumbar curve correction (43.4% vs. 56.4%) than did the nonselective-fusion group; however, coronal balance as measured by the distance between the plumbline from C7 to the CSVL was the same. The total SRS-24 scores preoperatively were the samein the two groups in the subanalysis, but the patients in the selective-fusion group had better total SRS-24 scores at 2 years (86.8 vs. 59.2), as well as better scores in each of the individual domains of the SRS-24. Further follow-up of these groups will be needed to see whether their coronal imbalance remains stable and whether the functional scores for the selective-fusion group continue to be higher than for the nonselective-fusion group.

## Conclusion

Within the case of a Lenke 1 curve with a B or C lumbar modifier, the ability to perform a selective thoracic fusion is based on careful consideration of the patient's clinical and radiographic characteristics. When the patient demonstrates a large rotational deformity and a truncal shift to the left, a satisfactory result is less likely to occur. Careful consideration of the magnitude and flexibility of both the thoracic curve and the lumbar curve, and of the ratios between the thoracic and lumbar curves with respect to the curve magnitude, apical translation, and rotation is critical to determining whether to perform a selective thoracic fusion. A selective thoracic fusion can be performed with either an anterior or a posterior approach with similar results with respect to improvement in thoracic curve and response of the lumbar curve. It is important to undercorrect the thoracic curve and leave some residual tilt of the LIV to allow spontaneous correction of the lumbar curve. When it is possible to perform selective thoracic fusion on curves with these patterns, the functional outcome scores on the SRS-24 questionnaire appear to be significantly better for all domains, most probably because of sparing of lumbar motion segments leading to better perceived results.

### References


1. Moe JH. A critical analysis of methods of fusion for scoliosis; an evaluation in two hundred and sixty-six patients. J Bone Joint Surg Am 1958;40A:529–554, passim
2. Moe JH. Methods of correction and surgical techniques in scoliosis. Orthop Clin North Am 1972;3:17–48
3. King HA, Moe JH, Bradford DS, Winter RB. The selection of fusion levels in thoracic idiopathic scoliosis. J Bone Joint Surg Am 1983; 65:1302–1313
4. Bassett GS, Hensinger MC, Keiper MD. Effect of posterior spinal fusion on spinal balance in idiopathic scoliosis. J Pediatr Orthop 1989;9:672–674
5. McCance SE, Denis F, Lonstein JE, Winter RB. Coronal and sagittal balance in surgically treated adolescent idiopathic scoliosis with the King II curve pattern. A review of 67 consecutive cases having selective thoracic arthrodesis. Spine 1998;23:2063–2073
6. Frez R, Cheng JC, Wong EM. Longitudinal changes in trunkal balance after selective fusion of King II curves in adolescent idiopathic scoliosis. Spine 2000;25:1352–1359
7. Bridwell KH, McAllister JW, Betz RR, Huss G, Clancy M, Schoenecker PL. Coronal decompensation produced by Cotrel-Dubousset "derotation" maneuver for idiopathic right thoracic scoliosis. Spine 1991;16:769–777
8. Lenke LG, Bridwell KH, Baldus C, Blanke K. Preventing decompensation in King type II curves treated with Cotrel-Dubousset instrumentation. Strict guidelines for selective thoracic fusion. Spine 1992;17(8, suppl):S274–S281
9. Richards BS, Birch JG, Herring JA, Johnston CE, Roach JW. Frontal plane and sagittal plane balance following Cotrel-Dubousset instrumentation for idiopathic scoliosis. Spine 1989;14: 733–737

10. Thompson JP, Transfeldt EE, Bradford DS, Ogilvie JW, Boachie-Adjei O. Decompensation after Cotrel-Dubousset instrumentation of idiopathic scoliosis. Spine 1990;15:927–931
11. Lenke LG, Betz RR, Harms J, et al. Adolescent idiopathic scoliosis: A new classification to determine extent of spinal arthrodesis. J Bone Joint Surg Am 2001;83A:1169–1181
12. Chang K-W, Chang K-I, Wu C-M. Enhanced capacity for spontaneous correction of lumbar curve in the treatment of major thoracic-compensatory C modifier lumbar curve pattern in idiopathic scoliosis. Spine 2007;32:3020–3029
13. Dobbs MB, Lenke LG, Walton T, et al. Can we predict the ultimate lumbar curve in adolescent idiopathic scoliosis patients undergoing a selective fusion with undercorrection of the thoracic curve? Spine 2004;29:277–285
14. Dobbs MB, Lenke LG, Kim YJ, Kamath G, Peelle MW, Bridwell KH. Selective posterior thoracic fusions for adolescent idiopathic scoliosis: Comparison of hooks versus pedicle screws. Spine 2006;31: 2400–2404
15. Suk S-I, Lee SM, Chung ER, Kim JH, Kim SS. Selective thoracic fusion with segmental pedicle screw fixation in the treatment of thoracic idiopathic scoliosis: More than 5-year follow-up. Spine 2005;30: 1602–1609
16. Wilk B, Karol LA, Johnston CE II, Colby S, Haideri N. The effect of scoliosis fusion on spinal motion: A comparison of fused and nonfused patients with idiopathic scoliosis. Spine 2006;31:309–314
17. Engsberg JR, Lenke LG, Reitenbach AK, Hollander KW, Bridwell KH, Blanke K. Prospective evaluation of trunk range of motion in adolescents with idiopathic scoliosis undergoing spinal fusion surgery. Spine 2002;27:1346–1354
18. Paonessa KJ, Engler GL. Back pain and disability after Harrington rod fusion to the lumbar spine for scoliosis. Spine 1992;17(8, suppl): S249–S253
19. Cochran T, Irstam L, Nachemson A. Long-term anatomic and functional changes in patients with adolescent idiopathic scoliosis treated by Harrington rod fusion. Spine 1983;8:576–584
20. Cochran T, Nachemson A. Long-term anatomic and functional changes in patients with adolescent idiopathic scoliosis treated with the Milwaukee brace. Spine 1985;10:127–133
21. Betz RR, Harms J, Clements DH III, et al. Comparison of anterior and posterior instrumentation for correction of adolescent thoracic idiopathic scoliosis. Spine 1999;24:225–239
22. Newton P, et al. Pulmonary function in anterior scoliosis surgery: Open vs. thoracoscopic approaches. Paper presented at: Annual Meeting of the Pediatric Orthopaedic Society of North America. 2004. St. Louis, MO
23. McCance SE, Winter RB, Lonstein JE. A King type II curve pattern treated with selective thoracic fusion: Case report with 44-year follow-up. J Spinal Disord 1999;12:262–265
24. Richards BS. Lumbar curve response in type II idiopathic scoliosis after posterior instrumentation of the thoracic curve. Spine 1992; 17(8, suppl):S282–S286
25. Lenke LG, Betz RR, Bridwell KH, Harms J, Clements DH, Lowe TG. Spontaneous lumbar curve coronal correction after selective anterior or posterior thoracic fusion in adolescent idiopathic scoliosis. Spine 1999;24:1663–1671, discussion 1672
26. Patel PN, Upasani VV, Bastrom TP, et al. Spontaneous lumbar curve correction in selective thoracic fusions of idiopathic scoliosis: A comparison of anterior and posterior approaches. Spine 2008;33: 1068–1073
27. Suk SI, Lee CK, Kim WJ, Chung YJ, Park YB. Segmental pedicle screw fixation in the treatment of thoracic idiopathic scoliosis. Spine 1995;20:1399–1405
28. Dobbs MB, Lenke LG, Walton T, et al. Can we predict the ultimate lumbar curve in adolescent idiopathic scoliosis patients undergoing a selective fusion with undercorrection of the thoracic curve? Spine 2004;29:277–285
29. Edwards CC II, Lenke LG, Peelle M, Sides B, Rinella A, Bridwell KH. Selective thoracic fusion for adolescent idiopathic scoliosis with C modifier lumbar curves: 2- to 16-year radiographic and clinical results. Spine 2004;29:536–546
30. Jansen RC, van Rhijn LW, Duinkerke E, van Ooij A. Predictability of the spontaneous lumbar curve correction after selective thoracic fusion in idiopathic scoliosis. Eur Spine J 2007;16: 1335–1342
31. McCall RE, Bronson W. Criteria for selective fusion in idiopathic scoliosis using Cotrel-Dubousset instrumentation. J Pediatr Orthop 1992;12:475–479
32. Lenke LG, Betz RR, Harms J, et al. Adolescent idiopathic scoliosis: A new classification to determine extent of spinal arthrodesis. J Bone Joint Surg Am 2001;83A:1169–1181
33. Liljenqvist UR, Bullmann V, Schulte TL, Hackenberg L, Halm HF. Anterior dual rod instrumentation in idiopathic thoracic scoliosis. Eur Spine J 2006;15:1118–1127
34. Schulte TL, Liljenqvist U, Hierholzer E, et al. Spontaneous correction and derotation of secondary curves after selective anterior fusion of idiopathic scoliosis. Spine 2006;31:315–321
35. Bullmann V, Fallenberg EM, Meier N, et al. Anterior dual rod instrumentation in idiopathic thoracic scoliosis: A computed tomography analysis of screw placement relative to the aorta and the spinal canal. Spine 2005;30:2078–2083
36. Goshi K, Boachie-Adjei O, Moore C, Nishiyama M. Thoracic scoliosis fusion in adolescent and adult idiopathic scoliosis using posterior translational corrective techniques (Isola): Is maximum correction of the thoracic curve detrimental to the unfused lumbar curve? Spine J 2004;4:192–201

# 13 Selection of Fusion Levels

*Daniel S. Mulconrey and Lawrence G. Lenke*

The selection of fusion levels for the surgical treatment of adolescent idiopathic scoliosis (AIS) has been debated since the inception of this surgical procedure. This debate began before the introduction of instrumentation for scoliosis [1–5] and has intensified during the modern era of segmental spinal fixation. After the introduction of posterior instrumentation, Harrington addressed the concept of the stable zone to identify the distal extent for a spinal fusion. Harrington defined the stable zone as the area between two parallel vertical lines running through the lumbosacral joint, and recommended that the end-vertebra of a spinal fusion be within that stable zone.[6,7] Moe introduced the practice of evaluating curve flexibility and vertebral rotation to select fusion levels; thus initiating the concept of giving flexible curves the ability to correct spontaneously while performing a selective fusion of the more rigid curvature.[4,8] Later, King and colleagues[9] categorized patients with AIS and created a classification system for it. Included in King's evaluation of patients with AIS was a description of the center sacral vertical line (CSVL), a vertical line that bisects the sacrum and is perpendicular to the level iliac crests. The CSVL falls in the middle of Harrington's stable zone[6,7] and bisects the stable vertebra (**Fig. 13.1**).

Lenke et al[10] further subdivided and analyzed patients with AIS to develop a comprehensive classification system. The Lenke classification included a two-dimensional (2D) evaluation of the scoliotic curvature with sagittal-plane emphasis, specific objective criteria for increasing interobserver reliability, and the ability to provide a template for spinal-fusion surgery.[11] The fundamentals of this classification system will be the focus of the remaining portion of this chapter. This classification system, as outlined in Chapter 9, provides an algorithm for assisting in the selection of spinal fusion levels. The selection of fusion levels is a complex decision-making process that focuses on both clinical and radiographic examination.

## History and Physical Examination

The history and physical examination is a critical facets in the process of spinal-fusion surgery. The patient's skeletal maturity, family history of scoliosis, medical comorbidities, activity level, and reported self-image influence the management of scoliosis. The clinical deformity (shoulder balance, trunk shift, thoracic and lumbar prominence) in addition to the radiographic deformity will determine the selection of fusion levels. The difficulty in fusion surgery is in predicting how the correction and fusion of the patient's scoliosis will affect this clinical deformity while maintaining coronal and sagittal balance.

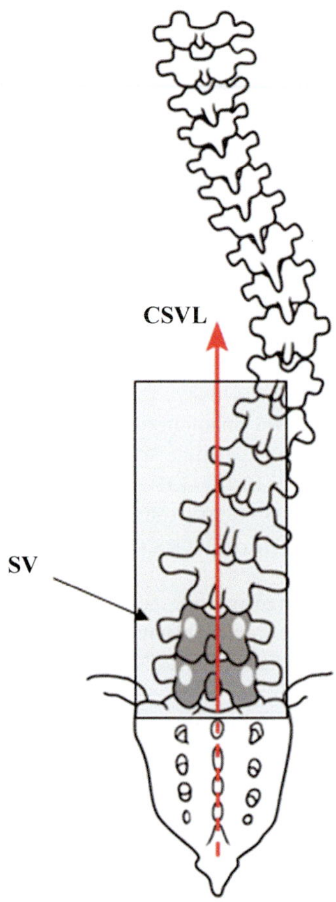


**Fig. 13.1** Illustration of the center sacral vertical line (CSVL). The figure has been modified to include the stable vertebra (SV) and Harrington's stable zone (*shaded area*). (From the Spinal Deformity Study Group Radiographic Measurement Manual, page 47, published by Medtronic, Inc., 2004.)

## ■ Radiographic Evaluation

Radiographic analysis of the patient with AIS should include long-cassette standing anteroposterior (AP) and lateral radiographs of the spine. The position of the patient's arms should also be noted on the radiograph, as different positions may lead to alterations in sagittal balance.[12] A set of flexibility films should also be collected, and may include right and left side-bending, push–prone, or traction radiographs.[13–16]

As discussed in Chapter 5, multiple radiographic measurements are needed to fully understand the patient's radiographic deformity. The magnitude and flexibility of each spinal curve will determine whether a curve is structural and should be included in the fusion. Identifying and measuring specific vertebrae will assist in selecting specific fusion levels. On the AP film, the C7 plumbline (C7PL) should be drawn as a vertical line from the center of C7 distally, and the CSVL should be drawn from the midpoint of the sacrum up to the proximal stable vertebra.[17] The apical vertebral translation (AVT) is the distance from the apical vertebrae to the CSVL in the lumbar spine or to the coronal C7PL in the thoracic spine. The apical vertebral rotation can be documented with the Nash–Moe index.[18]

The stable vertebra is the vertebra most bisected by the CSVL. The neutral vertebra is identified as the vertebra with a symmetrical location of the pedicle shadows within the outline of the vertebral body. The end-vertebra is the vertebra most tilted from the horizontal. The identification of these vertebrae has had poor interobserver and intraobserver reliability among reviewers. In one study, 50 consecutive surgically treated cases of AIS were reviewed by 16 scoliosis surgeons. Interobserver reliability for the end-, neutral, and stable vertebrae had kappa values of 0.45, 0.32, and 0.52, respectively.[19] Potter et al[20] reviewed the reliability of identifying of the end stable, and neutral vertebrae in plain radiographic studies. One hundred consecutive surgically treated cases of AIS were evaluated at several intervals by multiple spine surgeons. Intraobserver reliability was good-to-excellent for the stable, neutral, and end-vertebrae (kappa = 0.69 to 0.88, 0.65 to 0.73, and 0.74 to 0.91, respectively). However, interobserver reliability was poor (kappa = 0.26 to 0.39). The identification of these levels is crucial for selecting fusion levels. This variability in identifying the stable, end, and neutral vertebrae increases the variability seen in selecting fusion levels.

Certain clinical parameters, such as shoulder balance, can also be assessed on AP films. The radiographic interpretation of shoulder position is done in several ways including the measurement of the T1 tilt, coracoid height, and first rib clavicle height. Kuklo et al[21] reviewed 112 AIS patients with a proximal thoracic (PT) curve >20 degrees to identify radiographic parameters that would predict postoperative shoulder balance at 2 years of follow-up. The clavicle angle, as formed by the intersection of a horizontal line and the tangential line connecting the highest two points of each clavicle, provided the best preoperative radiographic prediction of postoperative shoulder balance (**Fig. 13.2**). How this translates into selecting the optimal proximal fusion level is still not clear.

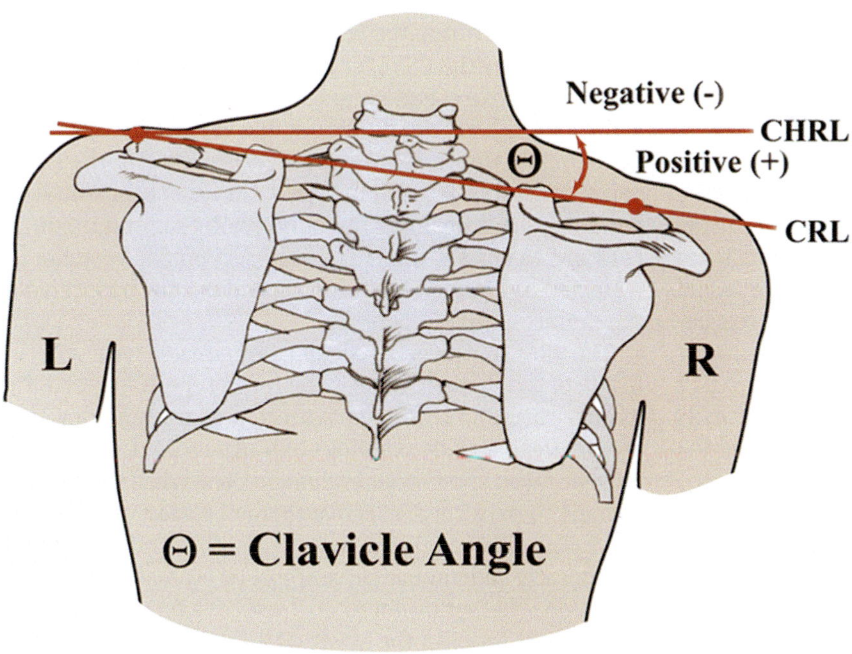


**Fig. 13.2** Illustration of the clavicle angle. (From the Spinal Deformity Study Group Radiographic Measurement Manual, page 56, published by Medtronic, Inc., 2004.) Abbreviations: CHRL, clavicle horizontal reference line; CRL, clavicle reference line.

# Operative Algorithm

The principles of surgical treatment for scoliosis are based on outcome measures including pulmonary function testing, radiography, cosmetic appearance, functional outcome, range of motion, and aerobic studies.[22-27] Classification and understanding of the patient's spinal-curve type is crucial in avoiding many postoperative complications, including decompensation. The system set forth by Lenke et al[10] provides a comprehensive classification of curve patterns and a template for the surgical management of AIS. A thorough understanding of the Lenke classification system is essential before determining the vertebral levels for spinal fusion.

# Selection of Fusion Levels

## Anterior Spinal Fusion

Anterior spinal fusion (ASF) with instrumentation is typically reserved for cases olf scoliosis in which only one curve is being treated; this specifically applies to cases of Lenke type 1 and type 5 curves. Awareness of the flexibility of the compensatory curve and its response to treatment of the main curve is critical in anterior surgery for scoliosis. The anterior approach, both open and thoracoscopic, has received increased attention in the past decade.[21,28-30] The anterior approach provides excellent curve correction and may facilitate the inclusion of fewer levels in the fusion mass than would a posterior approach.[4,31,32] Instrumentation of fewer levels is especially possible for flexible scoliotic curves.[33] Selection of fusion levels typically includes all segments within a curve, from the end vertebra cranially to the end-vertebra caudally.[34-36] Depending on the approach, either a single- or dual-rod technique can be utilized. We currently employ a dual-rod technique with screw fixation at every level in our open approach.

Hall and co-authors[33,37] advocated short instrumentation for flexible thoracolumbar/lumbar (TL/L) curves. If the apex of the curve is a vertebral body, they advocated fusing one vertebra above and one vertebra below the curve. If the apex is a disc space, the fusion and instrumentation would be performed two vertebral levels above and two levels below the apex. Using this technique, Hall and co-authors demonstrated an initial correction of 87%, declining to 67% at 2 years. The satisfaction rate in their study of 17 patients was 88%. To achieve these results, Hall et al recommended overcorrecting the instrumented vertebrae.

Application of any surgical technique requires assessment of the patient's overall coronal and sagittal balance as well as the clinical deformity. For example, an anterior procedure may lead to worsening of the kyphosis in kyphotic thoracic curves. If a patient has a high right shoulder preoperatively, selective anterior fusion of a left Lenke type 5 curve may increase the patient's shoulder asymmetry.

## Posterior Spinal Fusion

### Type 1: Main Thoracic Curves

Type 1 main thoracic (MT) curves are the most commonly treated form of AIS.[38] Although these curves can be treated with either ASF or posterior spinal fusion (PSF), posterior instrumentation and fusion remain the gold standard.[39] Although Chapter 17 provides an in-depth review of the Lenke type 1 curve, some basic principles and rules will be reviewed here.

To determine the upper instrumented vertebra (UIV), clinical shoulder balance needs to be assessed. As previously discussed, the clavicle angle appears to be the most reliable preoperative indicator for shoulder assessment. For a patient with a right MT curve and right shoulder elevation, proximal extension of spinal fixation to T4 or T5 is appropriate. Exclusion of the upper thoracic segments will allow left shoulder elevation to occur with correction, and will produce level shoulders postoperatively. For a patient with level shoulders, extension of fixation to T3 or T4 is often indicated. Cranial extension of the posterior spinal segmental instrumentation (PSSI) to include the upper thoracic segments will facilitate control over the left shoulder height and maintain shoulder balance postoperatively. For a patient with left shoulder elevation, extension of fixation to T2 is usually necessary to eliminate postoperative shoulder elevation. This proximal extension of the spinal fixation levels will allow intraoperative compression of the upper left thoracic segments to lower the left shoulder and correct the patient's preoperative imbalance.

The senior author of this chapter (L.L.) usually selects the lowest instrumented vertebra (LIV) as the lowest vertebra touched by the CSVL for lumbar curves with an A modifier in the Lenke classification system. Most commonly, this is the vertebra proximal to the stable vertebra (stable-1), or occasionally the vertebra two levels proximal to the stable vertebra (stable-2). PSSI in type 1 curves is best suited for patients with a normal or hyperkyphotic sagittal modifier. For type 1B curves, the LIV (the most cephalad vertebra intersected or bisected by the CSVL) will usually be located in the thoracolumbar junction.

The most controversial curve pattern treated with selective fusion of the thoracic spine is the Lenke type 1C pattern. The lumbar curves in this curve pattern are large and deviated, and are flexible (side-bending Cobb angle <25 degrees). Care must be taken and further evaluation done when the decision is made to perform a selective thoracic fusion on a type 1C curve. The Cobb-angle measurements, AVR, and AVT of both the thoracic and lumbar curves must be evaluated before deciding on whether or not to do a selective fusion. When the Cobb angles ratios of the MT-to-TL/L curves, and the respective ratios of their AVR and AVT values, are $>1.2$, a selective fusion is a possible surgical option, with a low incidence of lumbar decompensation or "adding-on" of caudal vertebral segments to the patient's spinal curvature.[40] Also, the thoracolumbar junction must lack kyphosis (i.e., the T10–L2 sagittal Cobb angle must be $<10$ degrees).[11] Clinical evaluation is also important in deciding whether or not to perform a selective fusion. The patient should have a thoracic-to-lumbar scoliometer ratio $>1.2$, and the right shoulder should be higher than or level with the left shoulder.[11] Additionally, the patient should demonstrate a significant clinical thoracic prominence and minimal flank deformity (**Fig. 13.3**).[40] With the patient erect, thoracic truncal shift should be much more visible than the lumbar shift. These findings on physical examination reinforce the concept of the thoracic curve being more structural than the lumbar curve. Skeletal maturity does not factor into this decision.[41]

Although these characteristics have been outlined in the literature, variability and differences in opinion remain with regard to surgical decisions. Newton et al[42] examined this variability by reviewing 203 patients with Lenke type 1B or 1C curves treated at five different sites of the Harms Study Group (HSG). The lumbar curve was included in from 6 to 33% of spinal fusions performed, depending on the study site. Factors that increased the performance of lumbar fusion included a larger preoperative lumbar curve, displacement of the apical vertebra from the CSVL, and a smaller thoracic-to-lumbar curve ratio (**Fig. 13.4**).

The advantages of ASF or PSF for Lenke type 1 curves have also been investigated. Potter et al[43] compared their results with ASF and PSF done with thoracic pedicle screws (TPS) for Lenke type 1 curves. The patients in this study were followed for an average of 3 years postoperatively. Patients who had PSF with TPS had ~1.2 more levels fused than did their

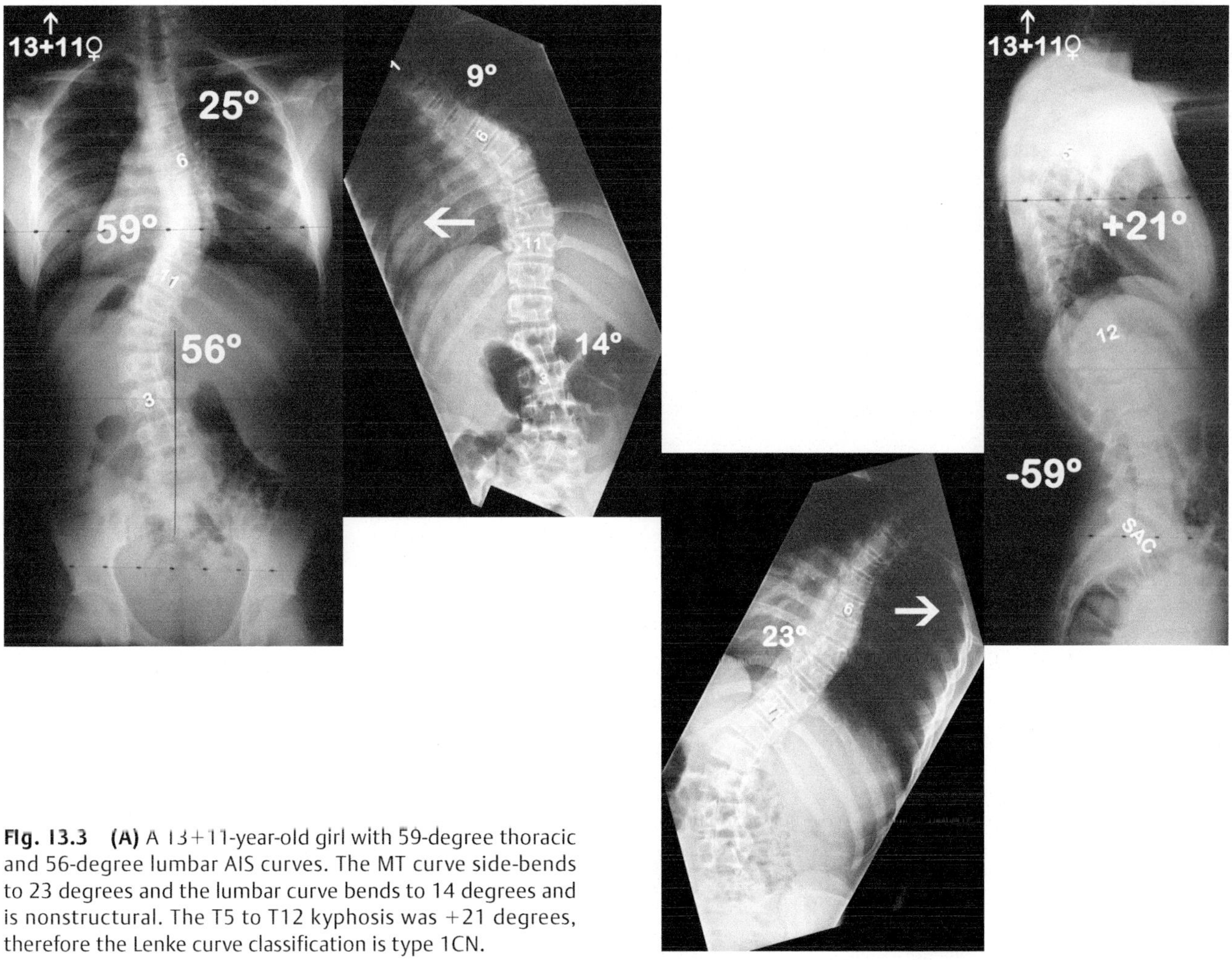


**Fig. 13.3 (A)** A 13+11-year-old girl with 59-degree thoracic and 56-degree lumbar AIS curves. The MT curve side-bends to 23 degrees and the lumbar curve bends to 14 degrees and is nonstructural. The T5 to T12 kyphosis was +21 degrees, therefore the Lenke curve classification is type 1CN.

A

(*Continued on page 154*)

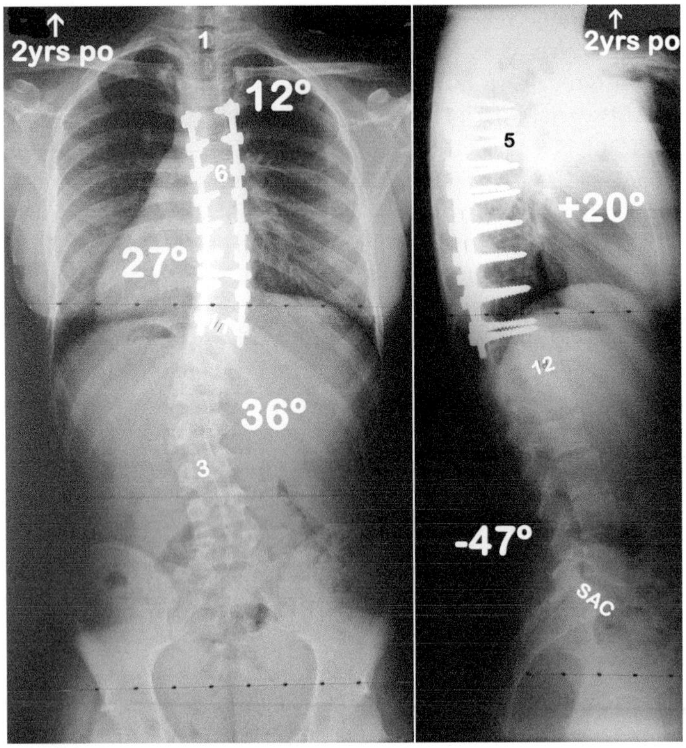


B

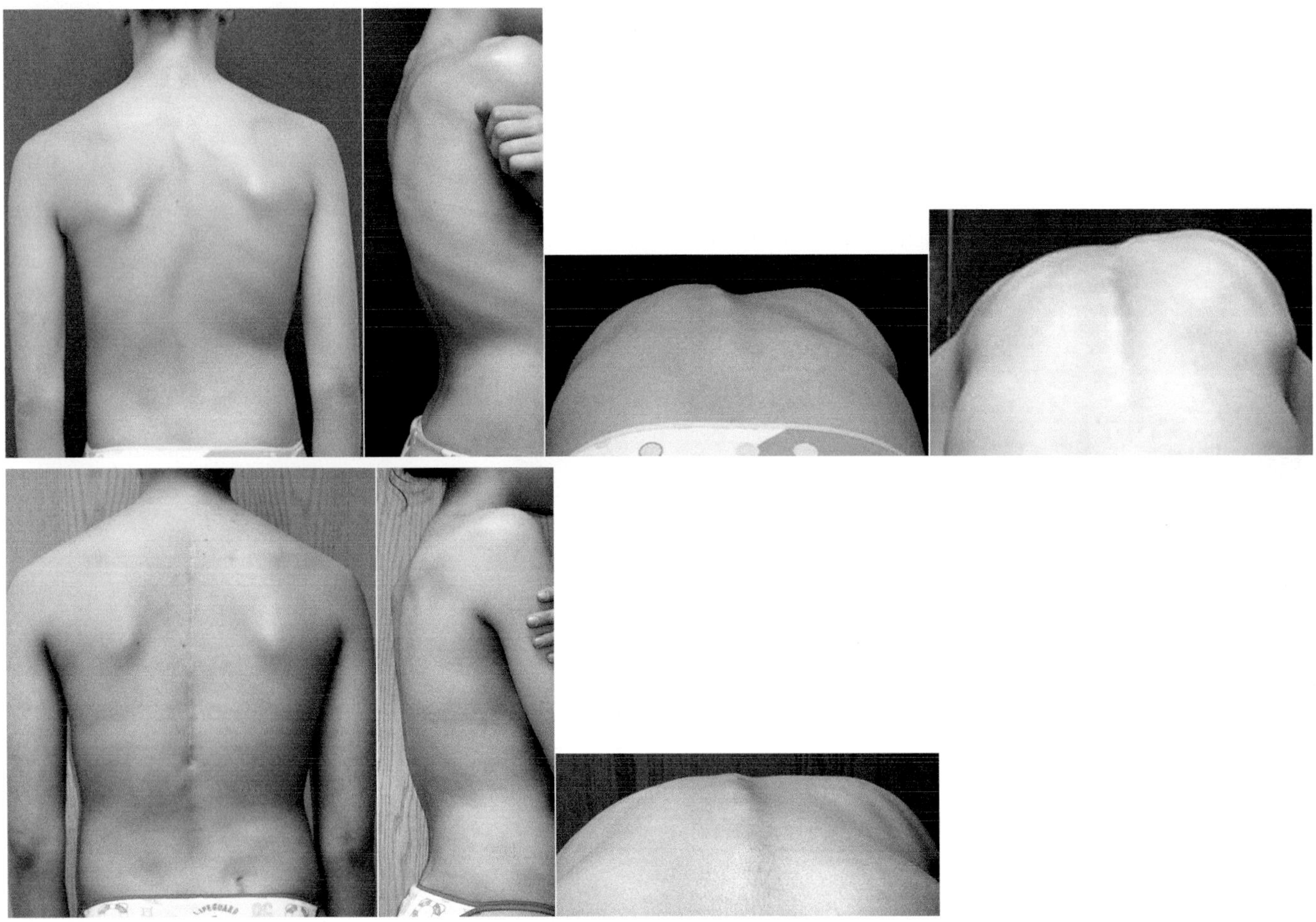

C

**Fig. 13.3** (*Continued*) **(B)** Although a very difficult decision to make, because of the nearly equal MT-to-lumbar curve Cobb-angle and AVT ratios, the patient underwent a selective posterior spinal fusion from T4 to T11. At 2 years postoperative, she had excellent alignment and balance. **(C)** Her pre- and postoperative photographs demonstrate her excellent truncal alignment.

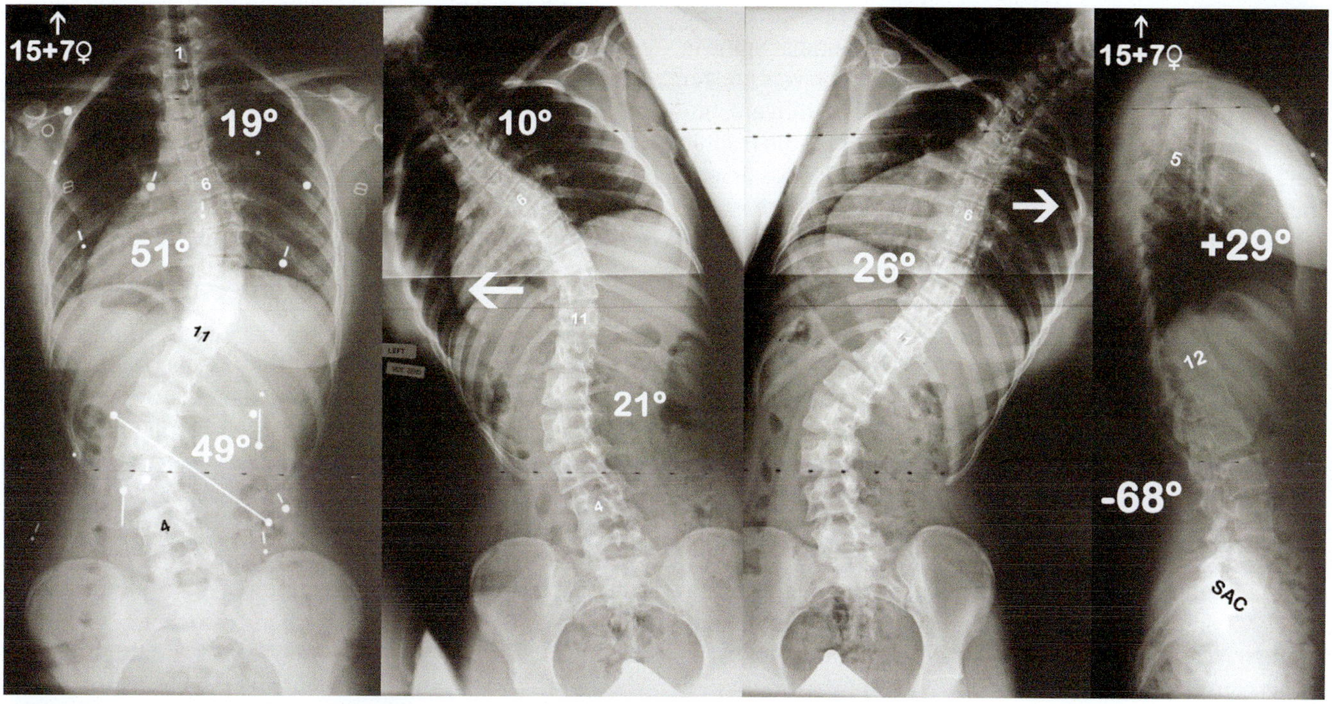


A

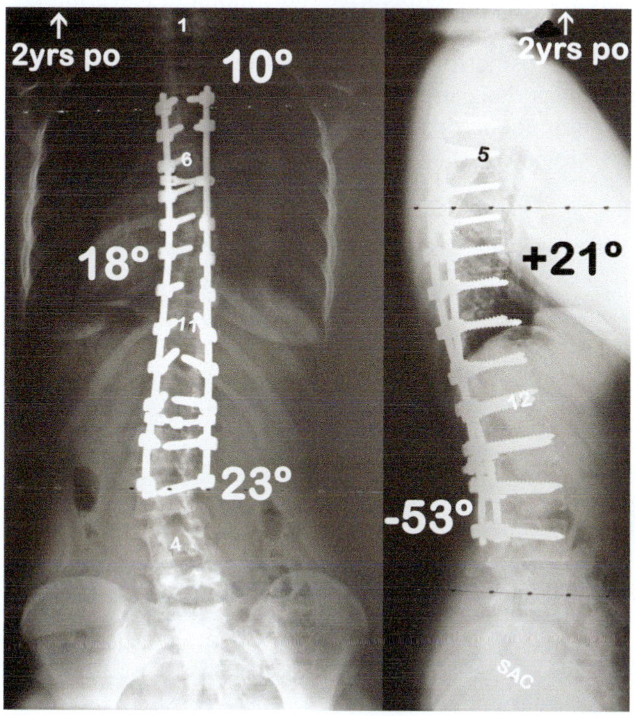


B

**Fig. 13.4** **(A)** A 15+7-year-old girl with a 19-degree PT, 51-degree MT, and 49-degree lumbar scoliosis. Both the PT and lumbar curves are nonstructural. There is +29 degrees of thoracic kyphosis, therefore the correct Lenke curve classification is type 1CN. **(B)** Because of the similar magnitude of the thoracic and lumbar Cobb angle measurements, AVRs, and AVTs, this patient underwent a posterior instrumentation and fusion from T4 to L3, with very reasonable realignment of her thoracic and lumbar curves and fractional lumbosacral curve at 2 years postoperative. The L3–L4 disc has remained relatively level over time.

matched cohorts who had ASF. However, a greater correction of scoliosis was achieved in the thoracic and lumbar spine in the group that had PSF. The rotational correction was greater in the PSF group with TPS. This yielded a significant improvement in the rib hump and other radiographic parameters in this group. However, PSF with TPS was associated with a decrease in thoracic kyphosis, whereas ASF tended to increase thoracic kyphosis in these patients.[44] Currently, we approach all Lenke type 1 curves posteriorly. By avoiding disruption of the chest wall, we obtain excellent corrections without the deleterious effects on pulmonary function seen with anterior approaches. Posterior techniques, such as Ponté osteotomies, are currently being investigated to determine their role in minimizing the tendency to increase the kyphosis effect of all pedicle screw thoracic constructs.

### Type 2: Double Thoracic Curves

Type 2 double thoracic (DT) curve includes a major structural MT and a structural minor PT curve.[45] The general guideline calls for posterior arthrodesis of both curves. The LIV is chosen in a manner similar to that for treating type 1 curves. The proximal level of fusion should be either T2 or T3. Consideration of the patient's clinical shoulder balance and radiographic clavicle angle is critical.[21] Patients with a high left shoulder preoperatively will require fusion extending to T2 (**Fig. 13.5**). This will allow greater control in balancing the shoulders. For patients with level shoulders, the UIV may be either T2 or T3. When assessing the patient's deformity to determine the UIV, the rigidity and magnitude of the PT curve will need to be considered. Large or inflexible curves will probably generate a significant shoulder imbalance as the MT curve is corrected. For patients with a high right shoulder, the UIV may be T3. Excluding the most proximal vertebrae will allow spontaneous left shoulder elevation with correction of the MT curve. Often, the PT curve is hyperkyphotic, and compression of the convexity is therefore applied first. In general, when correcting the PT curve, one must consider the correction that will be attained in the MT curve. Greater correction of the MT curve will further increase the elevation of the left shoulder.

Suk and colleagues[45] reviewed their results for patients with type 2 curves, analyzing the cases of 40 patients who had at least a 2-year follow-up. Eighteen of these patients were treated with fusion of both curves; 22 were treated with fusion of the MT curve. All of the patients' surgeries were performed before the inception of the Lenke classification system. All patients who had fusion of both curves had fusion extending to T1. A review of shoulder balance showed that right-shoulder elevation increased postoperatively when the preoperative right shoulder elevation was >12 mm in patients with fusion of the MT curve. Therefore, the best cosmetic result occurred when fusion of the PT curve was done in patients with left shoulder elevation, level shoulders, or right shoulder elevation <1.2 cm. Cil et al[46] reviewed the inclusion or exclusion of nonstructural

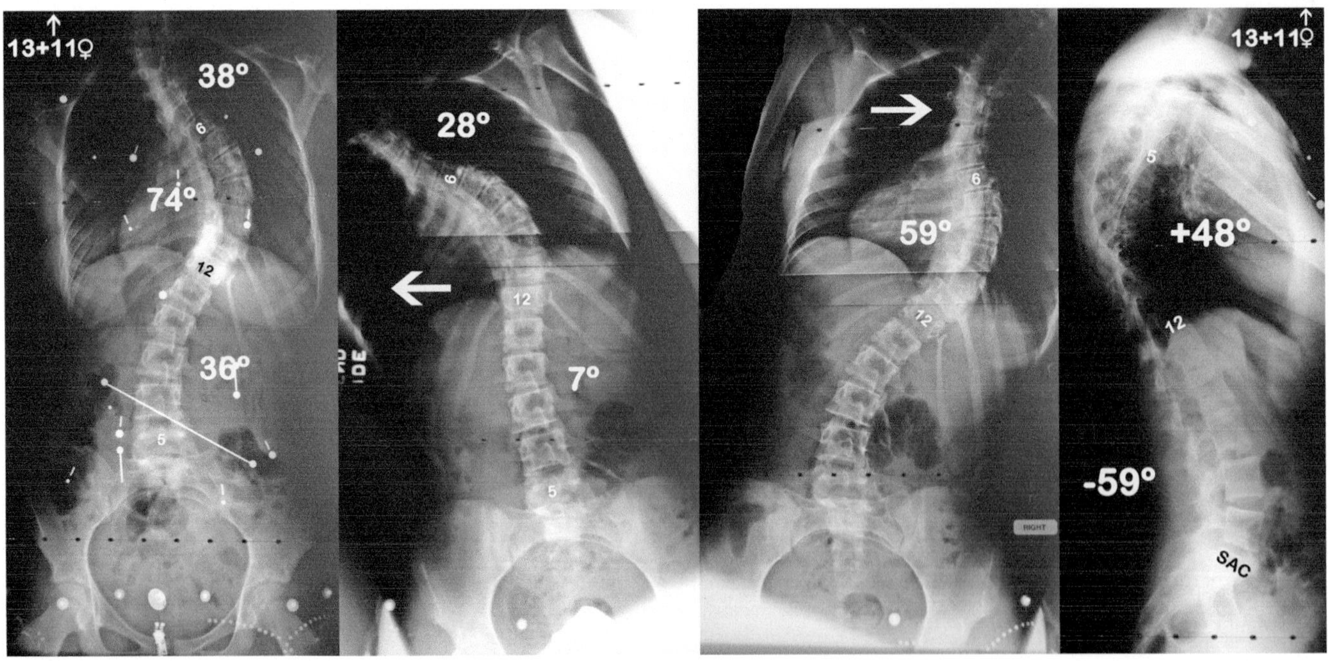


A

**Fig. 13.5 (A)** A 13+11-year-old girl with a 38-degree PT, 74-degree MT, and 36-degree lumbar scoliosis. The PT curve side bends to 28 degrees and is structural, whereas the lumbar curve bends to 7 degrees and is nonstructural. There is a +48-degree thoracic kyphosis, therefore the correct Lenke curve classification in this case is type 2A+.

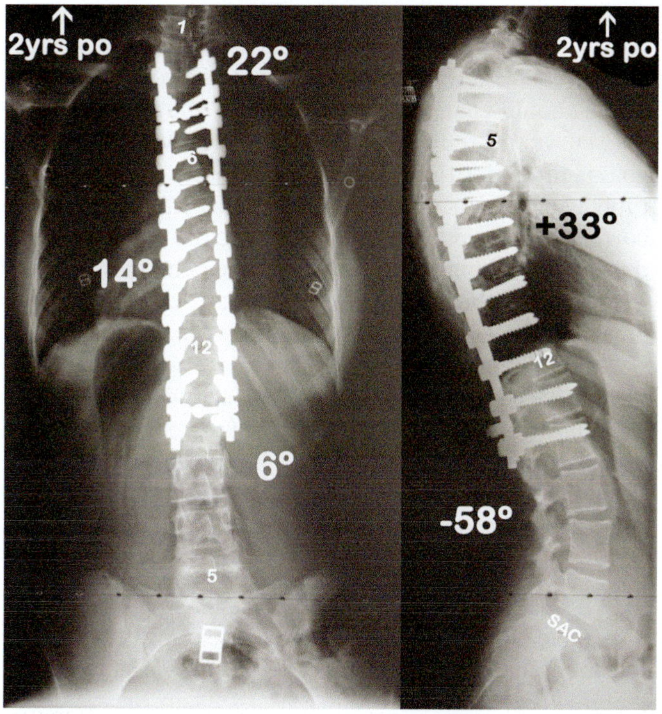


B

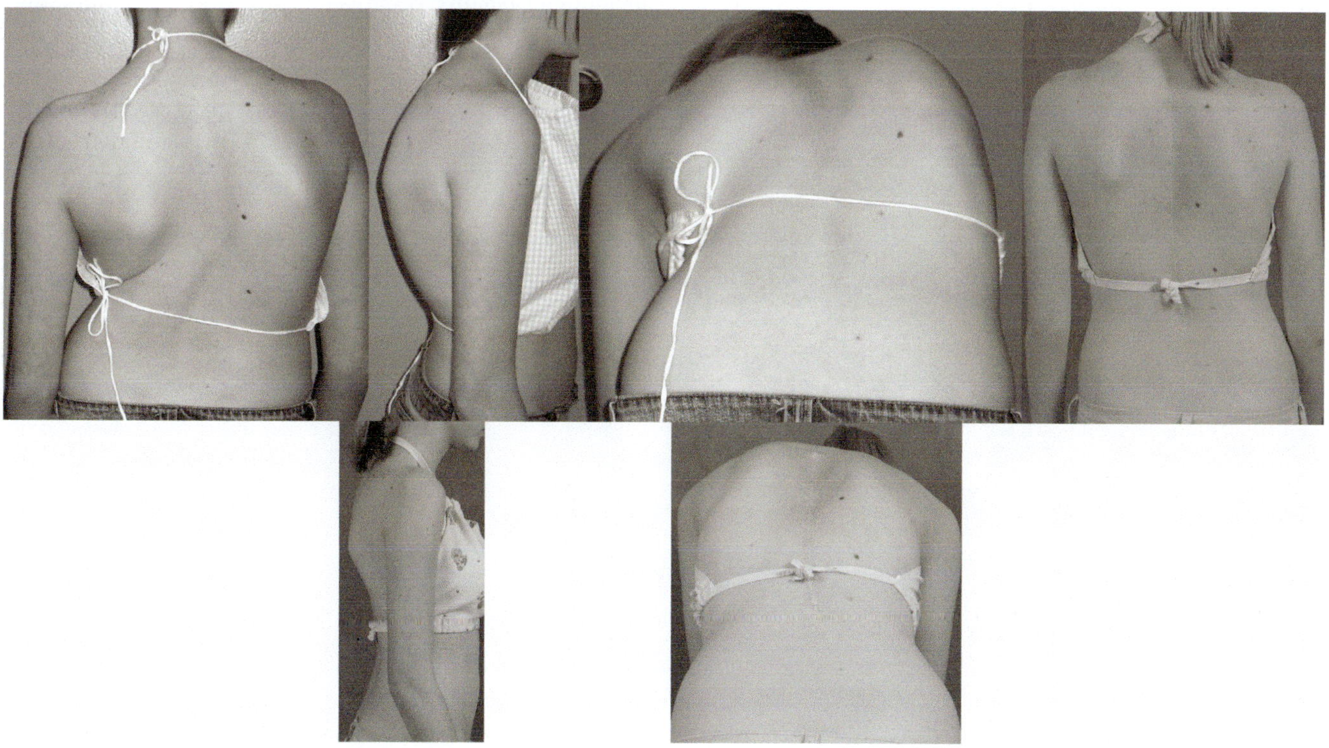

C

**Fig. 13.5** (*Continued*) **(B)** This patient underwent a posterior instrumentation and fusion from T2 to L2, with excellent radiographic alignment noted at 2 years postoperative. **(C)** Preoperative and postoperative clinical photographs demonstrate the patient's improved truncal realignment.

PT curves in patients with AIS classified according to Lenke's criteria. Thirty-eight of their patients underwent operative treatment for scoliosis before publication of the Lenke classification system. The mean follow-up of these patients was 54 months, and the UIV ranged from T2 to T4. Cil and coauthors evaluated shoulder balance and spontaneous correction of the PT curve. Spontaneous correction occurred in 41% of patients who had fusions extending to T4. Mild progression occurred postoperatively in 6 patients, but no curve reached a magnitude exceeding the preoperative Cobb-angle value. This study confirmed the Lenke classification system as a template for the selection of fusion levels.

### Type 3: Double Major Curves

Lenke type 3 double major (DM) curves involve a major structural TL/L MT curve and a minor structural TL/L curve. The general rule calls for posterior fusion of both curves (**Fig. 13.6**). Instrumentation begins at T3 to T5, depending on shoulder position, as with type 1 curves. The LIV is often the most cephalad lumbar vertebra touched by the CSVL when the lumbar curve is flexible and secure pedicle fixation is achieved, and is usually L3 or L4. The dilemma is in selecting the appropriate distal fusion level while attempting to maintain as many motion segments as possible in the lumbar spine. The LIV should have near-neutral rotation, the disc below the LIV preoperatively should be parallel or wedged at the convexity, and the apex of the lumbar curve should be at least one disc level above the LIV. The TL/L curve is often more flexible than the MT curve.[47] The goal is to render the LIV horizontal on the AP film. Often, type 3 curves will have TL kyphosis, and it is important to correct this regional deformity during the surgical procedure.[48] Instrumentation levels should not end in this area of kyphosis but should be extended distally to avoid postoperative sagittal decompensation.

A small percentage of type 3 curves show dominant thoracic curve characteristics. Careful evaluation of these curves may allow the surgeon to perform a selective thoracic fusion. Analysis of the variables discussed in the section on type 1C curves in this chapter will show that selective thoracic fusion is possible for a small set of patients with type 3 curves.

### Type 4: Triple Major Curves

The Lenke type 4 triple major curve pattern involves all three regions of the spine. The majority of patients with this pattern require fusion from T2 or T3 to L3 or L4. Again, the evaluation of shoulder balance is critical for determining the proximal level of fusion. Optimal horizontalization of the LIV is the

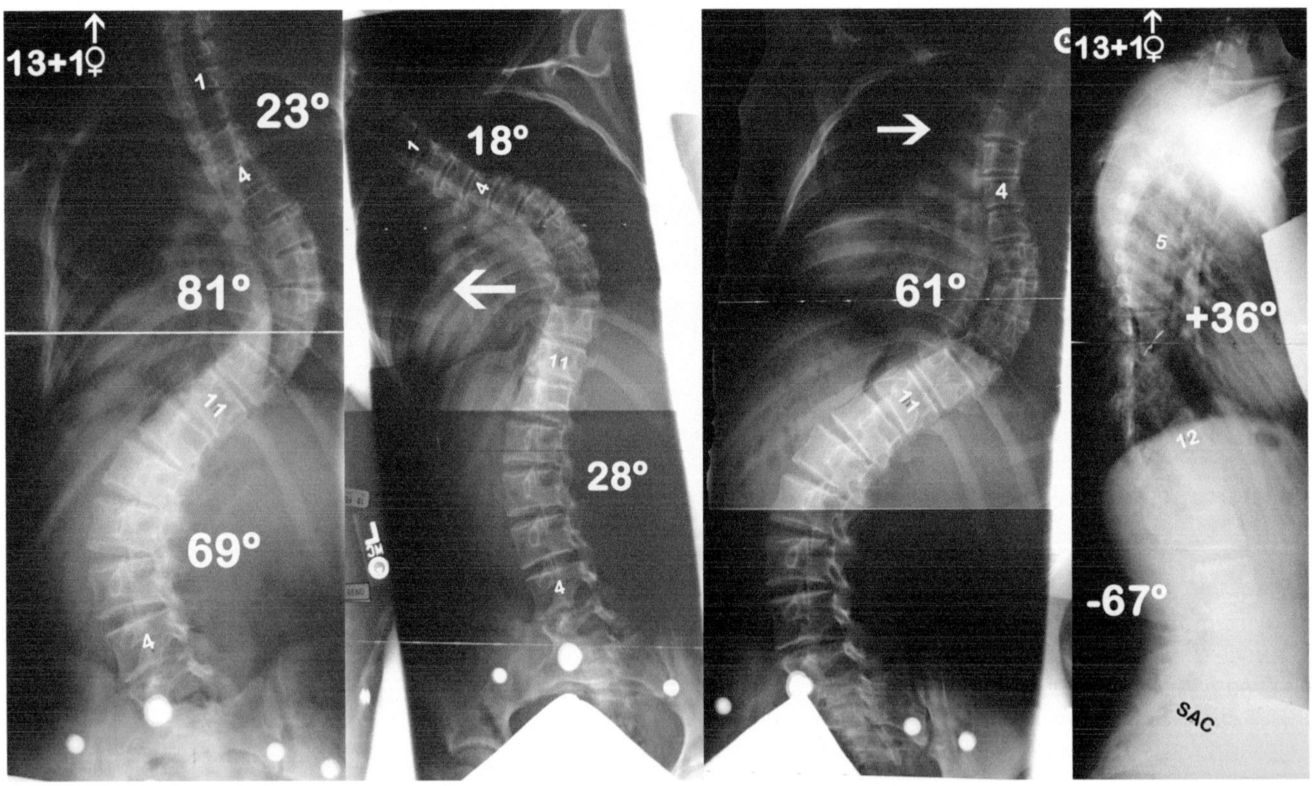


A

**Fig. 13.6** **(A)** A 13+1-year-old girl with a 23-degree PT, 81-degree MT, and 69-degree lumbar scoliosis. The PT curve is nonstructural at 18 degrees on side-bending, whereas the lumbar curve is structural at 28 degrees. There is a +36-degree thoracic kyphosis, and the correct Lenke curve classification in this case is type 3CN.

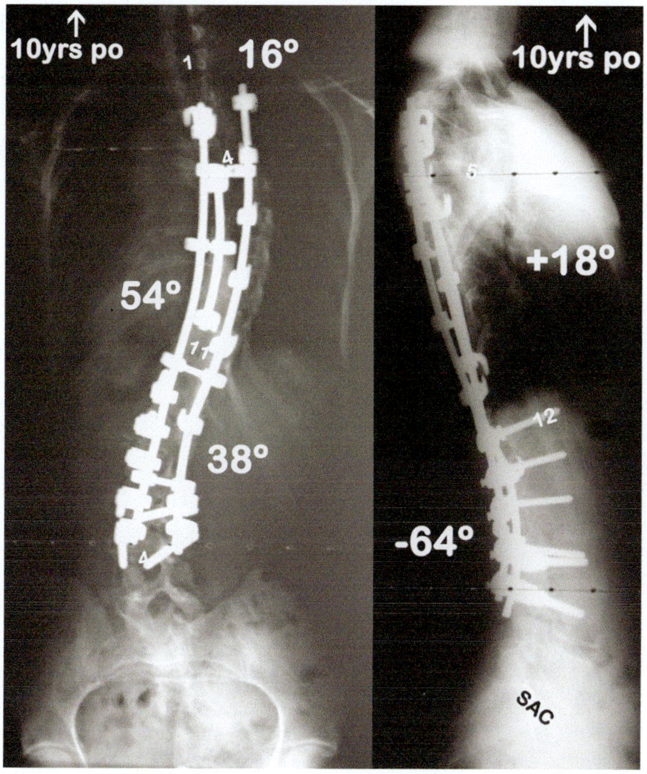


B

**Fig. 13.6** (*Continued*) **(B)** This patient underwent a posterior instrumentation and fusion utilizing a three-rod technique with a hybrid construct from T3 to L4, with excellent balance noted at 10 years postoperatively.

primary goal in the lumbar spine. The selection of both the proximal and distal levels of fusion corresponds with the previous discussion of type 1, 2, and 3 curves, respectively. Rarely, a selective thoracic or double thoracic fusion can be performed, leaving the lumbar curve unfused. In these cases the clinical and radiographic ratios of the thoracic-to-lumbar curve are >1.2 in favor of the larger thoracic curve, as discussed above for Lenke type 1C curves (**Fig. 13.7**).

## Type 5: Thoracolumbar/Lumbar Curves

The Lenke type 5 curve pattern demonstrates a major curve in the TL/L region with a minor nonstructural curve in the MT region. Curves of this pattern may be treated with either ASF or PSF. Occasionally, we still utilize an anterior spinal instrumentation and fusion from the upper to the lower end-vertebrae of the curvature. The surgical levels include all convex discs within the curve.[29,49] Instrumentation is achieved with a dual-rod system. Hurford et al[50] reviewed 48 TL/L curves treated with dual-screw/dual-rod constructs and found coronal correction of the TL/L curve averaging 75%, excellent sagittal alignment, and no instrumentation failure or pseudarthrosis at a minimum follow-up of 2-years. However, a trend toward posterior instrumentation is developing because of disadvantages of the anterior thoracolumbar approach. In selecting posterior fusion levels, the UIV and LIV are usually identical to those in ASF for the same curves. For small, very flexible curves, the minimal fusion technique of Hall and colleagues,[33] as previously described, may be used. It is extremely important to evaluate the MT and PT regions as well as shoulder balance. If the left shoulder is elevated, some residual tilt must be maintained at the UIV to aid with postoperative shoulder balance. Correction of the lumbar curve and secondary correction of the compensatory thoracic curve will cause further elevation of the left shoulder. Therefore, careful evaluation of shoulder balance is necessary, including examination of the scapulae and thoracic prominence. If there is no MT component to the curve, the UIV and LIV may be horizontalized for correction. The goal is minimal deformity above and below the thoracolumbar fusion levels.

Selective fusion of the TL/L spine requires careful clinical and radiographic evaluation. For successful selective fusion of this region of the spine, the Cobb angle and AVT and AVR ratios (TL/L:MT) should be >1.25. In addition, there must be greater flexibility of the MT than of the TL/L curve, and no evidence of TL junctional kyphosis.[11] Clinically, patients selected for such surgery must have level shoulders or a high left shoulder for optimal results. The TL/L truncal shift must be greater than the MT shift. The

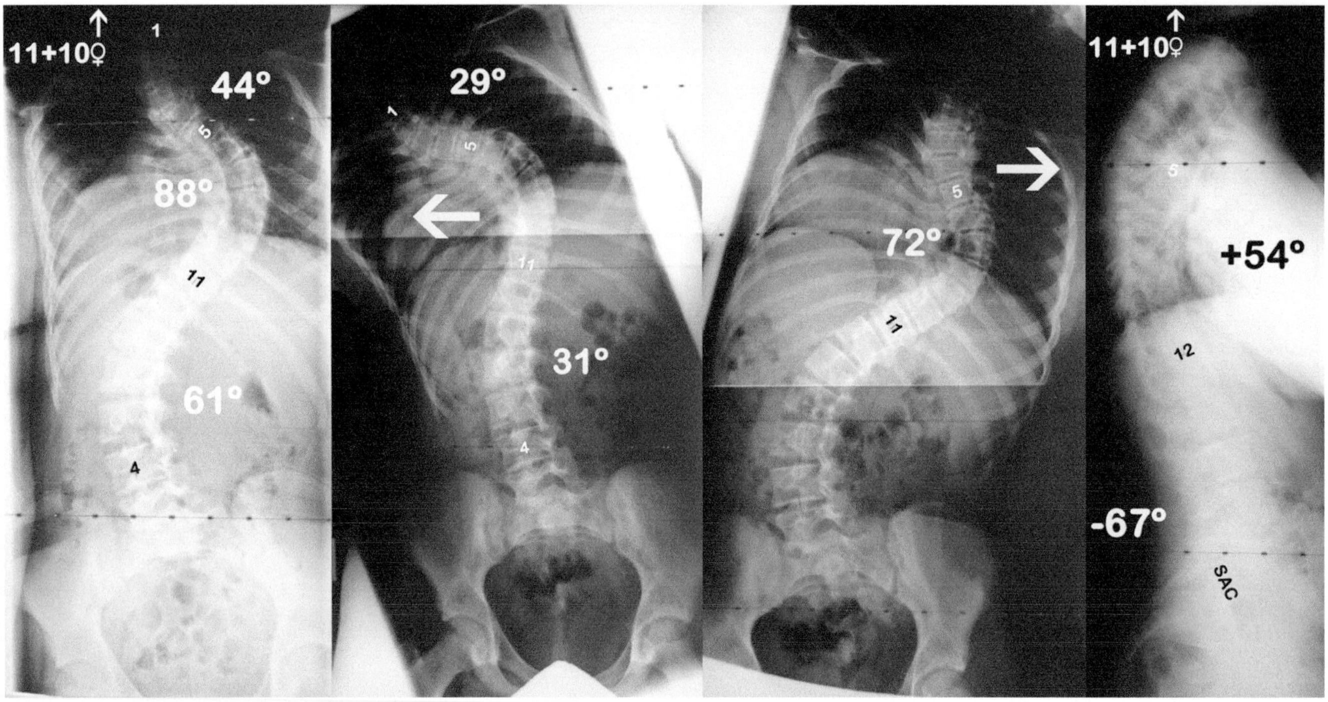


A

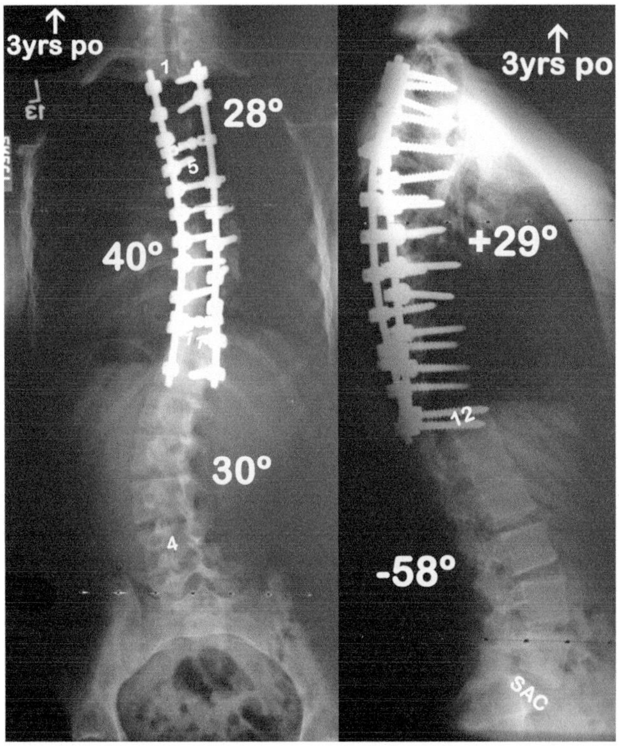


B

**Fig. 13.7** **(A)** An 11 + 10-year-old girl with a 44-degree PT, 88-degree MT, and 61-degree lumbar scoliosis. The PT curve is structural, in bending to 29 degrees, the lumbar curve is also structural, in bending to 31 degrees. There is a +54-degree thoracic kyphosis, therefore the correct Lenke curve classification is type 4C+. **(B,C)** Because of the marked difference in the thoracic-to-lumbar Cobb angle ratio, AVTs, and AVRs, this patient underwent a selective double thoracic ratio instrumentation and fusion from T2 to T12, with excellent coronal and sagittal correction and alignment at 3 years postoperative.

*(Continued)*

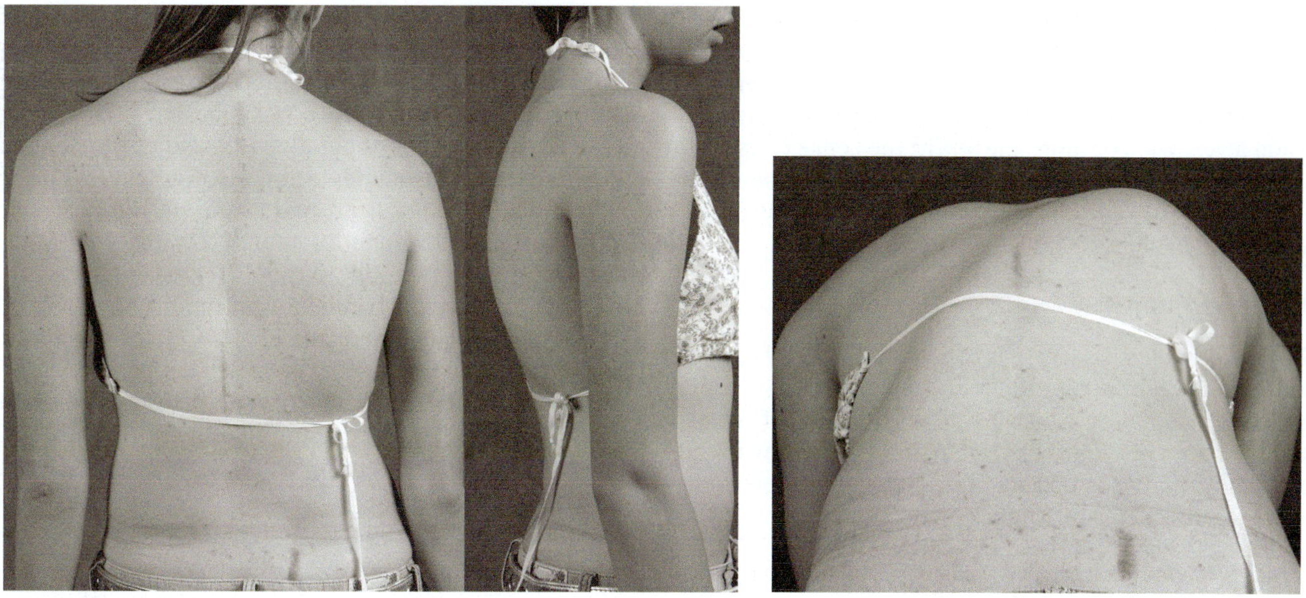

C

**Fig. 13.7** *(Continued)* **(C) (B,C)** Because of the marked difference in the thoracic-to-lumbar Cobb angle ratio, AVTs, and AVRs, this patient underwent a selective double thoracic ratio instrumentation and fusion from T2 to T12, with excellent coronal and sagittal correction and alignment at 3 years postoperative.

TL/L-to-MT scoliometer ratio should also be >1.2. Additionally, the rib prominence needs to be acceptable to the patient because little change in the rib deformity will occur postoperatively.

Excellent results can be achieved with selective lumbar fusion. Sanders et al[51] reviewed 49 AIS patients who had undergone selective fusion for TL/L curves of 30 to 55 degrees. All of the patients were followed for 2 years. Satisfactory results were achieved in patients with a TL/L-to-MT Cobb-angle ratio of >1.25 and a thoracic curve that bent to 20 degrees or less. These satisfactory results were defined as a thoracic curve at follow-up of <40 degrees, acceptable balance and sagittal alignment, and no need for further procedures.

### Type 6: Thoracolumbar/Lumbar Main Thoracic Curves

The Lenke type 6 thorocolumbar/lumbar-MT(TL/L-MT) curve pattern consists of a major structural TL/L curve with a minor structural MT curve. Most cases of this type require posterior arthrodesis of both structural curves. The UIV is usually from T2 to T5, but depends on shoulder balance, and the LIV is usually L3 or L4. This is usually determined by the most distal vertebra in the curve that touches the CSVL. Occasionally, a type 6 curve may undergo selective lumbar fusion if the radiographic and clinical characteristics of the thoracic curve are similar to those of the MT curve in the Lenke type 5 curve pattern.[52]

## Curve Classification

The general premise of treatment for AIS indicates that all structural curves are to be included in the spinal fusion, but that nonstructural curves should not be included.[41] In one retrospective study of 606 surgically treated cases of AIS, 90% of spinal-fusion procedures followed the recommendations of the Lenke classification system before its inception.[38] The Lenke classification system merely provides a guideline to assist in selecting curves and levels to be fused. Differences in surgeons' opinions and evaluation of the individual patient will ultimately affect the fusion levels chosen.

In another multicenter study, 1281 AIS patients who underwent surgery were evaluated with the Lenke classification system as a template for the selection of fusion levels. The classification guidelines were not followed in 15% of these surgical cases. The greatest deviation from the classification algorithm occurred with Lenke type 3 curves. Before the inception of the classification, the number of Lenke "rule-breakers" (curves not treated as recommended by the Lenke system) totaled 18%. This decreased to 12% after the inception of the Lenke system.[53]

A third multicenter study evaluated 543 patients who had surgery for AIS. In this study, the Lenke guidelines were followed in 74.2% of cases. The greatest agreement (84%) occurred with type 1 curves, whereas the poorest agreement (20%) occurred with type 4 curves. In 39% of cases in which the guidelines were not followed, side-bending measurements were the reason for bypassing the classification system. In 11% of cases, sagittal kyphosis (≥20 degrees) was present but not included in the fusion as recommended by the systematic guidelines.[54]

As instrumentation techniques evolve, refinements in the Lenke guidelines that facilitate the selection of spinal fusion levels will continue. Currently, the Lenke classification provides a reliable template for guiding the spine surgeon toward reproducible results of spinal fusion for patients with AIS.

## Decompensation

The goal of scoliosis surgery is to achieve balanced correction of a patient's deformity and halt its progression. Surgeons attempt to achieve this with fusion of fewest possible segments. Poor selection of fusion levels may lead to complications such as shoulder imbalance, persistent or progressive deformity, junctional kyphosis, or truncal decompensation.[10,45,55–57]

During selective fusion of a thoracic segment, the correctional forces occurring in the thoracic spine may generate torsional forces across the lumbar spine that exceed the flexibility of the nonstructural curve. Rod-rotation maneuvers appear to be associated with a higher incidence of this.[57] This unbalanced force with continued growth can lead to truncal decompensation. Often, this spinal imbalance requires revision surgery.[57] Treatment with selective thoracic fusion of a borderline Lenke type 3 (King type 2) curve may result in lumbar decompensation.[58] Ending a fusion in a region of kyphosis, or selecting fusion levels proximal to the appropriate LIV, may lead to progressive decompensation.[13,14,58] Lowe and colleagues[59] reviewed distal junctional kyphosis (DJK) after selective fusion in 375 AIS patients with MT curves, of whom 238 had anterior and 177 had posterior selective thoracic fusion and had DJK either pre- or postoperatively. DJK occurred preoperatively in 5% and postoperatively in 14.6% of patients in the posterior fusion group, with corresponding figures of 4.2% and 7.1% in the anterior fusion group. The authors identified preoperative TL kyphosis as a factor that increased the risk of postoperative DJK, and recommended the extension of instrumentation distal to the kyphotic segment. DJK also occurred more often in the posterior fusion group if instrumentation ended cranial to LEV+1. However, preoperative DJK in the TL region could be corrected by extending instrumentation and fusion to LEV+1 in the anterior fusion group and to LEV+2 in the posterior fusion group.

Bracing for mild to moderate degrees of decompensation may allow their eventual resolution. However, severe imbalance requires the extension of fusion to provide overall balance for the patient. Each case of decompensation is unique and requires individual evaluation and treatment.

## ■ Conclusion

The goals of spinal surgery for AIS are to achieve and maintain a stable spinal fusion, minimize spinal deformity, fuse as few segments as possible, and return patients quickly to their preoperative lifestyles. Selecting appropriate spinal levels for fusion is critical in achieving a successful surgical outcome. Radiographic and clinical examinations are essential in the evaluation of every patient with a spinal deformity. The guidelines provided by the Lenke classification system constitute a template for achieving a successful outcome in scoliosis surgery. Selection of the correct spinal segments for fusion during scoliosis surgery is a key factor in avoiding many postoperative complications, including truncal decompensation.

### References


1. Goldstein LA. Surgical management of scoliosis. J Bone Joint Surg Am 1966;48A:167–196
2. Hibbs RA. A report of fifty-nine cases of scoliosis treated by the fusion operation. J Bone Joint Surg (Amer) 1924;6:3–34
3. Hibbs RA, Risser JC, Ferguson AB. Scoliosis treated by the fusion operation. An end result study of three hundred and sixty cases. J Bone Joint Surg (Amer) 1931;13:91–104
4. Moe JH, Purcell GA, Bradford DS. Zielke instrumentation (VDS) for the correction of spinal curvature. Analysis of results in 66 patients. Clin Orthop Relat Res 1983;(180):133–153
5. Risser JC. Scoliosis: Past and present. J Bone Joint Surg Am 1964;46: 167–199
6. Harrington PR. Technical details in relation to the successful use of instrumentation in scoliosis. Orthop Clin North Am 1972;3:49–67
7. Harrington PR. Treatment of scoliosis. Correction and internal fixation by spine instrumentation. J Bone Joint Surg Am 1962;44A:591–610
8. Moe JH. A critical analysis of methods of fusion for scoliosis; an evaluation in two hundred and sixty-six patients. J Bone Joint Surg Am 1958;40A:529–554, passim
9. King HA, Moe JH, Bradford DS, Winter RB. The selection of fusion levels in thoracic idiopathic scoliosis. J Bone Joint Surg Am 1983; 65:1302–1313
10. Lenke LG, Betz RR, Harms J, et al. Adolescent idiopathic scoliosis: A new classification to determine extent of spinal arthrodesis. J Bone Joint Surg Am 2001;83A:1169–1181
11. Lenke LG, Edwards CC II, Bridwell KH. The Lenke classification of adolescent idiopathic scoliosis: How it organizes curve patterns as a template to perform selective fusions of the spine. Spine 2003; 28:S199–S207
12. Horton WC, Brown CW, Bridwell KH, Glassman SD, Suk SI, Cha CW. Is there an optimal patient stance for obtaining a lateral 36′ radiograph? A critical comparison of three techniques. Spine 2005; 30:427–433

13. Bridwell KH. Idiopathic scoliosis. In: Bridwell KH, DeWald RL, eds. The Textbook of Spinal Surgery, ed. 1. Philadelphia, PA: JB Lippincott; 1991:97–162
14. Bridwell KH. Spinal instrumentation in the management of adolescent scoliosis. Clin Orthop Relat Res 1997;(335):64–72
15. Polly DW Jr, Sturm PF. Traction versus supine side bending. Which technique best determines curve flexibility? Spine 1998;23:804–808
16. Takahashi S, Passuti N, Delécrin J. Interpretation and utility of traction radiography in scoliosis surgery. Analysis of patients treated with Cotrel-Dubousset instrumentation. Spine 1997;22:2542–2546
17. Lenke LG, Bridwell KH, Baldus C, Blanke K, Schoenecker PL. Cotrel-Dubousset instrumentation for adolescent idiopathic scoliosis. J Bone Joint Surg Am 1992;74:1056–1067
18. Nash CL Jr, Moe JH. A study of vertebral rotation. J Bone Joint Surg Am 1969;51:223–229
19. Dobbs MB, Glassman SD, Hedequist DJ, et al. Reliability analysis of end, neutral, stable, and lowest instrumented vertebrae selection in adolescent idiopathic scoliosis: surgeon versus digital software determination. Eur Spine J 2005;14:24S
20. Potter BK, Rosner MK, Lehman RA Jr, Polly DW Jr, Schroeder TM, Kuklo TR. Reliability of end, neutral, and stable vertebrae identification in adolescent idiopathic scoliosis. Spine 2005;30:1658–1663
21. Kuklo TR, Lenke LG, Graham EJ, et al. Correlation of radiographic, clinical, and patient assessment of shoulder balance following fusion versus nonfusion of the proximal thoracic curve in adolescent idiopathic scoliosis. Spine 2002;27:2013–2020
22. Kim YJ, Lenke LG, Bridwell KH, et al. Prospective evaluation of pulmonary function in adolescent idiopathic scoliosis relative to surgical approach: Minimum 5-year follow-up. J Bone Joint Surg Am 2005;87:1534–1541
23. Lenke LG, Bridwell KH, Blanke K, Baldus C, Weston J. Radiographic results of arthrodesis with Cotrel-Dubousset instrumentation for the treatment of adolescent idiopathic scoliosis. A five to ten-year follow-up study. J Bone Joint Surg Am 1998; 80(6):807–814
24. Rinella A, Lenke L, Peelle M, Edwards C, Bridwell KH, Sides B. Comparison of SRS questionnaire results submitted by both parents and patients in the operative treatment of idiopathic scoliosis. Spine 2004;29:303–310
25. Engsberg JR, Lenke LG, Reitenbach AK, Hollander KW, Bridwell KH, Blanke K. Prospective evaluation of trunk range of motion in adolescents with idiopathic scoliosis undergoing spinal fusion surgery. Spine 2002;27:1346–1354
26. Engsberg JR, Lenke LG, Uhrich ML, Ross SA, Bridwell KH. Prospective comparison of gait and trunk range of motion in adolescents with idiopathic thoracic scoliosis undergoing anterior or posterior spinal fusion. Spine 2003;28:1993–2000
27. Lenke LG, White DK, Kemp JS, Bridwell KH, Blanke KM, Engsberg JR. Evaluation of ventilatory efficiency during exercise in patients with idiopathic scoliosis undergoing spinal fusion. Spine 2002;27: 2041–2045
28. Betz RR, Harms J, Clements DH III, et al. Comparison of anterior and posterior instrumentation for correction of adolescent thoracic idiopathic scoliosis. Spine 1999;24:225–239
29. Sweet FA, Lenke LG, Bridwell KH, Blanke KM, Whorton J. Prospective radiographic and clinical outcomes and complications of single solid rod instrumented anterior spinal fusion in adolescent idiopathic scoliosis. Spine 2001;26:1956–1965
30. Lenke LG. Anterior endoscopic discectomy and fusion for adolescent idiopathic scoliosis. Spine 2003;28(15, suppl):S36–S43
31. Ogilvie JW. Anterior spine fusion with Zielke instrumentation for idiopathic scoliosis in adolescents. Orthop Clin North Am 1988;19: 313–317
32. Puno RM, Johnson JR, Ostermann PA, Holt RT. Analysis of the primary and compensatory curvatures following Zielke instrumentation for idiopathic scoliosis. Spine 1989;14:738–743
33. Hall JE, Mills MB, Snyder BD. Short segment anterior instrumentation for thoracolumbar scoliosis. In: Bridwell KH, DeWald RL, eds. The Textbook of Spinal Surgery, ed. 2. Philadelphia, PA: Lippincott-Raven; 1997:665–674
34. Betz RR, Harms J, Clements DH III, et al. Comparison of anterior and posterior instrumentation for correction of adolescent thoracic idiopathic scoliosis. Spine 1999;24:225–239
35. Dubousset J, Herring JA, Shufflebarger H. The crankshaft phenomenon. J Pediatr Orthop 1989;9:541–550
36. Harms J, Jeszenszky D, Beele B. Ventral correction of thoracic scoliosis. In: Bridwell KH, DeWald RL, eds. The Textbook of Spinal Surgery, ed. 2. Philadelphia, PA: Lippincott-Raven; 1997: 611–626.
37. Bernstein RM, Hall JE. Solid rod short segment anterior fusion in thoracolumbar scoliosis. J Pediatr Orthop B 1998;7:124–131
38. Lenke LG, Betz RR, Clements D, et al. Curve prevalence of a new classification of operative adolescent idiopathic scoliosis: Does classification correlate with treatment? Spine 2002;27: 604–611
39. Lenke LG, Bridwell KH, Baldus C, Blanke K. Analysis of pulmonary function and axis rotation in adolescent and young adult idiopathic scoliosis patients treated with Cotrel-Dubousset instrumentation. J Spinal Disord 1992;5:16–25
40. Lenke LG, Bridwell KH, Baldus C, Blanke K. Preventing decompensation in King type II curves treated with Cotrel-Dubousset instrumentation. Strict guidelines for selective thoracic fusion. Spine 1992;17(8, suppl):S274–S281
41. Edwards CC II, Lenke LG, Peelle M, Sides B, Rinella A, Bridwell KH. Selective thoracic fusion for adolescent idiopathic scoliosis with C modifier lumbar curves: 2- to 16-year radiographic and clinical results. Spine 2004;29:536–546
42. Newton PO, Faro FD, Lenke LG, et al. Factors involved in the decision to perform a selective versus nonselective fusion of Lenke 1B and 1C (King-Moe II) curves in adolescent idiopathic scoliosis. Spine 2003;28:S217–S223
43. Potter BK, Kuklo TR, Lenke LG. Radiographic outcomes of anterior spinal fusion versus posterior spinal fusion with thoracic pedicle screws for treatment of Lenke Type I adolescent idiopathic scoliosis curves. Spine 2005;30:1859–1866
44. Lenke LG, Bridwell KH, O'Brien MF, Baldus C, Blanke K. Recognition and treatment of the proximal thoracic curve in adolescent idiopathic scoliosis treated with Cotrel-Dubousset instrumentation. Spine 1994;19:1589–1597
45. Suk SI, Kim WJ, Lee CS, et al. Indications of proximal thoracic curve fusion in thoracic adolescent idiopathic scoliosis: Recognition and treatment of double thoracic curve pattern in adolescent idiopathic scoliosis treated with segmental instrumentation. Spine 2000; 25(18):2342–2349
46. Cil A, Pekmezci M, Yazici M, et al. The validity of Lenke criteria for defining structural proximal thoracic curves in patients with adolescent idiopathic scoliosis. Spine 2005;30:2550–2555

47. Klepps SJ, Lenke LG, Bridwell KH, Bassett GS, Whorton J. Prospective comparison of flexibility radiographs in adolescent idiopathic scoliosis. Spine 2001;26:E74–E79
48. Marsicano JG, Lenke LG, Bridwell KH, Chapman M, Gupta P, Weston J. The lordotic effect of the OSI frame on operative adolescent idiopathic scoliosis patients. Spine 1998;23: 1341–1348
49. Sweet FA, Lenke LG, Bridwell KH, Blanke KM. Maintaining lumbar lordosis with anterior single solid-rod instrumentation in thoracolumbar and lumbar adolescent idiopathic scoliosis. Spine 1999; 24:1655–1662
50. Hurford RK Jr, Lenke LG, Lee SS, Cheng I, Sides B, Bridwell KH. Prospective radiographic and clinical outcomes of dual-rod instrumented anterior spinal fusion in adolescent idiopathic scoliosis: Comparison with single-rod constructs. Spine 2006;31:2322–2328
51. Sanders AE, Baumann R, Brown H, Johnston CE II, Lenke LG, Sink E. Selective anterior fusion of thoracolumbar/lumbar curves in adolescents: When can the associated thoracic curve be left unfused? Spine 2003;28:706–713; discussion, 714
52. Clements DH, Marks MC, Newton PO, et al. Analysis of adherence to Lenke classification treatment algorithm recommendations. Paper presented at: 13th International Meeting on Advanced Spine Techniques (IMAST), Athens, Greece, July 12–15, 2006
53. Lenke LG, Sucato DJ, Emans JB, et al. Prospective multicenter evaluation of fusion level selection in adolescent idiopathic scoliosis: Are the Lenke classification rules still followed? Paper presented at: 13th International Meeting on Advanced Spine Techniques (IMAST), Athens, Greece, July 12–15, 2006
54. Bridwell KH. Adolescent idiopathic scoliosis: Surgical treatment. In: Weinstein SL, ed. The Pediatric Spine. Principles and Practice. New York: Raven Press; 1994:511–555
55. Hefti FL, McMaster MJ. The effect of the adolescent growth spurt on early posterior spinal fusion in infantile and juvenile idiopathic scoliosis. J Bone Joint Surg Br 1983;65:247–254
56. Mason DE, Carango P. Spinal decompensation in Cotrel-Dubousset instrumentation. Spine 1991;16(8, suppl):S394–S403
57. Bridwell KH, McAllister JW, Betz RR, Huss G, Clancy M, Schoenecker PL. Coronal decompensation produced by Cotrel-Dubousset "derotation" maneuver for idiopathic right thoracic scoliosis. Spine 1991;16:769–777
58. Lenke LG, Engsberg JR, Ross SA, Reitenbach A, Blanke K, Bridwell KH. Prospective dynamic functional evaluation of gait and spinal balance following spinal fusion in adolescent idiopathic scoliosis. Spine 2001;26:E330–E337
59. Lowe TG, Lenke L, Betz R, et al. Distal junctional kyphosis of adolescent idiopathic thoracic curves following anterior or posterior instrumented fusion: Incidence, risk factors, and prevention. Spine 2006;31:299–302

# 14 Posterior Correction Techniques in Late-onset Scoliosis

*Suken A. Shah*

Idiopathic scoliosis is a three-dimensional (3D) deformity with lateral deviation in the coronal plane, thoracic hypokyphosis in the sagittal plane, and rotation in the transverse plane. With pedicle-screw fixation and modern corrective techniques, true 3D correction of the spinal deformity in scoliosis can be accomplished. Intuitively, in typical thoracic adolescent idiopathic scoliosis (AIS) this would mean optimal coronal correction, restoration of normal thoracic kyphosis, and realignment of thoracic torsion by lifting of the thoracic rib concavity out of the chest and reducing the convex rib deformity without the need for thoracoplasty. There is no single technique for the surgical correction of scoliosis that will work in every situation. Careful preoperative planning to maximize the usefulness of implants, and observation of the correction intraoperatively, are mandatory for success. Criteria to be considered are spinal flexibility, the material properties of the implants being used, the type of vertebral fixation to be used, and the reduction techniques that are anticipated to be needed. With respect to spinal flexibility, an assessment should be made of how much correction is possible or necessary. Both coronal- and sagittal-plane flexibility should be considered. Hypokyphotic or lordotic thoracic deformities are often very difficult to reduce with posterior-only techniques. Is a release required to achieve the necessary correction? If so, what sort of release is needed? Is a simple intraspinous-ligament resection with facetectomy sufficient, or is some sort of osteotomy required? Flexible spines usually respond to any reduction maneuver. Stiff spines may defy all attempts at reduction until appropriately mobilized with a combination of techniques.

## Implant Properties

The material properties of implants are an important consideration in preoperative planning for the surgical treatment of scoliosis. By varying the diameter and composition of an implant rod, a surgeon can match the stiffness of the rod to the stiffness of the patient's spinal curve, the quality of the patient's bone, or both. Stainless steel (SS) has distinct advantages in correcting spinal deformities. The stiffness and strength of SS are benefits when reducing the spine to the rod because there is greater corrective power in conforming the spine to the rod and less potential for rod deformation. For example, for a stiff, lordotic thoracic scoliosis, SS would provide a better correction in both planes than would a titanium (Ti) rod, which would be expected to bend into the deformity and provide less corrective ability. However, there is such a thing as a rod that is too stiff; thus, if the stiffness of a rod exceeds the strength of the bone–implant interface, pullout of the implant is possible. The bending characteristics of SS allow its in situ contouring for challenging coronal- and sagittal-plane deformities because SS undergoes plastic deformation over a narrower range than Ti because of the latter's greater elasticity. Although SS is stiffer and stronger than Ti, whereas Ti is more elastic, both materials are acceptable once a construct is assembled because construct rigidity also depends on the number and type of anchors for the construct.

Titanium has other cited advantages in the areas of imaging, infection, corrosion, and sensitivity.[1,2] Because Ti does not create as many artifacts as SS, better postoperative computed tomography (CT) and magnetic resonance (MR) imaging with Ti has made it more popular than SS, especially in certain situations in which visualization within the spinal canal or evaluation of adjacent segment degeneration is valuable for clinical decision-making. Some centers favor the use of Ti for its resistance to infection in that it does not easily allow the formation of bacterial glycocalyx on its surface, which could permit it to harbor organisms that might cause deep late-onset infection. Moreover, the surface composition and ion charge of Ti are more friendly to osteoblasts than are those of SS. Explant corrosion studies cite less corrosion in Ti constructs, which may also be a factor in decreasing infection in that Ti tempers host immune responses.[3] Furthermore, Ti is a better choice of construct material for patients who have a known sensitivity to nickel, a component of the SS alloy.

For surgeons who favor Ti implants but are frequently disappointed by their lack of strength and stiffness in an application for treating a spinal deformity, cobalt chromium (CoCr) rods may offer a satisfactory compromise. The material properties of CoCr are close to those of SS in rods of the same diameter, and are compatible with Ti spinal anchors, with the result that a surgeon seeking to use Ti implants may not need to give up corrective capacity when using CoCr rods. Other materials that may be available in the future for use in corrective constructs are nitinol, a superelastic nickel–titanium alloy that has shape-memory properties, and dynamic rods made of polyetheretherketone (PEEK) or polyethylene polymers.

A properly contoured and applied rod provides most of the correction of a spinal deformity. Many reduction maneuvers can be applied during such correction. The most effective of these maneuvers are performed while only one rod is in place. The second rod adds stability and resistance to fatigue failure of the corrective construct. Occasionally, temporary or working rods may be required to facilitate reduction. These working rods will usually be placed on the side opposite that of the correcting or primary rod. Three-column osteotomy corrections, large curves with nonharmonious sagittal segments, or single long curves containing different sagittal contours are common indications for using temporary or working rods.

To a great degree, the techniques used to correct spinal deformities depend on the spinal implants used for the fixation of corrective constructs. Reduction techniques possible with first-generation implants using nonsegmental hooks (Harrington-rod constructs) were limited to the global en bloc distraction of multiple vertebral segments, correcting a deformity in the coronal plane, often at the cost of correcting it in the sagittal plane. Second-generation implant systems using "segmental hook" constructs (Cotrel–Dubousset constructs) allowed some flexibility in applying distraction as well as compressive forces across a deformity.[4] Although providing some additional options for reducing spinal deformities, hook-and-wire based systems fell short in several important ways. First, even segmental-hook systems did not allow truly segmental fixation (i.e., fixation at every vertebral level treated with a construct), and neither hook nor wire constructs provide rigid fixation, and therefore complete control, over the vertebral segments included in a corrective construct. Currently available pedicle-screw systems overcome both of these failings by allowing truly segmental spinal fixation at every level as well as direct control over each vertebral segment included in a construct. Now, with the ability to directly control each individual segment, the ability to reduce a spinal deformity has more to do with the adequacy of release (i.e., spinal mobilization), the creativity in designing reduction maneuvers that take into account the response of the spine during reduction, and the persistence of the surgeon in attempting to achieve complete reduction of the deformity.

The types of devices used for vertebral-body fixation will also dictate or influence reduction strategies. Monoaxial, uniplanar, and polyaxial reduction screws, hooks, and wires will lend themselves to specific reduction strategies. The type of implant and its position in a construct should be considered in the preoperative planning for its use.

## Correction Maneuvers

The following sections describe a variety of techniques and maneuvers that can be applied individually or in combination to achieve the reduction of spinal deformities. Although at one time the technique for reduction of scoliosis was dictated by the implants to be used or by philosophical constraints, multiple techniques can now be used to achieve the correction of a deformity. Because not every technique will work equally well in all situations, the success of a correction for scoliosis depends on the adequacy of spinal release and the skill and experience of the surgeon in applying the techniques used for the correction.

### 1. Compression–Distraction

Distraction on the concave rod of a construct decreases scoliosis. In the thoracic spine, distraction also increases thoracic kyphosis, which is generally desirable in view of the frequent loss of normal thoracic kyphosis noted in idiopathic scoliosis. Compression is useful to reduce hyperkyphotic thoracic deformities. Similarly, compression applied to implants along the rod on the convex side of the lumbar deformity both corrects scoliosis and restores or maintains lumbar lordosis. When compression and distraction are used as primary reduction maneuvers, it is important to remember the kyphosing and lordosing effects of these techniques so as not to negatively affect spinal balance in the sagittal plane. However, when compression–distraction is used primarily as a technique to refine a reduction after both rods of the corrective construct are in place and appropriately contoured, the positive and negative consequences of intrasegmental compression and distraction on the patient's sagittal profile are probably negligible. This segmental "fine-tuning" is particularly enhanced by using bilateral segmental pedicle screws.

The possible adverse effects of the compression–distraction technique include transmission of asymetric forces to adjacent levels of the spine, and especially to adjacent uninstrumented levels, resulting in junctional malalignment. The use of excessive forces may loosen implants. Fixed-angle or monoaxial screws do not lend themselves to this technique because they need to either plow through the pedicle or return to their previous orientation (precompression or distraction) when the set screws are tightened, and the screw head must be perpendicular to the rod for a secure connection. Uniplanar or polyaxial screws are effective in compression–distraction maneuvers. Distraction of the thoracic spine to induce kyphosis in the typical hypokyphotic situation in AIS is more effective when adequate releases of the facets and ligamentum flavum are achieved, but this should be done with caution.

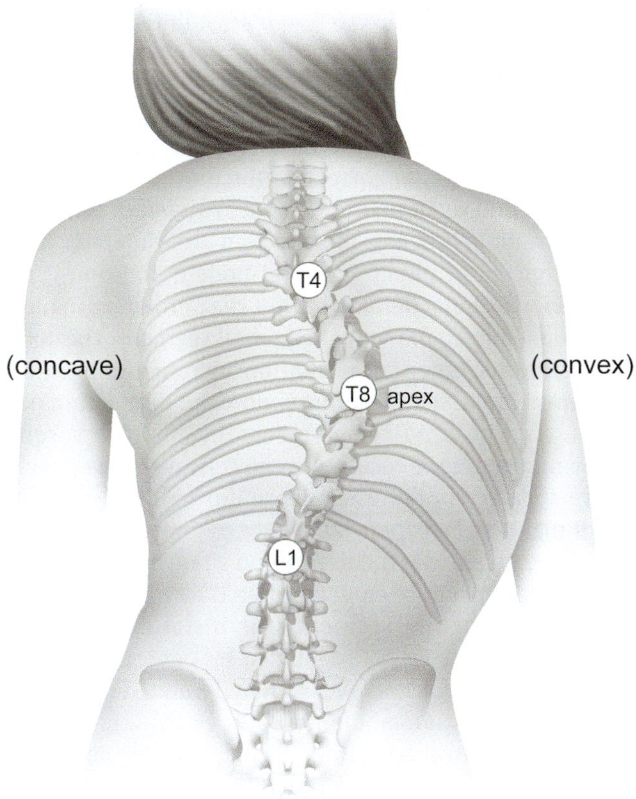


**Fig. 14.1** Posterior view of a patient with Lenke type 1 right thoracic scoliosis, showing the typical truncal shift, rib asymmetry, and convex rib prominence in this type of scoliosis. (From James Millerick, ©2006 DePuy Spine, Inc., used with permission.)

## 2. Rod-derotation Maneuver

For a typical lordotic thoracic curve (**Fig. 14.1**), the classic "derotation" maneuver of Cotrel and Dubousset may be applied.[4] A rod contoured for the coronal-plane deformity of the curve is placed in the screws on the concave side of the deformity. The set screws should be engaged within the screw head, but not tightened. The rod is then rotated into the correct position and the second rod is placed. This technique theoretically converts lateral deviation into deviation in the sagittal plane. Given that thoracic curvatures are often hypokyphotic, this maneuver can often both correct coronal plane deformity and restore natural thoracic kyphosis. However, some points should be made about this technique. Most important is that the derotation with this en bloc derotation maneuver really amounts to lateral translation or an in situ relocation of the apex of the treated curve. In addition, the desired sagittal contour is rarely concordant with the coronal plane of the scoliotic deformity. Hence, the conversion from a coronal-plane deformity to kyphosis or lordosis may occur at the wrong location. Moreover, the rod used for the derotation must be stiff enough to maintain its contoured shape, the bone must be strong enough to withstand screw pullout, and the spine must be flexible enough to be displaced posteriorly. This technique may not work well with Ti rods, which are more flexible than SS rods and have a tendency to "bend-out" and lose the sagittal contour that was created in them before their implantation.

Proponents of the Cotrel–Dubousset procedure believed that rotational correction of a scoliosis would occur with the rod-derotation maneuver. This was later disproved with pre- and postoperative CT scans of instrumented patients. Labele and colleagues used 3D digitizers intraoperatively and showed that the Cotrel–Dubousset rod-derotation maneuver did produce coronal- and sagittal-plane correction and relocated the instrumented portion of the spine, but with little axial-plane rotation.[5] Hook-and-wire fixation lacks the ability to derotate the spine because force is applied posterior to the instantaneous axis of rotation (IAR) and the moment arm is inadequate to apply sufficient torque. True correction of vertebral rotation in the axial plane, and consequently elimination of the convex thoracic or thoracolumbar (TL) prominence in scoliosis, is difficult to achieve without anterior diskectomy and chest-wall violation with thoracoplasty.

## 3. In-situ Contouring

With the use of appropriate bending tools for the rods used in a corrective construct, in situ contouring in both the coronal and sagittal planes can improve spinal alignment in scoliosis. This is a very useful technique for re-establishing the coronal contour of the spine if the rod used in the procedure bends out during rod rotation. It is much easier to effectively change the coronal than the sagittal plane once all the implants used with the rod are engaged on the rod. In situ sagittal rod benders are often very useful in working a rod into the vertebral implants for a corrective construct during difficult rod-to-implant reductions. Sagittal rod benders are also very helpful in creating lumbar lordosis. With the use of either technique, great care should be exercised to prevent the catastrophic failure of implant fixation in the vertebral body. This is especially a concern when using hooks for vertebral fixation. In situ contouring is not a useful technique with Ti rods because they require too much bend (deformation distance) to reach the plastic range to make this technique practical. The in situ contouring technique also does not work well for reducing thoracic hypokyphosis.

## 4. Coronal and Sagittal Translation

Pure translation is very effective for correcting thoracic curves. This can be achieved either with sublaminar wires or reduction screws on the concave side of the apical and periapical vertebrae of a thoracic curve. Reduction screws can be implanted in the four or five apical and periapical levels of a deformity to facilitate rod placement and correction of the deformity. The sequence of steps in reduction by translation involves first placing the rod in the distal or proximal implants, which are then closed loosely. Next, the rod is sequentially reduced into each adjacent implant, including the reduction implants. The reduction screws are initially left untightened. Rings should be placed on the reduction implants to prevent premature release of the flanges of the reduction screws. As a last step the rod is introduced into the most cephalad or distal implants, which are loosely closed. Following this the rod, which has been precontoured into the desired sagittal contour and left straight in the coronal plane, is rotated into the correct sagittal and coronal orientation. The inner screws on the reduction implants are then slowly and sequentially tightened to achieve reduction of the spine by pulling the spine to the rod. This results in correction of a scoliosis and produces posterior sagittal-plane translation, producing kyphosis. Among the benefits of this technique are that it allows slow reduction of the thoracic deformity in scoliosis, taking advantage of viscoelastic creep. It also allows the forces of reduction to be distributed over each segment of the deformity. The screws serve both as the final implants and the tools for reduction, eliminating the need for any additional instrumentation in the operative site. The extended tabs allow rotation of the rod into the final position with little stress applied to the rod. This helps to prevent rod "bend-out." Translation with reduction screws is not as effective with stiff curves or with Ti rods for the reasons mentioned above. Care must be taken to look for pullout of anchoring screws. To some degree this is prevented by assessing the flexibility of a curve and the strength of the patient's vertebral bone, and being satisfied with a reasonable reduction. Maximizing the diameter, length, and position of a screw within a vertebral body may also help prevent screw pullout.

## 5. En Bloc Vertebral Derotation

An alternative technique for reducing a scoliotic curve is regional vertebral derotation. This technique is used after the Cotrel–Dubousset procedure of rod derotation when the rod is in its final position. The maneuver involves the direct application of force to the entire periapical segment of a deformity from the convex side. This is achieved by placing devices on the convex pedicle screws that facilitate a derotation moment to be imparted to three or four of the periapical vertebrae of a deformity. This produces derotation around the concave rod. Once this is done, the set screws are tightened to hold the treated vertebrae in place.

## 6. Direct Vertebral-body Derotation

The challenges in the 3D correction of scoliosis with posterior-only surgery are well addressed with the use of segmental pedicle-screw fixation, and specifically the application of direct vertebral rotation, first described by Lee et al.[6] Pedicle screws extend into the vertebral body anterior to the IAR, and can be manipulated with the use of long derotator instruments attached to the screw heads to achieve true 3D correction of a scoliotic deformity. Segmental fixation with pedicle screws addresses the most rigid, rotated portion of the spine, spreads the corrective force over multiple implants, can pull the scoliotic rib concavity out of the chest, and will result in little loss of correction over time.

The concept of direct vertebral-body derotation is the same as for regional derotation, but the derotation maneuver is applied to an individual vertebral segment. This technique allows segmental derotation incrementally in the same way that repeated compression and distraction maneuvers can be used to incrementally improve coronal alignment. To use the technique, the concave-side screw in the treated vertebra must be loose during the derotation step. It may also be beneficial to have mobility of the vertebrae above and below the derotation site. The sequence of steps in the procedure can be initiated from either end of the treated vertebral segment. The distal and proximal ends of the construct are stabilized by tightening the set screws, and the adjacent level is then derotated by directly applying a derotation moment to the vertebra through the screw on the contralateral side. Once the desired derotation has been achieved, this set screw is tightened. This maneuver is repeated at each instrumented level. Additional derotation can be achieved by repeating the process at each level until a satisfactory result is achieved.

The goals of vertebral derotation are to achieve true 3D correction of a spinal deformity and reverse the torsional asymmetry induced by scoliosis. Intuitively, in typical thoracic AIS, this would mean optimal coronal correction, restoration of thoracic kyphosis, and the realignment of thoracic torsion by lifting the rib concavity out of the chest and reducing the convex rib deformity. The upper and lower instrumented vertebrae would be level, and along with the apex of the curve would be brought into the stable zone as defined by the center sacral vertical line (CSVL). The rib prominence would be virtually eliminated without thoracoplasty.

Some technical considerations are important in executing a direct vertebral-body derotation safely and effectively. Fixed-angle pedicle screws offer better axial-plane control of the vertebral segment being derotated than do polyaxial screws,[7] and an attempt should be made to use them in the strategic areas of the spine (i.e., the apex of the deformity). Recently, uniplanar screw technology has become available and allows the cephalad/caudad movement of a polyaxial screw, although the screw remains fixed in the coronal and axial planes for vertebral-body derotation maneuvers. Application of force to the screws in a construct being used for derotation should be slow, deliberate, and controlled, and depends on the bone mineral density of the patient's spine and integrity of the bone–screw interface. More force can be applied to the screws on the convex side of a deformity because the corresponding pedicles are typically larger than the concave-side pedicles in the apex of the scoliosis,[8] and the medial wall of the convex-side pedicle is thicker than the lateral wall of the pedicle.[9] When rotated to failure, the convex-side screws will fracture the medial wall of the pedicle and enter the spinal canal; the concave screws will fracture the lateral pedicle wall, rib/pedicle unit, and transverse process, and could injure the aorta.[10] Lastly, care must be taken not to transfer torsional forces beyond the instrumented segments and to compensatory curves or neutrally rotated vertebral levels to create iatrogenic torsion; the neutral end-vertebrae must be locked before derotation of the apical levels of the deformity being treated.[11]

## 7. Derotation via Differential Rod Contouring

To some degree, differential contouring in the sagittal plane between the convex and concave rod in a corrective construct can be used to apply some derotational force to the apical vertebrae in an instrumented curve. In a typical right-convex hypokyphotic or lordotic thoracic curve, the concave left side of the apical vertebrae needs to be displaced or rotated more posteriorly, whereas the convex right side of these vertebrae needs to be rotated anteriorly. To produce this derotation moment in the transverse plane, slight hyperkyphosis is contoured into the left rod of the treatment construct, with hypokyphosis contoured into the right rod.[11] Bilateral segmental pedicle-screw fixation can effectively be used to apply these moments to the vertebrae. This corrective torque may help in reducing a thoracic deformity in the sagittal plane (**Fig. 14.2**).

## 8. Cantilever Technique

Cantilever techniques find their greatest usefulness in kyphosis. In the hyperkyphotic thoracic curve or in the lumbar spine, however, a cantilever technique can be used to achieve correction in the coronal plane and induce relative or absolute lordosis as needed. In these cases the convex rod may be placed first. Bilateral screws are preferred as vertebral anchors in this circumstance. Rod insertion may be started either proximally or distally. The rod can then be sequentially reduced into each implant with a cantilever maneuver, and the screws loosely tightened. This is followed by appropriate compression and distraction to finalize the correction. If at this point there is no residual coronal deformity, the implant screws are simply retightened and the procedure completed. If there is a significant residual coronal or rotational deformity, the intervertebral derotation maneuver described above can be performed before placement of the second rod. As a final step, the second rod is inserted and the set screws are tightened.

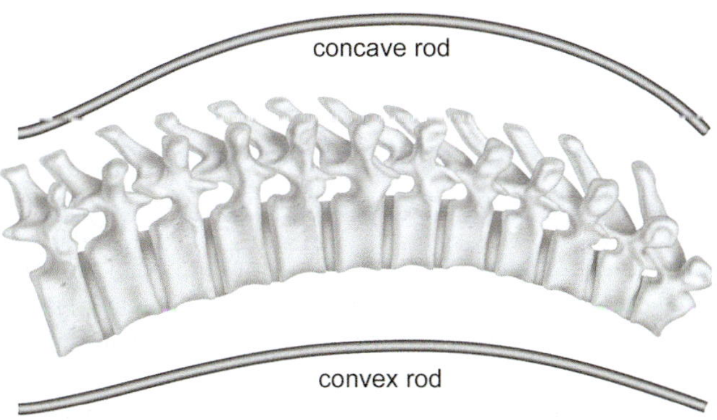


**Fig. 14.2** Differential rod contouring: The concave rod will pull the apical vertebrae dorsally out of the chest and the convex rod is relatively underbent to reduce the convex rib prominence. (From James Millerick, ©2006 DePuy Spine, Inc., used with permission.)

## 9. Traction

Traction was used extensively in the past to correct deformities, and had then fallen out of favor as a routine method as implant technology progressed, but has seen a resurgence in popularity as an option for treating rigid, severe curves and early-onset scoliosis. Halo-traction can be used preoperatively and is a safe, well-tolerated method of applying gradual, sustained traction to maximize the operative correction of spinal deformities in patients with severe idiopathic scoliosis (**Fig. 14.3**) and kyphosis. Traction can also be used intra-operatively and between staged procedures. Traction before instrumentation is facilitated by anterior and posterior releases. The releases can be performed in a staged fashion or together as the initial surgery for a deformity. This works well for large deformities or in patients who might not be able to tolerate a major anterior–posterior reconstruction in a single surgical operation. The technique for using traction can be found in Chapter 15. In a multicenter study, Sponseller and colleagues found a comparable frequency of the correction of deformity (62% vs. 59%) and of complications in the treatment of severe spinal deformities with and without traction, but patients given halo-traction had a less frequent need for vertebral-column resection.[12]

## 10. Temporary Working Rods

Working rods are rods that are placed temporarily to facilitate either partial reduction of an entire deformity or a segment of a deformity. The trick to using working rods is to apply them in such a way as to facilitate partial reduction of a deformity without blocking the ability to reduce the rest of it.

The most useful applications of the working-rod technique are in the reduction of double curves (double major curves consisting of structural main thoracic [MT] and thoracolumbar/lumbar [TL/L]curves, or double thoracic curves consiting of structural upper thoracic and MT curves) and temporary stabilization of spinal osteotomies or resections. If one or both of the curves in a double-curve deformity is

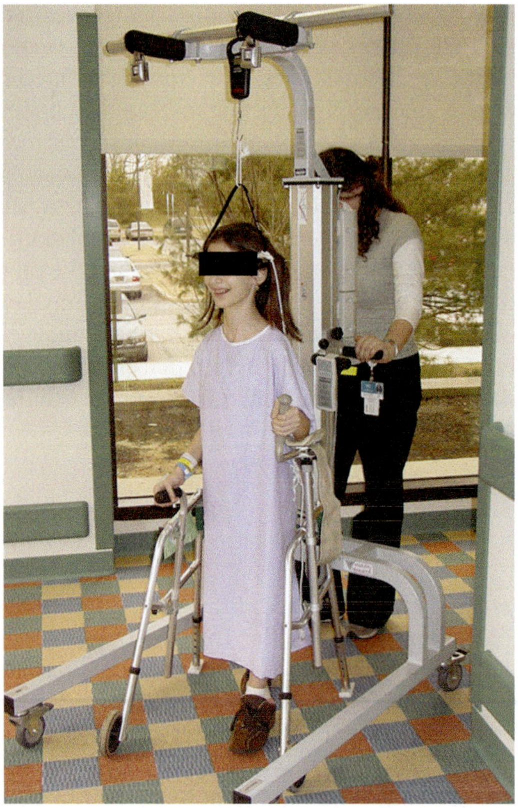

**Fig. 14.3** Clinical photograph of a patient ambulating with halo-gravity traction between phases of staged spinal surgery for severe scoliosis. This type of traction is well tolerated, safe, and effective for gentle reduction of severe scoliosis and kyphosis.

very stiff, or if the thoracic curves are very lordotic, it will be difficult if not impossible to place a single rod along the entire length of the deformity and to rotate the rod into a corrected position. Attempting to do so will usually result in bending-out of the rod with subsequent ineffective and incomplete reduction. The working-rod technique attempts to overcome this problem by maximizing the reductive forces exerted by a rod by applying them to a short segment of the spine, which can be more effectively manipulated. Once a segment is realigned, the rest of a deformity can be reduced. For example, placement of a concave lumbar rod in a double major deformity as a preliminary step in its reduction is especially useful in patients with large, highly rotated lumbar curves because coronal alignment, apical rotation, and lordosis can all be addressed independently of the thoracic spine. This part of the reduction often involves a simple derotation maneuver followed by segmental vertebral-body derotation and in situ rod bending if necessary. These maneuvers usually effect significant reduction of the lumbar component of a double major deformity. With the lumbar deformity reduced, the rod-bending, insertion sequence, and thoracic-reduction maneuvers can be applied to the thoracic convexity without the need for concern about the effect they will have on the lumbar deformity.

A more recently adopted technique involves placement of a rod into the thoracic convexity to achieve partial reduction of a thoracic scoliotic curve. This is a useful technique for stiff, lordotic, thoracic curves. The technique must be applied with reduction screws in the concave pedicles and polyaxial screws in the end-vertebrae of the thoracic deformity. The rod is contoured into a slightly greater kyphosis than is desired, anticipating that the rod will flatten out to some degree during reduction. The rod is inserted into the screw heads in a scoliotic alignment and rotated into the correct coronal alignment (i.e., straight in the coronal plane and kyphotic in the sagittal plane). The proximal and distal multiaxial screws are locked into place while the reduction screws remain loose. Since the rotation is performed with reduction screws in the apex of the deformity, only a small amount of stress is transferred to the rod and apical reduction screws during the rod-rotation maneuver. Once the rod is in the correct sagittal alignment, the reduction feature of the reduction screws is used to slowly translate the spine to the rod. This will affect both translation and derotation. If the curve is not too stiff, complete reduction may be achieved with this maneuver. If the rod begins to bend out or screw purchase becomes a concern, the reduction with the rod can be temporarily halted. The next step is to bend the contralateral rod into a hypokyphotic sagittal contour while leaving it straight in the coronal plane. This latter rod is inserted into the polyaxial screws on the convexity of the thoracic deformity. Using cantilever forces in both the coronal and sagittal planes, the scoliosis and the convex kyphosis (often caused by residual vertebral-body rotation) are pushed anteriorly and toward the midline, reducing the kyphosis and the scoliosis, respectively. This maneuver decreases the forces on the convex working rod. The concave working rod is now replaced with the permanent concave rod. Once the permanent concave rod is in place, the screw heads for the convex rod are loosened and final reduction is achieved through the reduction mechanisms on the screws.

## The Author's Preferred Technique of Direct Vertebral Rotation in Late-onset Idiopathic Scoliosis

- On the concave side of the thoracic curve: Insert monoaxial or uniplanar screws at every level. Consider using polyaxial reduction screws at the apex of the concavity, particularly for severe curves.
- On the convex side of the thoracic curve: Insert monoaxial or uniplanar screws into at least three or four convex pedicles at the apex of the curve, as well as into the proximal and distal foundations.

- Confirm placement of the screws and check screw length with fluoroscopy or plain X-ray films before rod insertion.
- Contour the concave rod to have extra kyphosis (anticipating that the rod will become flatter during the translation/reduction of the scoliosis) to pull the apical vertebrae dorsally out of the chest and correct apical lordosis (**Fig. 14.2**).
- Contour the convex rod to have less thoracic kyphosis so as to push down on the convex side of the vertebral bodies in the kyphosis, thus displacing them anteriorly and decreasing the associated rib prominence (**Fig. 14.2**).
- Insert the concave rod into the pedicle-screw anchors, leaving the set screws loose (**Fig. 14.4**).
- The rod can engage the anchors via one or both of the following:
    a. Translation maneuver: Insert the rod proximally and distally and tighten the set screws proximally and distally, leaving the rod in the correct sagittal plane. After the proximal and distal foundations are connected and locked, apical screw forces are translated to the rod segmentally by using reduction devices or reduction screws (**Fig. 14.5A**).
    b. Rod-rotation maneuver: Insert the rod and perform a rod-rotation maneuver as in the classic Cotrel–Dubousset technique.[4] In this case the rod rotates from the midline scoliotic position laterally to the left by ~90 degrees (**Fig. 14.5B**). During the 90-degree rotation, one must have control by pushing down over the convex ribs to avoid aggravating the rib prominence. This results in a translocation of the spine dorsally and medially, but rarely results in true axial-plane derotation.
- Proceed with one or both of the vertebral-body derotation techniques described below.

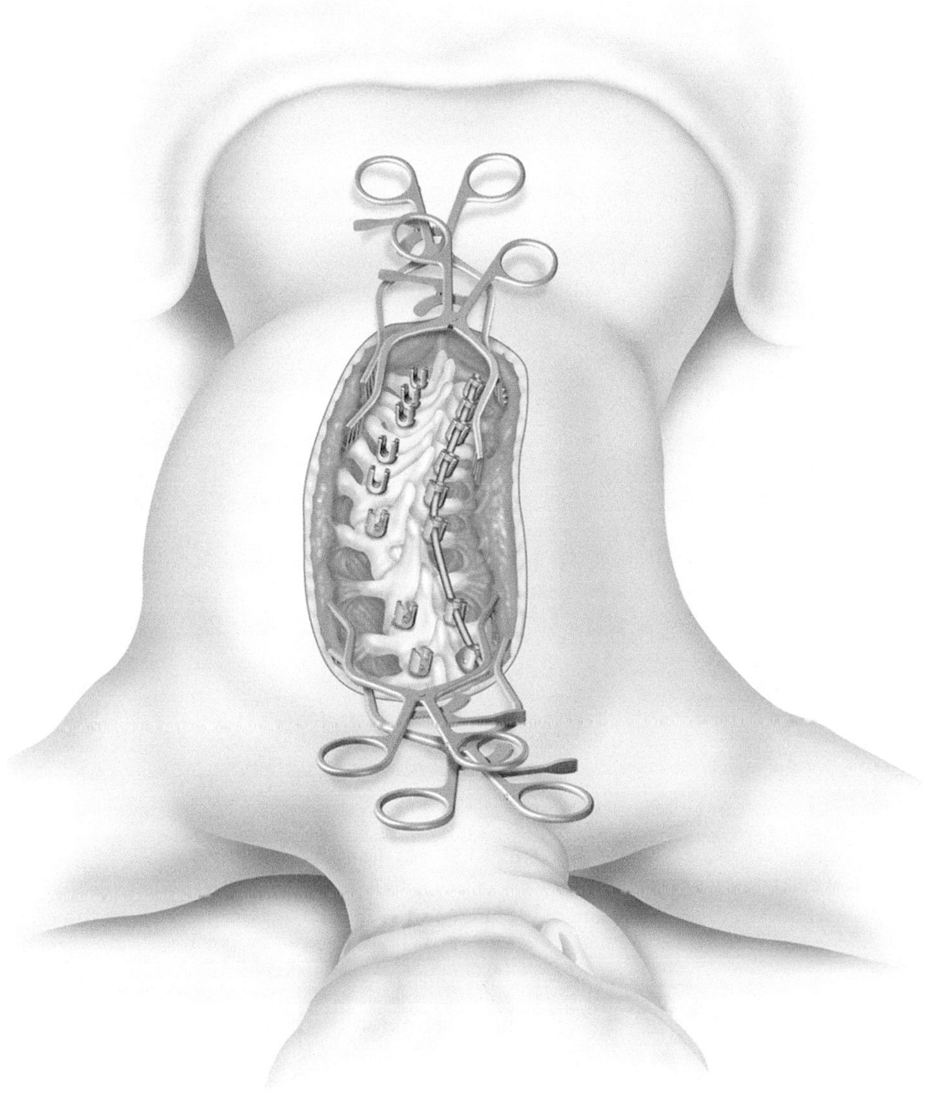

**Fig. 14.4** Concave rod inserted with the set screws left loose, before translation or derotation of a thoracic curve. (From James Millerick, ©2006 DePuy Spine, Inc., used with permission.)

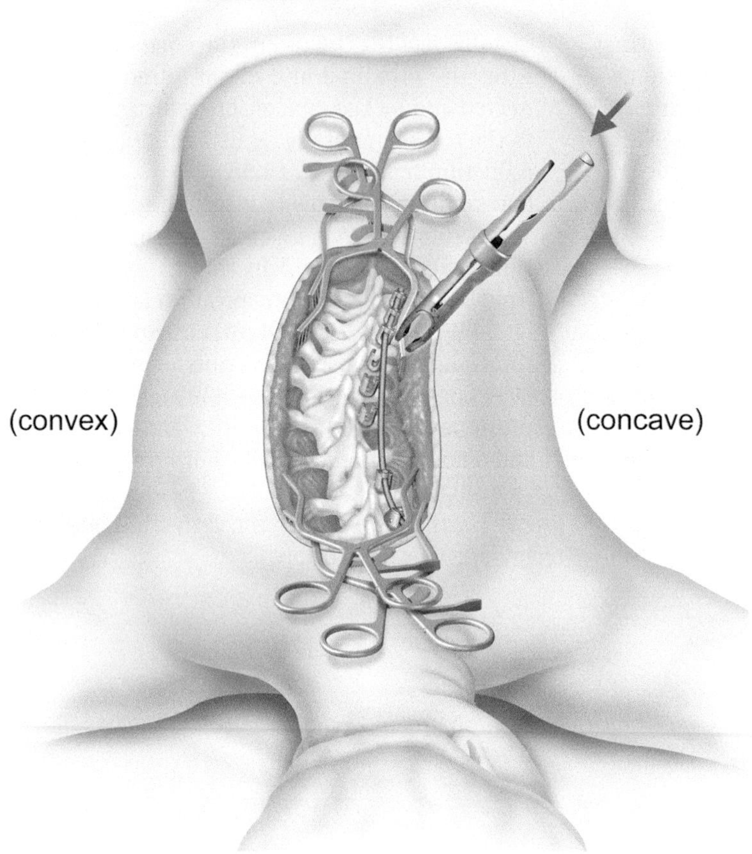


A

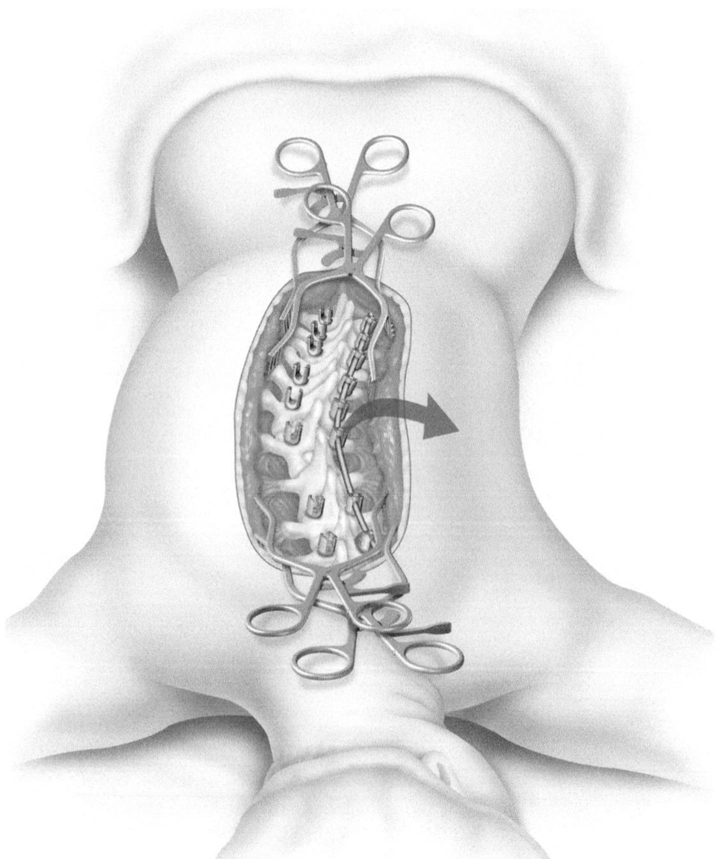

B

**Fig. 14.5** **(A)** Translational correction of scoliosis with a rod reduction device. **(B)** Alternate method of correction: Rod-derotation maneuver with *arrow* pointing in the direction of of a 90-degree rotation to correct scoliosis in the coronal plane and the set rod in the proper sagittal plane. (From James Millerick, ©2006 DePuy Spine, Inc., used with permission.)

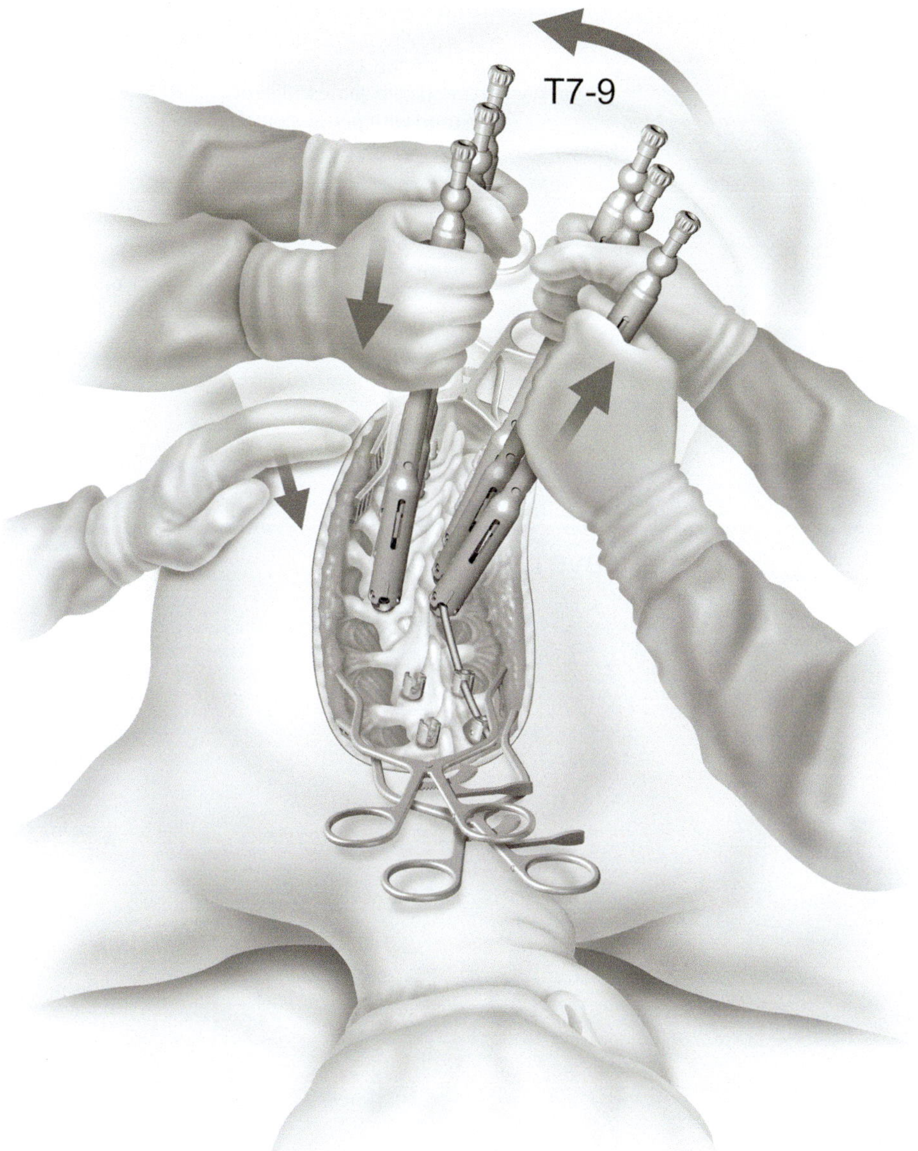


**Fig. 14.6** En bloc derotation of the thoracic apex of a coliotic curve with derotators attached to pedicle screws; only the concave rod is implanted at this point, and serves as the axis of rotation. (From James Millerick, ©2006 DePuy Spine, Inc., used with permission.)

## En Bloc Spinal Derotation

- After the concave rod is engaged in all anchors, attach derotation instruments to the apical screw heads on both the concave and convex sides (**Fig. 14.6**).
- An assistant pushes down on the convex ribs and the convex screws, and the surgeon rotates concave and convex screws in the direction that will reduce the rib prominence (counterclockwise in **Figs. 14.6** and **14.7**). The two maneuvers should be done simultaneously, to distribute strain and to limit loading of the bone–screw interface. The rotation of the concave screws will help decrease the torsion and will lift the rib concavity out of the patient's chest. A rehearsal of this maneuver before rod insertion can help in providing a sense of how much force is to be applied safely.
- Tighten the set screws on the concave rod, holding the curve in the position achieved (**Fig. 14.8A**).
- Implant the convex rod and tighten the set screws on the convex side of the curve (**Fig. 14.8B**).

## Segmental Spinal Derotation (Individual Vertebral Level)

Segmental vertebral-body derotation can be done as the sole derotation maneuver for a thoracic curve or in addition to the en bloc maneuver described above.

- Implant both the convex and concave rods and capture them with set screws. Most set screws should be left loose because lengthening of the spine is expected at

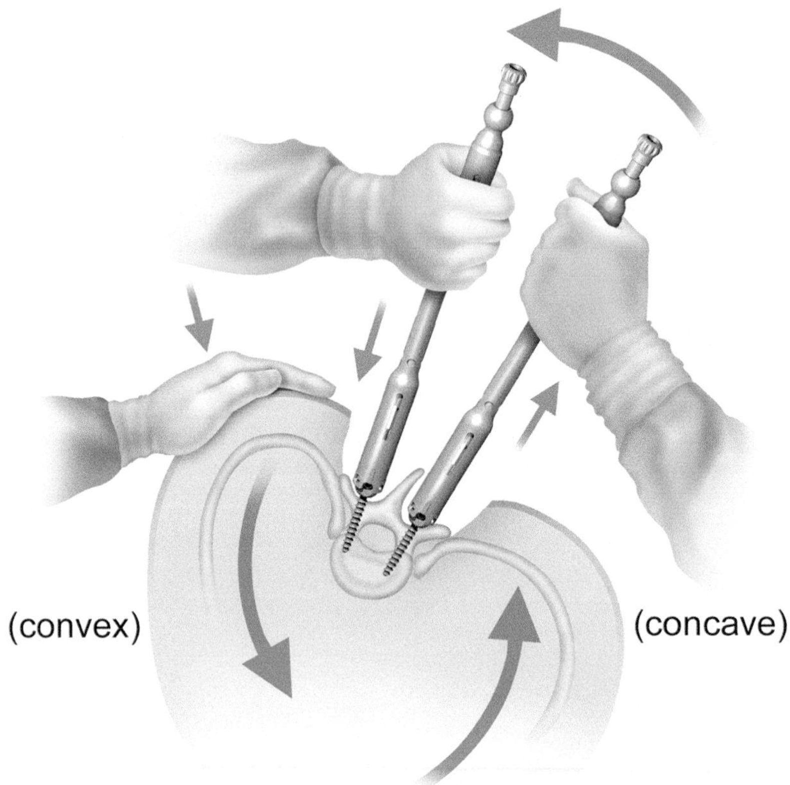


**Fig. 14.7** Axial view of the spinal-derotation concept: The screws on the concavity are pulled up and over, the screws on the convexity are pushed down and laterally from midline, and an assistant pushes down on the convex rib prominence to distribute forces. (From James Millerick, ©2006 DePuy Spine, Inc., used with permission.)

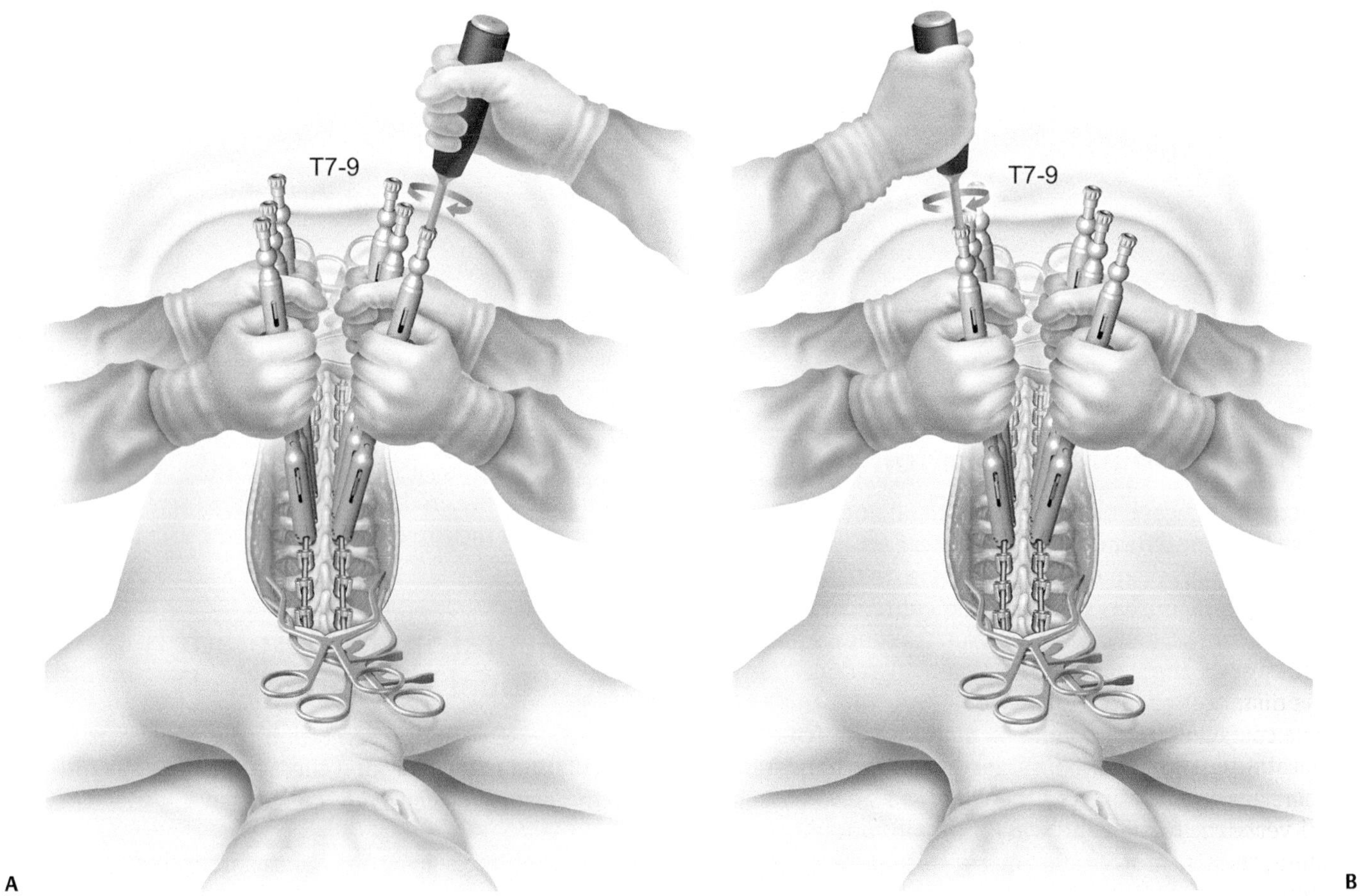


**Fig. 14.8** **(A)** En bloc derotation with concave rod implanted and set screws tightened. **(B)** The convex rod is then implanted and rotated, and is held in the corrected position while the set screws are tightened. (From James Millerick, ©2006 DePuy Spine, Inc., used with permission.)

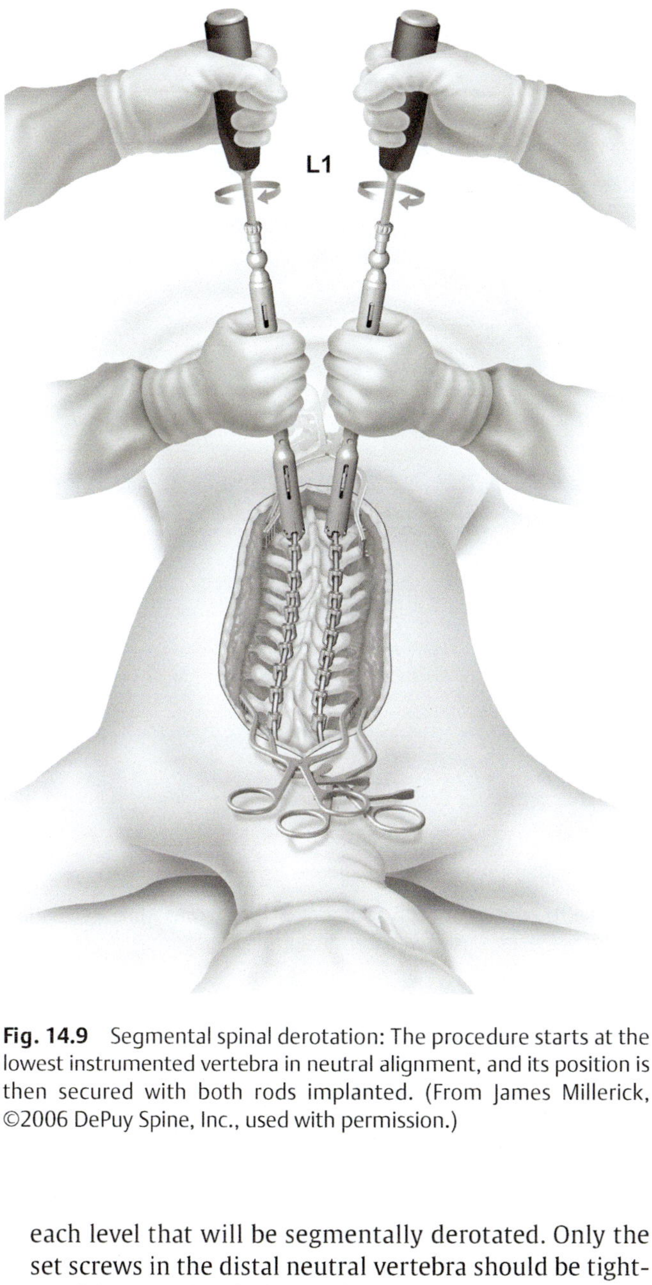


**Fig. 14.9** Segmental spinal derotation: The procedure starts at the lowest instrumented vertebra in neutral alignment, and its position is then secured with both rods implanted. (From James Millerick, ©2006 DePuy Spine, Inc., used with permission.)

each level that will be segmentally derotated. Only the set screws in the distal neutral vertebra should be tightened (e.g., L1 in **Fig. 14.9**), because derotation will be based on this neutral level and no torsional forces will be transmitted distally.

- Attach two derotators in the distal segment to lock the bottom neutral vertebra. Then attach derotators in the next proximal one or two vertebrae. The derotators on the distal vertebra must be held by an assistant to provide counter-rotation force.
- Derotate each proximal vertebral body sequentially to achieve a neutral position in reference to the neutral distal vertebra (**Fig. 14.10**). After derotation of each segment, the set screws are tightened. Repeat this process, moving along toward the apex of the curve. Complete neutral derotation might not be achieved at the apex relative to its torsion toward the axial plane. Revisiting the apical levels after a few minutes may allow additional correction owing to viscoelastic relaxation of the spine. Care must be taken not to loosen the bone–screw interface while performing the maneuver.
- Repeat the derotation for each segment until all vertebral levels nearly match the neutrally rotated distal vertebra. During segmental spinal derotation, segmental compression (convexity), distraction (concavity), or both may be applied simultaneously to effect maximal correction, just before the set screws are finally tightened.

## The Author's Preferred Technique for Reducing Spinal Deformity

For typical right-convex hypokyphotic scoliosis of late onset (**Fig. 14.1**), the author uses a 5.5-mm SS system and inserts bilateral segmental pedicle screws, most of which are uniplanar screws. In the periapical vertebra, polyaxial reduction screws are placed for larger deformities. On the convex side of the thoracic curve, uniplanar screws are placed at every level. The concave rod, which is overbent in kyphosis to affect the sagittal plane (technique 7, above) is placed and a rod derotation is performed to align the rod in the proper sagittal plane (technique 2, above). Because of the use of periapical reduction screws, this maneuver does not typically produce significant correction. Coronal translation is achieved as described above using reduction screws (technique 4, above). If this maneuver results in rod deformation, corrective coronal and sagittal in-situ contouring is performed (technique 3, above). Next, gentle compression and distraction are applied to further reduce the deformity by lengthening of the curve concavity and shortening of the convexity (technique 1, above); this will result in some establishment of thoracic kyphosis as well. En bloc vertebral derotation is then performed (technique 5, above). If additional derotation is necessary, direct vertebral-body derotation is performed (technique 6, above) and usually revisited after both rods are implanted and sufficient time for creep and viscoelastic relaxation has passed. If any residual apical rotation persists after this maneuver has been applied differential rod contouring is used during placement of the convex rod (technique 7, above). During this maneuver the concave periapical screws must be loosely applied to the rod to allow derotation of the apical vertebra around the concave rod. The derotation force results from a posterior-to-anterior cantilever force that is applied as the hypokyphotic convex rod is being seated into the apical screws at the convex apical kyphosis. Once both rods are in place, a final round of compression and distraction is applied to finely adjust the segmental correction (technique 1, above) and to horizontalize the upper and lower instrumented

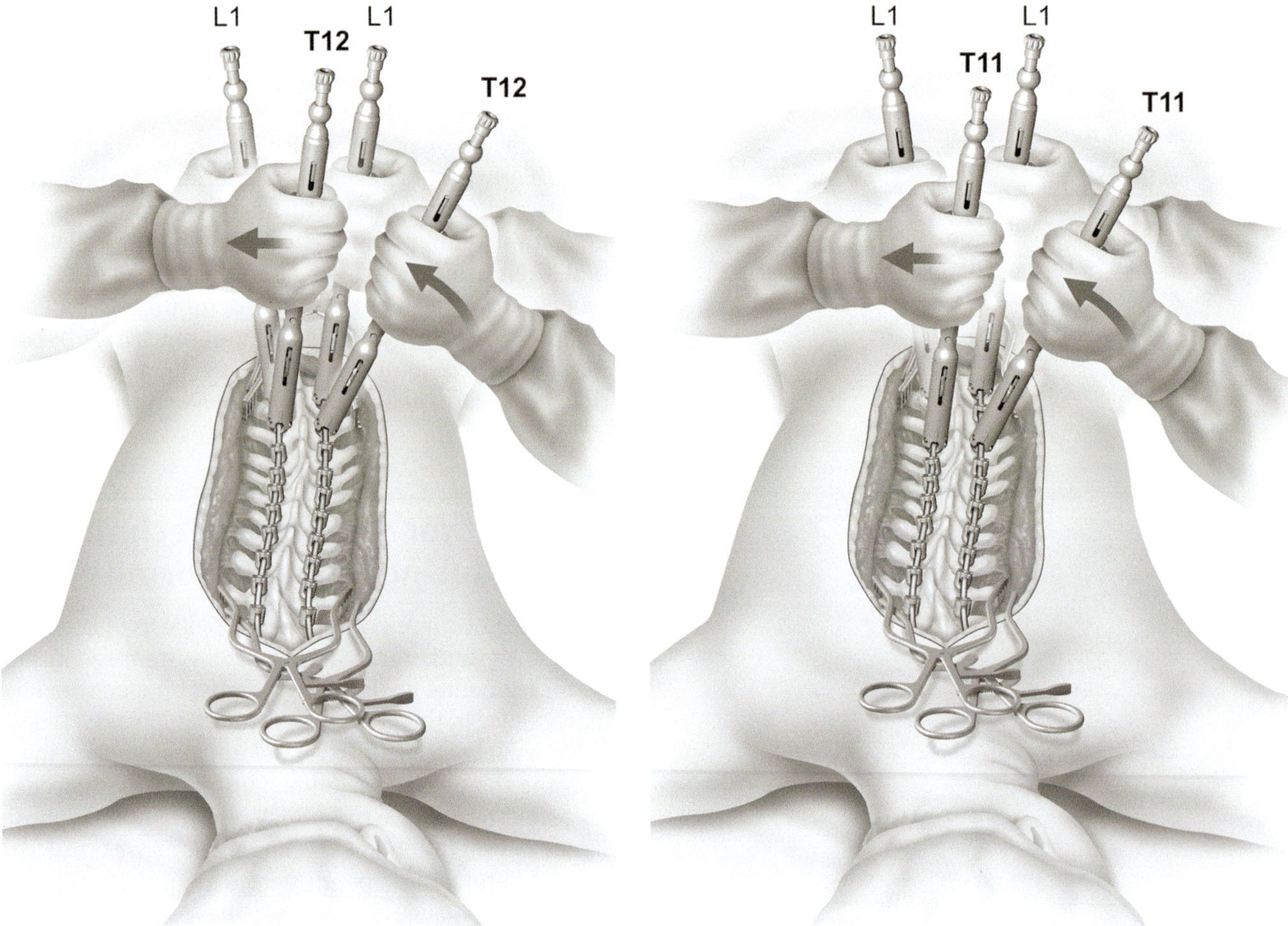


A B

**Fig. 14.10 (A,B)** Segmental spinal derotation: With the lowest instrumented vertebra held in countertorsion, derotators are used sequentially, proceeding cephalad and adjusting the axial-plane rotation relative to neutral at each segment. (From James Millerick, ©2006 DePuy Spine, Inc., used with permission.)

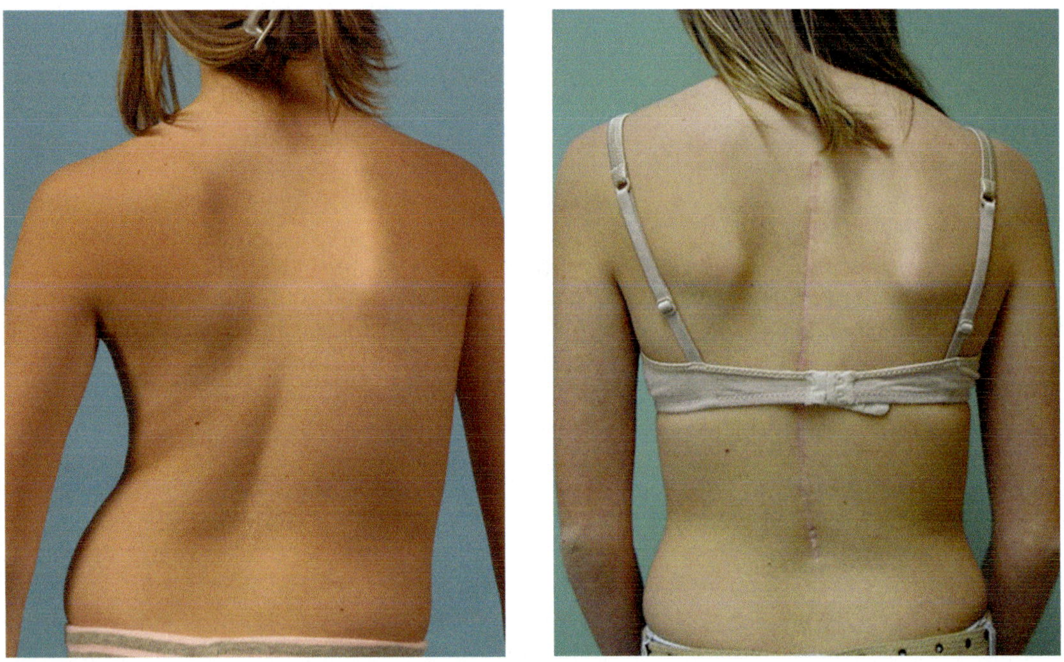

A B

**Fig. 14.11** Clinical photographs and radiographs pre- and postoperatively ( at 2-year follow-up) of a 13-year-old girl with AIS. Note the correction of truncal shift, thoracic torsion, rib asymmetry, and rib prominence on forward bending after surgery with segmental pedicle-screw fixation and vertebral derotation without thoracoplasty. **(A)** Preoperative clinical photograph. **(B)** Two-year postoperative clinical photograph.

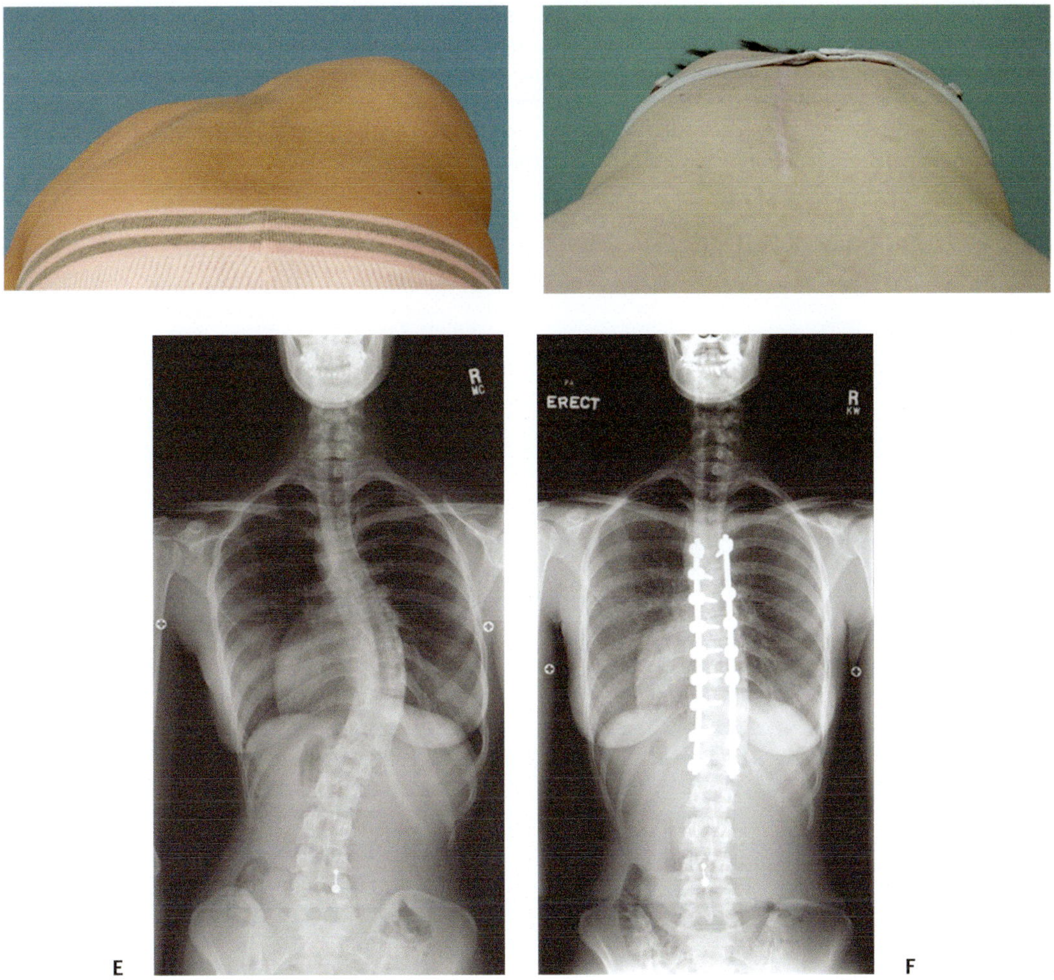


C D E F

**Fig. 14.11** *(Continued)* **(C)** Preoperative photograph of the patient in the forward-bend position. **(D)** Two-year postoperative of the patient in the forward-bend position. **(E)** Preoperative posteroanterior (PA) X-ray film. **(F)** Two-year postoperative PA X-ray film.

vertebral bodies, when this is desirable. Once all the instrumentation is in place, the alignment of the spine should be checked radiographically. Careful attention should be given to the end-instrumented segments to assess how they influence the alignment of the uninstrumented spine, particularly at the junction of instrumented and uninstrumented segments. This will help prevent unacceptable postoperative junctional rotation or tilt.

## Conclusion

Many techniques are available from which to select the design of a construct and correct a scoliotic deformity. Multiple methods can ultimately be chosen, and this will depend upon the requirements of the patient's deformity, the preference of the surgeon, and the available implants (**Fig. 14.11**).

## References


1. Wang JC, Sandhu HS, Yu WD, Minchew JT, Delamarter RB. MR parameters for imaging titanium spinal instrumentation. J Spinal Disord 1997;10:27–32
2. Soultanis KC, Pyrovolou N, Zahos KA, et al. Late postoperative infection following spinal instrumentation: Stainless steel versus titanium implants. J Surg Orthop Adv 2008;17:193–199
3. Kirkpatrick JS, Venugopalan R, Beck P, Lemons J. Corrosion on spinal implants. J Spinal Disord Tech 2005;18:247–251
4. Dubousset J, Cotrel Y. Application technique of Cotrel-Dubousset instrumentation for scoliosis deformities. Clin Orthop Relat Res 1991;264:103–110
5. Labelle H, Dansereau J, Bellefleur C, de Guise J, Rivard CH, Poitras B. Peroperative three-dimensional correction of idiopathic scoliosis with the Cotrel-Dubousset procedure. Spine 1995;20: 1406–1409

6. Lee SM, Suk SI, Chung ER. Direct vertebral rotation: A new technique of three-dimensional deformity correction with segmental pedicle screw fixation in adolescent idiopathic scoliosis. Spine 2004;29:343–349
7. Kuklo TR, Potter BK, Polly DW Jr, Lenke LG. Monaxial versus multiaxial thoracic pedicle screws in the correction of adolescent idiopathic scoliosis. Spine 2005;30:2113–2120
8. Parent S, Labelle H, Skalli W, Latimer B, de Guise J. Morphometric analysis of anatomic scoliotic specimens. Spine 2002;27: 2305–2311
9. Kothe R, O'Holleran JD, Liu W, Panjabi MM. Internal architecture of the thoracic pedicle. An anatomic study. Spine 1996;21:264–270
10. King A. Derotation of the thoracic spine using pedicle screws, a comparison of concave to convex screws. Paper presented at: 39th Annual Meeting of the Scoliosis Research Society, Buenos Aires, Argentina, 2004
11. Shah SA. Derotation of the spine. Neurosurg Clin North Am 2007; 18:339–345
12. Sponseller PD, Takenaga RK, Newton PO, et al. The use of traction in the treatment of severe spinal deformity. Spine 2008;33:2305–2309

# 15 The Use of Traction in Treating Large Scoliotic Curves in Idiopathic Scoliosis

*Paul D. Sponseller and Ryan Takenaga*

Large or rigid spinal deformities are challenging to correct safely, and their rapid or extensive correction can increase the risk of neurological compromise.[1] Additionally, instrumentation anchor sites may fail when extreme corrective forces are applied to achieve correction of such deformities.[2] Methods of traction have been devised to more slowly and completely correct severe deformities. A primary benefit of traction is that correction of a severe curve is done gradually so that less demand is put on the bone–anchor interface when instrumentation is applied to the curve. Also, except for periods of sleep, the patient is awake while in halo-gravity traction, which allows rapid and easy neurological monitoring. External and internal traction are two types of traction available in the surgeons' armamentarium.

## ■ External Traction

### Halo-Femoral Traction

External traction is applied by affixing to the patient's head a halo and effecting countertraction through a device extending from the halo and affixed to the femur, tibia, or pelvis, or by using the patient's body weight to provide the countertractive force (halo-gravity traction). The literature contains reports of the use of these methods in series of patients without untreated controls. In general, more significant corrective forces are generated by halo-femoral and halo-tibial traction than by halo-gravity traction.

Originally described by Kan and colleagues,[3] halo-femoral traction is one form of gaining control of severe curves in neuromuscular and idiopathic scoliosis. In their 1967 study, Kan and colleagues described achieving correction through halo-femoral traction over a period of 2 to 6 weeks and then maintaining the correction with casting, bracing, fusion, or instrumented fusion. The average correction they achieved was 48% (preoperative average curve of 112 degrees corrected to an average of 58 degrees). All complications were transient, but included paresthesias, hypertension, and an abducent nerve palsy.[3] There have been a few more modern studies of the efficacy of halo-femoral traction. Mehlman et al studied 24 patients who had halo-femoral traction with a pretraction spinal release and post-traction posterior fusion.[4] Eleven of these patients had idiopathic scoliosis with an average preprocedure curve of 85 degrees; these 11 patients had a 55% curve correction after release and traction and a 67% curve correction after fusion. Only one of Mehlman and colleagues' 24 patients experienced an adverse event in the form of a transient, bilateral lower-extremity sensory deficit, which resolved with reduction of the traction weight. Qiu and colleagues described a series of 30 patients with idiopathic scoliosis who underwent halo-femoral traction before posterior instrumented fusion. In a group in which the average coronal deformity was 91 degrees, Qiu et al noted an average 58% correction after fusion, as well as an average 33% correction of thoracic kyphosis. Transient brachial plexus palsy was seen in 10% of the patients.[5] Other complications associated with halo-femoral traction are pin-site infections, triceps palsy, deep vein thromboses, and hip dislocation.[1,6]

### Halo-Pelvic Traction

Halo-pelvic traction has the benefit of allowing more direct tension to be applied to the spine without crossing the hip joint; however, the constant, high level of traction in this technique is associated with several complications. In the initial description by O'Brien and coworkers in 1971, halo-pelvic traction was used primarily for patients with severe spinal deformities of neuromuscular or tuberculous pathology.[7] Ransford and Manning described a series of 114 patients treated with halo-pelvic traction that included 72 patients with infantile, juvenile, and adolescent idiopathic scoliosis (AIS). An average correction of 55% was achieved; however, the treatment course was long, with 4 to 6 weeks in traction and 3 months of bed rest following fusion, and was fraught with complications including pin-site problems, cranial-nerve palsies, and spinal-cord paraplegia.[8] Despite the powerful correction effected by this method, the prevalence of complications has driven halo-pelvic traction out of favor. Wilkins and MacEwen noted cranial nerve palsy in 6 of 70 patients treated with halo-femoral or halo-pelvic traction.[9] The abducent nerve was the most commonly affected, with involvement of the glossopharyngeal, hypoglossal, and vagus nerves being less common. Other complications of halo-pelvic traction are avascular necrosis of the tip of the dens, peritoneal penetration or intestinal perforation by traction pins, and hip dislocation.[10,11]

## Halo-Gravity Traction

In contrast to halo-femoral and halo-pelvic traction, halo-gravity traction appears to be a simpler and safer method to correct severe scoliotic curves. This method, which was popularized by Stagnara, uses the weight of the patient's body as the counterforce.[12] Correction occurs in the frontal and sagittal planes, and truncal decompensation improves. In addition, in contrast to the case with halo-femoral traction, which requires prolonged bed rest, the forces in halo-gravity traction can be applied while a patient is in bed, a wheelchair, or a walking frame. Contraindications to halo traction include cervical kyphosis or stenosis, significant instability, or ligamentous laxity. A few case series have investigated the success of halo-gravity traction in correcting severe scoliotic curves. Rinella and coworkers conducted a retrospective analysis of 33 patients with severe scoliosis, kyphoscoliosis, or kyphosis.[1] Four of the 33 patients had idiopathic scoliosis, and in these patients the main coronal curve ranged from 84 to 131 degrees with a mean of 101 degrees. In the patients with idiopathic scoliosis, traction resulted in an average 54% decrease in the main coronal curve. The only complication associated with the four cases of idiopathic scoliosis was rod migration.

Sink et al conducted a retrospective review of 19 children with severe scoliosis who underwent spinal fusion surgery after 6 to 21 weeks of preoperative halo-gravity traction.[2] Only 4 of the 19 patients had idiopathic scoliosis. Preoperative traction lasted from 14 to 18 weeks and postoperative traction ranged from 0 to 4 weeks. One patient had posterior spinal fusion complemented by traction, which yielded a 22% decrease (from 97 to 76 degrees) in the main coronal curve immediately after traction and a 26% decrease (from 97 to 72 degrees) after fusion. Three patients had anterior and posterior spinal fusion complemented by traction. This resulted in an average decrease in the main coronal curve of 43% immediately after traction and of 51% after fusion. Although halo-gravity traction is primarily used for neuromuscular scoliosis, Sink and colleagues' study described it as an effective method of correcting rigid idiopathic scoliosis. Seller et al conducted one of the few studies done of the safety and efficacy of halo traction with a comparison control group; however, the patients in this study had neuromuscular spinal deformities.[13] In the group not treated with halo traction the main Cobb angle decreased by an average of 57% (from 77 to 33 degrees). In the halo-traction group the average decrease in the main Cobb angle was 61% (from 85 to 33 degrees). The difference was not significant ($P = 0.19$), and Seiler and colleagues herefore concluded that unless there are specific indications for halo traction, it is not needed as a standard procedure in treating neuromuscular deformities.

Although halo-gravity traction is not without complications, it has a lower incidence of neurological complications. Sink et al[2] reported a 30% complication rate, which came mainly from pin loosening and pin-site infections, but also a case of cervical paresthesia in a child with Klippel–Feil syndrome. Rinella and colleagues[1] reported pin loosening, pin-site infection, nausea, nystagmus, cervical discomfort, and trapezial soreness as complications and symptoms associated with halo-gravity treatment. In a study of 300 cases of halo-gravity and halo-femoral traction combined with posterior fusion of severe scoliosis, Qian and coworkers described three cases of treatment with halo-gravity traction in which brachial-plexus palsy lasting up to 3 months was discovered.[14] A temporary hypoglossal nerve injury with halo-gravity traction, manifested as difficulty in swallowing, difficulty in speaking, or protrusion of the tongue has been reported.[15] Although halo-gravity traction is a powerful tool in the treatment of rigid scoliosis, its associated risks and discomforts should be discussed thoroughly with the patient and patient's family before treatment is begun.

### Technique of Halo-Gravity Traction

In the authors' experience, patients with unusually stiff curves (bony apical fusions or flexibility of <20% on radiographs made during traction), pretraction release can be a useful adjunct in allowing traction to correct extraspinal tissue contractures. Most patients, however, begin traction without a release, which probably results in the lowest risk of eventual infection. Usually, the halo is applied with sedation and local anesthesia. Six to eight pins are used in children under the age of 6 years, to minimize the risk of loosening of the halo. The pins are tightened to 4 inch-pounds of torque in children under 6 years of age, or to 6 to 8 inch-pounds for older children or adults (assuming normal cranial bone density). The halo is placed just below the equator of the skull, above the eyebrows and the pinnae of the ears. The anterior pins are placed laterally to the mid-portion of the eyebrows to avoid the supra-orbital nerves. Every effort is made to place the posterior pins diametrically opposite the anterior pins. After 24 to 48 hours the pins may be retightened. If there is clinical indication of loosening after this, the pin should be relocated. Traction is started immediately with 5 lbs of weight for young children and 10 lbs for those closer to maturity. The traction weight is gradually increased by 2 to 3 lbs/day as tolerated, with the goal being a weight of 33 to 50% of the patient's body weight. The bed is inclined downward caudally. The patient's skin should be inspected regularly, because bony prominences are common in this patient population and pressure sores are a risk. This is especially true of patients who have significant kyphosis or who have difficulty in turning over. The traction is applied continuously throughout the day. Patients should be in an upright position in a halo wheelchair or walker during part of the day. For a patient sitting in a wheelchair, the goal is to suspend the patient's

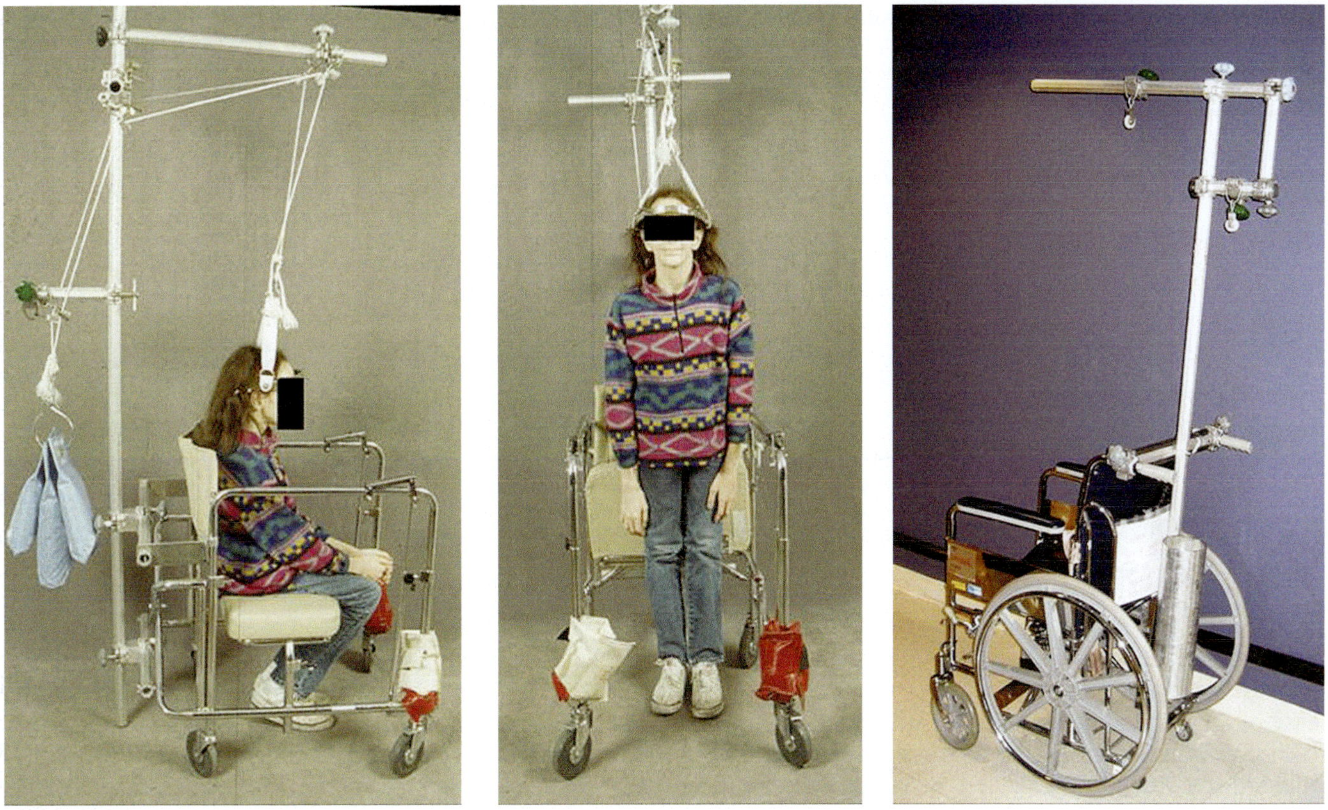
A–C

**Fig. 15.1** **(A,B)** Halo walker and **(C)** halo wheelchair. (**[A,B]** Courtesy of Kathy Blanke and Larry Lenke.)

trunk as much as possible (**Fig. 15.1**). Traction may also be applied while the patient is standing in a specially constructed walker. The traction weight may be decreased when the patient is sleeping, especially when the weight nears its maximum.

Given the various forces involved, traction has different implications according to the body's position. Neurological assessments of the patient's upper and lower extremities are done three times per day and cranial nerve function is checked daily. The duration of preoperative halo-gravity traction may vary from 2 to 12 weeks depending on the magnitude of the patient's curve, its response to traction, and the patient's overall medical condition. Radiographs should be obtained approximately every week for assessing the improvement in the patient's spinal curve. Patients with borderline pulmonary or nutritional reserve may benefit from long periods of traction to optimize their nutrition and minimize their pulmonary restrictive defect.

## A Multicenter Retrospective Case–Control Study of Halo-Gravity Traction in Adolescent Idiopathic Scoliosis

On the basis of the studies described above, it appears that halo-gravity traction is a safe, well-tolerated method of applying gradual, sustained traction to maximize postoperative spinal-curve correction in patients with severe scoliosis and kyphosis. However, these studies have primarily involved patients with neuromuscular and congenital scoliosis and only a relatively small number of patients with idiopathic scoliosis. and only one of the studies had a comparison control group. Because of the limitations of these studies, the Harms Study Group (HSG) conducted a multicenter, retrospective, nonrandomized comparison-group study. The primary goal of the study was to compare the surgical correction of large scoliotic curves in patients with idiopathic scoliosis with and without traction. The HSG collected retrospective data at the group's nine study sites.

### *Methods*

The halo-traction group had large rigid curves that were selected by the operating surgeon for a period of traction. Patients in the control group, who were operated on without a period of traction, were included if they had a main coronal curve of >100 degrees, their sagittal curve was >120 degrees, or their curve flexibility was <25%. The etiology of the spinal deformity in every patient was idiopathic scoliosis, and all of the patients had a minimum of 2 years of follow-up. Four types of data were collected: demographic, perioperative and operative, postoperative, and radiographic.

**Table 15.1 Characteristics of Patients with Adolescent Idiopathic Scoliosis***

| Patient Characteristic | Traction Group (*n* = 15) | Control Group (*n* = 8) | *P*-value |
|---|---|---|---|
| Age at time of surgery, years (SD) | 14 (2) | 15 (2) | 0.583 |
| Weight, kg (SD) | 43 (9) | 41 (6) | 0.635 |
| Height, cm (SD) | 154 (10) | 152 (11) | 0.664 |
| Pretreatment curves, degrees (SD) | | | |
| Main coronal curve | 97 (19) | 93 (12) | 0.536 |
| Compensatory curve | 58 (18) | 61 (17) | 0.705 |
| Kyphotic curve | 50 (26) | 42 (21) | 0.491 |
| Mean flexibility, % (SD) | 19 (14) | 20 (9) | 0.825 |
| Spinal length, cm (SD) | 37 (5) | 38 (3) | 0.643 |

*$n = 23$

### Results

Twenty-nine patients with idiopathic scoliosis were studied. Of these patients, two had scoliosis of infantile onset, four had disease of juvenile onset, and the remaining 23 had disease of adolescent onset. Fifteen of the patients received halo-gravity traction (Tx group) and 8 did not, and constituted the control group. Patient demographics were similar in the two groups. The mean ages at surgery in the treatment and control groups were 14 and 15 years, respectively (**Table 15.1**). The mean weight and height of the treatment group were 43 kg and 154 cm, respectively, and for the control group were 41 kg and 152 cm, respectively. The average pretreatment magnitudes of curvature in the treatment and control groups were 97 and 93 degrees for the main curve, 58 and 61 degrees for the compensatory curve, and 50 and 42 degrees for the kyphotic curve, respectively. The traction and control groups had mean curve flexibilities of 19% and 20%, respectively. The two groups also had similar spinal lengths (37 cm vs. 38 cm, respectively). However, the group that underwent traction tended to have a longer average hospital stay, at 41 versus 21 days (nonsignificant difference: $P = 0.2$), and also tended to have shorter operative times (405 minutes vs. 496 minutes) and less blood loss (2057 mL vs. 2975 mL). At 2 years postoperatively, there were statistically insignificant differences in the mean curve corrections in the two groups (**Table 15.2**).

The mean percent correction of the main coronal curve was 64% in the halo-traction group and 61% in the control group (**Figs. 15.2, 15.3**). Scoliotic kyphosis decreased by 3 degrees in the treatment group and 22 degrees in the control group. The control group showed better improvement of the coronal compensatory curve. The mean percent correction was 56% in the control group but only 17% in the treatment group. The unusually low percent correction and high standard deviation of the compensatory curve in the traction group was the result of a patient whose compensatory curve actually increased, from 11 degrees to 52 degrees. If this outlier is excluded, the percent correction and standard deviation for the compensatory curve would be 59% and 24%, respectively. Overall, these

**Table 15.2 Operative and Postoperative Data for Patients with Adolescent Idiopathic Scoliosis***

| Patient Characteristic | Traction Group (*n* = 15) | Control Group (*n* = 8) | *P*-value |
|---|---|---|---|
| *2-Year postoperative mean correction* | | | |
| Main coronal curve, % (SD) | 64 (19) | 61 (14) | 0.725 |
| Compensatory curve, % (SD) | 17 (100) | 56 (24) | 0.451 |
| Kyphosis curve (post- vs. preoperative) | −3 (12) | −22 (23) | 0.260 |
| Operative time, minutes (SD) | 405 (160) | 496 (104) | 0.220 |
| Surgical blood loss, mL (SD) | 2057 (1981) | 2975 (2526) | 0.346 |
| Average hospital stay, days (SD) | 41 (35) | 21 (38) | 0.212 |
| Vertebral-column resection, % | 0 | 25 | 0.043 |

*$n = 23$

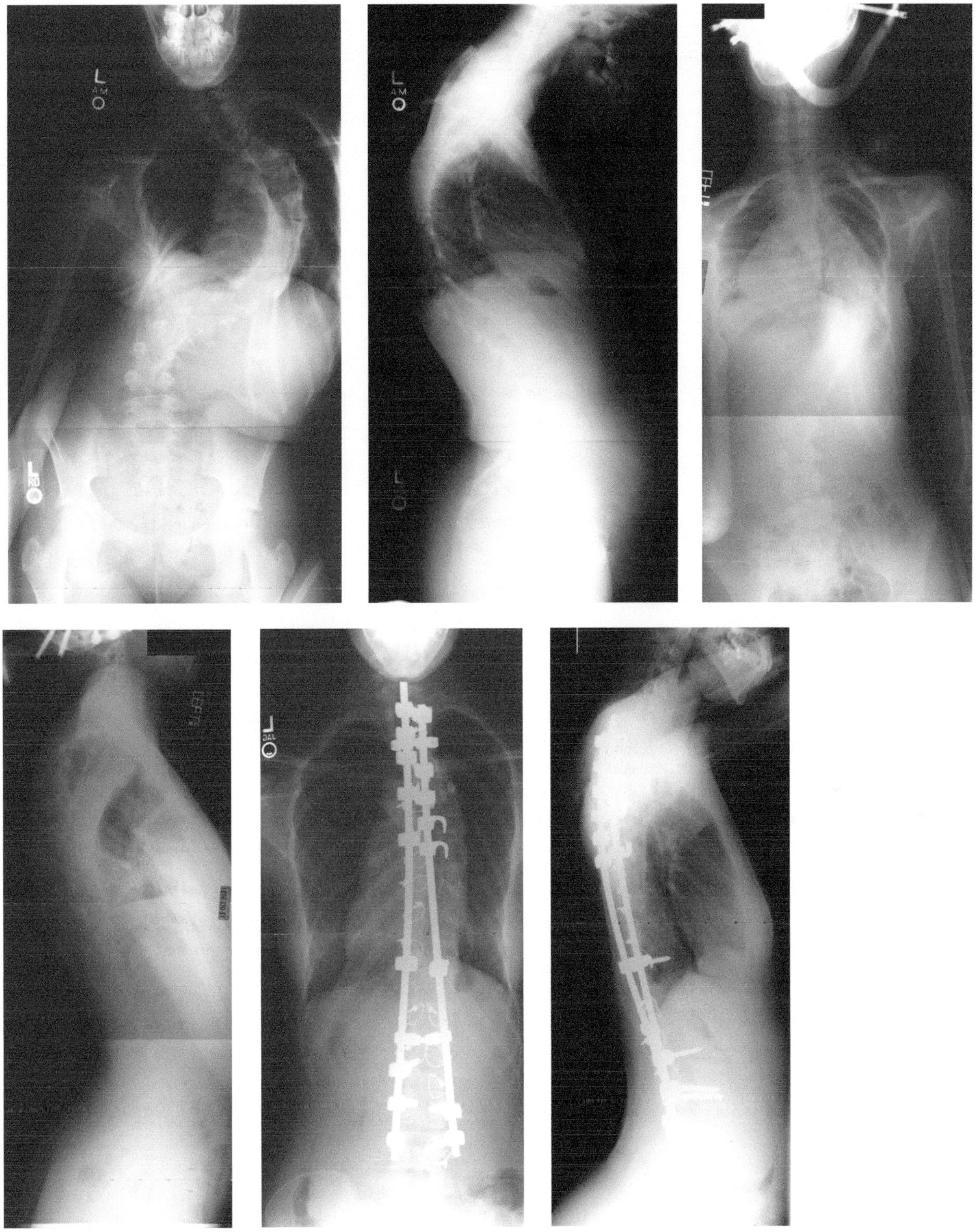

A–C

D–F

**Fig. 15.2** Severe Idiopathic scoliosis in an 11+2-year-old girl. **(A,B)** (The patient's preoperative scoliosis was 125 degrees and her preoperative kyphosis was 75 degrees). The patient was treated with anterior release and 1 week of traction, and her scoliosis decreased to 48 degrees; and kyphosis to 51 degrees. **(C,D)** Radiographs made at the patient's last follow-up visit at maturity, 3 years postoperatively. **(E,F)** The patient's scoliosis had been reduced to 20 degrees and her kyphosis to 40 degrees.

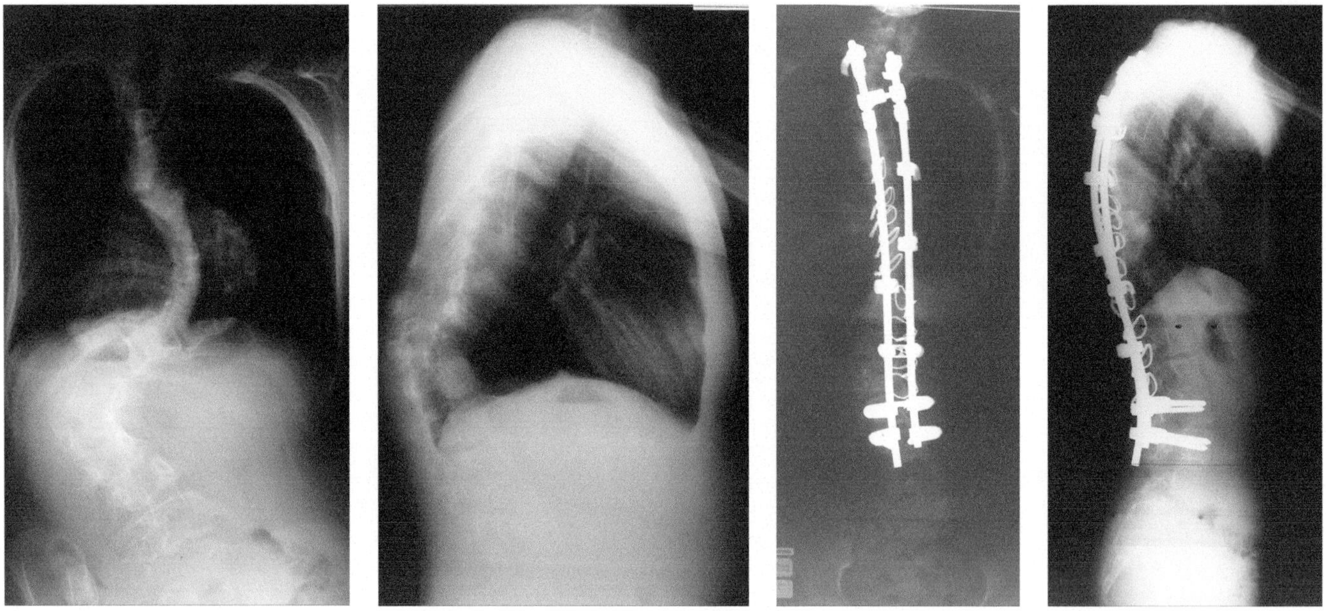

A–D

**Fig. 15.3** A 12-year-old girl with 111-degree idiopathic double curves **(A,B)** treated without traction. She underwent a one-stage anterior release and posterior fusion. **(C,D)** Follow-up at 2.5 years revealed 35- and 38-degres curves and a 49-degree kyphosis.

slight differences in operative and radiographic data for the halo-traction as compared with the nontraction control group were not statistically significant. However, during the surgery for scoliosis, vertebral-column resection was more commonly performed in the control (25%) than in the treatment (0%) group, and this difference was statistically significant ($P = 0.04$).

Complications occurred in 27% of the halo-traction group and 25% of the control group, and the difference was not statistically significant (**Table 15.3**). Each group had one instance of an intraoperative respiratory complication. The halo-traction group also had one instance of an intraoperative instrumentation complication and one instance of an ischial pressure sore. Additionally, a dural tear occurred in one of the patients in the traction group and dilutional coagulopathy in a patient in the control group. At 2 years postoperatively the halo-traction group had had one case of reoperation requiring four rib excisions and revision of a

**Table 15.3 Complications in Halo-traction and Control Groups of Patients with Adolescent Idiopathic Scoliosis***

| Complication | Traction Group ($n = 15$) | Control Group ($n = 8$) | $P$-value |
|---|---|---|---|
| Intraoperative | | | |
| Respiratory | 1 | 1 | |
| Instrumentation | 1 | 0 | |
| Other | 1 | 1 | |
| Postoperative | | | |
| Ischial lesion | 1 | 0 | |
| Reoperation | 1 | 0 | |
| Total complications (%) | 33 | 25 | 0.68 |
| Complications causing neurological damage | 0 | 0 | |
| Complications causing reoperation | 1 | 0 | |

*$n = 23$

hypertrophic chest scar. No neurological complications were associated with the correction of idiopathic scoliosis in either group.

### *Discussion*

Axial traction is used with the goal of achieving safer and more effective correction of severe spinal deformities. The gradual increase in traction over a period of weeks allows partial correction of the large curvature and associated extraspinal contractures in such deformities, so that surgical correction is done on a less pronounced spinal deformity. Theoretically, this should allow better overall correction without the complications associated with one-stage surgical correction of large spinal curves.

Although the halo-gravity traction group in our study showed a trend toward shorter operative time, less blood loss, and improved correction of main coronal and sagittal kyphotic curves, none of these differences was statistically significant. The study was limited by the small sample size and by its retrospective nature. Yet given the rarity of the severe scoliotic curves in the study population, it is uncertain whether a controlled prospective study of halo-traction for such curvature can be done. In light of these limitations, the message of the study is that good results may be obtained with or without halo-gravity traction in the treatment of severe scoliotic curves in patients with AIS. The use of halo traction may permit the surgery to be completed with a reduced need for vertebral-column resection, which may be important for more medically challenged patients, such as those who are more frail or have a lower pulmonary reserve. On the other hand, if excessive distraction is needed to correct a curve to an acceptable level of balance, bone resection may be preferable to halo traction. The surgeon should use his or her own judgment about what will produce the best result for these severe curves on the basis of their flexibility and medical and technical factors.

## ■ Intraoperative Traction

Cranial traction also has a role in the operating room. This may be a continuation of preoperative traction or it may be applied only during the surgical procedure. In either case it helps to assure global body-pelvic alignment in large curves that include major pelvic obliquity or truncal shift. Such alignment is difficult to obtain and assess from the limited perspective of the surgical field. Intraoperative traction is useful for curves that exceed ~80 degrees. It bears repeating that the surgeon should image the patient's cervical spine before application of traction, and avoid traction in patients with cervical stenosis or instability. If the patient has a halo in place, traction can be applied through this. If there is no halo, we prefer to use Gardner–Wells tongs. Patients with osteogenesis imperfecta or Marfan syndrome, and others with abnormal bone density or dural enlargement, should be given a halo with more pins at lower torque.

The amount of weight used in itraoperative cranial traction should be 25 to 35% less than the maximum weight used when the patient is awake, to avoid overdistraction of the relaxed patient. Countertraction may be obtained by inclining the operating table (reverse Trendelenburg position) in cases of a proximal curve, or by traction through the lower extremities for distal curves. If lower-extremity traction is needed, we prefer to use traction tape over a single layer of soft roll, extending at least up to the knee (**Fig. 15.4**). Alternatively, a traction boot

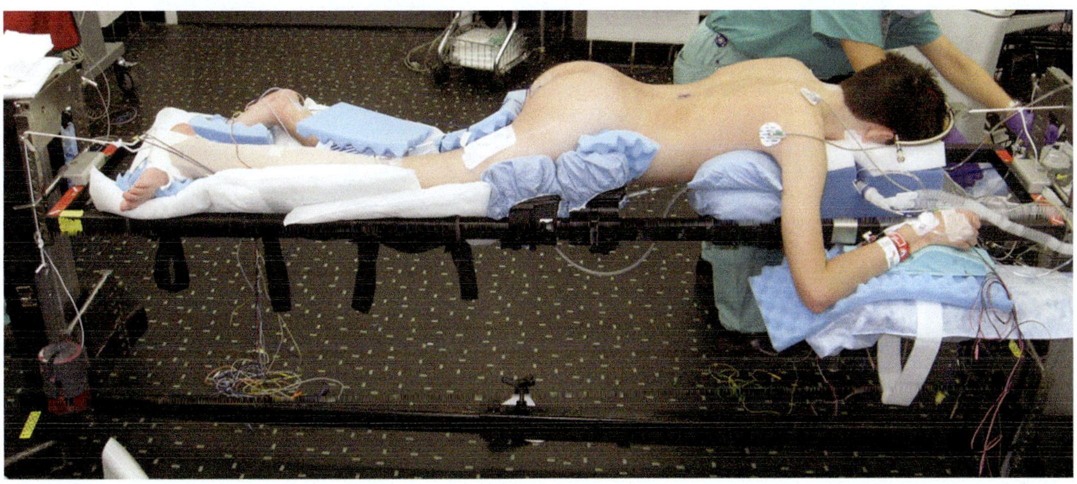

**Fig. 15.4** Intraoperative traction. Cranial traction is applied via Gardner–Wells or Mayfield tongs. The patient is positioned as straight as possible. Distally, skin traction is shown here applied to the "high" side, but femoral traction and bilateral traction are other options. Traction in the presence of flexion contractures may produce more lordosis.

may be used. This arrangement allows the use of 10 to 15 lbs of traction. In patients with pelvic obliquity, the counter traction may be applied just to the "high" side. If more force is desired, some surgeons have used skeletal traction through the distal femur. Lower extremity traction is less effective in the presence of hip or knee flexion contractures, and may impart unwanted lordosis.

The surgeon should be sure that the position of the patient's head and face is re-checked once the final traction system is in place. It is also important to ensure that the traction rope rides freely and easily over the pulley(s) in the system. The spinal cord should be monitored from the time of initial positioning of the patient onward. The traction may be discontinued when the instrumented spinal correction is maintained.

## ■ Temporary Internal Distraction

Temporary internal distraction has emerged as an alternative to external traction. It consists of inserting temporary internal rods to provide maximal longitudinal distraction over the area of greatest deformity. Absolute indications for this technique include patients for whom cervical traction is contraindicated, such as those with cervical deformity, laxity, or instability. Relative indications for temporary internal distraction include lumbar deformity or patients for whom greater mobility is desired. The technique involves a posterior release over the rigid portion of the deformity curve and anchor placement near the intended upper and lower end-vertebrae of the curve. At least one pair of anchors is needed for each rod. If possible, placement of the anchors slightly short of the final end-vertebrae of fusion will preserve the sites for the final fusion. In the presence of spinal-cord monitoring, careful distraction of the deformation curve(s) is done to the limits of the surgeon's discretion, which usually exceed what is achieved in the preoperative films of the patient in traction. The anchors of the traction device are then locked and the incision closed. The patient may be mobilized and even discharged if desired. A second, final correction is scheduled for 1 to 3 weeks later (**Fig. 15.5**). At this stage the spine is noted to have significantly greater flexibility,

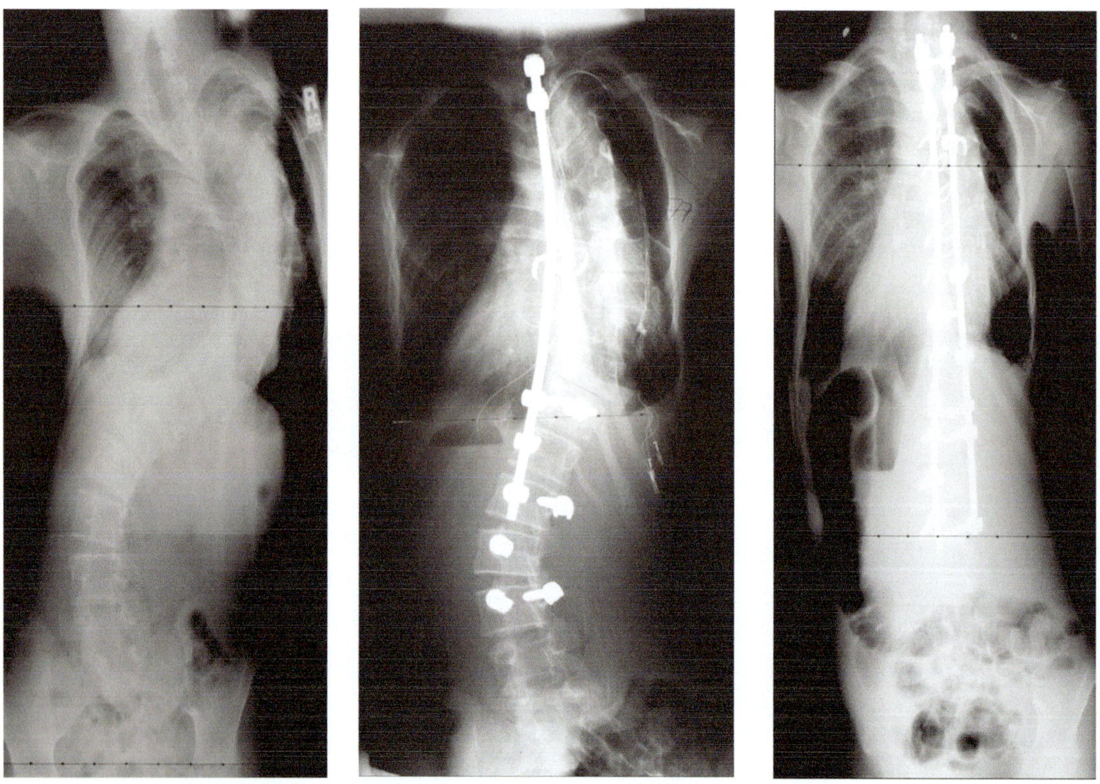

A–C

**Fig. 15.5** **(A)** A 131-degree idiopathic scoliosis in a 12-year-old boy, which decreased only to 107 degrees on bending. **(B)** Because of a forced vital capacity that was only 30% of predicted, the patient underwent a posterior release and temporary fixation with an internal rod. **(C)** This was followed 1 week later by definitive posterior fusion. The patient's final curve, 2 years later, was 30 degrees. (Courtesy of David Skaggs.)

and more correction may be obtained. Buchowski and colleagues described a series of 10 patients undergoing this procedure, 2 of whom were patients with AIS. These two patients attained 73% and 78% correction of their curves, respectively, which exceeded 100 degrees preoperatively. The authors reported only one instance of pneumothorax and no instances of infection. This approach may allow the benefits of perioperative traction with less time spent in the hospital. Further studies will be needed to analyze the efficacy and safety of temporary internal distraction as compared with external traction.[16]

## Conclusion

In summary, there are several options for using mechanical measures to assist in correcting severe scoliotic curves. Concerns in using these measures include minimizing neurological risk and blood loss while optimizing curve correction. Greater use of operative release and bone resection appears to reduce the need for traction, but with potentially more technically demanding surgeries. Precise knowledge of the patient's preoperative baseline status and high-quality intraoperative monitoring are essential. The surgeon should consider all of these factors in deciding whether or not to use traction.

### References

1. Rinella A, Lenke L, Whitaker C, et al. Perioperative halo-gravity traction in the treatment of severe scoliosis and kyphosis. Spine 2005;30:475–482
2. Sink EL, Karol LA, Sanders J, Birch JG, Johnston CE, Herring JA. Efficacy of perioperative halo-gravity traction in the treatment of severe scoliosis in children. J Pediatr Orthop 2001;21:519–524
3. Kane WJ, Moe JH, Lai CC. Halo-femoral pin distraction in the treatment of scoliosis. J Bone Joint Surg Am 1967;49:1018–1019
4. Mehlman CT, Al-Sayyad MJ, Crawford AH. Effectiveness of spinal release and halo-femoral traction in the management of severe spinal deformity. J Pediatr Orthop 2004;24:667–673
5. Qiu Y, Liu Z, Zhu F, et al. Comparison of effectiveness of Halo-femoral traction after anterior spinal release in severe idiopathic and congenital scoliosis: A retrospective study. J Orthop Surg 2007;2:23
6. Leslie IJ, Dorgan JC, Bentley G, Galloway RW. A prospective study of deep vein thrombosis of the leg in children on halo-femoral traction. J Bone Joint Surg Br 1981;63B:168–170
7. O'Brien JP, Yau AC, Smith TK, Hodgson AR. Halo pelvic traction. A preliminary report on a method of external skeletal fixation for correcting deformities and maintaining fixation of the spine. J Bone Joint Surg Br 1971;53:217–229
8. Ransford AO, Manning CW. Complications of halo-pelvic distraction for scoliosis. J Bone Joint Surg Br 1975;57:131–137
9. Wilkins C, MacEwen GD. Cranial nerve injury from halo traction. Clin Orthop Relat Res 1977;(126):106–110
10. Toledo LC, Toledo CH, MacEwen GD. Halo traction with the Circolectric bed in the treatment of severe spinal deformities: A preliminary report. J Pediatr Orthop 1982;2:554–559
11. Tredwell SJ, O'Brien JP. Avascular necrosis of the proximal end of the dens. A complication of halo-pelvic distraction. J Bone Joint Surg Am 1975;57:332–336
12. Stagnara P. [Cranial traction using the "Halo" of Rancho Los Amigos] Rev Chir Orthop Repar Appar Mot 1971;57:287–300
13. Seller K, Haas S, Raab P, Krauspe R, Wild A. [Preoperative halo-traction in severe paralytic scoliosis]. Z Orthop Ihre Grenzgeb 2005;143:539–543
14. Qian BP, Qiu Y, Wang B. Brachial plexus palsy associated with halo traction before posterior correction in severe scoliosis. Stud Health Technol Inform 2006;123:538–542
15. Ginsburg GM, Bassett GS. Hypoglossal nerve injury caused by halo-suspension traction. A case report. Spine 1998;23:1490–1493
16. Buchowski JM, Bhatnagar R, Skaggs DL, Sponseller PD. Temporary internal distraction as an aid to correction of severe scoliosis. J Bone Joint Surg Am 2006;88:2035–2041

# 16 The Treatment of Rigid Adolescent Idiopathic Scoliosis: Releases, Osteotomies, and Apical Vertebral Column Resection

*Lynn Letko, Rubens G. Jensen, and Jürgen Harms*

Rigid adolescent idiopathic scoliosis (AIS), defined as AIS showing less than 25% periapical correction on bending films, often requires more extensive surgical intervention than is otherwise needed to achieve the goals of scoliosis surgery. Adequate mobilization of this rigid deformity is necessary to achieve maximal correction, with care taken to avoid neurological complications. The number of vertebral levels fused in cases of complete correction of deformity with releases, osteotomies. or apical vertebral resection (AVR), alone or in combination, should be the same or fewer than in cases of incomplete correction. The sagittal profile should be restored and the end-instrumented vertebra (EIV) should be horizontal. Halo-gravity traction, various releases, osteotomies, and apical vertebral resection are often used in combination to achieve the desired results.

## Spinal-Column Releases

When inflexibility of a spinal curve is a limiting factor in the surgical correction of AIS, anterior or posterior releases or both can improve curve flexibility and allow greater correction with the possibility of fusing fewer motion segments of the spine. These releases are often a component of extensive surgeries, and require meticulous surgical planning that includes consideration of the curve location and degree of curvature, the sagittal and coronal balance, and the patient's overall medical condition and ability to tolerate such extensive surgery. Available techniques for releases and osteotomies include anterior, posterior, and combined approaches, which will be discussed individually.

### Anterior Release

Complete anterior release as performed in our institution is done through an open approach to the thoracic or lumbar spine or both, to allow improved mobilization of a curve and correction of sagittal and coronal deformities. In the thoracic spine, the convex rib heads are resected and an attempt is made to rupture the concave costovertebral joints. In both the thoracic and lumbar spine the disc and posterior annulus are removed, with release of the posterior longitudinal ligament. The convex inferior endplate is then resected with or without resection of the convex superior endplate. This allows mobilization and correction in the coronal plane. In addition, the sagittal profile of the thoracic spine, which is often hypokyphotic in thoracic AIS, can be corrected to its normal degree of kyphosis by essentially shortening the anterior column. Anterior structural support is often recommended in the lumbar spine and at the thoracolumbar junction to prevent the development of kyphosis. After complete anterior release, the patient may be instrumented anteriorly if the curve is not too large or rigid. Generally, thoracic curves of up to 70 degrees that have flexibility of >25% may be corrected well with anterior release and instrumentation. An additional posterior release with instrumentation may be required in more rigid deformities.

### Posterior Release

First described by Hibbs in 1924, the posterior facetectomy involves removal of the inferior articular process of the facet joint with curretage of the joint cartilage.[1] The technique has become a standard in posterior scoliosis surgery because it allows some increased mobility, facilitating curve correction while improving the fusion bed. Howarth, in 1943, added resection of intraspinous ligaments and spinous processes to this technique, further improving curve mobility and the amount of local bone available for fusion.[2]

## Posterior Osteotomies

Some spinal deformities involve bony changes that cannot be corrected through the release of soft tissue alone. Bone resection by means of osteotomies is necessary for improved correction. The type of osteotomy used depends on the amount of correction needed, the location of the deformity, the sagittal and coronal imbalance, and the patient's condition. Transverse osteotomies, including those of the Smith–Peterson and Ponte types, were originally designed to correct deformity in the sagittal plane. Pedicle subtraction osteotomy (PSO) is a sagittal-plane, closing-wedge osteotomy. Opening-wedge osteotomies are not recommended because of lengthening of the thecal sac and increased potential for neurological problems. Often used in combination with posterior spinal instrumentation, these surgeries require careful preparation and planning. The patient characteristics and the technical abilities of the surgeon need to be assessed realistically preoperatively. Collaboration with a multidisciplinary team including intensivists and anesthesiologists is essential for success with these difficult and often lengthy surgeries.

## Smith–Petersen Osteotomy

This osteotomy was described by Smith–Petersen and colleagues in 1945 for use in treating the deformity in lumbar flexion that can result from ankylosing spondylitis ("rheumatoid arthritis").[3,4] A modified posterior resection is now used in treating spinal deformity of many etiologies. Smith–Peterson osteotomies (SPOs) allow mobilization and correction primarily of deformities in the sagittal profile, but may be useful in obtaining coronal mobilization as well. The SPO procedure closes the posterior column, hinges on the middle column, and lengthens the anterior column of the spine. This results in a posterior shift of the gravity line, shortening the moment arm for posteriorly applied corrective forces. As originally described, the SPO required a fracture of the ankylosed anterior column. The modified SPO in common use today requires a mobile anterior column; the resultant lengthening of the anterior column may require anterior structural support.

The procedure in SPO produces a "V"-shaped osteotomy with the "V" directed caudally. The spine is exposed through a standard posterior approach. The spinous processes are resected. The ligamentum flavum is detached from the inferior margin of the lamina and the inferior articular process. An oblique osteotomy is made through the superior articular process of the caudal vertebra and inferior articular process of the cephalad vertebra, directed 45 degrees to the frontal plane. The intervening facet joint is excised. An extension or posterior compression force is applied gradually to the posterior elements to obtain correction. One millimeter of bone resection corresponds to roughly one degree of sagittal plane correction. From 5 to 15 degrees of sagittal-plane correction can be expected per osteotomy (**Fig. 16.1**). Although SPO is primarily used for sagittal-plane correction, coronal correction can be achieved with asymmetric osteotomies, especially when multiple SPOs are used. It has been noted by some that asymmetric PSOs may be more effectively used for this purpose.[5]

When applying the SPO to fixed coronal deformities, care must be taken to prevent worsening of the deformity. Intervertebral-body fusion by means of a transverse intervertebral

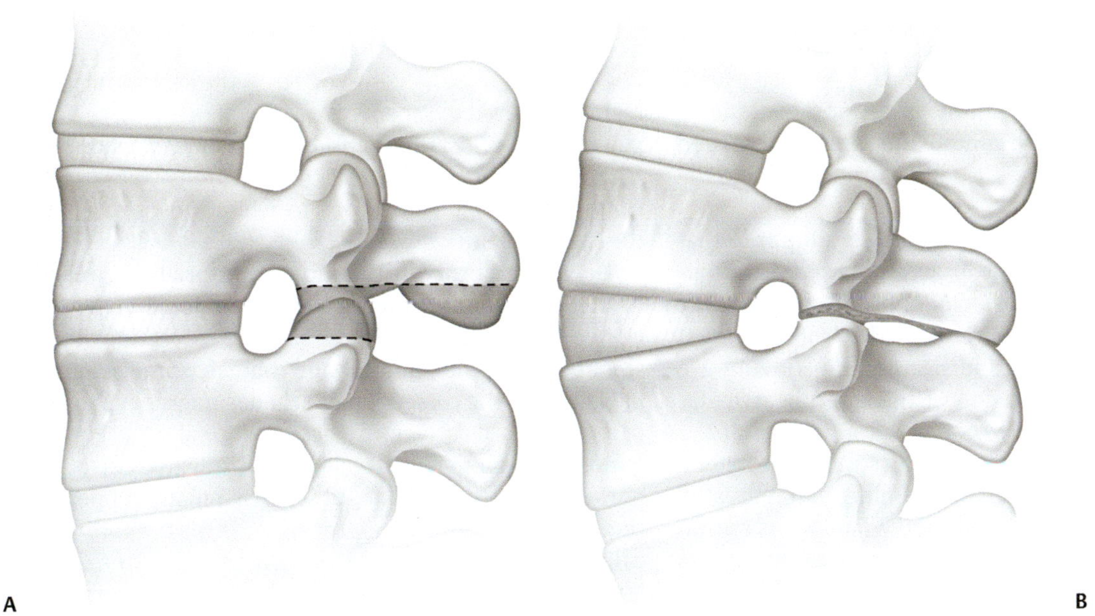


**Fig. 16.1** **(A)** Lateral view of the bone to be removed (highlighted) for an SPO. **(B)** The correction expected after closure of the SPO.

approach may be useful in correcting the deformity. Asymmetric placement of an interbody spacer may help in correcting a coronal deformity. By using the interbody spacer as a fulcrum, one may obtain the same amount (or more) of correction of a sagittal deformity with less neuroforaminal compromise.[6]

Reported complications of SPO include pseudarthrosis, which may result from creating a gap in the disc space. This alters the integrity of the anterior column, which bears 80 to 90% of the compressive forces on the spine in the standing position. Degeneration of adjacent segments has also been reported. Neurological complications can be significant, and have been reported in as many as 30% of patients undergoing SPO.[3,6] Radiculopathy may result from compression of nerve roots as they exit the foramina narrowed by closure of the SPO. Care must be taken to perform wide foraminotomies at the level of an SPO. Pedicle fractures may occur with overzealous compression during the closing of an SPO.

## Ponte Osteotomies

The osteotomy described by Alberto Ponte allows mobilization and correction of the sagittal profile.[7] It was initially described for use in the thoracic spine in cases in which no ankylosis exists, such as in Scheuermann's kyphosis and osteoporosis. In contrast to the originally described SPO, Ponte osteotomies are posterior shortening procedures associated with minimal lengthening of the anterior column of the spine. This is achieved through a generous posterior resection of the superior and inferior laminae as well as the facet joint. It has been suggested that the center of rotation moves anteriorly in Ponte osteotomies, lengthening the moment arm of the posterior corrective forces.[8] Because of the compression exerted on the middle column of the spine, it is also imperative to rule out the presence of disc herniation before using this purely posterior technique, to prevent possible spinal-cord compression from a herniated disc when posterior compressive forces are applied to the spine.

The technique of the Ponte osteotomy is similar to that of the modified SPO commonly utilized today, in that it initially involves a standard posterior approach to the spine and resection of the spinous processes. The soft tissues of the interspinous ligaments and ligamentum flavum are removed. The standard excision of the inferior articular process is complemented by removal of a portion of the superior articular process as well. Thus, at each level of a Ponte osteotomy, a 4- to 6-mm interlaminar gap is created (**Fig. 16.2**). Generous undercutting of the laminae is crucial to prevent spinal-cord compression when the resulting interlaminar gaps are closed by means of compression. Resection is performed laterally into the neural foramen (**Fig. 16.3**). Compression forces are applied across the

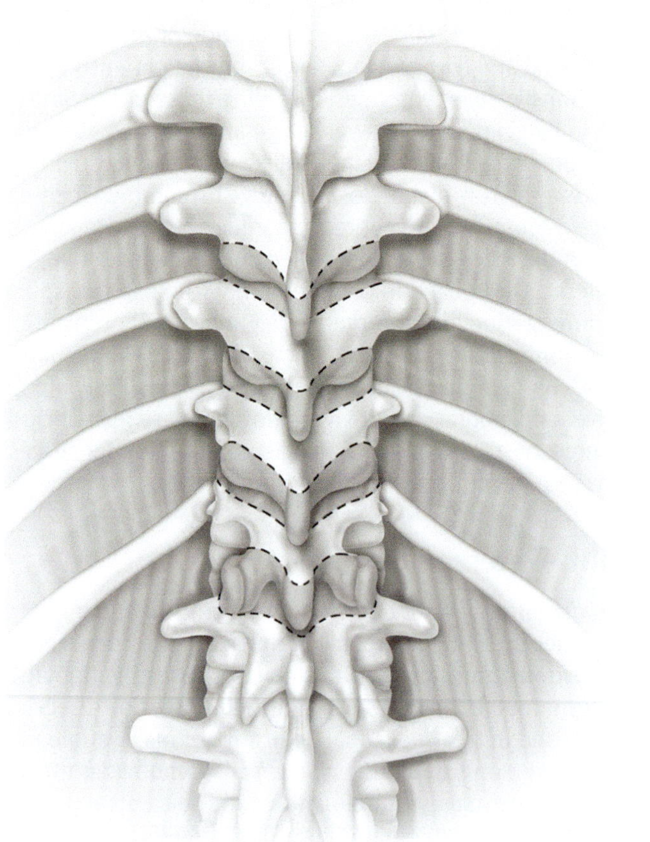

**Fig. 16.2** Outline of the structures (ligamentum flavum, inferior and superior articular processes, and spinous process) to be excised for a Ponte osteotomy.

instrumentation; segmental multiple compressions may be needed to obtain the desired correction (**Fig. 16.4**).

Geck and co-workers[9] reported on the sagittal-plane correction achieved in Scheuermann's kyphosis with segmental pedicle-screw instrumentation and Ponte osteotomies in 17 patients. No neurological complications were reported. However, care should be given to avoiding overcorrection in the sagittal plane.

Debate exists about the most appropriate terminology for the procedure involving complete release of the posterior vertebral elements in the surgical correction of a rigid spinal curve. When done in the thoracic spine over multiple levels for the correction of Scheuermann's kyphosis, the procedure is clearly most accurately called a Ponte osteotomy. When a single level, 30- to 45-degree correction is performed in the lumbar spine with a marked opening of the anterior column, the procedure is most appropriately called an SPO. Unfortunately, the terms are often used interchangeably for the often multilevel thoracic or lumbar excision of the inferior and superior articular processes as well as all intervertebral posterior soft tissues. These

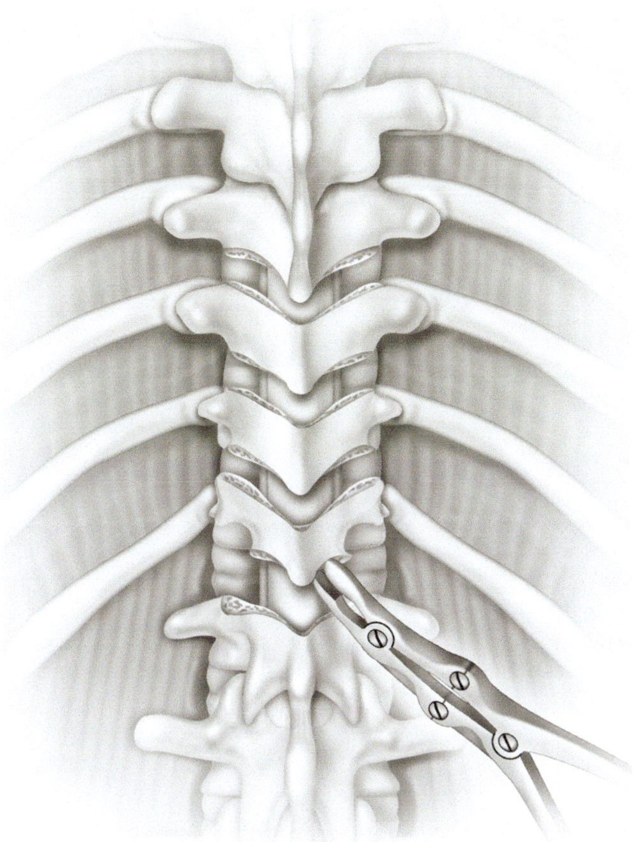

**Fig. 16.3** Technique for a multilevel Ponte osteotomy.

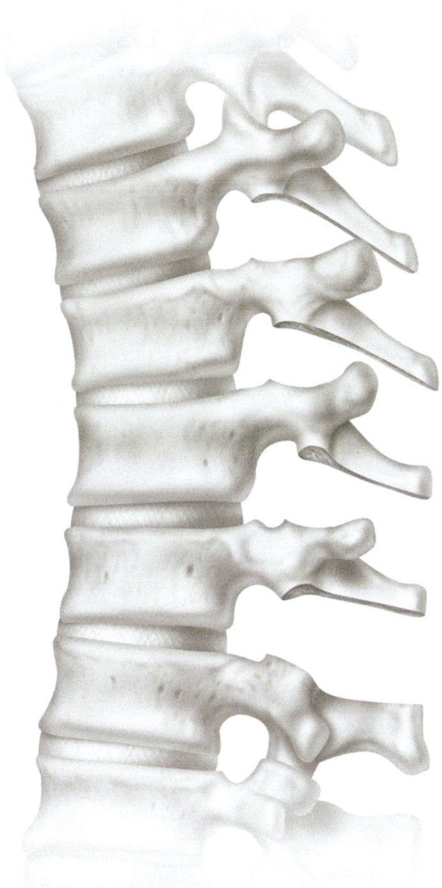

**Fig. 16.4** Defects left after a multilevel Ponte osteotomy. Closure of these defects allows for shortening of the posterior column and correction of the kyphosis.

releases may also be used for coronal-plane correction, for which they were not initially described.

## Pedicle Subtraction Osteotomy

The PSO originates from a technique first described by Michele and Krueger in 1949.[10] Also known as the eggshell procedure, it was originally developed as a purely posterior treatment for vertebral ostomyelitis. Over time, the technique has been modified to become a closing-wedge osteotomy. Use of a dorsally based wedge with symmetrical pedicle subtraction results in correction and mobilization of a deformity in the sagittal plane. Generally done in the lumbar spine, the PSO involves shortening of the middle and posterior columns, with the anterior longitudinal ligament acting as the hinge for realignment. Approximately 2.5 to 3.5 cm of posterior bone resection results in correction of 30 to 35 degrees; however, more than one closing-wedge osteotomy may be required to attain the desired correction. The amount of bone resection needed to attain the desired degree of correction can be calculated preoperatively, depending on the vertebral level(s) at which the osteotomy is undertaken (**Fig. 16.5**). An asymmetrical PSO (APSO) is a laterally based wedge resection that allows mobilization in the coronal and sagittal planes and correction of 25 to 40 degrees of curvature per level. Either procedure maintains the length of the anterior column because the anterior cortex is left intact. Generally, the disc spaces above and below the level of treatment are not disturbed; however, additional correction can be achieved if a portion of the superior disc is also resected.

The exposure for a PSO is a standard posterior approach to the spine. Before any boney resection is done, pedicle-screw instrumentation is placed above and below the level(s) to be resected. Resection of the posterior elements begins with a laminectomy of the selected level and undercutting of the laminae of adjacent levels. The transverse processes are then resected.

The lateral vertebral-body walls at the vertebral level selected for treatment are exposed in preparation for the osteotomy. In a PSO, both of the vertebral pedicles are excised; in an APSO, only the pedicle on the convex side is excised. An osteotome is used to create a symmetrical, dorsally based

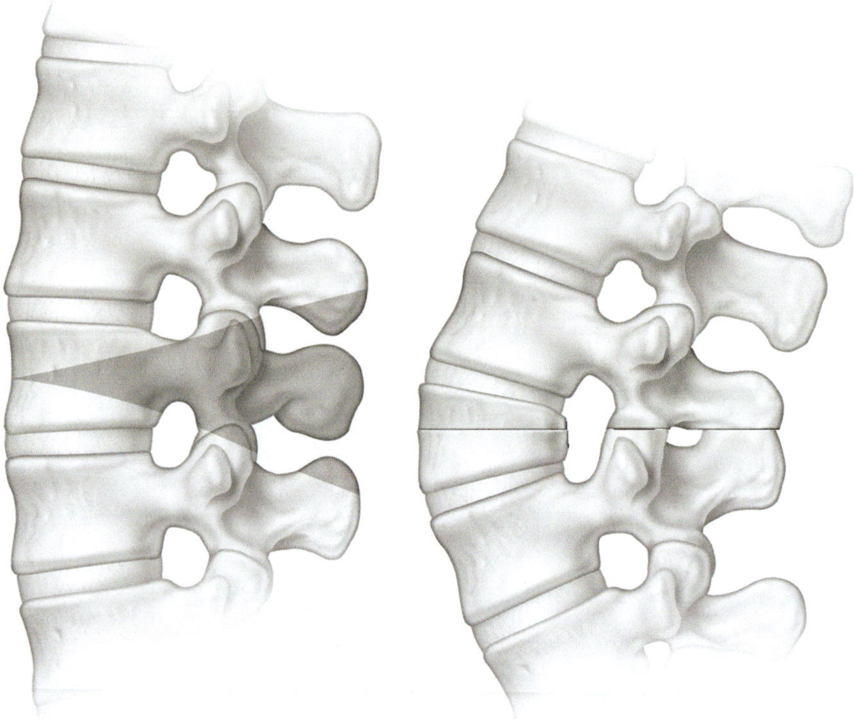


**Fig. 16.5** **(A)** Outline of a PSO. **(B)** The correction expected after closing the PSO.

wedge in the vertebral body or a three-dimensionally asymmetrical wedge in the case of an APSO. After the bone wedge is removed, compression across segmental pedicle-screw instrumentation closes the osteotomy. Care must be taken to undercut the adjacent laminae to avoid nerve-root compression. The wedge cuts should be symmetrical to avoid posterior overhang, which may impinge on the thecal sac and its contents as the wedge is closed.

Yamin et al[11] studied 21 cases of rigid scoliosis with a mean curvature of 80 degrees. These were treated with anterior release followed by halo-pelvic traction and a second-staged posterior fusion. In those cases with a preoperative curve flexibility <10% and a remaining scoliosis of >70 degrees, Yamin and colleagues recommended PSO in the second procedure to increase the correction of these rigid curves.

## Apical Vertebral Resection

Although PSOs can provide 40 degrees or more of correction in both the sagittal and/or coronal planes, some deformities are not amenable to correction with osteotomies alone. Initially described for the treatment of hemivertebrae, spondyloptosis, spinal cord tumors, and congenital kyphosis, AVR involves the resection of one or more vertebral levels. Also known as vertebral column resection (VCR), the procedure can be done through a combined anterior–posterior approach or a posterior-only approach. Combined anterior–posterior AVR was first described in the treatment of deformity secondary to congenital hemivertebra by von Lackum[12] between 1924 and 1933. Combined anterior vertebrectomy and posterior fusion was used to treat fixed lateral deformities in congenital scoliosis and "ordinary scoliosis." VCR is indicated for fixed rigid spinal deformities in which spinal balance cannot be achieved by osteotomies alone.

The procedure for AVR has been modified over the years by a number of surgeons including Luque[13] and Bradford.[14] In the first description of a posterior-only approach by MacLennan[15] in 1922, the vertebral body was excavated through the apex of the deformity, with partial resection above and below the resected vertebra. Postoperatively, the uninstrumented fusion was allowed to solidify in a cast.

The number of vertebral bodies to be resected in an AVR is based on the rigidity and characteristics of the patient's curve. The goal of the procedure is optimal correction in the coronal and sagittal planes, with the avoidance of neurological compromise. Generally, resection of one or two vertebrae suffices for correction. In rare cases, as needed, three vertebrae have been resected. Segmental pedicle-screw instrumentation is required three levels above and three levels below the resection to adequately stabilize the spine.

Modern techniques of AVR use pedicle-screw instrumentation to allow the application of adequate corrective forces and to insure maintenance of the correction achieved with the procedure. In contrast to the osteotomies described earlier in this chapter, VCRs do not produce bone-on-bone contact or require structural allografts or autografts or a metal cage to reconstruct the vertebral column after resection. Apical rib-head resection must be done in conjunction with both complete and incomplete AVR. Enough of the periapical convex or concave rib heads or both should be resected to allow safe access to the vertebral bodies that will be resected. Rib-head resection also allows improved spinal mobilization and better correction of rib asymmetry. The extent of correction of a deformity depends on the amount of resection. In 2002, Suk et al[16] reported the correction of ~40 of scoliosis per vertebra resected in cases of adult scoliosis. In a review of VCRs done for AIS by the Harms Study Group, a mean correction of 53 degrees per vertebra resected was noted.

The description that follows is of the posterior only approach to AVR. After the standard posterior approach, segmental instrumentation is applied to the three vertebral levels cephalad and three levels caudad to the proposed site of resection. A wide lateral dissection is done to allow resection of the transverse processes in the lumbar spine or of the concave rib and rib head in the thoracic spine. This allows access for the vertebral-body resection (**Fig. 16.6**).

The thecal sac is then exposed by means of a laminectomy, with removal of the posterior elements in the area to be resected. The laminae of vertebrae at adjacent levels are generously undercut to avoid nerve-root and thecal-sac compression. In the thoracic spine, nerve roots in the area to be resected are tied off to avoid traction on the spinal cord. The soft tissues anterior to the treated vertebral body and the great vessels are protected. After preparation of the lateral vertebral body, the concave pedicle is resected, in a piecemeal fashion, using pituitary rongeurs, curettes, osteotomes, or a high-speed drill alone or in combination (**Fig. 16.7**). This is followed by resection of the concave vertebral body and disc. The concave side is then stabilized by placing and securing the concave rod to prevent undesired vertebral translation (**Fig. 16.8**). The same procedure

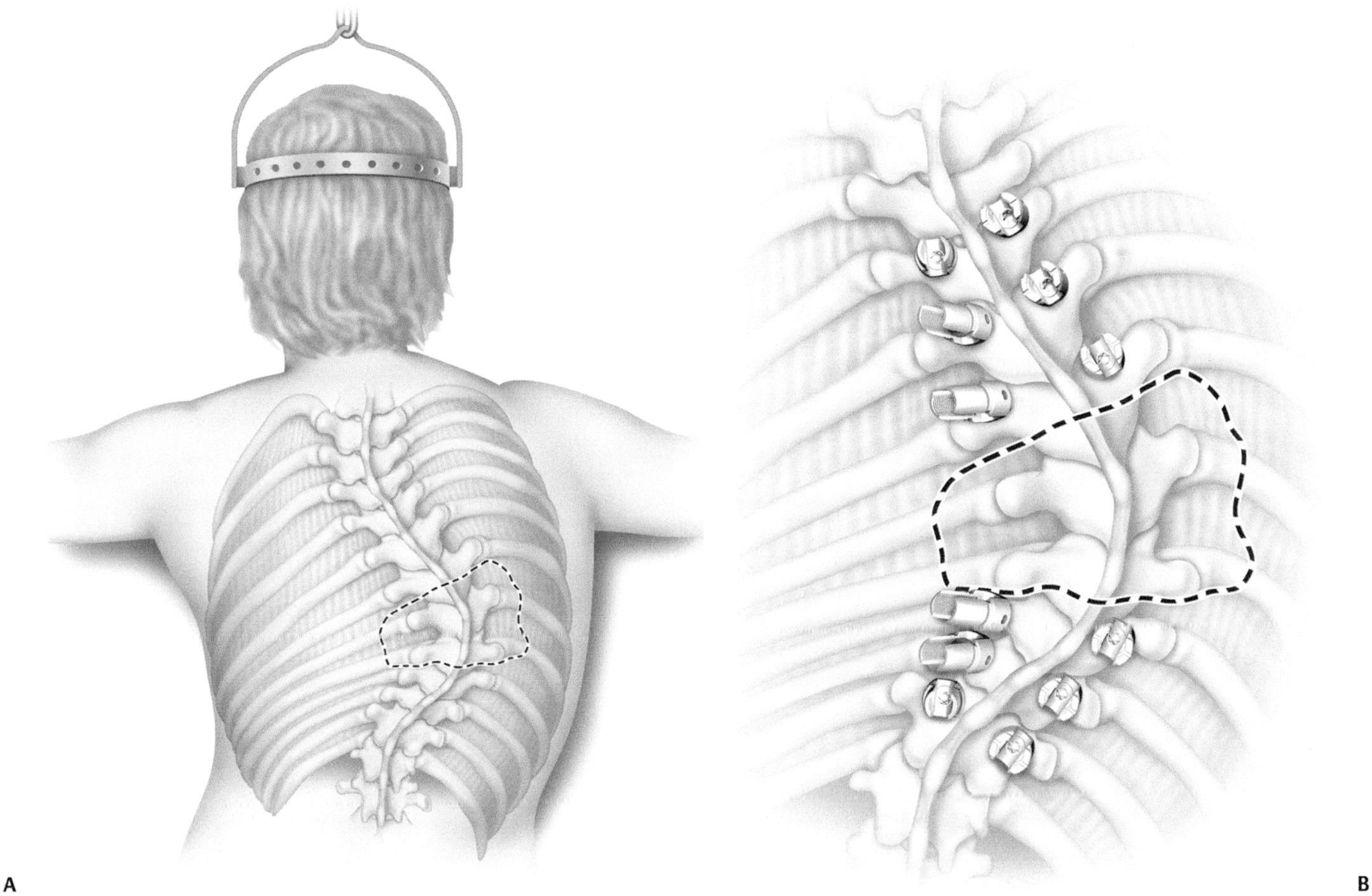


**Fig. 16.6** **(A)** Outline of the vertebrae to be resected with an apical vertebral excision for this rigid scoliosis. **(B,C)** Placement of the pedicle screws (three levels above and three levels below the region of resection) prior to the apical vertebral excision.

(*Continued on page 194*)

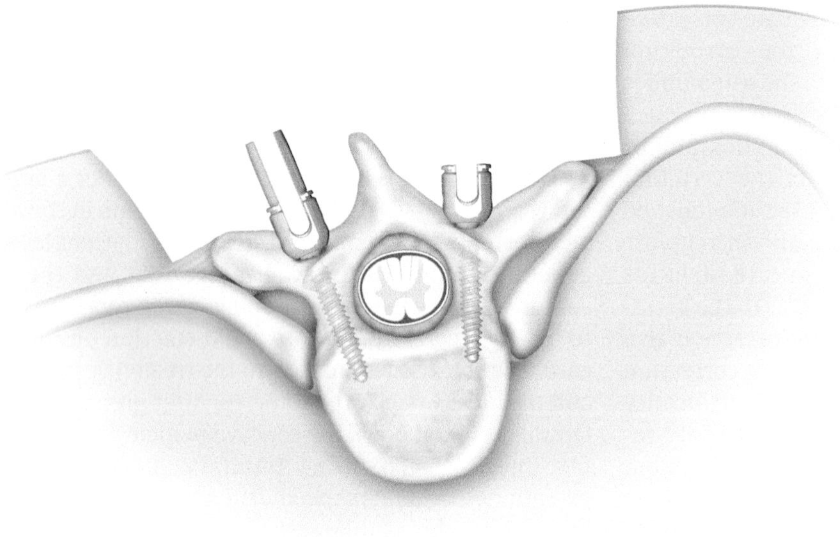

C

Fig. 16.6 (*Continued*) **(C)** Placement of the pedicle screws (three levels above and three levels below the region of resection) prior to the apical vertebral excision.

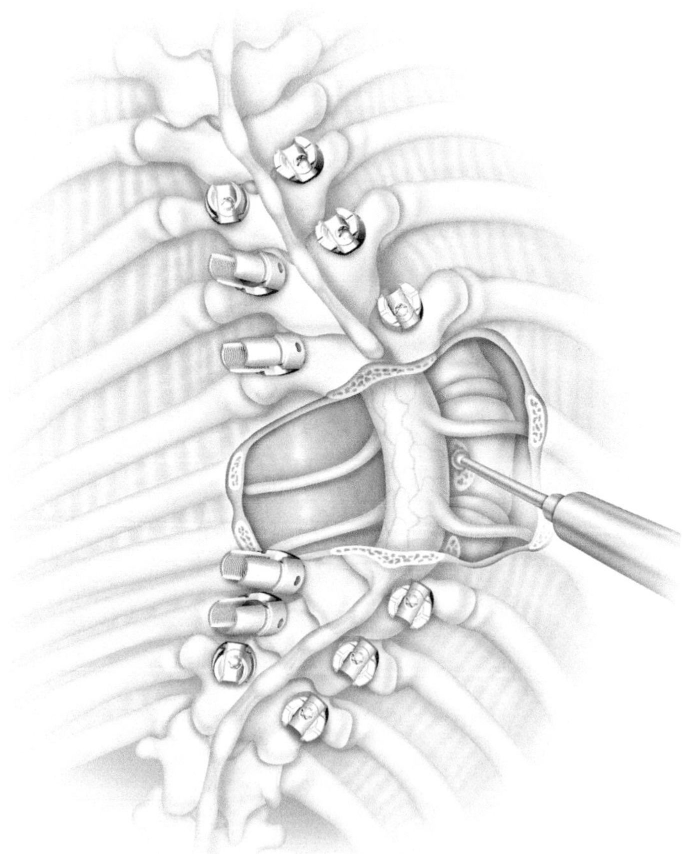

A

**Fig. 16.7 (A,B)** Excision of the posterior elements and concave pedicle. Wide decompression of the thecal sac and nerve roots is needed to prevent neurological injury.

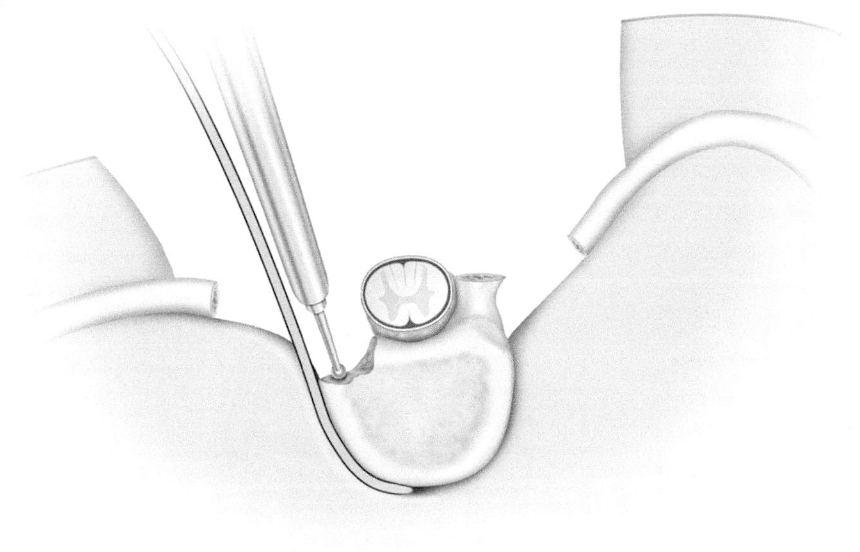

B

**Fig. 16.7** (*Continued*) **(B)** Excision of the posterior elements and concave pedicle wide decompression of the thecal sac and nerve roots is needed to prevent neurological injury.

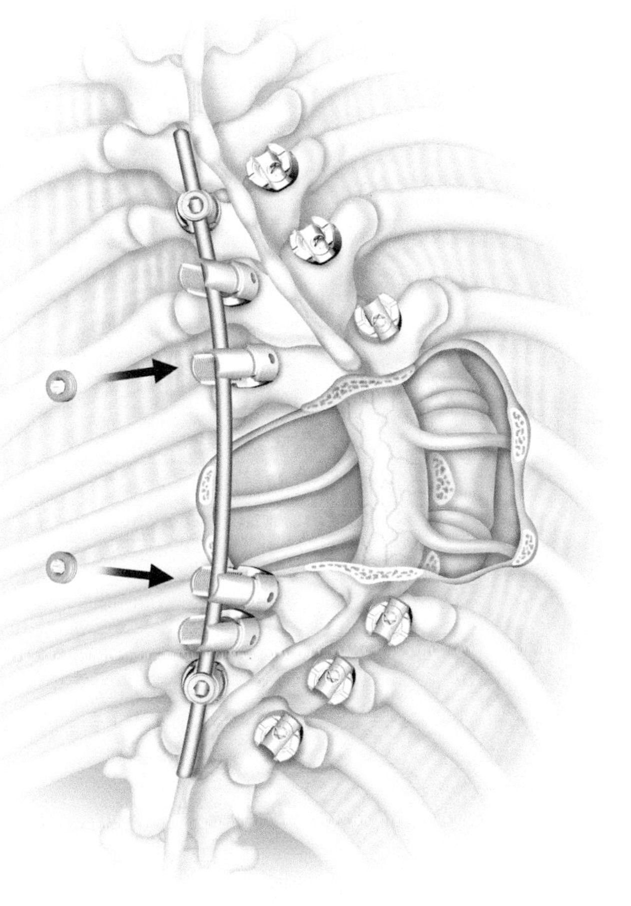

**Fig. 16.8** Placement of the concave rod before excessive anterior- or middle-column removal or both is needed to prevent instability and neurological injury.

is done on the convex side (**Fig. 16.9**). Correction is obtained gradually through repeated compression and shortening of the vertebral column with temporary rods. This is followed by rod rotation (**Fig. 16.10**) and compression of the convex side of the deformity (**Fig. 16.11**). A small anterior cage or structural graft may be required in the gap left after resection, to prevent overshortening of the spinal column, which may create the risk of dural or spinal-cord buckling or both (**Fig. 16.12**). Spinal-cord monitoring is critical during such corrections.

Postoperative hemothorax frequently follows AVR; it may be prophylactically treated with chest-tube placement or as needed with pleural taps. Patients undergoing AVR are generally mobilized as soon as possible, without the need for immobilization with a brace.

Review of the literature reveals several studies of the correction of large deformities with AVR at the expense of a high rate of complications. Suk and colleagues[17,18] reviewed 16 patients with severe, rigid fixed scoliosis who underwent VCR. All of the patients' curves measured >80 degrees and had an apical flexibility of less than 25%. From one to three vertebrae were removed per patient, with a total of 21 vertebral resections. Mean estimated blood loss was 7035 mL, and mean correction was 59%. Four complications were reported, including one complete paralysis, one hematoma, one proximal junctional kyphosis, and one hemothorax. Jensen et al[19,20] reported on 32 curves in 23 patients with fixed coronal deformities. From one to three vertebrae were resected per patient, with a mean estimated blood loss of 3400 mL. The mean primary curve correction was 78%, with a mean segmental apical correction of 81%. Complications included two

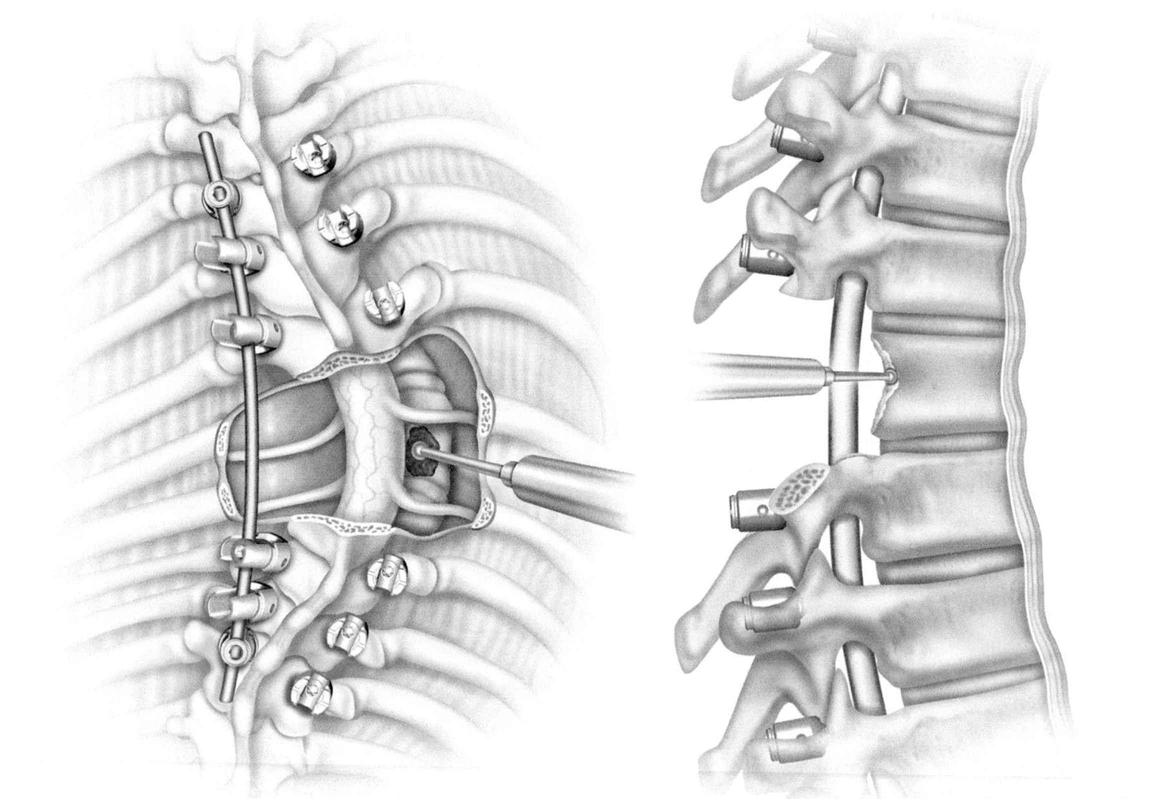

A B

**Fig. 16.9 (A,B)** Removal of vertebral body from the convex side. This is completed with the use of a burr and pituitary rongeur.

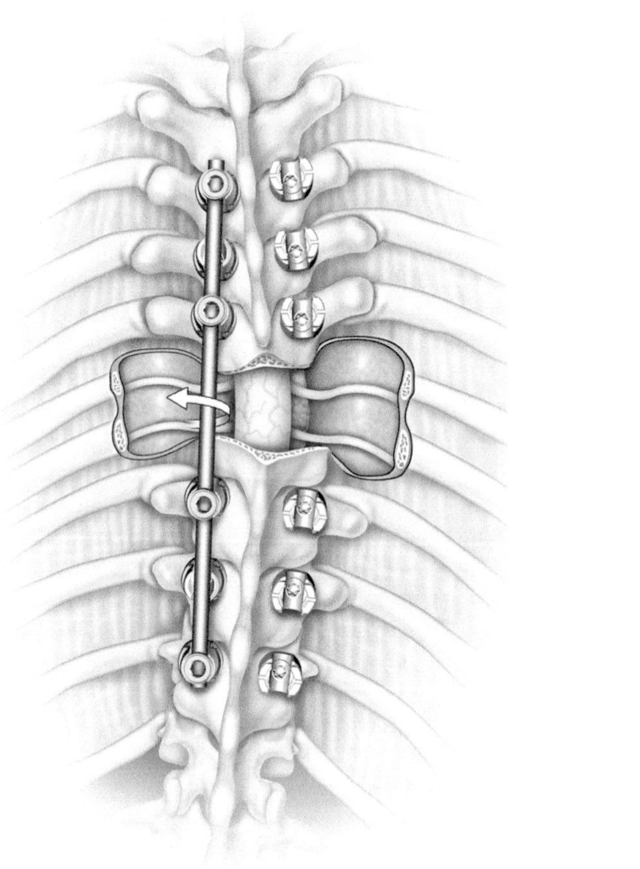

**Fig. 16.10** Reduction of the deformity in rigid AIS by rod rotation.

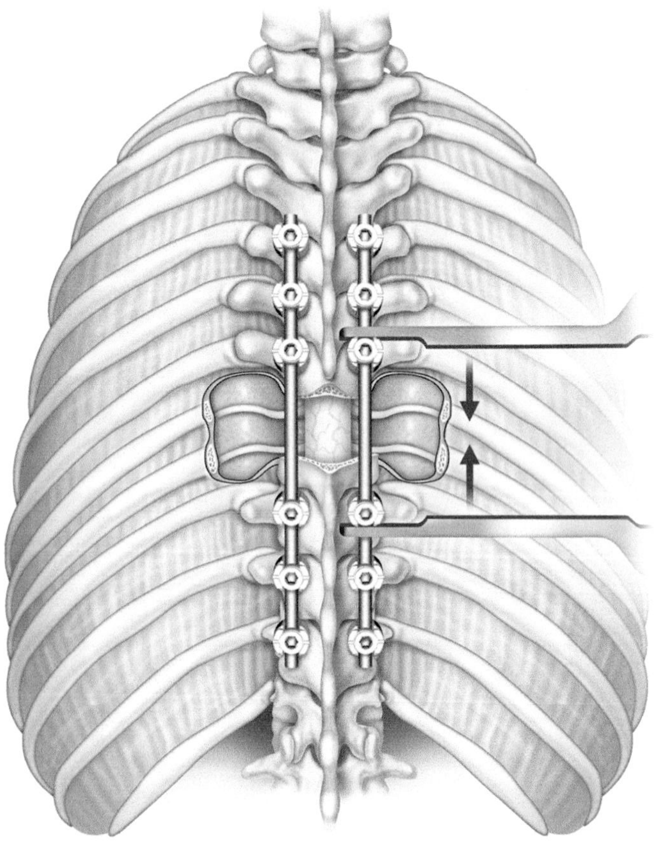

**Fig. 16.11** Further reduction of the deformity in AIS by compression across the convex rod.

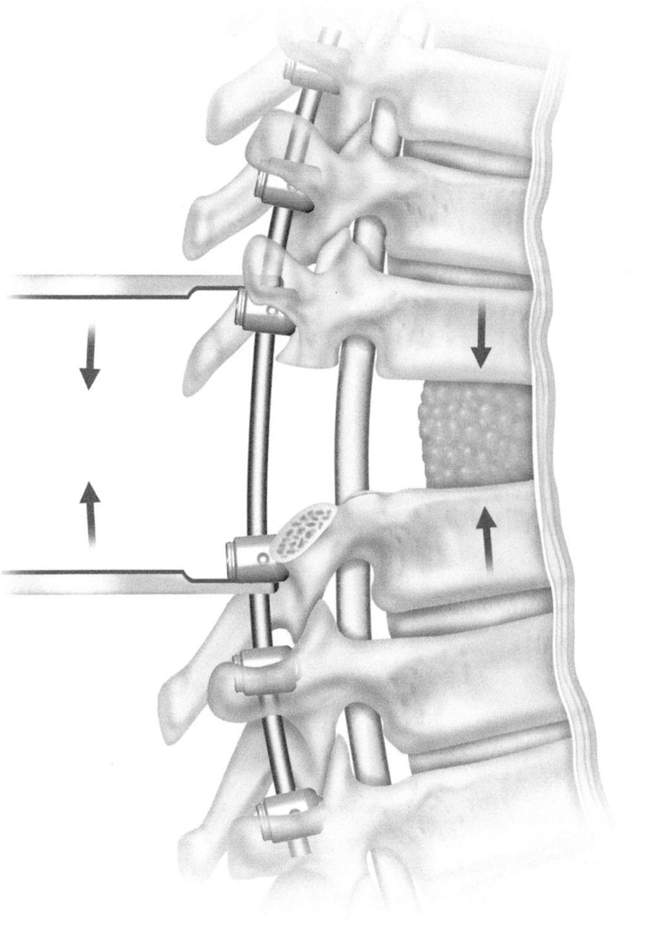

Fig. 16.12 Incomplete closure following correction of a deformity requires the addition of anterior support (a cage or graft). Compression with the graft or cage as a fulcrum can further reduce the deformity.

wound infections, two pneumonias, two hemothoraxes, one transient brachial plexus lesion, one transient paraparesis, one lumbar curve decompensation, and one death as the result of hypovolemic shock. Of the 23 patients treated with AVR, 43% had at least one complication.

Letko and co-workers[21] have additionally retrospectively studied 16 patients with previously untreated idiopathic scoliosis who underwent complete or incomplete AVR with a total of 23 vertebrae being resected. Ten thoracic vertebrae were completely resected in the apical region. Asymmetric wedge resection was undertaken 13 times in 11 patients.

**Table 16.1 Curve Magnitude***

| | Mean | Range |
|---|---|---|
| Preoperative, degrees | 887.2 | 70–110 |
| Postoperative, degrees | 8.1 | 0–20 |
| Last follow-up, degrees | 8.5 | 0–20 |
| % Correction | 90% | 75–100% |

*$n = 20$

One complete vertebral resection with partial excision of an additional vertebra was done in 2 of the 16 patients. In 13 patients, halo traction was also used. Eight of the 16 patients had a preceding anterior release. The patients' mean time in the operating room was 6 hours 6 minutes (range: 6 to 15.6. hours). Mean estimated blood loss was 7062 mL. The mean preoperative curve magnitude was 87 degrees, which was corrected and maintained at a mean of 8 degrees postoperatively and at last follow-up (a mean correction of 90%) (**Table 16.1**). The mean preoperative apical angulation in these patients, as measured one level above and one level below the apex of the deformity curve, was 60 degrees. This corrected and was maintained at a mean of 5 degrees at last follow-up (a mean correction of 92%) (**Table 16.2**). There were no intraoperative complications. Fourteen postoperative complications occurred in 11 patients, including two wound infections, two wound-healing problems, seven hemothoraxes or pleural effusions, one pneumothorax, one urinary tract infection, and one transient peroneal nerve palsy.

**Figure 16.13** illustrates a case study of severely rigid AIS in which the techniques described in this chapter were used.

**Table 16.2 Apical Curve Angulation***

| | Mean | Range |
|---|---|---|
| Preoperative, degrees | 60.1 | 40–90 |
| Bend, degrees | 57.5 | 30–80 |
| Last follow-up, degrees | 4.7 | 0–10 |
| % correction | 92.4% | 80–100% |

*$n = 20$

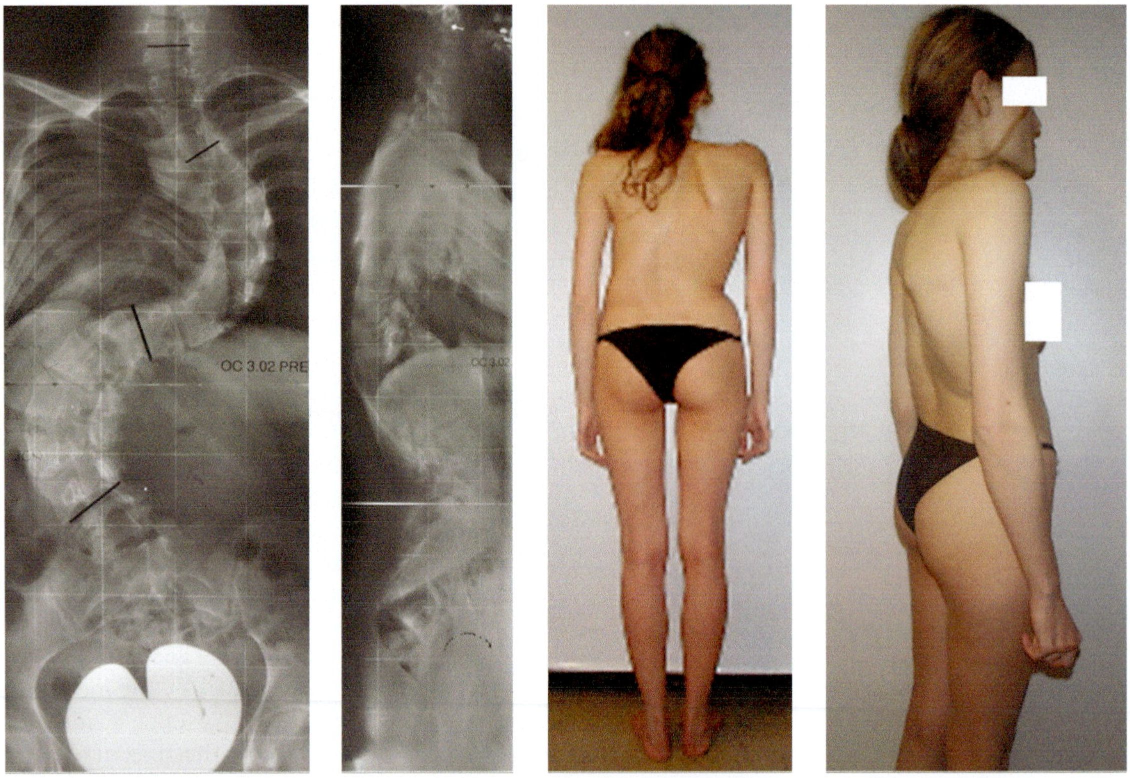


A–D

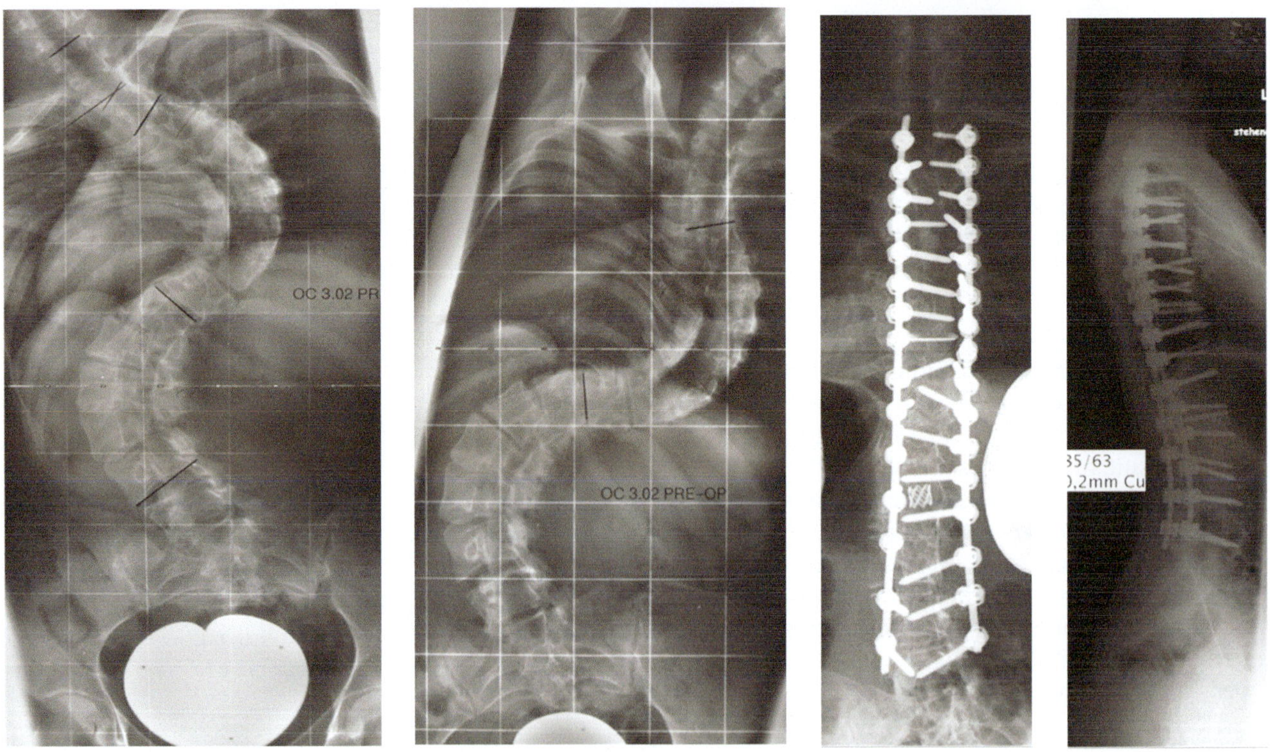


E–H

**Fig. 16.13** **(A,B)** Anteroposterior and sagittal X-ray films of a 21-year-old woman with a Lenke type 3CN scoliosis. The curve from T5 to T11 measures 110 degrees and the curve from T12 to L4 measures 95 degrees. **(C,D)** Preoperative clinical photographs of the patient. **(E,F)** Bending films demonstrate 12% flexibility (94 degrees) in the thoracic curve and 19% flexibility (80 degrees) in the lumbar curve. **(G,H)** The patient underwent preoperative halo traction. She then underwent a staged anterior release from T4 to L1, followed by a posterior release with multiple transverse (Ponte) osteotomies, resection of periapical concave and convex rib heads, asymmetric PSOs of T8, T9, and L2, and instrumentation from T2 to L4.

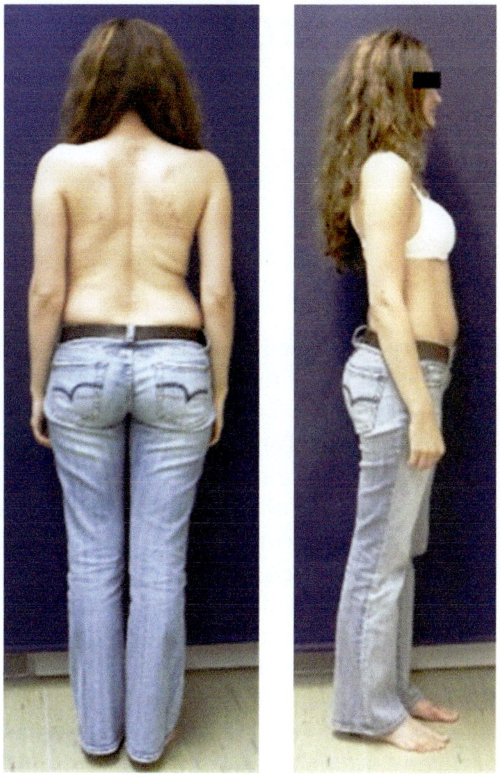

I J

**Fig. 16.13** *(Continued)* **(I,J)** Postoperative clinical photographs of the patient.

## Conclusion

PSO, APSO, and AVR have proven highly efficacious in the treatment of scoliosis of various etiologies. AVR allows excellent deformity correction in moderate and severely rigid AIS. These techniques may need to be combined with transverse osteotomies to achieve optimal correction. PSO, APSO, and AVR are technically demanding procedures with the potential for neurological and vascular complications. Monitoring of somatosensory evoked potentials and motor evoked potentials is essential during these procedures. At present, the major disadvantages of PSO, APSO, and AVR are extensive blood loss and the potential risk of neurological injury.

## References


1. Hibbs RA. A report of fifty-nine cases of scoliosis treated by the fusion operation. J Bone Joint Surg 1924;6:3–37
2. Howorth MB. Evolution of spinal fusion. Ann Surg 1943;117:278–289
3. Burton DC. Smith-Petersen osteotomy of the spine. Instr Course Lect 2006;55:577–582
4. Smith-Petersen MN, Larson CB, Aufranc OE. Osteotomy of the spine for correction of flexion deformity in rheumatoid arthritis. J Bone Joint Surg 1945;27:1–11
5. Bridwell KH. Decision making regarding Smith-Petersen vs. pedicle subtraction osteotomy vs. vertebral column resection for spinal deformity. Spine 2006;31(19, suppl):S171–S178
6. La Marca F, Brumblay H. Smith-Petersen osteotomy in thoracolumbar deformity surgery. Neurosurgery 2008; 63(3, suppl):163–170
7. Ponte A. Posterior column shortening for Scheuermann's kyphosis: an innovative one-stage technique. In: Haher TR, ed. Surgical Techniques for the Spine. New York: Thieme Medical Publishers; 2003:107–113.
8. Ponte A. Personal communication, 2006
9. Geck MJ, Macagno A, Ponte A, Shufflebarger HL. The Ponte procedure: Posterior only treatment of Scheuermann's kyphosis using segmental posterior shortening and pedicle screw instrumentation. J Spinal Disord Tech 2007;20:586–593
10. Michele A, Kreuger FJ. A surgical approach to the vertebral body. J Bone Joint Surg Am 1949;31:873–878
11. Yamin S, Li L, Xing W, Tianjun G, Yupeng Z. Staged surgical treatment for severe and rigid scoliosis. J Orthop Surg 2008;3:26
12. Von Lackum HL, Smith AD. Removal of vertebral bodies in the treatment of scoliosis. Surg Gynecol Obstet 1933;57:250–256
13. Luque ER. Vertebral column transposition. Orthop Trans 1983;7:29
14. Bradford D. Vertebral column resection. Orthop Trans 1985; 9:130
15. MacLennan A. Scoliosis. BMJ 1922;2:864–866
16. Suk SI, Kim JH, Kim WJ, Lee SM, Chung ER, Nah KH. Posterior vertebral column resection for severe spinal deformities. Spine 2002; 27:2374–2382
17. Suk SI, Chung ER, Kim JH, et al. Posterior vertebral column resection (PVCR) for rigid scoliosis. 39th Annual Meeting, Scoliosis Research Society, Buenos Aires, Argentina, Sept 6–9, 2004
18. Suk SI, Chung ER, Kim JH, Kim SS, Lee JS, Choi WK. Posterior vertebral column resection for severe rigid scoliosis. Spine 2005;30:1682–1687
19. Jensen R, Letko L, Melcher R, et al. Posterior resection of the apical vertebra allows excellent correction in rigid scoliosis. 40th Annual Meeting Of the Scoliosis Research Sociity, Miami, FL, Oct 27–30, 2005
20. Jensen R, Letko L, Melcher R, et al. Posterior resection of the apical vertebral allows excellent correction in rigid scoliosis. 12th International Meeting on Advanced Spine Techniques, Banff, Canada, July 7–9, 2005
21. Letko K, Jensen R, Harms J. Partial or complete apical vertebral resection in the treatment of cases of moderate and severe rigid AIS. 13th International Meeting on Advanced Spine Techniques, Athens, Greece, July 12–15, 2006

# 17 Surgical Treatment of the Right Thoracic Curve Pattern

*Peter O. Newton and Vidyadhar V. Upasani*

The right main thoracic (MT) curve pattern is the prototypic scoliotic deformity seen in adolescent idiopathic scoliosis (AIS), being found in almost 50% of all cases treated surgically. By definition, the MT curve in AIS has an apex between T2 and T11, and has the largest coronal deviation of any of the curves in this condition as measured by the Cobb-angle method. Measuring apical deviation, relative apical lordosis, and transverse-plane rotation provides a further means of describing the major curve and captures some of the three-dimensional (3D) nature of this deformity that is lost in the largely two-dimensional (2D) imaging of it. Characteristics of the minor curves proximal and distal to the MT curve are as important as the features of the 3D thoracic deformity. Many of the decisions to be made in the treatment of MT curves depend on these minor-curve characteristics. Understanding how minor curves will "respond" to surgical correction of the MT curve is critical in the treatment of scoliosis. This chapter addresses the characteristics of the right MT curve pattern in AIS and discusses the criteria used to decide when and how to address this spinal deformity. Options for selective versus nonselective fusion are discussed, as are the surgical approaches currently used for the correction of right MT curves. Specifically, the particular indications and contraindications for each approach are evaluated, and recommendations are made for surgical technique and for the selection of fusion levels in correcting such curves.

## ■ Deformity Classification

When the Harms Study Group (HSG) was instituted, the King classification of scoliotic curves did not work for new instrumentation strategies beyond pure distraction. Both the King [1] and Lenke [2] classification systems for AIS have been useful in characterizing the classic right thoracic curve pattern. Three of the five types of curve in the King classification describe a major thoracic spinal deformity: King II, King III, and King IV. These roughly correlate with the following types of curve in the Lenke system: Lenke 1B/1C, Lenke 1A/1B, and Lenke 1A, respectively. Although neither system is perfect, both provide insight into choosing the appropriate treatment for this common pattern of scoliosis.

The major feature distinguishing right MT curves from one another is the nature of the lumbar deformity. It is the varying degree of apical deviation of the lumbar curve that the lumbar modifier in the Lenke system describes. The "A" modifier is used when the center sacral vertical line (CSVL) falls medial to the pedicle of the lumbar apical vertebra, and describes both lumbar curves with no apical deviation (King IV) and lumbar curves with slight apical deviation (King III). The "B" lumbar modifier is applied when the minor lumbar curve has moderate apical deviation as defined by the CSVL falling between the medial pedicle wall and the lateral edge of the apical vertebral body. The "C" modifier represents a more substantial lumbar curve with the entire apical vertebral body deviated lateral to the CSVL. These distinctions are important when choosing the lumbar curve that may need to be included in the fusion in a case of AIS, as well as in selecting the lowest instrumented vertebra (LIV) for each type of curve.

The definitions of type 1 or MT curve patterns Lenke classification system are largely reproducible. The original study that described the Lenke classification system[2] reported high interobserver (0.92) and intraobserver (0.83) kappa values among the five investigators who developed the system. An independent analysis[3] in 2002 reported lower kappa values with the Lenke system than with the King classification system (0.62 and 0.73, respectively), however, they were still noted to be significantly higher than those historically reported for the King system.[4,5] Despite the relatively high level of agreement in the classification of scoliotic curves, variability exists in both the selection of an operative approach and fusion levels for treating these deformities, confirming the current lack of standardized treatment paradigms in scoliosis surgery.[6]

The Lenke system works because it has relatively simple rules that define the curve patterns in scoliosis. The system was developed to aid in choosing surgical treatment for AIS, and therefore does not necessarily distinguish among truly different curve patterns. As suggested above, this is most obvious for Lenke type 1A curves. In an analysis of these curves done on the HSG database, two distinct curve patterns emerged.[7] The Lenke type 1A curve with L4 tilted to the right, denoted as type 1AR, is a long thoracic curve similar to the King IV pattern (**Fig. 17.1**). The fusion level for

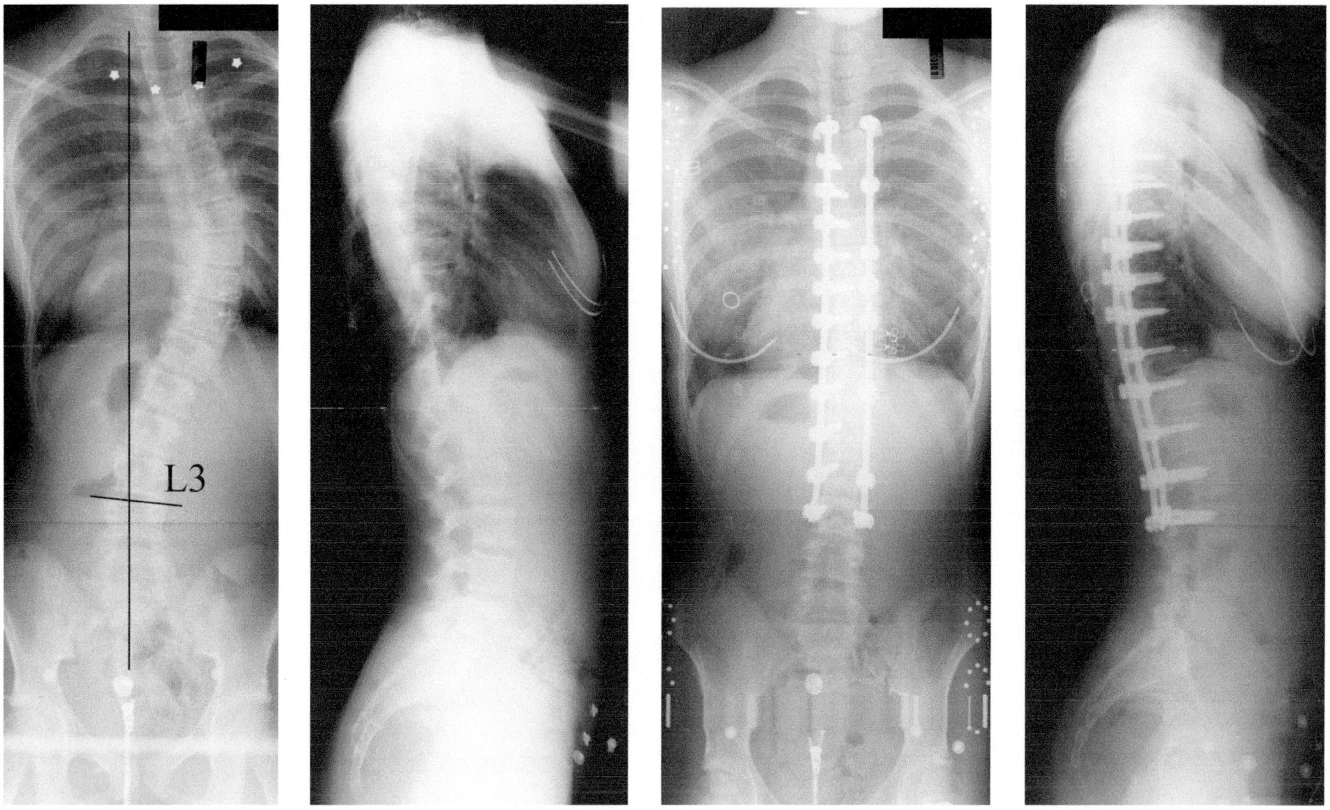


**Fig. 17.1** Preoperative posteroanterior (PA) and lateral radiographs of a 15-year-old girl demonstrate a 51-degree thoracic and 24-degree thoracolumbar curve (Lenke type 1AR deformity). **(A,B)** The patient underwent posterior spinal instrumentation and fusion with segmental pedicle screws from T4 to L3. The LIV was selected as the most proximal lumbar vertebra "substantially touched" by the CSVL. **(C,D)** Postoperative PA and lateral radiographs demonstrate an 18-degree thoracic and 5-degree thoracolumbar curve.

this curve is more distal than when L4 is tilted to the left (type 1AL) (**Fig. 17.2**). The type 1AL curve resembles the Lenke type 1B/C pattern, especially from the standpoint of choosing the LIV (**Fig. 17.3**).

Another area of controversy with regard to the classification of right thoracic curves relates to the sagittal and axial planes. The Lenke classification has added a sagittal modifier, bringing attention to this important aspect of the deformity in scoliosis. However, the T5-to-T12 sagittal measure used to grade the sagittal alignment as hyperkyphotic, normal, or hypokyphotic does not characterize the sagittal deformity at the thoracic apex, which is nearly always less kyphotic than is normal. This apical "lordosis" has been suggested for years by numerous authors[8–12] as a common feature of thoracic scoliosis, and can be difficult to appreciate on standard lateral radiographs because of the presence of vertebral rotation. Stagnara and Quencau[11] suggested a rotated anteropoaterior (AP) and lateral view to identify the "true" nature of the deformity in both planes. However, this rotated view does not capture the global deformity or the 3D relationship of the thoracic curve to the other regions of the spine. Three-dimensional imaging is an obvious but costly solution to the adequate imaging of the scoliotic spine. An analysis of the apical segments of 66 patients, done with software and 3D reconstructions at St. Justine Hospital (Montreal, Quebec), demonstrated consistent reduction in kyphosis.[13] It is clear that an understanding of all three planes of deformity in each patient with AIS is required to optimize surgical treatment. Additionally, an axial rotational deformity that in many cases represents the primary deformity in the eyes of the patient is associated with the apical lordosis (whether relative or absolute). Clinical deformity of trunk shape as determined by coronal decompensation, truncal shift, difference in shoulder height, a thoracic rib hump, and lumbar prominence varies among patients with right thoracic curves (unpublished HSG data, 2008) (**Table 17.1**). These clinical findings, as well as radiographic measures, have to be incorporated into the surgical plan for each patient. Those with a lumbar curve to the left, of varying magnitude (Lenke types 1AL, 1B, 1C), whose heads may be relatively balanced over their pelves (**Fig. 17.4**), and those with an isolated thoracic curve (Lenke type 1AR) who tend to have a greater right-sided truncal shift and a larger thoracic rib hump (**Fig. 17.5**), require different treatment strategies. At this time, the best strategy is to combine 2D radiographic information with clinical information to develop a best treatment plan.

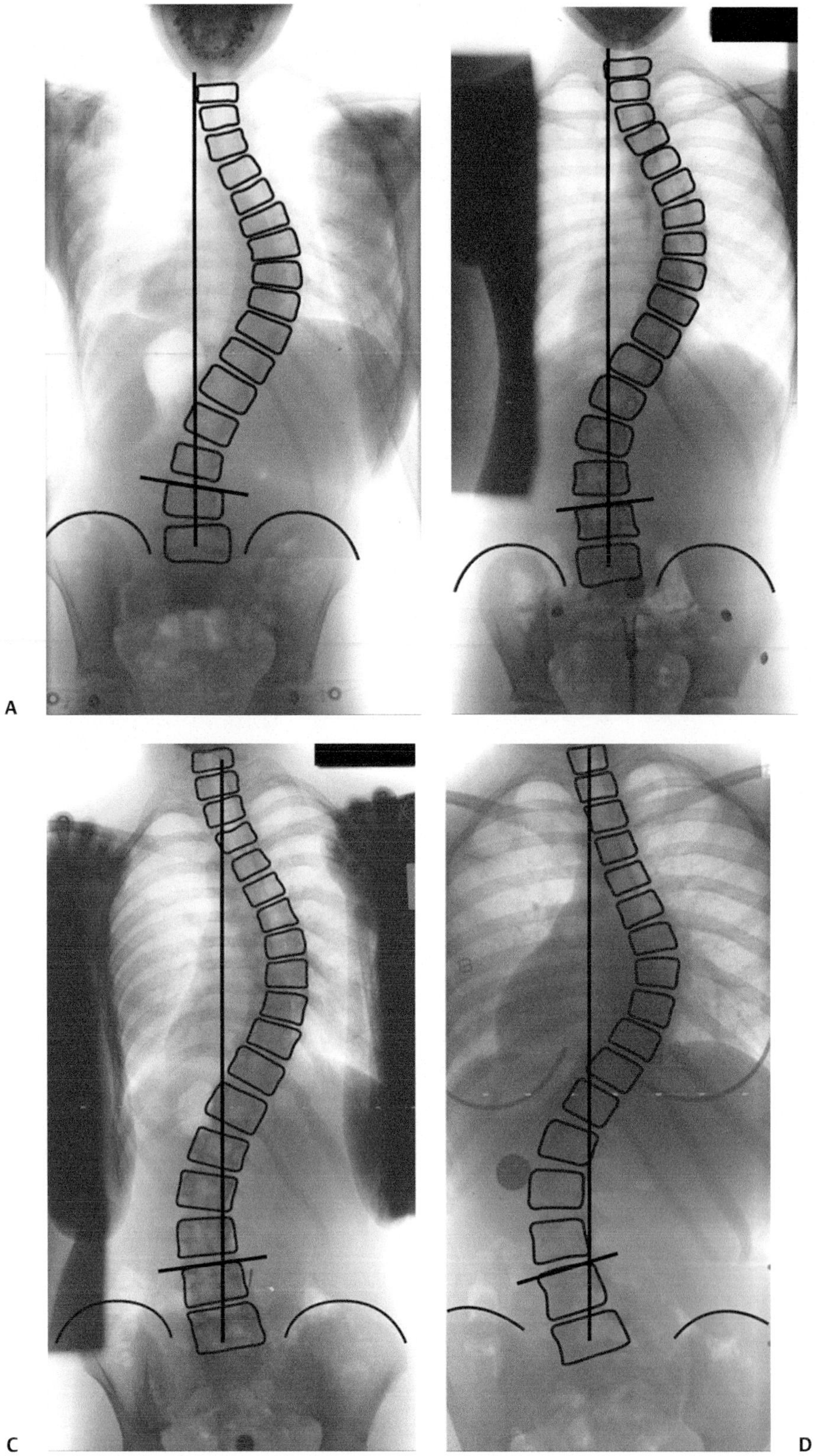


**Fig. 17.2** Radiographic PA images with outlined vertebral bodies, CSVL, and L4 tilt for **(A)** a Lenke type 1AR curve (L4 tilts to the right); **(B)** a Lenke type 1 AL curve (L4 tilts to the left); **(C)** a Lenke type 1B curve; and **(D)** a Lenke type 1C curve.

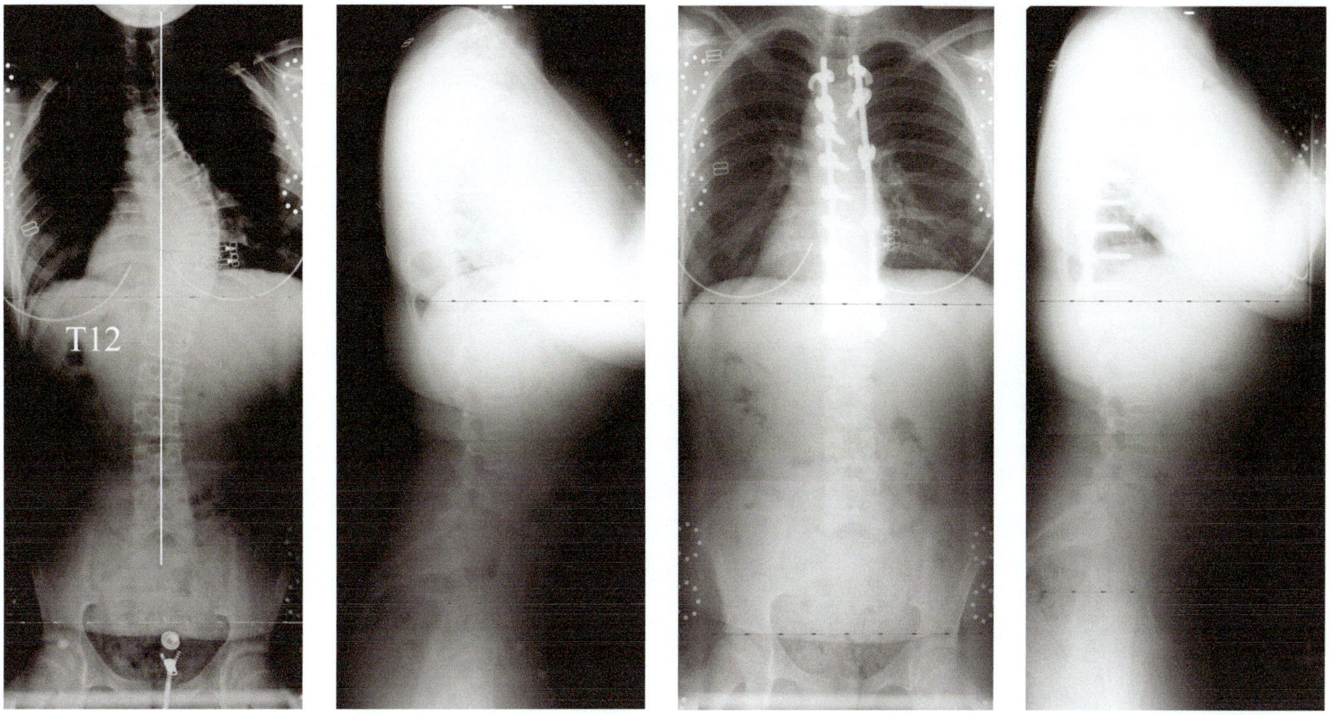


**Fig. 17.3** **(A,B)** Preoperative PA and lateral radiographs of a 15-year-old girl demonstrate a 45-degree thoracic and 21-degree thoracolumbar curve (Lenke type 1AL deformity). The patient underwent posterior spinal instrumentation and fusion with segmental pedicle screws from T4 to T12. The stable vertebra was selected as the LIV to prevent decompensation to the left. **(C,D)** Postoperative PA and lateral radiographs demonstrate a 12-degree thoracic and 7-degree thoracolumbar curve.

## Decisions Relating to Surgical Treatment

A number of decisions must be made before and during the surgical correction of right MT curves in scoliosis. The questions to be addressed in each case are listed below and will frame the discussion that follows.

1. Is an instrumented fusion indicated?
2. Which, if any, of the minor curves should be included in the fusion?
3. To what extent should the thoracic curve be corrected for ideal global balance?
4. What vertebral levels should be included in the fusion?
5. What is the best approach?
6. Is an anterior release indicated?

### Is a Surgically Instrumented Fusion Indicated?

Whether a surgically instrument fusion is indicated in a case of AIS remains one of the more controversial questions in its treatment. This is particularly so for curves in the 40- to 50-degree range. Treatment assumes that both the short- and long-term outcomes will be better with a fused spine than with the untreated natural history of AIS. It is the lack

**Table 17.1 Preoperative Trunk-Shape Measurements in Patients with Lenke Type 1 Curves**

| | Curve Type | | |
|---|---|---|---|
| | Lenke Type 1A | Lenke Type 1B | Lenke Type 1C |
| Number of patients | 98 | 52 | 38 |
| Coronal decompensation | 1.2 ± 1.0 cm | 1.1 ± 1.0 cm | 1.4 ± 1.0 cm |
| Trunk shift | 2.1 ±1.5 cm | 1.6 ±1.4 cm | 1.4 ±1.3 cm |
| Shoulder height | 1.4 ± 1.0 cm | 1.4 ± 1.0 cm | 1.7 ± 1.1 cm |
| Thoracic rib hump (scoliometer) | 14.4 ± 4.6° | 13.6 ± 3.9° | 13.0 ± 4.2° |
| Lumbar prominence (scoliometer) | 5.5 ± 3.7° | 6.8 ± 3.8° | 7.3 ± 4.5° |

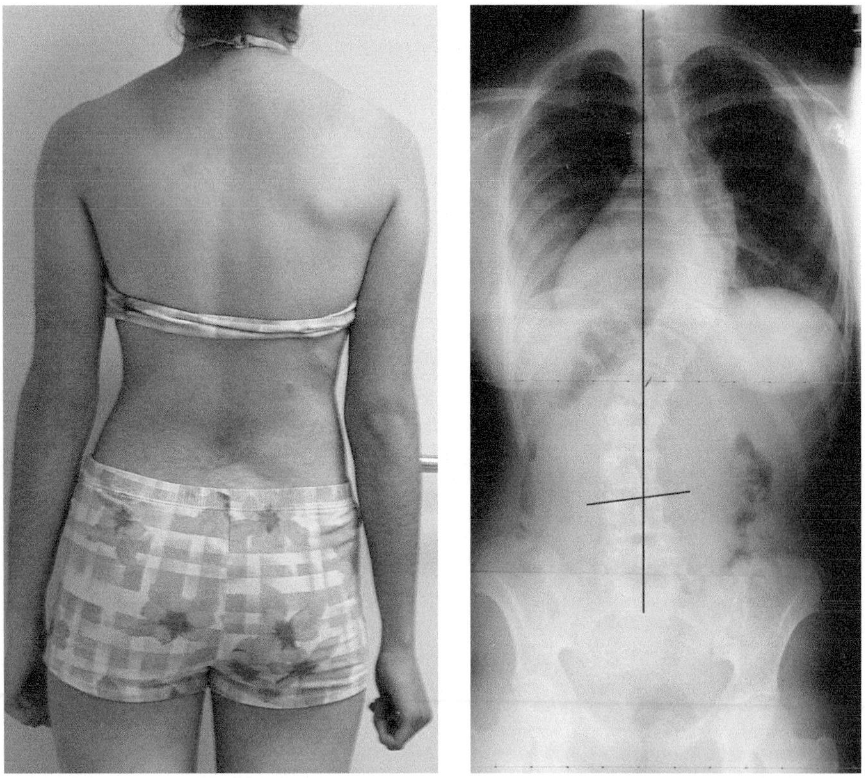

A B

**Fig. 17.4 (A)** Preoperative PA clinical photograph and **(B)** PA radiograph of a patient with a Lenke type 1B deformity, demonstrating a well-balanced standing posture with the head over the pelvis.

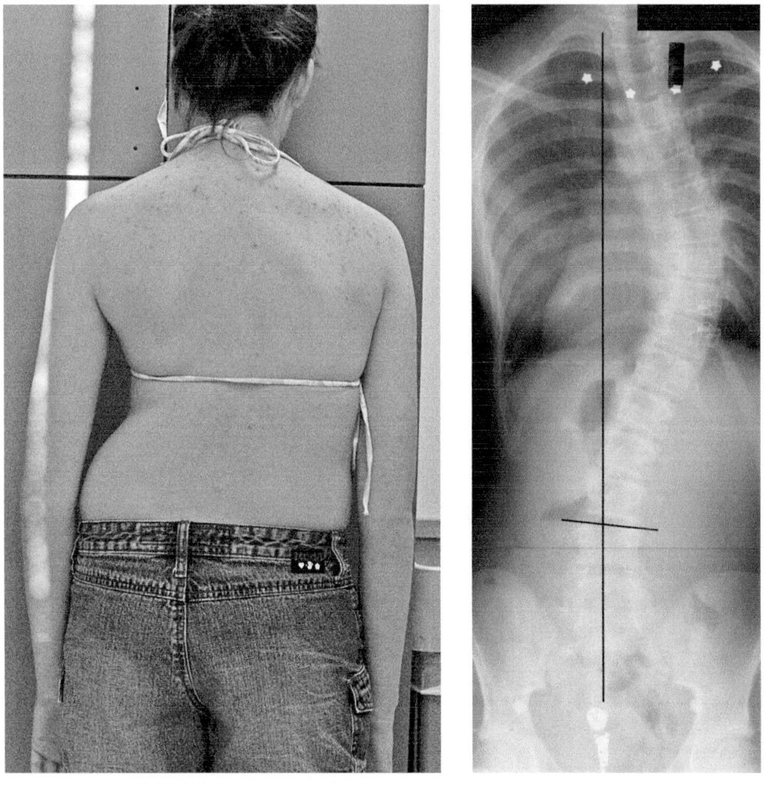

A B

**Fig. 17.5 (A)** Preoperative PA clinical photograph and **(B)** PA radiograph of a patient with a Lenke type 1AR deformity, demonstrating a right-sided truncal shift.

of knowledge in both of these situations over the long term that leaves the need for surgical treatment of these patients open to debate.

Traditionally, the magnitude of the spinal curvature in AIS as reflected by the Cobb angle has been the primary determinant of risk for curve progression in adulthood. Weinstein and colleagues[14,15] suggested the tidemark of 50 degrees as the criterion for this in thoracic curves. With curvature greater than this there is a significant risk for progression. The risk with curves between 40 and 50 degrees is less clear, and with curves of <40 degrees the risk of adult progression appears low. There are, however, various other ways to define the qualities of a spinal curve besides the Cobb angle, and it seems almost certain that there are more precise ways to predict late progression.[16–18] Until these are identified, we use limited data and prudent judgment to make this most critical decision. With excellent instrumentation systems available, surgery for AIS in adults is less problematic. Therefore, it is more common in practice to recommend observation for a thoracic curve of up to 60 degrees accompanied by minimal cosmetic disfigurement and normal results of pulmonary function tests (PFTs).

Another unproven variable used in the decision to operate in cases of AIS relates to the length of the curve. The more vertebra within the Cobb angle the more severe the clinical deformity. Coronal balance is also an important variable, and when a lumbar curve exists that matches or balances the thoracic deformity, as in many curves of Lenke type 1C, the curve magnitude suggesting fusion increases. In addition, for patients who have not completed growth, the remaining growth potential may weigh into the decision about whether or not to operate, with surgery often being indicated for younger patients with curves >40 degrees, as compared with the traditional 50-degree indication for those who have completed growth.

## The Inclusion of Minor Curves in the Fusion

In the MT curve pattern of AIS, the MT curve will clearly be surgically treated because it is the dominant deformity in this pattern of the condition. However, debate continues about when to include the minor lumbar curve. Selective thoracic fusion for the MT curve pattern of AIS was suggested by Moe more than 50 years ago,[19] and for the most part this concept remains as valid today as it was then. The difficulty has been to find a reliable way to determine the structurality of the minor lumbar curve. The Lenke classification system was designed with the goal of answering this specific question, and suggests that minor nonstructural curves (which side-bend to <25 degrees) can be spared from fusion if there is no appreciable junctional kyphosis.

Several recent studies have supported the guidelines provided by the Lenke classification as appropriate for the majority of cases of AIS, supporting the use of selective thoracic fusion in King type II and Lenke type 1C curves (**Fig. 17.6**). In 2003, Lenke and colleagues[20] reported that selective thoracic fusion of the major curve could be successfully accomplished even when the minor lumbar curve deviated completely from the midline (lumbar modifier C), thus optimizing the postoperative number of mobile lum-

A

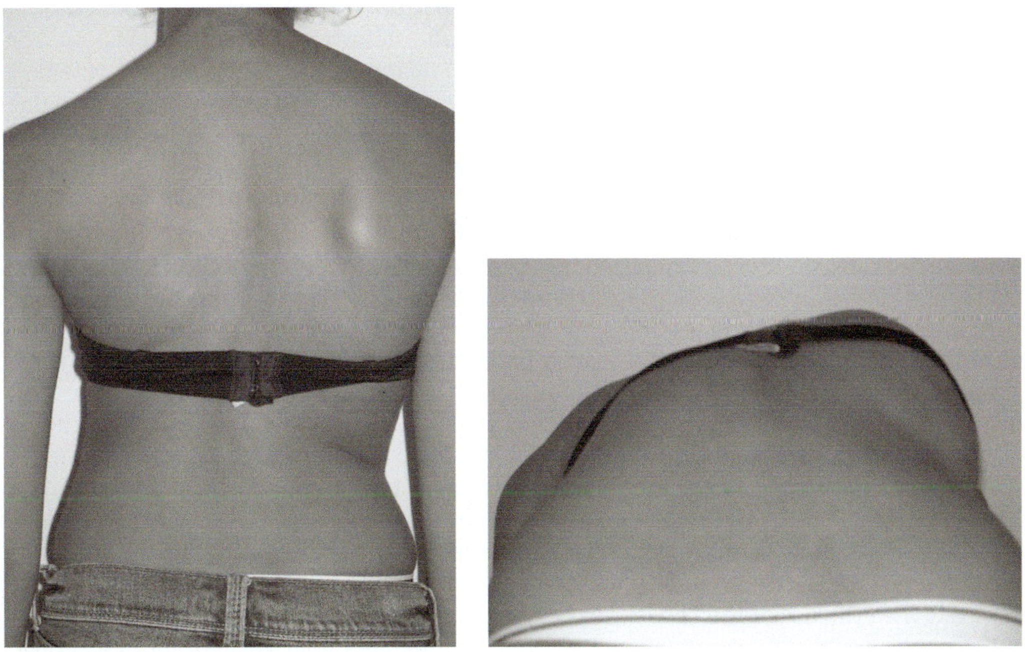

B

**Fig. 17.6 (A,B)** Preoperative PA and forward-bending clinical photographs.

(Continued on page 206)

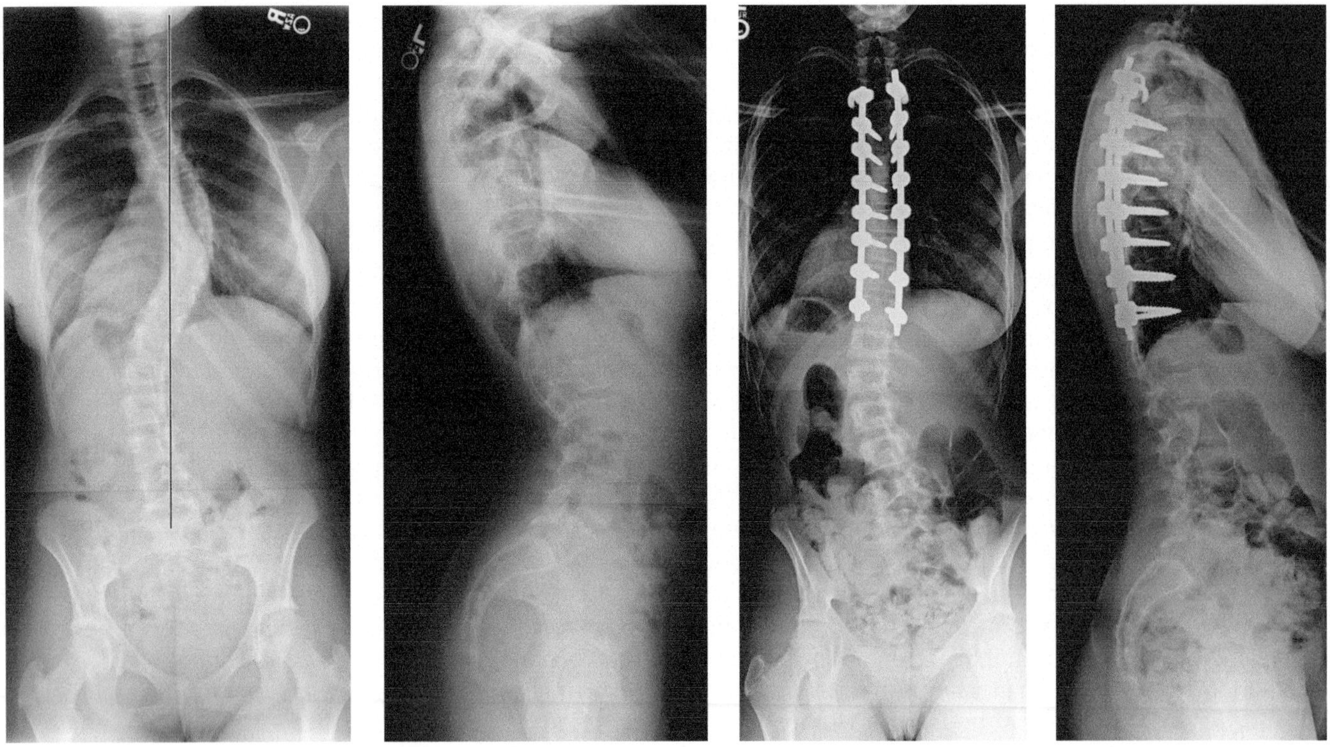

C–F

**Fig. 17.6** (*Continued*) **(C,D)** PA and lateral radiographs of a 15-year-old girl demonstrate a 52-degree thoracic and 40-degree thoracolumbar curve (Lenke type 1C deformity). The thoracic curve bends to 32 degrees (38% flexibility) and the lumbar curve bends to 10 degrees (75% flexibility). Selective posterior spinal instrumentation and fusion with segmental pedicle screws from T4 to T11 was done in this case because of a low clinical lumbar prominence (8 degrees), high lumbar curve flexibility, and low lumbar curve apical (L1) deviation from the CSVL (1.8 cm). **(E,F)** Postoperative PA and lateral radiographs demonstrate a well-balanced 18-degree thoracic and 26-degree lumbar curve.

bar segments. In 2004, Edwards et al[21] also described satisfactory results after selective thoracic fusion of properly selected curves with a Lenke C lumbar modifier. These latter authors concluded that mild coronal imbalance was well tolerated and did not necessitate distal extension of the fusion in such cases. On the basis of these studies of selected fusion in cases of the MT curve pattern of scoliosis with the most deviated lumbar apices, it appears that apical deviation alone does not dictate structurality. The biggest problem in what is considered a satisfactory result of surgery in such cases varies in the viewpoints of surgeons and patients.

Clements and co-workers[22] reviewed the surgical procedures used for the cases in the HSG database before and after the Lenke classification was developed. The Lenke classification was applied retrospectively to cases treated before 2001, and was found to correctly predict which curves were actually fused in 82% of the cases. After the HSG adopted the use of the Lenke classification, the system predicted the curves actually fused in a significantly greater percentage of cases (88%; $P = 0.001$). Thus, the uniformity of treatment improved with the use of the Lenke classification system, but the system did not completely explain the practice of this group of experienced scoliosis surgeons. "Rule-breakers" were defined as patients whose treatment did not follow the recommendations of the Lenke classification system. From 6 to 29% of the time (depending on the curve pattern), other aspects of a patient's clinical and radiographic deformity suggested deviation from the recommended treatment paradigm. From this rule-breaking, it can be concluded that the classification system does not identify the structural lumbar curve in 100% of cases of AIS.

Breaking the "rules" of the Lenke classification system for choosing the minor curves to treat or not to treat in patients with AIS is appropriate; the trick is to know when to break the rules and to understand why they are broken. Being wrong 10% of the time is not good enough when addressing the motion of a child's spine over its lifetime. Puno et al[23] evaluated the usefulness of the Lenke classification system in providing treatment recommendations for idiopathic scoliosis. They compared the postoperative Cobb-angle correction and truncal shift in patients who were either treated or not treated according to the Lenke classification system, and reported better radiographic results when the Lenke classification system was used to select fusion levels with avoidance of the unnecessary fusion of nonstructural lumbar or thoracic curves and avoidance of the undercorrection of structural secondary curves. However, the distinction between different types of curves in the Lenke classification can be difficult (i.e., types 1C, 3C, and 6C curves with large thoracic and large thoracolumbar/lumbar [TL/L] spinal deformities), and can influence treatment decisions. Differentiation of these types of curves according to the Lenke classification system is based on arbitrary values for the magnitude and flexibility of the TL spine, and does not address 3D and clinical aspects of deformity.

Not surprisingly, the debate about when to include the lumbar curve in the fusion levels in cases of Lenke types 1C and 3C curves is most controversial (**Fig. 17.7**). In 1992, Lenke and co-workiers[24] described strict criteria for preventing lumbar decompensation in the performance of selective thoracic fusion. The rules were based on ratios of the magnitudes of the thoracic and lumbar Cobb angles,

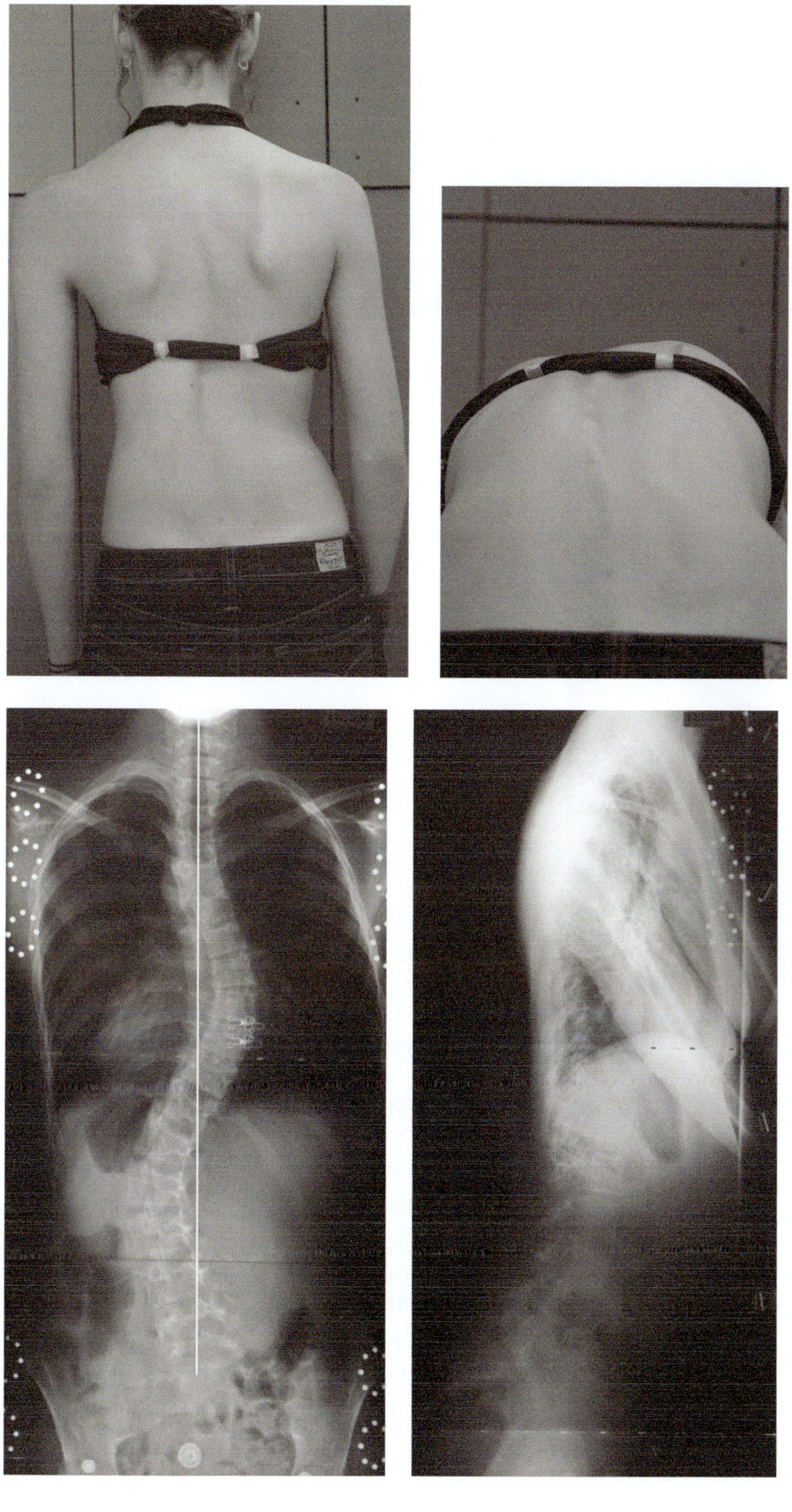

A B C D

**Fig. 17.7** **(A,B)** Preoperative PA and forward-bending clinical photographs and **(C,D)** PA and lateral radiographs of a 14-year-old girl demonstrate a 49-degree thoracic and 44-degree thoracolumbar curve (Lenke type 1C deformity). The thoracic curve bends to 17 degrees (65% flexibility) and the lumbar curve bends to 13 degrees (70% flexibility). Nonselective posterior spinal instrumentation and fusion with segmental pedicle screws from T5 to L4 was done in this case because of the large apical (L2) deviation of the lumbar curve from the CSVL (4.0 cm), large preoperative clinical lumbar prominence (17 degrees), and low ratio of the thoracic-to-lumbar curve magnitude (1.1).

(*Continued on page 208*)

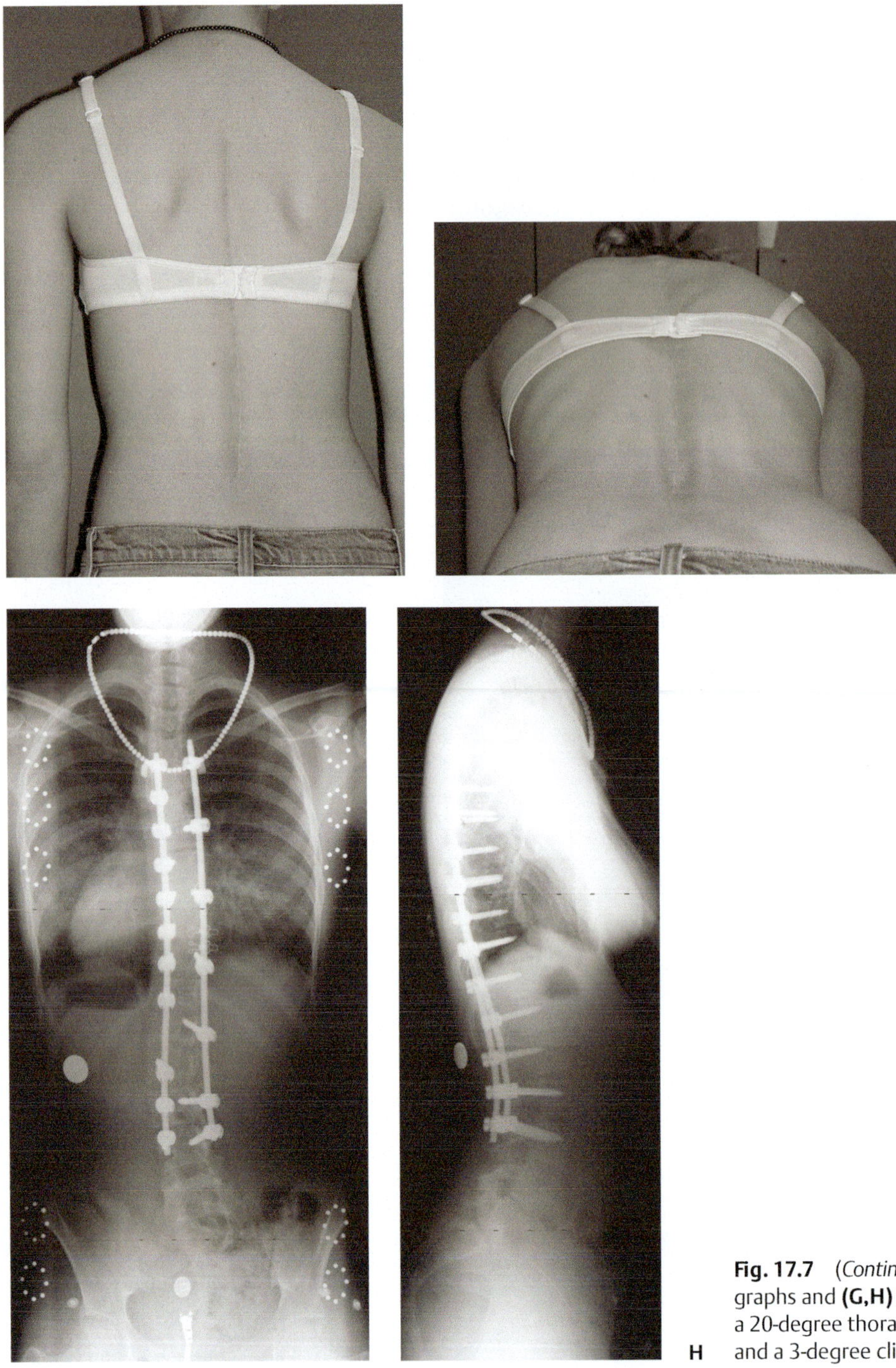

E F G H

**Fig. 17.7** *(Continued)* **(E,F)** Postoperative clinical photographs and **(G,H)** PA and lateral radiographs demonstrate a 20-degree thoracic and 19-degree thoracolumbar curve, and a 3-degree clinical lumbar prominence.

apical vertebral deviation from the midline, and apical vertebral rotation on the standing coronal radiograph. Despite these guidelines, a review by Newton et al[25] of the frequency with which surgeons in the HSG included the lumbar curve in fusion in cases of Lenke types 1B and 1C curves found a substantial variation in the frequency of nonselective fusion into the lumbar curve (6 to 33%). Excluding cases of junctional kyphosis, the lumbar curve was included in the fusion for Lenke type 1B curves in only a few cases (2%). However, the incidence of inclusion of the lumbar spine in fusions of Lenke 1C curves varied from a low of 6% for one surgeon to a high of 67% for another. Disparity of this magnitude suggests a void in the knowledge base about the current definition of the structural lumbar curve. Factors associated with nonselective fusion in Newton and colleagues' review included a lumbar curve of larger preoperative magnitude (42 ± 10 degrees vs. 37 ± 7 degrees, $P < 0.01$), greater lumbar apical deviation,

(3.1 ± 1.4 cm vs. 2.2 ± 0.8 cm, $P < 0.01$), and a smaller ratio of thoracic-to lumbar-curve magnitude (1.31 ± 0.29 vs. 1.44 ± 0.30, $P = 0.01$). In addition, selective fusions were also performed if the trunk and chest wall were clinically more prominent than the corresponding features of the lumbar spine on examination in both the upright and forward-bending positions.

The concept underlying the initial analysis of a patient with a Lenke type 1 curve should be to fuse only the thoracic curve. With this approach the surgeon seeks a reason to include the lumbar spine in the fusion rather than a reason not to do so. One of the predictors of success of a selective thoracic fusion is a preoperative thoracic Cobb-angle to lumbar Cobb-angle ratio >1.2. Similarly, if the preoperative thoracic apical translation from the C7 plumbline is at least 1.2 times the lumbar apical translation from the CSVL, a selective thoracic correction will probably be acceptable.[20] Ratios of relative rotation can also be considered, but when based on plain radiography will yield a less reliable assessment of axial deformity. Lastly, relative clinical deformity continues to be one of the most useful determinants of success in fusion surgery. The outcome of a selective thoracic fusion will not be favorable if the clinical deformity associated with the lumbar curve is more severe than that of the thoracic curve.

If a selective thoracic fusion for a Lenke 1C curve is attempted and the patient's spine decompensates to the left, the opportunity exists to add the lumbar spine to corrective surgery at any time in the future. If the surgeon "plays it safe" and includes the lumbar spine unnecessarily, the patient may be predisposed to a greater risk of lumbar degenerative disease that might have been avoided. At some point the contrary argument can be made, that in the long term, a large residual lumbar deformity would be better fused but straight. The degree of lumbar deformity with intact motion that in the long term would yield the best outcome if treated by fusion at an early point is ill-defined and undetermined. Even the strongest proponents of preserving motion in the lumbar region would in most cases prefer lumbar curves of <40 degrees after selective thoracic fusion.

The balance between maximizing correction and maintaining lumbar motion is critical. A recent study[26] defined values for quantifying this postoperatively. The deformity–flexibility quotient (DFQ) consists of the postoperative residual lumbar deformity divided by the number of unfused motion segments (**Fig. 17.8**). All other aspects being equal, a lower DFQ implies a better outcome (less deformity and more motion). This concept has been validated in two ways within the HSG.

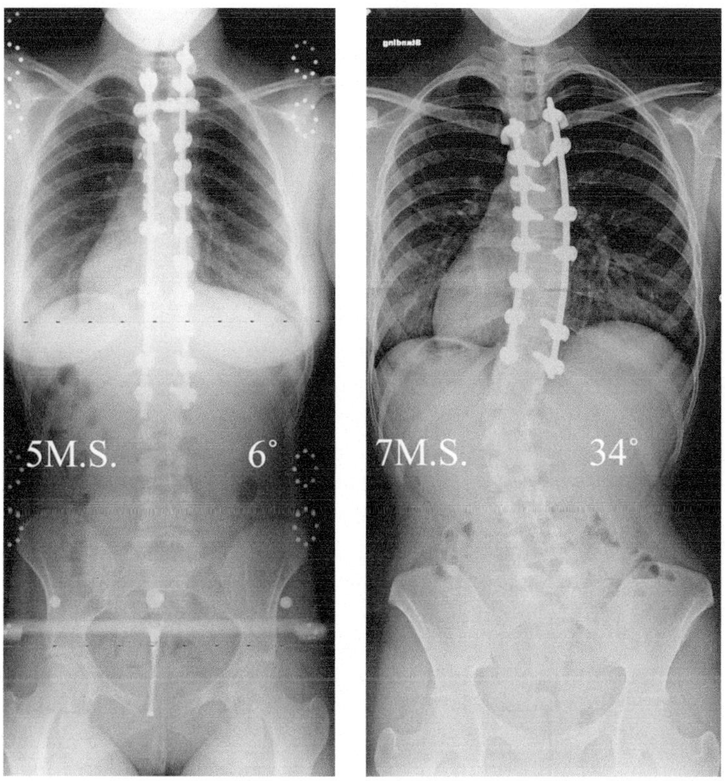


A B

**Fig. 17.8** Two-year postoperative PA radiographs of patients with four different deformity-flexibility quotients (DFQ = residual lumbar deformity divided by number of unfused motion segments). **(A)** A 6-degree curve divided by 5 motion segments yields a DFQ of 1.2. **(B)** A 34-degree curve divided by 7 motion segments yields a DFQ of 4.9.

*(Continued on page 210)*

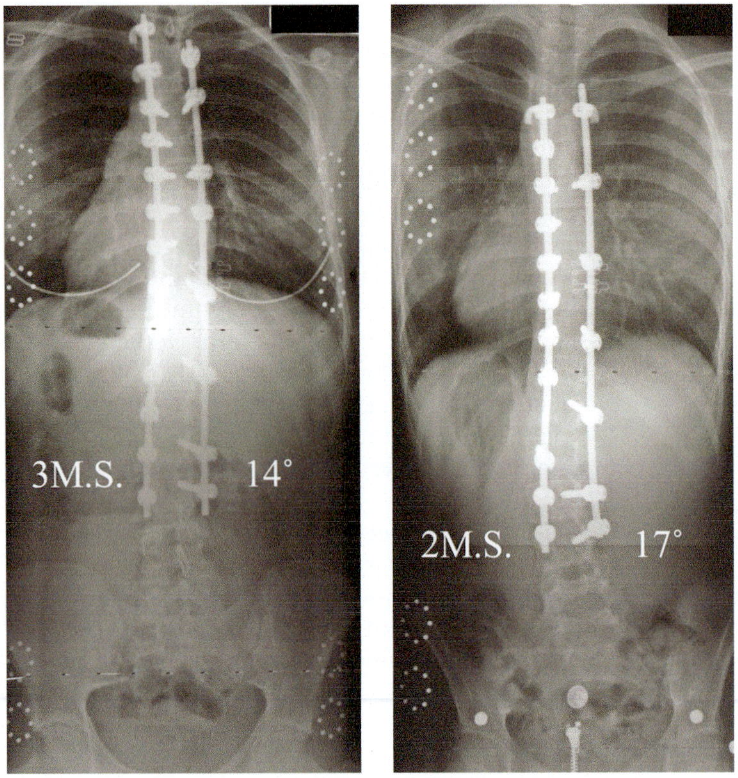


C D

**Fig. 17.8** (*Continued*) Two-year postoperative PA radiographs of patients with four different deformity-flexibility quotients (DFQ = residual lumbar deformity divided by number of unused motion segments). **(C)** A 14-degree curve divided by 3 motion segments yields a DFQ of 4.7. **(D)** A 17-degree curve divided by 2 motion segments yields a DFQ of 8.5.

First, the members of the HSG were asked to compare pairs of postoperative radiographs of varying degrees of lumbar deformity and lowest instrumented vertebrae. Use of the DFQ predicted with high probability those radiographs that the group considered "most ideal." Additionally, the DFQ was calculated retrospectively for 155 AIS patients in the HSG database, and a lower DFQ was statistically correlated with greater satisfaction scores on the SRS-24 instrument at 2 years postoperatively. Following patient outcomes over a longer period is critical to assessing the success of a fusion, and correlating a patient's DFQ with these outcomes may be of future value in deciding whether to do a selective or nonselective fusion.

With this in mind, some idea of the factors that predict spontaneous lumbar curve correction is required in preoperative decision-making. In a recent review of the HSG database, Patel et al[27] found an average 50% spontaneous lumbar-curve correction (SLCC) after selective thoracic fusion. Radiographic features that correlated with the percent SLCC included the level of the LIV, lumbar-curve flexibility, and percent thoracic-curve correction. In no case did the SLCC reach the degree of correction seen on the lumbar bending film, which always exceeded the correction ultimately obtained.

## To What Extent Should the Thoracic Curve Be Corrected for Ideal Balance?

Ideal balance is defined as existing when the head and trunk are centered over the pelvis in the coronal and sagittal planes. If both lumbar and thoracic curves are present in a case of scoliosis, they are generally of similar magnitude when the trunk is coronally balanced. The greater the lumbar curve as compared with the thoracic curve, the greater the risk of decompensation to the left. If the patient's trunk is preoperatively shifted to the left, it is hard to imagine how a selective thoracic fusion could do anything but worsen this; yet in fact this is not always the case. Lumbar-curve correction following selective fusion is not always predictable.

The safest approach to selective thoracic fusion in the treatment of Lenke type 1C curves is to limit the degree of coronal-plane correction of the thoracic curve obtained during surgery. Correcting the thoracic curve to 50% of the magnitude of the preoperative lumbar curve, and assuming an average 50% spontaneous lumbar-curve correction, should limit the risk of decompensation. Intraoperative radiographs can assist in determining the amount of correction. However, this may overestimate the SLCC, because it does not include the effect of gravity. In theory, correction of a thoracic apical lordosis should be maximized because this relieves the torsional pressures that result from relative anterior overgrowth of the spine after fusion, and may in fact improve SLCC. This concept requires further investigation with 3D data sets.

Through the years there have been conflicting data about whether an anterior or a posterior approach yields the greatest SLCC. Early studies suggested more SLCC with an anterior approach. More recent analyses, using third-generation instrumentation, suggest better correction with posterior methods. A comprehensive review of the HSG database, using a multivariate regression analysis, determined that the LIV was important in determining the percent SLCC.[27] Because posterior instrumentation was traditionally longer than that used in anterior procedures, some of the "spontaneous" correction with the use of posterior techniques was in fact to the result of instrumented correction of the upper vertebra of the lumbar curve. When controlling for the LIV, there was no difference in SLCC in 28 cases treated with an anterior approach and 28 matched cases treated with a posterior approach.

The response of the upper thoracic curve to thoracic-curve correction should also be considered. Whether appropriate or not, relatively little value is given to the upper thoracic motion segments in selective fusion. Rather, the trend seems to be to include more of the upper thoracic spine, especially with increasing correction of the MT curve. Suk and colleagues[28] have stated that the upper thoracic curve should be included if the right shoulder is less than 1 cm higher than the left. The upper thoracic spine is one area in which side-bending to <25 degrees does not give enough information about when to include this region in a fusion. It is not clear whether a greater attempt should be made to preserve upper thoracic motion segments, limiting thoracic correction to preserve both balance (of the shoulders) and motion. Some nonstructural upper thoracic curves should be treated. Management strategies for these curves can be found in the discussion of Lenke type 2 curves in Chapter 18.

## What Levels Should Be Included in the Fusion?

After the curves to be instrumented have been chosen in planning a selective fusion, selection of the precise upper and lower limits for fusion of a given curve remains a major challenge. There is often disagreement about this among surgeons; the most appropriate levels may depend on the surgeon and the surgeon's particular techniques of correction. As previously discussed, there are two patterns of right thoracic curves, those with a lumbar curve (Lenke types 1AL, 1B, and 1C) and those without a true lumbar curve (Lenke type 1AR). We believe that these two patterns require different rules for selecting the vertebral levels for caudal fusion.

For the more common thoracic curves with an accompanying minor lumbar curve, the LIV is chosen as the stable vertebra[29,30] of the thoracic curve, and is generally between T11 and L1 (**Fig. 17.3**). The concern with these types of curves is extending fusion more distally than the stable vertebra, which increases the risk of decompensation to the left. In contrast, for Lenke type 1AR curves, the LIV is selected as the most proximal lumbar vertebra that is substantially "touched" by the CSVL (**Fig. 17.1**). This is generally one to two levels proximal to the stable vertebra, most frequently at L2 and L3, and always at or distal to the end-vertebra. Thus, in all cases the entire measured Cobb angle should be included in the instrumentation. These rules are applied to posterior instrumentation with pedicle screw implants at the distal extent. For anterior constructs, the levels fused are the levels included in the Cobb angle, with the exception that if there is a parallel disc at the distal end of the curve, the level below the parallel disc should also be included (**Fig. 17.9**).

As mentioned earlier, the selection of the distal level of fusion remains controversial. Suk et al evaluated the relationship of the LIV to the neutral vertebra. Their facility reviewed 42 patients with major thoracic curves who were followed for a minimum of 2 years after fusion. When the end-vertebra of the Cobb angle and the neutral vertebra were within two levels of each other, they recommended fusing to the neutral vertebra. However, when the neutral vertebra was more than two levels from the end-vertebra, fusion extending to the neutral vertebra-1 was recommended. In cases in which the fusion was extended to neutral vertebra-2, unsatisfactory results were more frequent. Unsatisfactory results were described as a truncal shift of >2.0 cm, decompensation, or extension of the primary curvature (adding on).

In determining fusion levels, it is also important to consider any sagittal deformity. Consideration should be given to crossing a TL junctional kyphosis >10 to 15 degrees. Similarly, the occasional globally hyperkyphotic patient may require a more distally extensive fusion to L2 or L3, resembling what is done in a patient with Scheuermann's kyphosis. Choosing the proximal extent of fusion is also controversial, and is often less emphasized than choosing the distal level. However, given the frequency of proximal junctional kyphosis and shoulder imbalance in scoliosis, the importance of this decision should not be underestimated. Certainly the proximal end-vertebra should be included in the fusion. However, the appropriate levels to include above the proximal end-vertebra depend on the degree of planned correction of the MT curve, preoperative shoulder balance, and proximal sagittal alignment. When the right shoulder is elevated preoperatively and correction of the thoracic curve will be limited (to preserve balance with a lumbar curve), the upper instrumented vertebra may be safely chosen as the uppermost level of the Cobb

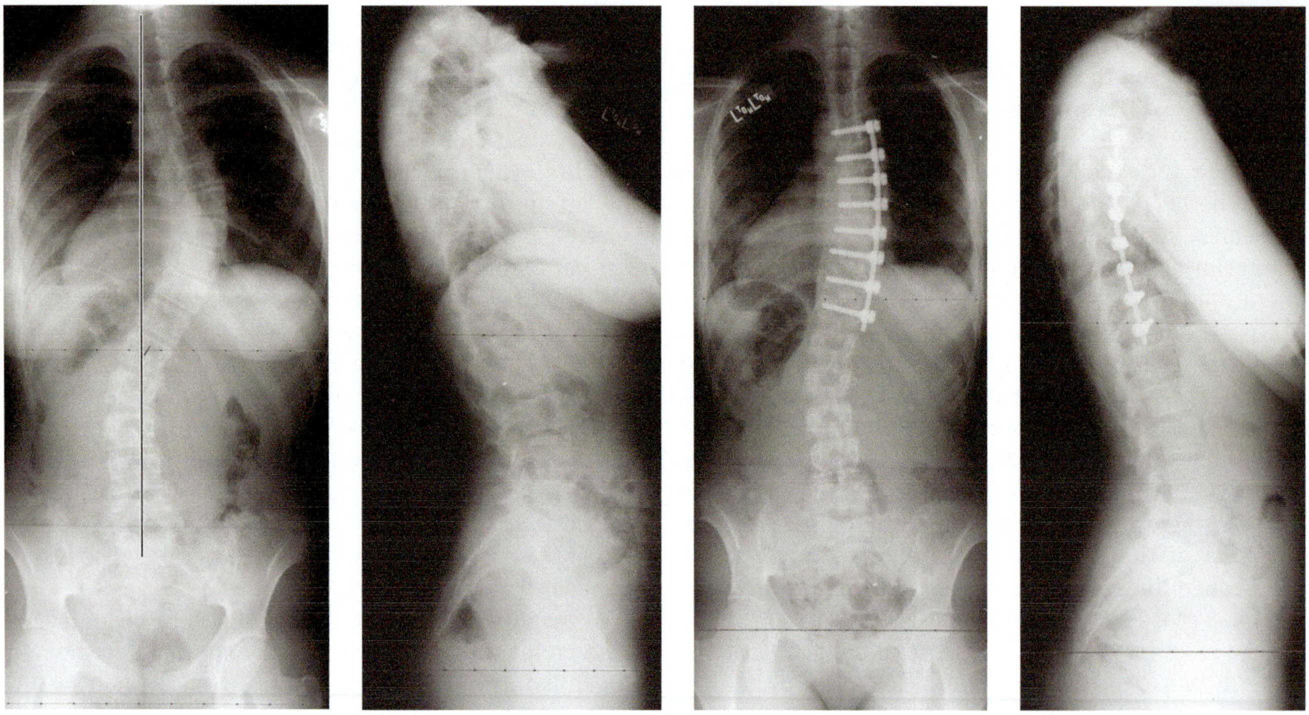

A–D

**Fig. 17.9** **(A,B)** Preoperative PA and lateral radiographs of a 15-year-old girl demonstrate a 51-degree thoracic and 32-degree thoracolumbar curve (Lenke type 1B deformity). Thoracoscopic anterior spinal instrumentation and fusion from T5 to T12 was done in this case because the thoracic curve had a preoperative flexibility of 53% (reducing to 24-degrees on the right-bending film) and the entire thoracic region comprising the Cobb angle could be instrumented without entering the lumbar spine. **(C,D)** Postoperative PA and lateral radiographs demonstrate a well-balanced 22-degree thoracic and 19-degree thoracolumbar curve.

angle. Level shoulders preoperatively require inclusion of some portion of the PT curve to limit postoperative left-shoulder elevation. Similarly, patients with preoperative left-shoulder elevation will have even greater shoulder asymmetry if most of the PT curve is not instrumented. These concepts apply when maintaining shoulder balance is a surgical goal, and are discussed in further detail in Chapter 18. The "physiological cost" of fusion in this region of the spine is poorly understood.

## What Is the Best Approach?

In general, the spine can be fused from either an anterior or a posterior approach or both. Three surgical options exist for Lenke type 1 curves: (1) open anterior spinal fusion (OASF); (2) thoracoscopic anterior spinal fusion (TASF); and (3) posterior spinal fusion (PSF). Several years ago the HSG began a prospective study designed to identify the optimal surgical approach for Lenke type 1 curves (unpublished HSG data, 2008). As of February 2008, 188 patients (28 OASF; 63 TASF; 97 PSF) had been enrolled in this study at eight spinal-deformity treatment centers in Europe and North America. Most of the enrolled patients (98/ of 188, or 52%) had a Lenke type 1A spinal deformity. Another 52 patients (28%) had a Lenke type 1B deformity, and 38 patients (20%) had a Lenke type 1C deformity. As of this writing,143 patients (76%) had had at least a 2-year follow-up and 171 patients (91%) at least a 1-year follow-up.

Selected radiographic parameters for the patients with a 2-year follow-up are shown in **Table 17.2**. The average magnitude of the thoracic curve decreased for the entire cohort from a preoperative value of 50.6 ± 8.1 degrees to a 2-year postoperative value of 17.7 ± 8.5 degrees (an average maintained correction of 65%), without any significant differences in the percent correction maintained at 2 years among curves treated with the three surgical approaches ($P = 0.29$). Of note is that patients in the PSF group had a significantly smaller thoracic kyphosis at 2 years postoperatively (19.5 ± 8.1 degrees) than did patients in the OASF or TASF groups (25.5 ± 12.1 degrees and 25.3 ± 9.4 degrees, respectively) ($P = 0.003$). Patients who underwent an anterior procedure tended to have a more hypokyphotic spine preoperatively and gained ~7 degrees of kyphosis postoperatively. On the other hand, patients who underwent a posterior procedure were more kyphotic preoperatively (23.1 ± 13.1 degrees) and lost ~4 degrees of kyphosis postoperatively. Although these decreases in the post-versus preoperative difference in thoracic kyphosis seem minor, evaluation of the cervical spine for loss of cervical lordosis, even in cases of kyphosis with thoracic

**Table 17.2 Preoperative and 2-Year Postoperative Radiographic Outcomes for the Three Surgical Approach Options for Patients with Lenke Type 1 Curves**

| | APPROACH | | | |
|---|---|---|---|---|
| | Open Anterior | Thoracoscopic Anterior | Posterior | *P*-value |
| *n* | 21 | 48 | 74 | |
| Preoperative thoracic Cobb angle | 49.5 ± 5.3° | 51.0 ± 8.9° | 50.7 ± 8.3° | 0.75 |
| 2-Year postoperative thoracic Cobb angle | 14.9 ± 7.5° | 18.6 ± 7.7° | 18.1 ± 9.5° | 0.21 |
| Preoperative thoracolumbar Cobb angle | 30.6 ± 7.4° | 33.5 ± 9.0° | 30.7 ± 10.6° | 0.26 |
| 2-Year postoperative thoracic Cobb angle | 14.9 ± 7.5° | 18.6 ± 7.7° | 18.1 ± 9.5° | 0.21 |
| Preoperative thoracic kyphosis | 19.7 ± 9.7° | 18.3 ± 10.8° | 23.1 ± 13.1° | 0.11 |
| 2-Year postoperative thoracic kyphosis | 25.5 ± 12.1° | 25.3 ± 9.4° | 19.5 ± 8.1° | **0.003** |
| Preoperative lumbar lordosis | 57.5 ± 9.4° | 60.0 ± 13.0° | 61.3 ± 13.4° | 0.49 |
| 2-Year postoperative lumbar lordosis | 64.4 ± 10.2° | 62.1 ± 11.8° | 57.2 ± 12.0° | **0.03** |
| Preoperative thoracic apical translation | 3.7 ± 2.8 cm | 4.1 ± 2.2 cm | 4.2 ± 3.0 cm | 0.76 |
| 2-Year postoperative thoracic apical translation | 1.0 ± 1.5 cm | 0.7 ± 1.4 cm | 1.0 ± 1.5 cm | 0.54 |
| Percent correction aintained | 69.8 ±15.6% | 63.8 ± 13.3% | 64.3 ± 18.3% | 0.29 |
| 2-Year postoperative lumbar Cobb angle | 11.6 ± 7.9° | 16.6 ± 10.3° | 12.6 ± 8.3° | 0.08 |
| 2-Year postoperative lumbar lordosis | 64.4 ± 10.2° | 62.1 ± 11.8° | 57.2 ± 12.0° | **0.03** |

**Boldface type** indicates that this value is statistically significant ($p < 0.05$).

hypokyphosis, may indicate long-term junctional outcomes. Consequentially, patients in the PSF group also had a significantly smaller 2-year postoperative lumbar lordosis (57.2 ± 12.0 degrees) than did patients in the OASF or TASF groups (64.4 ± 10.2 degrees and 62.1 ± 11.8 degrees, respectively; $P = 0.03$).

Scores on the SRS-24 questionnaire for 95 patients at 2-years of follow-up are shown in **Table 17.3**. Scores in all

**Table 17.3 Preoperative and 2-Year Postoperative Scores on the Scoliosis Research Society-24 Questionnaire for the Three Surgical Approach Options in Patients with Lenke Type 1 Curves**

| | | APPROACH | | | |
|---|---|---|---|---|---|
| | | Open Anterior | Thoracoscopic Anterior | Posterior | *P*- value |
| | *n* | 19 | 37 | 39 | |
| | Pain | 3.9 ± 0.7 | 3.9 ± 0.7 | 3.7 ± 0.6 | 0.33 |
| | General self- image | 3.8 ± 0.7 | 3.8 ± 0.8 | 3.7 ± 0.8 | 0.84 |
| **Preoperative Score** | General function | 4.0 ± 0.7 | 4.0 ± 0.7 | 3.9 ± 0.5 | 0.91 |
| | Level of activity | 4.3 ± 0.8 | 4.5 ± 0.7 | 4.6 ± 0.7 | 0.29 |
| | Total | 4.0 ± 0.6 | 4.0 ± 0.6 | 3.9 ± 0.5 | 0.63 |
| | Pain | 4.4 ± 0.4 | 4.4 ± 0.5 | 4.3 ± 0.5 | 0.68 |
| | General self-image | 4.2 ± 0.8 | 4.2 ± 0.7 | 4.4 ± 0.6 | 0.69 |
| | General function | 4.3 ± 0.4 | 4.4 ± 0.4 | 4.2 ± 0.5 | 0.28 |
| | Level of activity | 4.7 ± 0.4 | 4.8 ± 0.4 | 4.7 ± 0.4 | 0.25 |
| **2- Year Postoperative Score** | Self-image after surgery | 3.5 ± 0.6 | 3.5 ± 0.6 | 3.4 ± 0.9 | 0.94 |
| | Function after surgery | 3.1 ± 0.9 | 3.4 ± 0.6 | 2.7 ± 1.3 | **0.01** |
| | Patient satisfaction | 4.5 ± 0.5 | 4.5 ± 0.5 | 4.4 ± 0.6 | 0.48 |
| | Total | 4.2 ± 0.3 | 4.3 ± 0.3 | 4.1 ± 0.4 | 0.29 |

**Table 17.4 Postoperative Time Required for Right Shoulder Function to Return to 80% of Preoperative Value***

| | | APPROACH | | | |
|---|---|---|---|---|---|
| | | **Open Anterior (Weeks)** | **Thoracoscopic Anterior (Weeks)** | **Posterior (Weeks)** | ***P*-value** |
| **Strength** | Flexion | 52 | 6 | 6 | **0.02** |
| | Abduction | 24 | 12 | 6 | **0.001** |
| | Forward flexion | 6 | 6 | 6 | NS |
| **Range of Motion** | Extension | 6 | 1 | 6 | **0.01** |
| | Abduction | 12 | 6 | 6 | **0.003** |

*Patients who underwent an open anterior spinal fusion required a significantly longer time to regain right shoulder strength and range of motion than did patients treated through the other two surgical approaches.

*Abbreviation:* NS, not significant.

four preoperative domains (pain, general self-image, general function, and level of activity) improved significantly from the preoperative to the 2-year postoperative point regardless of surgical approach ($P < 0.05$). At 2-years postoperatively, patients who underwent PSF were noted to have a significantly lower function-after-surgery score on the SRS-24 ($2.7 \pm 1.3$) than patients in the TASF group ($3.4 \pm 0.6$; $P = 0.01$). However, all other 2-year postoperative scores on the SRS-24, including those for patient satisfaction and level of activity, were not significantly different among the three surgical-approach groups.

Measurements of shoulder function (range of motion and strength) were made on all patients enrolled in the HSG study at selected intervals (preoperatively, at discharge [approximately 1 week postoperatively], and at 6 weeks, 3 months, 6 months, 1 year, and 2 years postoperatively).[31] Shoulder range of motion was evaluated in active abduction, forward flexion, and extension, with a goniometer. Shoulder strength was evaluated in forward flexion and abduction with the use of a hand-held digital dynamometer. **Table 17.4** shows the time required for shoulder function to return to 80% of its preoperative value in each of the three surgical-approach groups. The open anterior approach was found to significantly delay the return of shoulder strength (flexion and abduction) and range of motion (abduction) as compared with the posterior and anterior thoracoscopic approaches.

In summary (unpublished HSG data, 2008), all three approaches resulted in similarly satisfactory outcomes for most of these patients undergoing selective thoracic fusion, with specific advantages to each technique. For example, the patients in the PSF group had more vertebral levels fused, yet had the shortest average operative time ($P \leq 0.001$), whereas those in the TASF group had the smallest incisions and the lowest estimated blood loss ($P \leq 0.014$) (**Table 17.5**).

During the time of this prospective study, the use of thoracic pedicle screws became more popular and accepted. This improvement in posterior techniques seems to have swung the pendulum back in favor of posterior methods among many surgeons. Clearly, this has come at some cost to thoracic kyphosis. Old techniques such as distraction and new techniques such as Ponte-type releases are being used to lengthen the posterior spinal column in corrective surgery for scoliosis. Further evaluation is needed to determine whether their use can overcome the lordosing effect of thoracic pedicle screws.

The isolated open anterior approach to fusion in thoracic scoliosis has been nearly abandoned because of its approach-related morbidity in terms of both trunk musculature and pulmonary function. Posterior instrumentation remains the

**Table 17.5 Selected Perioperative Data for the Three Surgical Approach Options Used in Treating Patients with Lenke Type 1 Curves**

| | APPROACH | | | |
|---|---|---|---|---|
| | **Open Anterior** | **Thoracoscopic Anterior** | **Posterior** | ***P*-value** |
| *n* | 28 | 63 | 97 | |
| Levels fused (vertebrae) | $8 \pm 1$ | $7 \pm 1$ | $10 \pm 2$ | $\leq$ **0.001** |
| Surgical time (minutes) | $378 \pm 99$ | $359 \pm 124$ | $227 \pm 82$ | $\leq$ **0.001** |
| Estimated blood loss (mL) | $921 \pm 798$ | $443 \pm 430$ | $877 \pm 856$ | **0.014** |
| Incision length (cm) | $27 \pm 9$ | $11 \pm 3$ | $28 \pm 6$ | $\leq$ **0.001** |

accepted standard, although some surgeons and patients continue to choose thoracoscopic correction in select situations. The thoracoscopic approach remains the least invasive option but continues to make with substantial technical demands. Correction of scoliosis c without a posterior incision is possible but requires more operative time and is associated with a high rate of pseudarthrosis (~5 to 10%), particularly in the earlier phase of a surgeon's learning curve.

## When Is an Anterior Release Indicated?

Traditionally, anterior release and fusion followed by posterior instrumentation has been utilized in treating severe scoliosis (curves ≥70 degrees) to increase curve flexibility and improve the correction of deformity; and in younger patients at risk for developing a crankshaft deformity.[32–36] However, the indications for an anterior release in right thoracic scoliosis have been changing, particularly with the increasing use of pedicle screws in the thoracic spine.

In 2005, Luhmann and co-workers[37] reviewed 84 patients with MT curves of 70 to 100 degrees in a comparison of anterior–posterior spinal fusion (APSF) with purely PSF. They concluded that APSF allowed greater coronal correction than did posterior thoracic hook or hybrid constructs; however, the correction was similar with the use of posterior constructs having only pedicle screws. In terms of postoperative sagittal alignment, no differences were found in the treatment groups. In 2007, Suk and colleagues[38] reported obtaining >60% correction of deformity in AIS and maintenance of the correction at 2 years of follow-up with the use of posterior segmental constructs having only pedicle screws in patients with curves of 70 to 100 degrees. They also found no evidence of the development of crankshaft deformity in immature patients older than 9.8 years, proposing that pedicle screws were better able to control all three columns of the spine than were other anchors as growth continued. Suk and colleagues recommend changing the indications for anterior release to curves ≥110 degrees having a flexibility ≤20% when using segmental pedicle screws.

There is little doubt that thoracic pedicle screws can apply a greater corrective force to the spine in all three planes of motion than can other anchors, and prevent the cardiopulmonary complications of an anterior approach; however, the indication for an anterior release is to some extent based on the desired result. It is simple enough to say that with current posterior methods an anterior release is never required; and in the strict sense this is true. For severe curves, a purely posterior approach will either result in less but still satisfactory correction or be associated with a more aggressive posterior procedure consisting of pedicle subtraction or vertebral resection osteotomies. The ideal treatment should balance the risk of the procedures used with the benefit of the correction achieved.

Although there is clearly support for avoiding an anterior release for many curves that in the past would have been treated with one, it is open to question whether the overall result would in fact be better if an anterior release were used in addition to the powerful posterior techniques now available. The use of an anterior approach should be based on the 3D thoracic deformity that exists in addition to the flexibility of the thoracic curve. Thoracic curves >70 degrees that are associated with severe apical lordosis and an angle of trunk rotation >20 degrees as measured with a scoliometer remain an indication for thoracoscopic anterior release in the view of some surgeons (**Fig. 17.10**).

Beyond the initial learning curve,[39] thoracoscopic procedures for anterior release are associated with little morbidity.

A,B

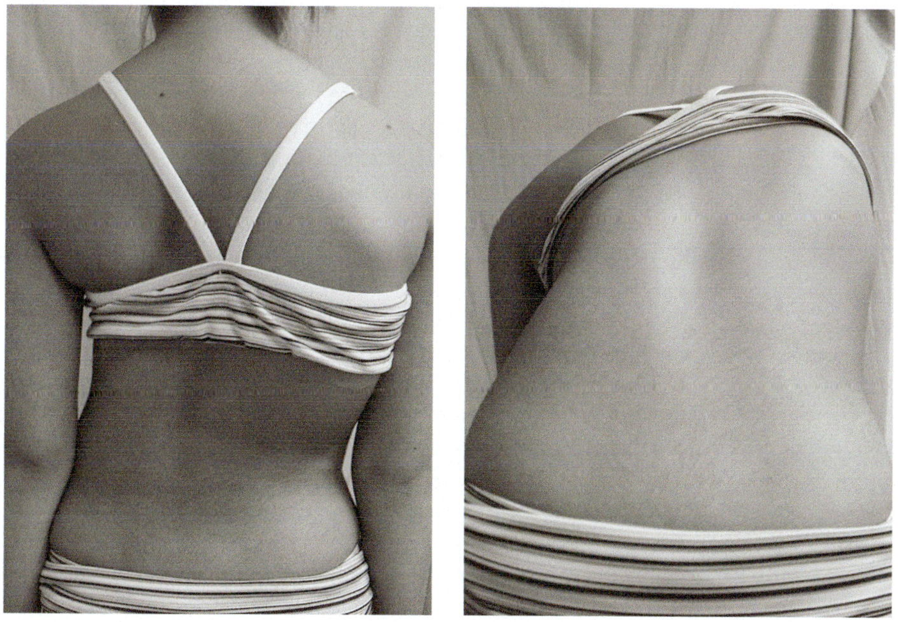

**Fig. 17.10 (A,B)** Preoperative PA and forward-bending clinical photographs.

(*Continued on page 216*)

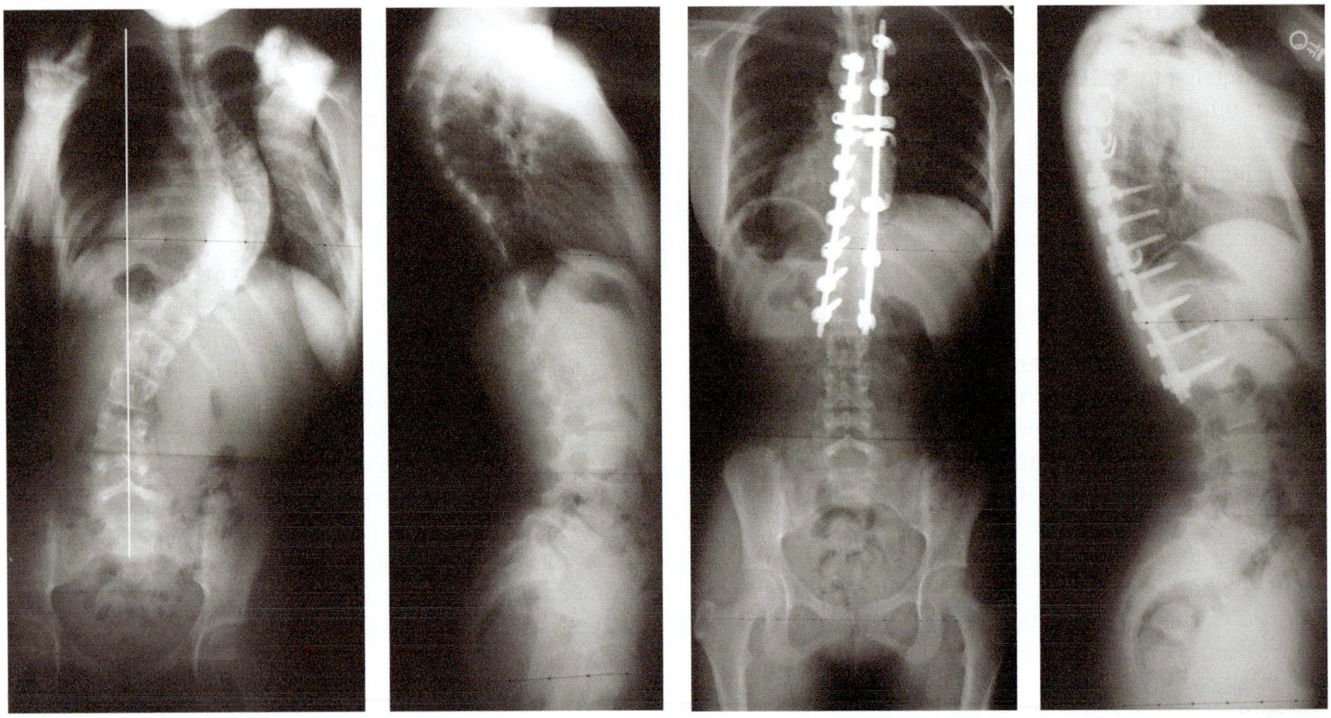

C–F

**Fig. 17.10** (*Continued*) **(C,D)** PA and lateral radiographs of an 11-year-old girl demonstrate a 70-degree thoracic and 45-degree thoracolumbar curve (Lenke type 1AR deformity). The thoracic curve bends to 36 degrees (49% flexibility) and the lumbar curve bends to 14 degrees (69% flexibility). A thoracoscopic anterior release from T5 to T11 was first performed to increase the flexibility of the thoracic curve and address the lordotic thoracic sagittal profile (T5 to T12: 4 degree lordosis). Postoperative PA and lateral radiographs **(E,F)** demonstrate a 15-degree thoracic and 7-degree thoracolumbar curve. Most importantly, the sagittal profile is well restored, with a thoracic kyphosis of 23 degrees.

Disc removal in these cases allows the shortening of the anterior column that is critical in achieving both axial-plane correction and the restoration of thoracic kyphosis, particularly at the apex of the thoracic curve. Derotation in the transverse plane is associated with increasing anterior spinal length. Without an anterior column shortening (by disc excision), and often a posterior apical lengthening (by Ponte-type osteotomies), complete 3D correction of a scoliotic curve is impossible. Ultimately, the decision to include an anterior procedure should be made on a case-by-case basis according to the time, risk, and morbidity entailed by either an open or a thoracoscopic release.

# Surgical Techniques

## Posterior Spinal Instrumentation and Fusion

Posterior instrumentation and fusion is currently the gold standard for the surgical treatment of AIS. Segmental pedicle screws, although more expensive than other anchors, permit significantly better major and minor curve correction, and require a shorter fusion length than do historically used posterior spine implants.[40,41] The exact number of screws required is currently debated. In general, after the fusion levels have been determined, a pedicle screw is placed in every level on the concave side of the deformity. On the convex side, screws are placed in the two most distal and proximal vertebrae and in two or three vertebrae around the apex of the thoracic deformity. Pedicle-screw options include monoaxial, polyaxial, and uniaxial screws. The advantage of each in coronal-, sagittal-, and axial-plane correction is discussed in Chapter 14. Transverse-process hooks can be used at the upper instrumented vertebra with the goal of reducing the soft-tissue exposure required to insert screws at this level and its potential for soft-tissue damage, and to decrease construct stiffness at the proximal junction.

Focusing on the number of pedicle screws required in a fusion procedure is ill advised because this aspect of curve correction, although important, does not define the amount of correction obtained. Increasing apical thoracic kyphosis, while maximizing apical vertebral derotation, is largely determined by the degree of posterior (and anterior) soft-tissue and bone release in the surgical procedure for correcting a deformity. This under-reported feature of the surgical technique for curve correction is likely to have a substantial effect on the global correction achieved. For some surgeons, the use of Ponte-type osteotomies has become standard in the treatment of thoracic scoliosis. The resulting release of the posterior column permits establishment of the relative lengths of the anterior and posterior columns during apical derotation maneuvers. Complete segmental release of the vertebrae allows the posterior column to lengthen with correction.

Rods of varying material properties and diameters afford an array of options, each offering different capacities for the transfer of corrective to the spine. Differential rod contouring is a helpful technique for achieving the 3D correction of a deformity, particularly with regard to apical rotation in the transverse plane (**Fig. 17.11**). In this technique

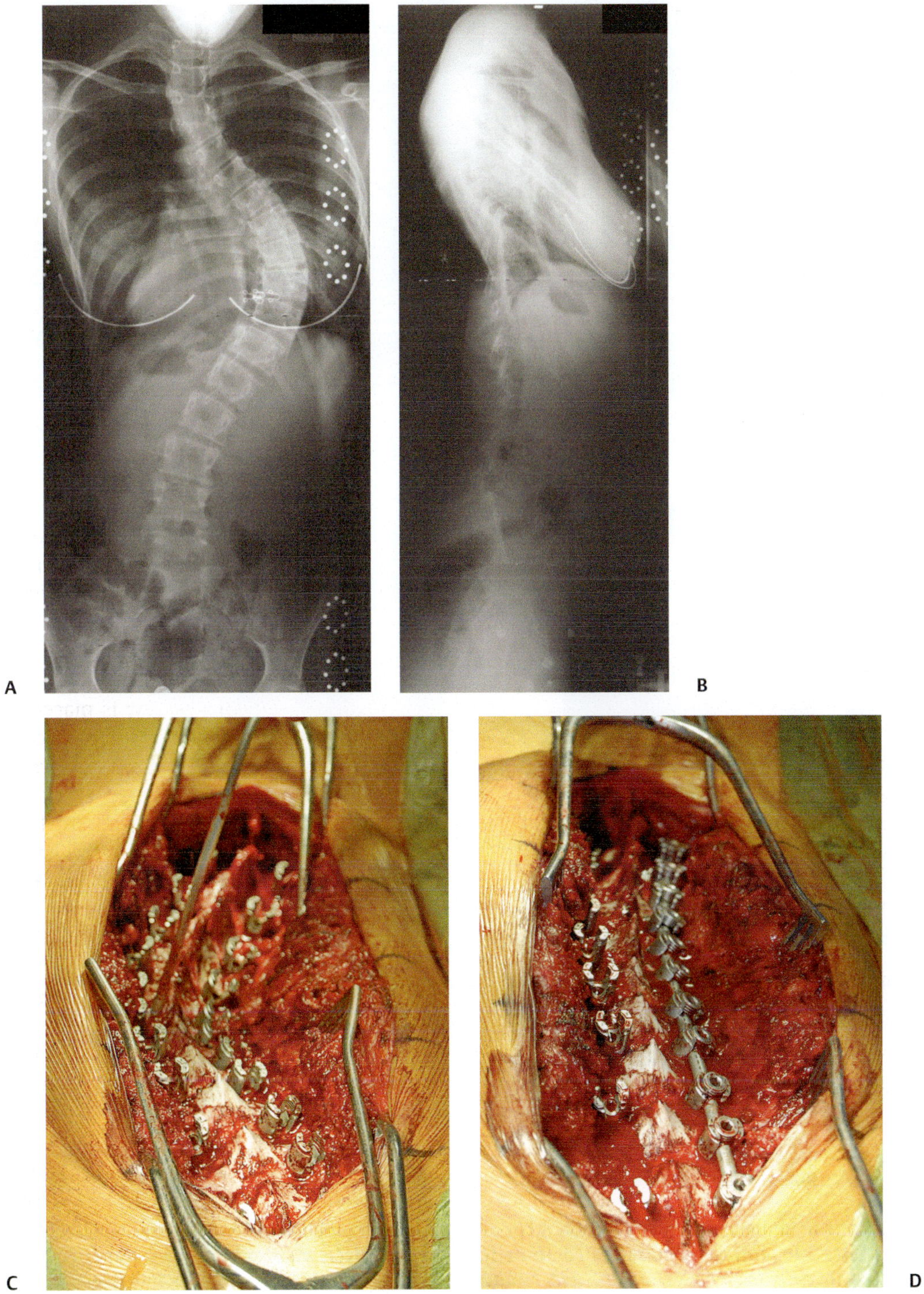

**Fig. 17.11** **(A,B)** Preoperative PA and lateral radiographs of a 15-year-old girl demonstrate a 53-degree thoracic and 29-degree thoracolumbar curve (Lenke type 1AR deformity). L2, the lowest level touched by the CSVL, was selected as the LIV. **(C,D)** Intraoperative photographs of posterior spinal instrumentation and fusion in this case. **(C)** Bilateral pedicle screws are instrumented segmentally. **(D)** The overcontoured (see technique 7 in Chapter 14) concave rod is inserted first and rotated to optimize thoracic kyphosis (although this maneuver tends to extenuate apical vertebral rotation).

(*Continued on page 218*)

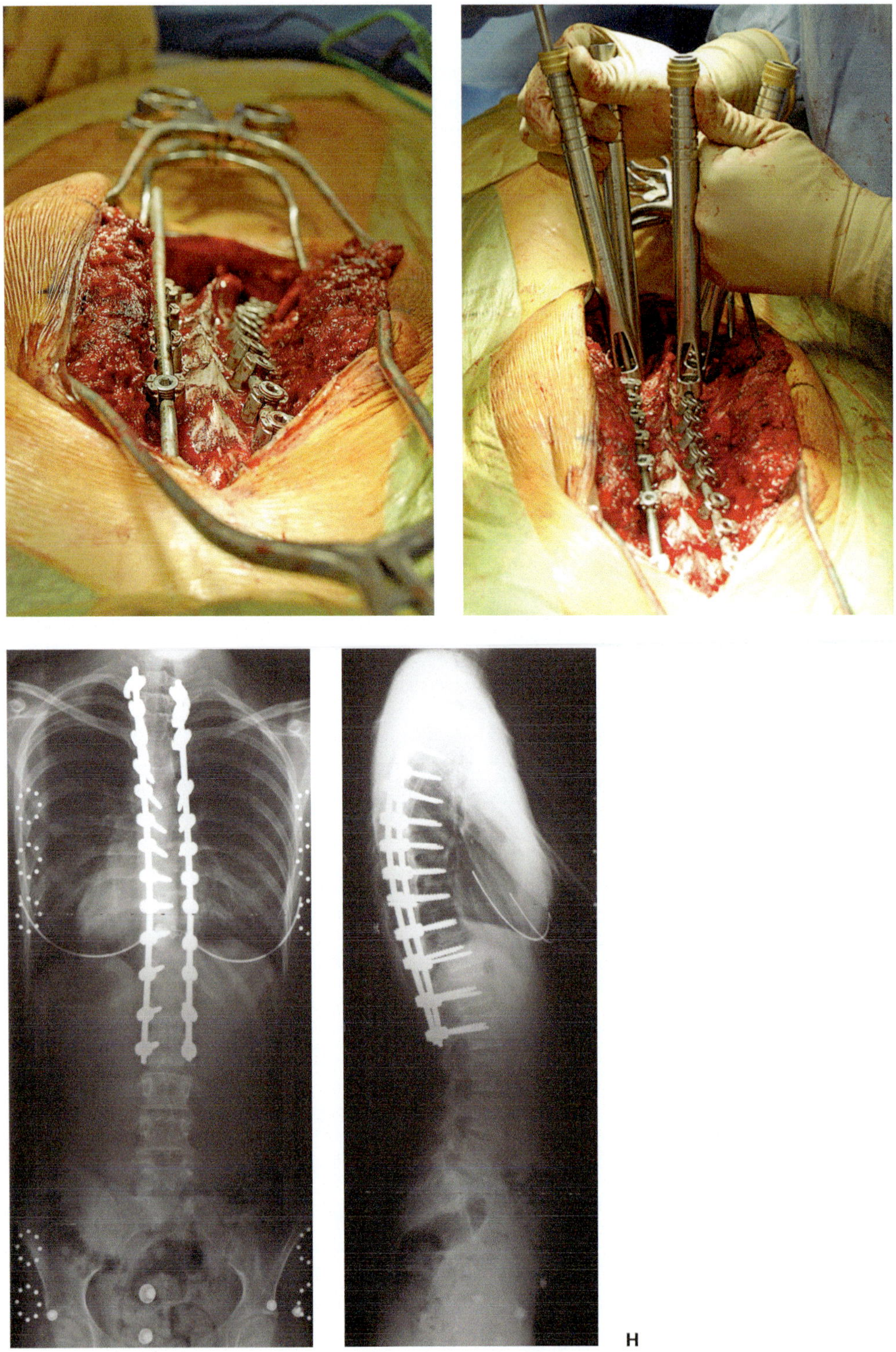

E F

G H

**Fig. 17.11** (*Continued*) **(E)** The second or undercontoured (see technique 7 in Chapter 14) rod is then attached proximally and cantilevered over the convex apex of the thoracic curve, exerting a derotational force at the thoracic apical vertebra. **(F)** The transverse-plane deformity is then addressed further with segmental vertebral derotation, compression/distraction, or both. **(G)** On the lateral postoperative radiograph, the concave (preoperatively overcontoured) rod is now flatter, whereas the convex (preoperatively undercontoured) rod has a greater contour. **(H)** As these rods attempt to return to their preoperative shapes, they will continue to exert a derotational force on the spine.

the concave rod is overcontoured and the convex rod is undercontoured. The concave rod is inserted first and rotated to optimize thoracic kyphosis. It is important to push down on the convex rib hump during the rod-derotation procedure because this can create a torque in the thoracic spine that eases the axial rotational deformity. The convex rod is then inserted into and cantilevered over the apex to affect additional derotation. The neutral vertebra in the lumbar spine is locked and segmental vertebral derotation is performed sequentially in the cephalad direction to optimize the individual axial-plane correction of each vertebra. Selective distraction and compression is used as needed to adjust coronal and sagittal alignment.

## Open Anterior Spinal Instrumentation and Fusion

Open anterior surgical techniques for the correction of spinal deformity were first described in the late 1960s. Current implant systems use rigid single- or dual-rod constructs to achieve spinal realignment and stabilization. Special indications for anterior procedures include patients with decreased kyphosis and the potential to save fusion levels.[42,43] The anterior approach is contraindicated in patients with preoperatively impaired pulmonary function and in those who have comorbidities associated with intrathoracic or intra-abdominal visceral abnormalities.

In the anterior approach, the thoracic spine is most commonly accessed through a single or double anterolateral thoracotomy from the convexity of the thoracic curve. After circumferential exposure of the spine, a thorough discectomy is performed at each subsequent level, with excision of the annulus and the anterior longitudinal ligament (ALL). Visualization of the posterior disc may require resection of the rib head down to the base of the transverse process. The cartilaginous superior and inferior endplates must be completed separated, and the bony endplates should be exposed. Screw placement next to the endplate provides better fixation than screw placement in the traditional midvertebral location.[44] Pronged staples and bicortical screw fixation can be used to increase construct stiffness. Derotation, translation, and compression maneuvers may all be used during rod insertion to correct a deformity. Vertebral body derotation can be achieved either directly by cantilevering of the vertebral screws or by rotating the precontoured rod from scoliosis into the sagittal plane. After tightening of the proximal screws, further coronal correction can be obtained by sequential compression between screws along the convexity of the instrumented curve.

## Thoracoscopic Anterior Spinal Instrumentation and Fusion

In the early 1990s, anterior spinal surgery evolved with the reintroduction of video-assisted thoracoscopy by Regan and Mack and their coworkers.[45,46] In the past decade early experience has been gained with endoscopic techniques for instrumenting the anterior spine through a minimally invasive approach that is less detrimental to pulmonary function and more favorable in terms of postoperative pain and cosmesis.[47–49] Early studies reported high rates of pseudarthrosis, implant failure, and loss of fixation with thoracoscopic anterior procedures,[50–52] but after the initial steep learning curve in this approach was passed,[39,53] comparable results have been reported with thoracoscopic anterior procedures and with alternative spinal surgical techniques.[54–58]

Anterior thoracoscopic techniques are more applicable to the treatment of curves with certain characteristics than to others (**Fig. 17.12**). For example, smaller curves, usually <70 degrees and with more than 50% flexibility, can be

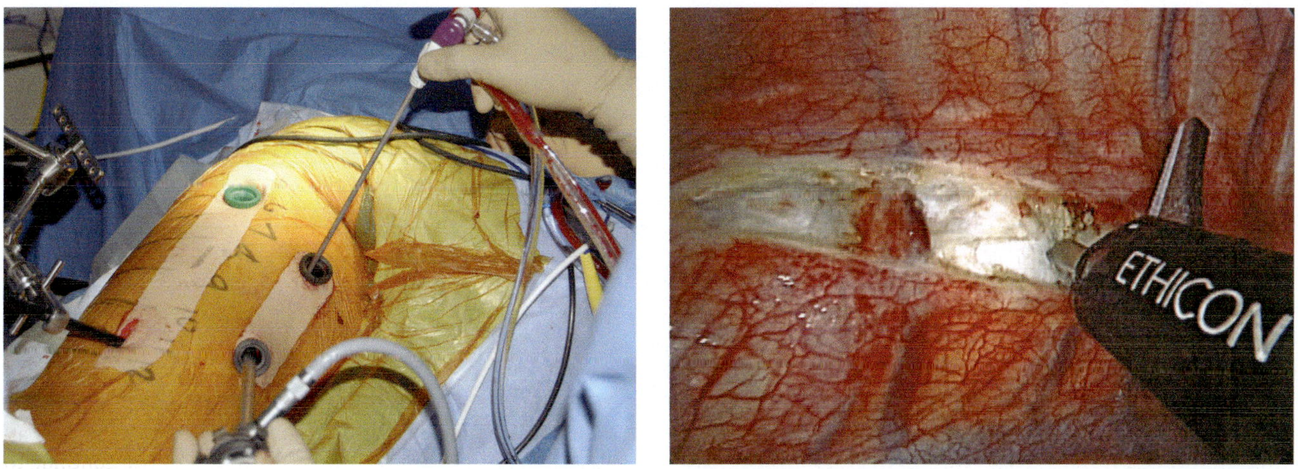


A B

**Fig. 17.12** Intraoperative photographs of thoracoscopic anterior instrumentation and fusion (refer to Fig. 17.9). **(A)** Operating room setup with recommended port placement (two ports along the anterior axillary line and two or three along the posterior axillary line). **(B)** A harmonic scalpel creates a longitudinal opening of the pleura and is used to coagulate the segmental vessels.

(*Continued on page 220*)

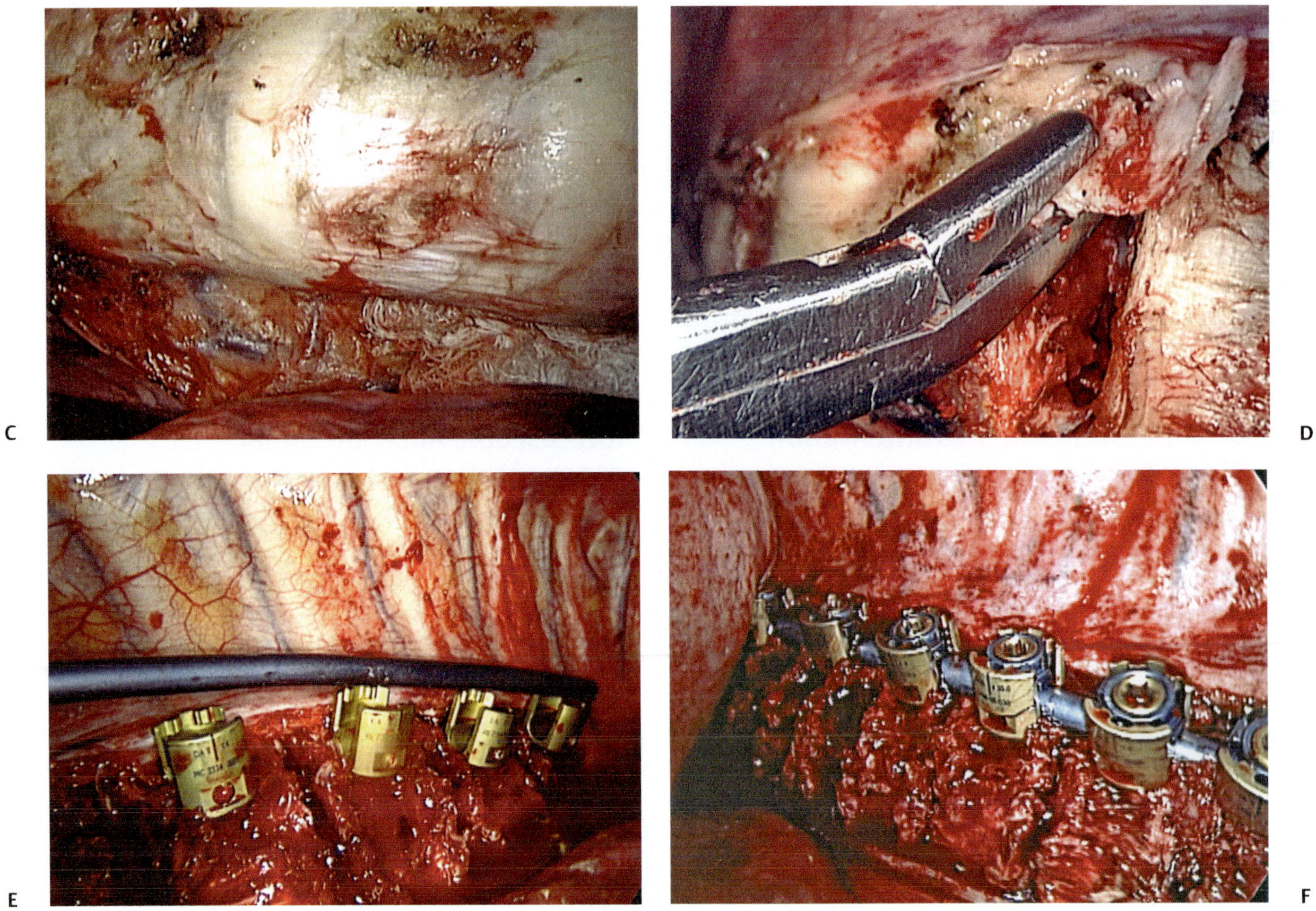

Fig. 17.12 (*Continued*) Intraoperative photographs of thoracoscopic anterior instrumentation and fusion. **(C)** A packing sponge is used to protect adjacent neurovascular structures. **(D)** A complete discectomy is performed and the posterior longitudinal ligament is visualized by opening of the disc space. **(E)** Juxta-endplate screw placement is performed and a precontoured rod is cantilevered into position to obtain of the spinal deformity. **(F)** Completed instrumentation with disc spaces filled with bone graft.

appropriately treated with a single rod–screw construct. The presence of intrathoracic pleural adhesions from prior thoracotomies or pulmonary infections should be considered relative contraindications to anterior thoracoscopic surgery. In addition, even though children weighing less than 30 kg have been safely treated with the anterior thoracoscopic approach, the relative benefit of this minimally invasive technique seems to be reduced in very small patients. A rigid spinal deformity or one that is too closely approximated to the rib cage would also be difficult to treat with an anterior thoracoscopic procedure.[59]

A complete discectomy requires optimal visualization deep into the disc space, ensuring that the integrity of the PLL is maintained and that the neural elements are protected. Each screw used in an anterior thoracoscopic procedure should be started in the mid-aspect of the vertebral body, just anterior to the rib-head articulation, and should achieve bicortical purchase. A tubular plunger device is used to pack the intervertebral spaces with bone graft. Correction of the spinal deformity is accomplished by cantilevering a precontoured rod into position and applying segmental compression after insertion of the rod.

## Summary of Treatment Recommendations

### Lenke Type 1AR Curves

The surgeon should carefully assess the lumbar deformity of Lenke type 1A curves. When L4 tilts to the right the patient is at risk for continued truncal shift to the right postoperatively if the fusion is too short. The distal end-vertebra is often too short in this curve pattern and the LIV should be intersected within the pedicle by the CSVL. When the so-called distal end vertebra touches the CSVL, the result is a moderate tilt below the LIV. It is also important that the disc below the LIV reverse by 5 degrees, in accord with the guidelines established by Cotrel–Dubousset. Posterior instrumentation with segmental pedicle screws offers maximal correction. The goal of complete coronal, sagittal, and axial realignment is often achievable with little risk of decompensation. Thoracoscopic instrumentation is rarely indicated for curves with the Lenke type 1AR pattern because the LIV is often distal to L1 (the last practical level reachable by a thoracoscopic approach).

## Lenke Type 1AL/1B Curves

There is little value in distinguishing curves with a Lenke 1AL or 1B pattern from one another, and both are at little risk of decompensation after a selective thoracic fusion, which should be the treatment in essentially all patients with these curves. Selection of the LIV is based on the stable vertebra at the thoracolumbar junction unless a thoracolumbar kyphosis precludes selection of such a vertebral level. The coronal correction sought may need to be limited to a slight degree for some patients with larger lumbar curves, but postoperative decompensation in these patients is rarely a problem. Posterior constructs are reliable in treating Lenke 1AL or 1B curves, and their use is straightforward, but selected patients with these curves are also amenable to thoracoscopic instrumentation.

## Lenke Type 1C Curves

The vast majority of Lenke type 1C curves are candidates for selective thoracic fusion with the LIV as the stable vertebra at the TL junction. Patients with these curves are at much greater risk for coronal imbalance if the thoracic curve is overcorrected. Leaving deformity in the thoracic and lumbar spine may be the best long-term strategy in treating these curves. However, the lumbar curve in some patients bends to <25 degrees (defining these patients as having a Lenke type 1 as opposed to a Lenke type 3 curve), but these patients still seem to be best treated with a fusion below the lumbar apex (most often to L3). Lumbar rotation and clinical lumbar prominence enter as factors in this assessment when the lumbar curve is >40 degrees, and are unfortunately poorly measured with current 2D radiographic techniques. Advances in the 3D assessment of scoliosis may allow better definition of those patients who are best treated with selective thoracic fusion as opposed to those who require inclusion of the lumbar curve in a fusion.

## Conclusion

The right thoracic curve pattern is common in AIS, but in most cases a reliable outcome of its treatment is achievable with careful preoperative assessment. The Lenke 1C curve remains the most troublesome and controversial scoliotic curve pattern. Balancing the correction of a scoliotic deformity with preservation of motion of the lumbar spine is critical. With more long-term data, the DFQ may help quantify these variables in a given patient and guide treatment decisions about selective versus nonselective fusions in patients with scoliosis.

Posterior instrumentation has over the past decade become the standard for the surgical treatment of nearly all thoracic curves, and pedicle screws seem to be at the root of the change from prior practice, in which anterior instrumentation was more common. Although careful prospective assessment of the thoracoscopic approach suggests that it is a viable option for some patients, it appears to be impractical for the vast majority of surgeons. With similar radiographic and patient-reported outcome measures, the additional operative time and technical challenges of the thoracoscopic approach do not seem to be worth the effort for most patients.

Finally, it is essential to be realistic with regard to the increasing use of purely posterior techniques, even for the most severe thoracic deformities. Aggressive posterior osteotomies and vertebral-column resections have a role in treating scoliosis, but there may be situations in which an anterior release and a simpler posterior procedure may be safer and less morbid for the patient. As spine surgeons strive for the increasing correction of scoliosis, it is necessary to always remember the primary goal of surgery of safely achieving a balanced spinal fusion that will limit the risk of curve progression and late sequelae.

### References


1. King HA, Moe JH, Bradford DS, Winter RB. The selection of fusion levels in thoracic idiopathic scoliosis. J Bone Joint Surg Am 1983; 65:1302–1313
2. Lenke LG, Betz RR, Harms J, et al. Adolescent idiopathic scoliosis: A new classification to determine extent of spinal arthrodesis. J Bone Joint Surg Am 2001;83A:1169–1181
3. Ogon M, Giesinger K, Behensky H, et al. Interobserver and intraobserver reliability of Lenke's new scoliosis classification system. Spine 2002;27:858–862
4. Cummings RJ, Loveless EA, Campbell J, Samelson S, Mazur JM. Interobserver reliability and intraobserver reproducibility of the system of King et al. for the classification of adolescent idiopathic scoliosis. J Bone Joint Surg Am 1998;80:1107–1111
5. Lenke LG, Betz RR, Bridwell KH, et al. Intraobserver and interobserver reliability of the classification of thoracic adolescent idiopathic scoliosis. J Bone Joint Surg Am 1998;80:1097–1106
6. Lenke LG, Betz RR, Haher TR, et al. Multisurgeon assessment of surgical decision-making in adolescent idiopathic scoliosis: Curve

classification, operative approach, and fusion levels. Spine 2001; 26:2347–2353
7. Miyanji FNP, Pawelek JB, Van Valin SE, Upasani VV, Newton PO. Is the lumbar modifier useful in surgical decision making?: Defining two distinct Lenke 1A curve patterns. Spine 2008;33:2545–2551
8. Roaf R. Rotation movements of the spine with special reference to scoliosis. J Bone Joint Surg Br 1958;40B:312–332
9. Somerville EW. Rotational lordosis; the development of single curve. J Bone Joint Surg Br 1952;34B:421–427
10. Dickson RA, Lawton JO, Archer IA, Butt WP. The pathogenesis of idiopathic scoliosis. Biplanar spinal asymmetry. J Bone Joint Surg Br 1984;66:8–15
11. Stagnara P, Queneau P. [Evolutive scoliosis in period of growth: Clinical and radiological aspects, therapeutic suggestions.]. Presse Med 1953;61:1490–1491
12. Perdriolle R, Vidal J. [A study of scoliotic curve. The importance of extension and vertebral rotation (author's transl)]. Rev Chir Orthop Repar Appar Mot 1981;67:25–34
13. Hayashi K, Upasani VV, Pawelek JB, Aubin CE, Labelle H, Lenke LG. Jackson R. Newton PO. Three-dimensional analysis of thoracic sagittal alignment in adolescent idiopathic scoliosis. Spine 2009; 34(8):792–797
14. Weinstein SL. Idiopathic scoliosis. Natural history. Spine 1986; 11:780–783
15. Weinstein SL, Ponseti IV. Curve progression in idiopathic scoliosis. J Bone Joint Surg Am 1983;65:447–455
16. Biondi J, Weiner DS, Bethem D, Reed JF III. Correlation of Risser sign and bone age determination in adolescent idiopathic scoliosis. J Pediatr Orthop 1985;5:697–701
17. Lonstein JE, Carlson JM. The prediction of curve progression in untreated idiopathic scoliosis during growth. J Bone Joint Surg Am 1984;66:1061–1071
18. Peterson LE, Nachemson AL. Prediction of progression of the curve in girls who have adolescent idiopathic scoliosis of moderate severity. Logistic regression analysis based on data from The Brace Study of the Scoliosis Research Society. J Bone Joint Surg Am 1995;77: 823–827
19. Moe JH. A critical analysis of methods of fusion for scoliosis; an evaluation in two hundred and sixty-six patients. J Bone Joint Surg Am 1958;40A:529–554, passim
20. Lenke LG, Edwards CC II, Bridwell KH. The Lenke classification of adolescent idiopathic scoliosis: How it organizes curve patterns as a template to perform selective fusions of the spine. Spine 2003; 28:S199–S207
21. Edwards CC II, Lenke LG, Peelle M, Sides B, Rinella A, Bridwell KH. Selective thoracic fusion for adolescent idiopathic scoliosis with C modifier lumbar curves: 2- to 16-year radiographic and clinical results. Spine 2004;29:536–546
22. Clements D, Marks M, Newton P, et al. Analysis of adherence to Lenke classification treatment alogrithm recommendations. Paper presented at:13th International Meeting on Advanced Spine Techniques, July 12–15, 2006, Athens, Greece
23. Puno RM, An KC, Puno RL, Jacob A, Chung SS. Treatment recommendations for idiopathic scoliosis: An assessment of the Lenke classification. Spine 2003;28:2102–2114, discussion 2114–2115
24. Lenke LG, Bridwell KH, Baldus C, Blanke K. Preventing decompensation in King type II curves treated with Cotrel-Dubousset instrumentation. Strict guidelines for selective thoracic fusion. Spine 1992;17(8, Suppl):S274–S281
25. Newton PO, Faro FD, Lenke LG, et al. Factors involved in the decision to perform a selective versus nonselective fusion of Lenke 1B and 1C (King-Moe II) curves in adolescent idiopathic scoliosis. Spine 2003;28:S217–S223
26. Patel P, Upasani V, Bastrom T, et al. Spontaneous lumbar curve correction in selective thoracic fusions of idiopathic scoliosis. A comparison of anterior and posterior approaches. Paper presented at: 74th American Academy of Orthopedic Surgeons Annual Meeting, February 14–18, 2007, San Diego, CA
27. Newton PO, Upasani VV, Bastrom TP, Marks MC. The deformity-flexibility quotient predicts both patient satisfaction and surgeon preferance in the treatment of Lenke 1B or 1C curves for adolescent idiopathic scoliosis. Spine 2009;34(10):1032–9
28. Suk SI, Kim WJ, Lee CS, et al. Indications of proximal thoracic curve fusion in thoracic adolescent idiopathic scoliosis: Recognition and treatment of double thoracic curve pattern in adolescent idiopathic scoliosis treated with segmental instrumentation. Spine 2000;25: 2342–2349
29. Lenke LG, Bridwell KH, Baldus C, Blanke K, Schoenecker PL. Ability of Cotrel-Dubousset instrumentation to preserve distal lumbar motion segments in adolescent idiopathic scoliosis. J Spinal Disord 1993;6:339–350
30. Lenke LG, Bridwell KH, Blanke K, Baldus C, Weston J. Radiographic results of arthrodesis with Cotrel-Dubousset instrumentation for the treatment of adolescent idiopathic scoliosis. A five to ten-year follow-up study. J Bone Joint Surg Am 1998;80:807–814
31. Ritzman T, Upasani VV, Bastrom T, Pawelek J, Betz R, Newton PO. Return of shoulder girdle function after anterior versus posterior adolescent idiopathic scoliosis surgery. Paper presented at: 42nd Annual Meeting of the Scoliosis Research Society, Edinburgh, Scotland, September 5–8, 2007
32. De Giorgi G, Stella G, Becchetti S, Martucci G, Miscioscia D. Cotrel-Dubousset instrumentation for the treatment of severe scoliosis. Eur Spine J 1999;8:8–15
33. Lenke LG. Anterior endoscopic discectomy and fusion for adolescent idiopathic scoliosis. Spine 2003;28(15, suppl):S36–S43
34. Newton PO, White KK, Faro F, Gaynor T. The success of thoracoscopic anterior fusion in a consecutive series of 112 pediatric spinal deformity cases. Spine 2005;30:392–398
35. Niemeyer T, Freeman BJ, Grevitt MP, Webb JK. Anterior thoracoscopic surgery followed by posterior instrumentation and fusion in spinal deformity. Eur Spine J 2000;9:499–504
36. Upasani VV, Newton PO. Anterior and thoracoscopic scoliosis surgery for idiopathic scoliosis. Orthop Clin North Am 2007;38: 531–540, vi vi
37. Luhmann SJ, Lenke LG, Kim YJ, Bridwell KH, Schootman M. Thoracic adolescent idiopathic scoliosis curves between 70 degrees and 100 degrees: Is anterior release necessary? Spine 2005;30: 2061–2067
38. Suk SI, Kim JH, Cho KJ, Kim SS, Lee JJ, Han YT. Is anterior release necessary in severe scoliosis treated by posterior segmental pedicle screw fixation? Eur Spine J 2007;16:1359–1365
39. Newton PO, Shea KG, Granlund KF. Defining the pediatric spinal thoracoscopy learning curve: Sixty-five consecutive cases. Spine 2000;25:1028–1035
40. Kim YJ, Lenke LG, Cho SK, Bridwell KH, Sides B, Blanke K. Comparative analysis of pedicle screw versus hook instrumentation in posterior spinal fusion of adolescent idiopathic scoliosis. Spine 2004; 29:2040–2048

41. Kim YJ, Lenke LG, Kim J, et al. Comparative analysis of pedicle screw versus hybrid instrumentation in posterior spinal fusion of adolescent idiopathic scoliosis. Spine 2006;31:291–298
42. Sweet FA, Lenke LG, Bridwell KH, Blanke KM. Maintaining lumbar lordosis with anterior single solid-rod instrumentation in thoracolumbar and lumbar adolescent idiopathic scoliosis. Spine 1999;24:1655–1662
43. Sweet FA, Lenke LG, Bridwell KH, Blanke KM, Whorton J. Prospective radiographic and clinical outcomes and complications of single solid rod instrumented anterior spinal fusion in adolescent idiopathic scoliosis. Spine 2001;26:1956–1965
44. Horton WC, Blackstock SF, Norman JT, Hill CS, Feiertag MA, Hutton WC. Strength of fixation of anterior vertebral body screws. Spine 1996;21:439–444
45. Mack MJ, Regan JJ, Bobechko WP, Acuff TE. Application of thoracoscopy for diseases of the spine. Ann Thorac Surg 1993;56: 736–738
46. Regan JJ, Mack MJ, Picetti GD III. A technical report on video-assisted thoracoscopy in thoracic spinal surgery. Preliminary description. Spine 1995;20:831–837
47. Landreneau RJ, Hazelrigg SR, Mack MJ, et al. Postoperative pain-related morbidity: Video-assisted thoracic surgery versus thoracotomy. Ann Thorac Surg 1993;56:1285–1289
48. Landreneau RJ, Wiechmann RJ, Hazelrigg SR, Mack MJ, Keenan RJ, Ferson PF. Effect of minimally invasive thoracic surgical approaches on acute and chronic postoperative pain. Chest Surg Clin N Am 1998;8:891–906
49. Newton PO. The use of video-assisted thoracoscopic surgery in the treatment of adolescent idiopathic scoliosis. Instr Course Lect 2005;54:551–558
50. Picetti GD III, Ertl JP, Bueff HU. Endoscopic instrumentation, correction, and fusion of idiopathic scoliosis. Spine J 2001;1:190–197
51. Picetti GD III, Pang D, Bueff HU. Thoracoscopic techniques for the treatment of scoliosis: Early results in procedure development. Neurosurgery 2002;51:978–984, discussion 984
52. Sucato DJ. Thoracoscopic anterior instrumentation and fusion for idiopathic scoliosis. J Am Acad Orthop Surg 2003;11:221–227
53. Lonner BS, Scharf C, Antonacci D, Goldstein Y, Panagopoulos G. The learning curve associated with thoracoscopic spinal instrumentation. Spine 2005;30:2835–2840
54. Graham EJ, Lenke LG, Lowe TG, et al. Prospective pulmonary function evaluation following open thoracotomy for anterior spinal fusion in adolescent idiopathic scoliosis. Spine 2000;25:2319–2325
55. Grewal H, Betz RR, D'Andrea LP, Clements DH, Porter ST. A prospective comparison of thoracoscopic vs open anterior instrumentation and spinal fusion for idiopathic thoracic scoliosis in children. J Pediatr Surg 2005;40:153–156, discussion 156–157
56. Lonner BS, Kondrachov D, Siddiqi F, Hayes V, Scharf C. Thoracoscopic spinal fusion compared with posterior spinal fusion for the treatment of thoracic adolescent idiopathic scoliosis. J Bone Joint Surg Am 2006;88:1022–1034
57. Muschik MT, Kimmich H, Demmel T. Comparison of anterior and posterior double-rod instrumentation for thoracic idiopathic scoliosis: Results of 141 patients. Eur Spine J 2006;15:1128–1138
58. Newton PO, Parent S, Marks M, Pawelek J. Prospective evaluation of 50 consecutive scoliosis patients surgically treated with thoracoscopic anterior instrumentation. Spine 2005; 30(17, suppl):S100–S109
59. Early SD, Newton PO, White KK, Wenger DR, Mubarak SJ. The feasibility of anterior thoracoscopic spine surgery in children under 30 kilograms. Spine 2002;27:2368–2373

# 18 Diagnosis, Treatment, and Outcomes of Treatment of the Double Thoracic Curve Pattern in Adolescent Idiopathic Scoliosis

*Shay Bess, Frances Faro, and Thomas G. Lowe*

The double thoracic (DT) or Lenke type 2 curve pattern, defined as the combination of a structural proximal thoracic (PT) and structural main thoracic (MT) curve, is one of the later-defined deformity patterns in adolescent idiopathic scoliosis (AIS). Depending upon the classification used, however, surveys have indicated that DT curves may be the second or third most common pattern of curvature in AIS that present to physicians.[1–3] The prevalence of DT curves underscores the importance of identifying this curve pattern and understanding the options for effective treatment. The goal of this chapter is to review the definition and incidence of DT curves, provide an overview of the clinical and radiographic features, and describe effective treatment modalities for DT curve pattern.

## Definition and Incidence of Double Thoracic Curves

The reported incidence of the DT curve pattern depends upon the classification scheme used to categorize curve types for AIS. Moe and Kettleson, in their early series of 166 patients treated with braces, found that the DT pattern was the third most common curve pattern treated, occurring in 14% of patients.[4] Recognition of AIS patterns that contained more than one major curve was facilitated by Moe's routine use of 36-inch-long films.

King et al described the DT curve pattern that the authors defined as the King V pattern.[2] Left PT curves that had an elevated left first rib and a positive T1 tilt (defined as the left upper corner of T1 being higher than the right upper corner generating a tilt of T1 into the concavity of the PT curve) were thought to be complete curves with structural characteristics that needed to be included in fusion procedures (**Fig. 18.1**). PT curves that did not have a positive T1 tilt were believed to be fractional curves and did not require inclusion in fusion procedures. The King V pattern was the fourth most common of five patterns of curvature in AIS, and occurred in 11.6% of patients.

King and colleagues recognized the importance of curve flexibility as determined from side-bending radiographs. However, they applied an analysis of curve flexibility and a flexibility index only to the MT and thoracolumbar/lumbar (TL/L) curves to help differentiate between true double major and false double major patterns. Therefore, curve flexibility did not play a role in the criteria used to define the King V DT pattern. Although the King classification calls attention to the PT curve, it provides the physician with a somewhat vague guide for assessing the PT curve. This,

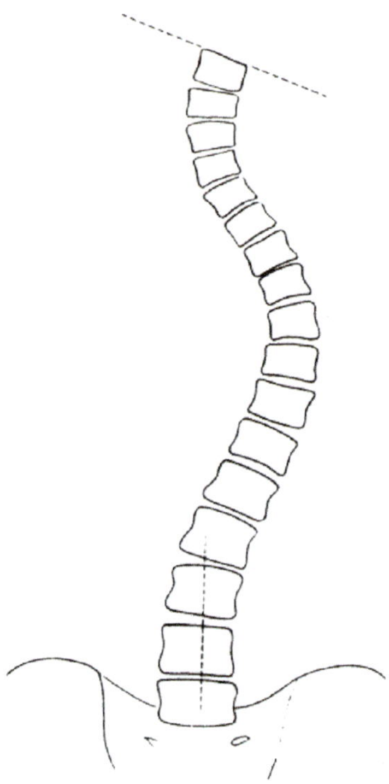

**Fig. 18.1** DT curve or Lenke type 2 curve, demonstrating positive T1 tilt. (From King HA, Moe JH, Bradford DS. The selection of fusion levels in thoracic idiopathic scoliosis. J Bone Joint Surg 1983. 65A: 1302-13. Reprinted with permission.)

together with poor inter- and intraobserver validity, reliability, and reproducibility in defining curves according to the King classification system, motivated Lenke and coworkers to develop a more comprehensive classification scheme for AIS that utilized curve magnitude, curve flexibility, and sagittal profile to differentiate structural from compensatory curves.[5–6] The Lenke classification defines the major curve as the largest measured curve on standing 36-inch posteroanterior (PA) radiographs. The smaller minor curves are defined as structural if they remain at ≥25 degrees on side-bending radiographs or if they have a hyperkyphotic sagittal profile with ≥20 degrees of focal kyphosis. For DT curves in the Lenke classification, the MT curve is always larger than the PT curve, and is the major curve. If the PT curve remains at ≥25 degrees on side-bending radiographs or if the T2-to-T5 focal kyphosis on lateral radiographs is ≥20 degrees, the PT curve is considered structural. This, in combination with a nonstructural thoracolumbar or lumbar curve, denotes a DT or Lenke 2 curve pattern. Using the Lenke classification with more refined criteria to delineate structural curves, Lenke and colleagues reported a 20% prevalence of DT curve patterns in a multicenter retrospective review of 606 operatively treated AIS patients.[3]

Looking to the future, further attention has been directed to establishing more reliable measures for differentiating structural from nonstructural minor curves. Criticisms of using side-bending radiographs to define a curve include variable patient effort during side-bending radiographs and inconsistent technique. This motivated Cheh et al to compare the reliability of supine 36-inch anteroposterior (AP) radiographs with that of side-bending films when predicting curve flexibility.[8] Cheh and coworkers reported that PT curves that remained at ≥30 degrees on supine radiographs were highly likely to be structural curves, and concluded that supine radiographs are a reproducible means for defining curve structurality and may eventually replace side-bending radiographs.

## Clinical Evaluation

The clinical evaluation of a patient with scoliosis, regardless of age or etiology, should include a frontal view of the shoulders and posterior view of the entire spine, unobstructed by hair and clothing, to permit assessment of shoulder balance and trapezial fullness. Left trapezial fullness and an elevated left shoulder in the presence of a right MT rotational prominence should alert the physician to the possibility of a structural left PT curve and DT curve pattern.[9,10] Patients with PT kyphosis may have a midline upper thoracic prominence, a forward-protruding cervical spine, or both. This may also indicate a structural PT curve, secondary to kyphosis, as part of a DT curve pattern.

## Radiographic Evaluation

The radiographic evaluation of a patient with scoliosis should include upright 36-inch PA and lateral radiographs that allow the surgeon to visualize the spine at least from the C7 vertebra to the pelvis, including the femoral heads. The size of all curves should be routinely measured on the PA film so as not to ignore a potentially structural minor curve in the presence of a large major curve. PT focal kyphosis is measured from T2 to T5. As previously indicated, PT focal kyphosis ≥20 degrees is indicative of a structural PT curve and is consistent with a DT curve pattern in the presence of a structural MT curve and nonstructural TL/L curve.[6] Side-bending and supine radiographs are obtained to evaluate curve flexibility and provide further criteria for curve structurality. PT curves of ≥25 degrees on side-bending radiographs or of ≥30 degrees on supine radiographs are structural. The angle of T1 tilt is measured from the intersection of a line drawn along the T1 cephalad endplate and a line parallel to the horizontal (or perpendicular to the vertical edge of the radiograph) (**Fig. 18.2**).[11] A positive T1 tilt (elevation of the left upper corner) and

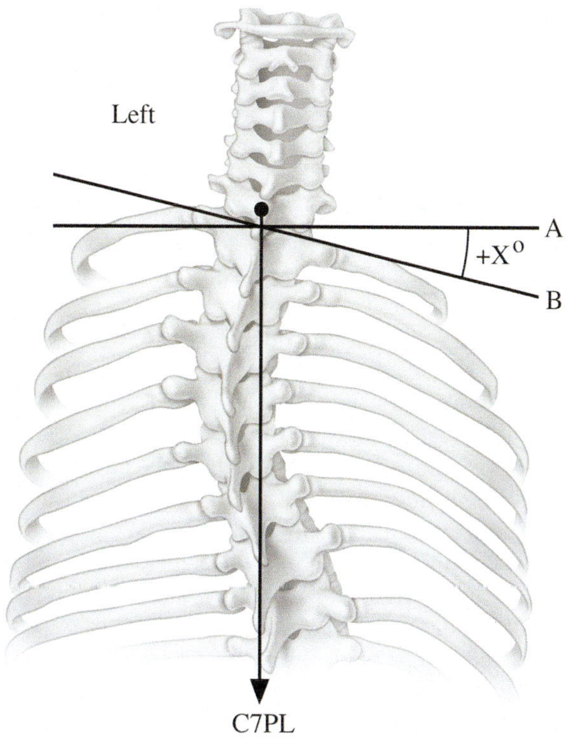


**Fig. 18.2** T1 tilt angle. The T1 tilt angle is measured at the intersection of a line drawn along the T1 cephalad endplate (line B) and a line parallel to the horizontal (or perpendicular to the vertical edge of the radiograph; line A). A positive T1 tilt angle is denoted when the left upper corner of T1 is higher than the right upper corner. A negative T1 tilt angle is denoted when the right upper corner of T1 is higher than the left upper corner.

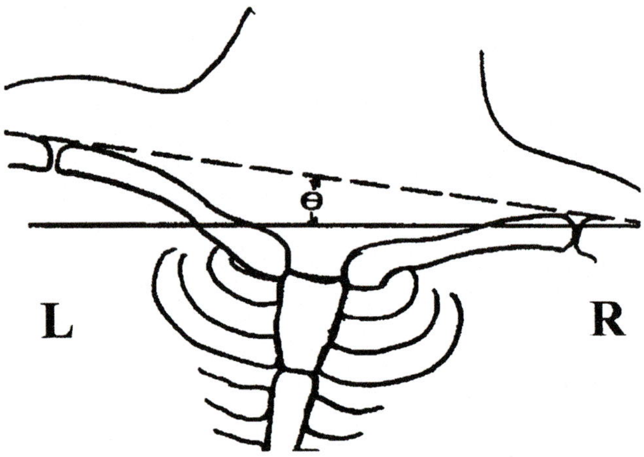


Fig. 18.3 The clavicle angle is measured at the intersection of a tangential line touching the two highest points of the clavicle and another line that is perpendicular to the horizontal. A positive clavicle angle is defined as the left clavicle being higher than the right clavicle. (From O'Brien MF, Kuklo TR, Blanke K. Spinal Deformity Study Group Radiographic Measurement Manual. Memphis, TN: Medtronic Sofamor Danek, 2004. Reprinted with permission.)

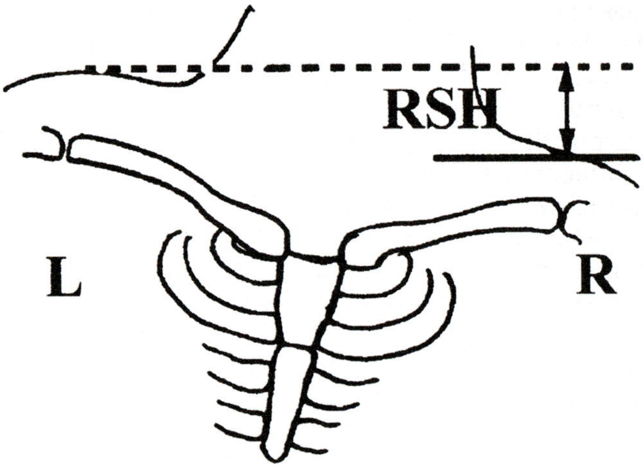


Fig. 18.4 The radiographic shoulder height is determined by the difference in the soft- tissue shadow directly superior to each acromioclavicular joint on standing PA radiograph (a positive result is defined as the left shoulder being higher than the right shoulder). (From O'Brien MF, Kuklo TR, Blanke K. Spinal Deformity Study Group Radiographic Measurement Manual. Memphis, TN: Medtronic Sofamor Danek, 2004. Reprinted with permission.)

angulation of the T1 endplate into the concavity of the PT curve on standing PA radiographs may be considered indicative of a complete PT curve, whereas a neutral or negative T1 tilt may be indicative of a fractional PT curve. However, some studies have supported curve flexibility and shoulder measurements as more accurate than T1 tilt in predicting the structural behavior of a PT curve.[2,12–14]

Measures of shoulder balance include clavicle angle, radiographic shoulder height, coracoid height difference, and first rib–clavicle height difference. These measures allow preoperative assessment of shoulder balance and can be used to predict postoperative shoulder balance.[13] The clavicle angle is formed by the intersection of a tangential line touching the two highest points of the clavicle with another line perpendicular to the horizontal (**Fig. 18.3**).[14] Radiographically determined shoulder height is the difference in the soft-tissue shadow directly superior to each acromioclavicular joint as measured on a standing PA radiograph (**Fig. 18.4**).[14] The difference in coracoid height is measured as the difference between the horizontal lines traced along the superior edge of each of the two coracoid processes. A positive value is denoted when the left coracoid process is higher than the right.[15] The first rib–clavicle height is defined as the vertical distance from the apex of the first rib to the immediately overlying superior clavicle.[13]

Several features of a DT curve are associated with central nervous system (CNS) abnormalities. Chiari malformation, hydrosyringomyelia, and other CNS abnormalities are uncommon in AIS, with a reported incidence ranging from 2 to 4%.[16–20] Focal and global hyperkyphosis has been associated with an increased incidence of CNS abnormalities found on magnetic resonance imaging (MRI) in patients with presumed AIS.[16,19] Davids et al reported a 2% incidence of CNS abnormalities among 274 patients with presumed AIS who had an MRI scan.[16] Absence of thoracic apical lordosis was the most valuable indicator of a potential CNS abnormality on MRI scanning. Speigel and colleagues reported that in addition to an atypical curve pattern (e.g., left MT curve), the DT curve pattern was independently associated with an increased incidence of CNS abnormality on MRI scanning.[19] In light of these reports, physicians evaluating a patient with a DT curve pattern and associated focal PT kyphosis should consider obtaining a screening MRI of the neural axis to rule out an underlying CNS abnormality that may require neurosurgical intervention before the definitive treatment of scoliosis.

## Nonoperative Treatment

As in all patterns of AIS, the primary treatment goal is to prevent curve progression. It has been established that the risk of curve progression depends on the magnitude of the curve, the amount of growth that the patient has remaining, and where the patient's remaining growth will occur in relation to the rapid phase of the adolescent growth spurt.[21] The decision to observe, brace, or surgically treat the condition is based on these factors. The specifics of bracing can be found in Chapters 7 and 8 of this book. With regard to the DT curve pattern, the main challenge of bracing is controlling the PT curve. A thoraco-lumbo-sacral orthosis (TLSO) brace is effective only for curves with an apex at T7 or caudally, because the TLSO brace fits beneath the arms and cannot generate the appropriate reduction forces for controlling high thoracic curves. Consequently, a Milwaukee-type cervical–thoracic–lumbar–sacral (CTLSO) brace with an attached chin piece is recommended for treating the PT curve. Poor compliance with Milwaukee-type brace-wearing and poor efficacy of bracing in controlling PT curves have been documented.[22–25] Lonstein and Winter reported that 26% of 218 patients with a DT curve pattern treated with a brace went on to surgical treatment, as compared with an average of 22% progression to surgery for patients with all other curve patterns.[26] They acknowledged that the PT curve is difficult to control with external bracing. Lonstein and Winter also indicated that the PT curve is rarely progressive, and that this portion of the DT curve pattern plays less of a role in progression to surgery than does the MT curve. They therefore believed that the DT pattern is amendable to bracing with a Milwaukee brace. Documentation of the PT curve size, flexibility, and T1 tilt angle before bracing is essential because worsening of the PT curve can be a perceived complication of bracing when in fact a structural PT curve was present before bracing.

## Operative Treatment

Challenges encountered in surgically treating the DT curve pattern include deciding on the approach, whether to include the PT curve in the fusion procedure, selecting the proximal level for fusion, correcting an elevated shoulder, and preventing postoperative shoulder decompensation. As indicated above, the King classification provided vague criteria for what constitutes a structural PT curve. King and colleagues recommended fusing both the PT and the MT curves if the PT curve was a complete curve with structural characteristics indicated by a positive T1 tilt.[2] Lee and coworkers evaluated the efficacy of Harrington instrumentation for treating the PT curve in DT patterns.[27] They recommended including the PT curve in the fusion if the left shoulder was elevated on clinical or radiographic examination, or if the patient showed left trapezial fullness or a left PT rotational prominence.

In contrast to the King classification, Lee et al reported that positive T1 tilt did not correlate with postoperative shoulder balance, and that what correlated most with postoperative shoulder balance was the pattern of preoperative shoulder imbalance and the magnitude of intraoperative MT curve correction. In their series, most unfused PT curves corrected spontaneously and did not progress after selective fusion of the MT curve. Lee and colleagues reported that because correction of the right MT curve elevates the left shoulder, patients with an elevated right shoulder preoperatively were more likely to have balanced shoulders postoperatively if the PT curve was not fused and the MT curve was not overcorrected. Overcorrection of the MT curve put the patient at risk for postoperative left-shoulder elevation. If the patient had balanced shoulders, postoperative shoulder balance depended on relative curve flexibility. If the PT curve was more rigid than the MT curve, Lee et al recommended fusing both curves. If the flexibility of the PT and MT curves was equal, or if the PT curve was more flexible than the MT curve, they recommended fusing only the MT curve, with the caveat, again, to avoid overcorrection of the MT curve. Greater attention to overcorrection of the MT curve is needed with pedicle-screw systems, because pedicle screws allow greater curve correction than hook-and-wire instrumentation techniques. Lee and colleagues found that among patients with an elevated left shoulder preoperatively, spontaneous PT curve correction could not match the correction obtained after instrumenting the MT curve. Consequently, patients with a preoperatively elevated left shoulder were most at risk for postoperative shoulder imbalance if the PT curve was not included in the fusion. On the basis of these findings, Lee and colleagues recommended including the PT curve in the fusion in patients with an elevated left shoulder.

Lenke et al evaluated shoulder balance after the treatment of DT curves using Cotrel–Dubousset instrumentation.[28] They hypothesized that 90-degree rod rotation with Cotrel–Dubousset instrumentation generated more powerful corrective forces than did Harrington instrumentation, and could therefore magnify the deformity of an unrecognized or uncorrected PT curve. Consequently, Lenke and coworkers recommended the inclusion of all PT curves with structural characteristics in the instrumented fusion, even if the patient's shoulders were balanced or the right shoulder was high. Characteristics indicative of a structural PT curve included:

1. A curve size >30 degrees that remained >20 degrees on side-bending radiographs
2. Nash–Moe apical rotation above grade I
3. More than 1 cm of apical translation from the C7 plumbline
4. Transitional vertebra from the left PT to the right MT curves at T6 or caudally
5. Positive T1 tilt
6. Clinically elevated left shoulder

Lack of side-bending flexibility was the most consistent criterion for a structural PT curve. This is consistent with the definition of a structural curve according to the Lenke classification. If a structural PT curve was identified, Lenke and colleagues recommended fusion and instrumentation to T2 posteriorly. They also believed that the sagittal contour of the PT curve was most commonly hyperkyphotic. Corrective maneuvers included convex compression across the PT curve, to reduce focal kyphosis and depress the elevated left shoulder, followed by rod derotation across the MT curve to correct the MT coronal deformity and reduce MT hypokyphosis.

Cil et al further supported the use of curve flexibility to define a structural PT curve.[29] In a retrospective analysis of patients undergoing posterior spinal fusion (PSF) for a Lenke type 1 curve (structural MT curve, nonstructural PT and TL/L curves), they divided the patients into two groups. In Group 1 the PT curve was included in the fusion levels (proximal fusion to T2 or T3); Group 2 had selective MT fusion (proximal fusion to T4 or caudally). Both groups had statistically similar preoperative PT, MT, and side-bending curve values and equivalent preoperative shoulder-height measurements. Postoperative PT and MT curve values and curve correction were similar between both groups. Postoperative shoulder balance was similar in the two study groups, and no patient demonstrated postoperative shoulder or PT curve decompensation. Cil and colleagues concluded that the curve flexibility and the Lenke criteria for defining a structural curve were valid for identifying PT curves for inclusion in or exclusion from fusion. They also hoped that their findings would provide guidelines for the upper instrumented vertebra (UIV) (e.g., stopping at T3, T2, or T1) as the end-vertebra, but neither their data nor a literature review could delineate the criteria for the safe UIV.

Since the advent of thoracic pedicle-screw instrumentation (TPS), several authors have reported greater segmental curve correction with TPS than with hook-and-wire constructs.[30,31] Suk and colleagues reported the results of treatment of DT curves with segmental TPS.[32] In this series, they segmentally instrumented all PT curves to T1, and extended the instrumentation distally to the caudal neutral vertebra of the MT curve. Corrective maneuvers included placement of a short concave rod along the PT curve, 90-degree clockwise rod rotation to the desired sagittal contour, and securing of the concave PT rod to the pedicle screws. They then placed another short concave rod along the MT curve, rotated the short MT rod by 90 degrees counterclockwise to the desired sagittal contour, and locked the rod into the pedicle screws. Convex rods were then inserted and secured to the concave rods with rod connectors. Suk and colleagues found that TPS further increased the risk for postoperative shoulder decompensation, and recommended that the PT curve be included in a fusion only if PI curves were >25 degrees and the patient's shoulders were level or the left shoulder was high. If the patient had an elevated right shoulder, inclusion of the PT curve was considered optional, but if the right shoulder was ≥12 mm higher than the left, the authors recommended fusing only the MT curve.

Kuklo et al evaluated the fate of the PT curve after selective anterior spinal fusion (ASF) or PSF of the MT curve.[14] All of the patients in their study had preoperative PT curves ≥20 degrees. All patients undergoing ASF were instrumented to T4 or caudally, and all patients undergoing PSF were instrumented to T3 or caudally. Patients undergoing ASF had significantly greater spontaneous PT curve correction than did patients undergoing PSF. However, Kuklo and colleagues cautioned that the flexibility of the PT curve must be carefully assessed before committing to an anterior approach, and that in contrast to the situation with a posterior approach, the instrumentation used in an anterior approach cannot be extended proximally into the PT curve if intraoperative radiographs show a large residual PT curve and associated shoulder imbalance or coronal imbalance. Curves with a positive T1 tilt angle ≥5 degrees and a clinically elevated left shoulder were reported to be a contraindication for ASF. Patients who had equal right and left shoulder heights, a neutral T1 tilt, and a PT curve that reduced to ≤25 degrees on side-bending radiographs, selective MT fusion via ASF or PSF was feasible, provided that residual tilt was retained in the UIV of the MT curve, to accommodate the residual PT curve. Subsequent analysis by Kuklo et al of various radiographic parameters of shoulder height demonstrated that the preoperative clavicle angle and coracoid height were the best predictors of postoperative shoulder balance.[12] Factors not predictive of postoperative shoulder balance in any of the treatment groups were T1 tilt, trapezius length, first rib-clavicle height, and radiographic shoulder height (RSH). The magnitude of the PT curve, PT apical vertebral translation, and side-bending measures were also not predictive of shoulder balance. On the basis of these findings, Kuklo and colleagues recommended that patients with a positive clavicle angle and an elevated left shoulder should have their PT curve instrumented at least to T3, whereas patients with a neutral clavicle angle (balanced shoulders) or a negative clavicle angle (correlating with right shoulder elevation) were candidates for selective MT fusion even if they had a positive T1 tilt or rigid PT curve. The authors maintained that ASF should not be attempted unless the PT curve reduces to ≤20 degrees.

The Harms Study Group (HSG) has conducted a review of prospectively collected data for 102 patients with DT curves treated with either posterior spinal instrumented fusion (PSF) of both the curves ($n = 77$) (**Fig. 18.5**) or selective anterior spinal instrumented fusion of the MT curve ($n = 25$) (**Fig. 18.6**). Radiographic, clinical, and functional outcomes scores for the two groups were evaluated and compared (**Table 18.1**). As in previous studies, selective fusion of the MT curve in the ASIF group resulted in some spontaneous PT-curve correction, but this was significantly less than the correction provided by inclusion of the PT curve in the PSIF group (37.6% vs. 49.9%, $P < 0.001$). However, 30% of ASIF patients with a T1 tilt <5 degrees developed unacceptable shoulder imbalance after fusion. Of the 48 patients with acceptable shoulder balance before

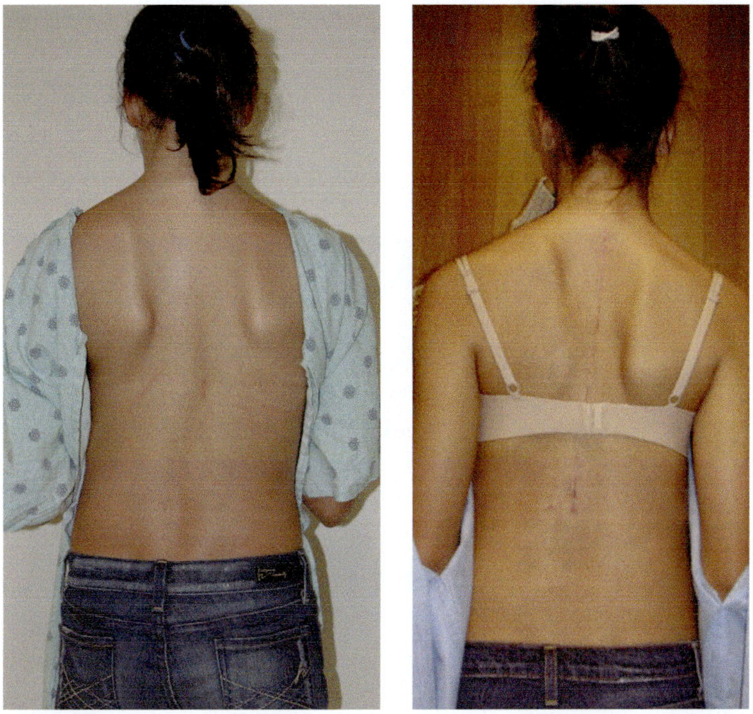

A,B

**Fig. 18.5** **(A)** This clinical photograph demonstrates features typical of Lenke type 2 curves. Note the elevated left shoulder, a feature of the left high thoracic curve. Also note the fullness in the left cervicothoracic junction. **(B)** After surgical correction of both thoracic curves, the shoulders are level and the fullness of the left cervicothoracic junction is diminished. The waist is symmetrical and the scapular prominences are symmetrical. **(C)** The MT curve is noted on the preoperative radiographs. The high left thoracic curve here measures 35 degrees, and on bending 30 degrees. The Lenke classification of this pattern of curvature is type 2AN. **(D)** The lateral radiograph is not remarkable. **(E)** After instrumentation from T2 to T12, essentially complete correction of both curves is attained. The clavicles are level and the lumbar spine is straight. **(F)** This postoperative lateral radiograph demonstrates physiological sagittal contours.

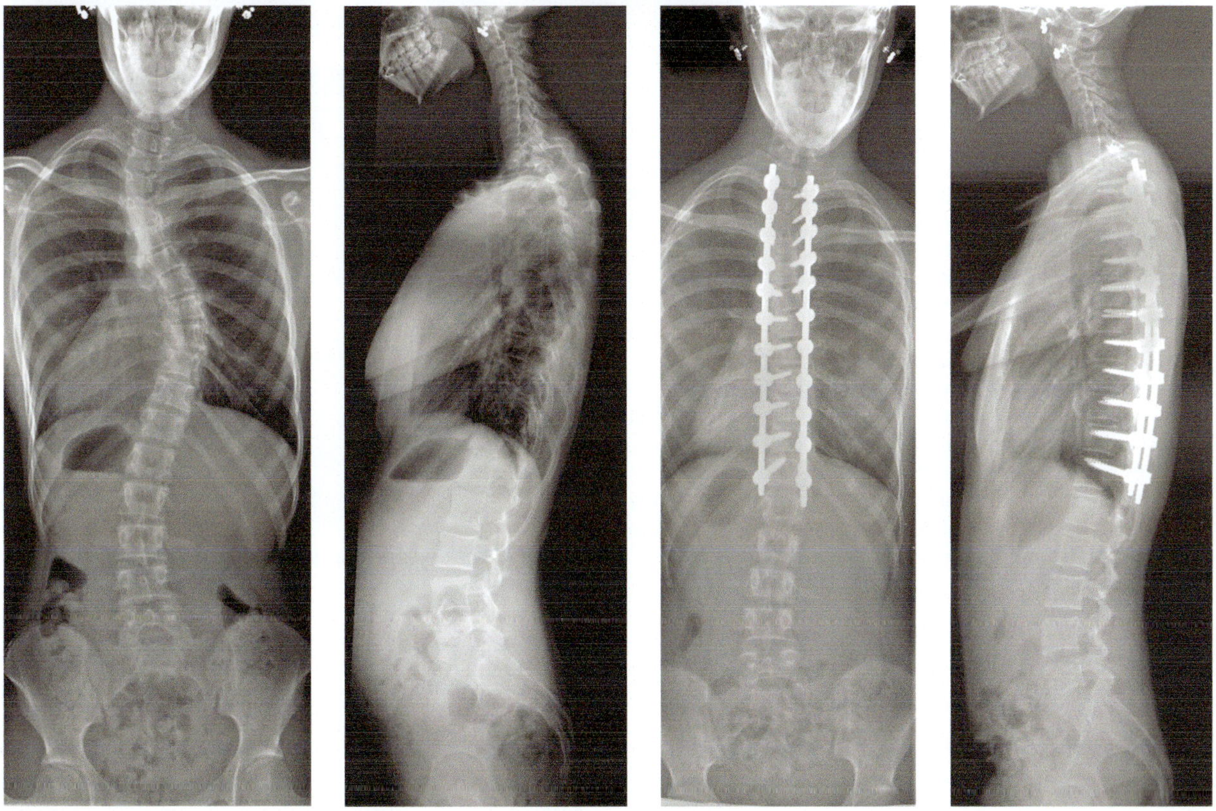

C–F

surgery, 33% of those in the PSIF group developed shoulder imbalance, and 41% of patients with a shoulder imbalance preoperatively showed correction to a T1 tilt <5 degrees after PSIF (**Table 18.2**). There was no correlation between T1 tilt and the UIV. Loss of shoulder balance in both the PSIF and ASIF groups was associated with a lower MT-to-PT curve-size ratio. Although these data do not specifically delineate what leads to a loss of shoulder balance, the

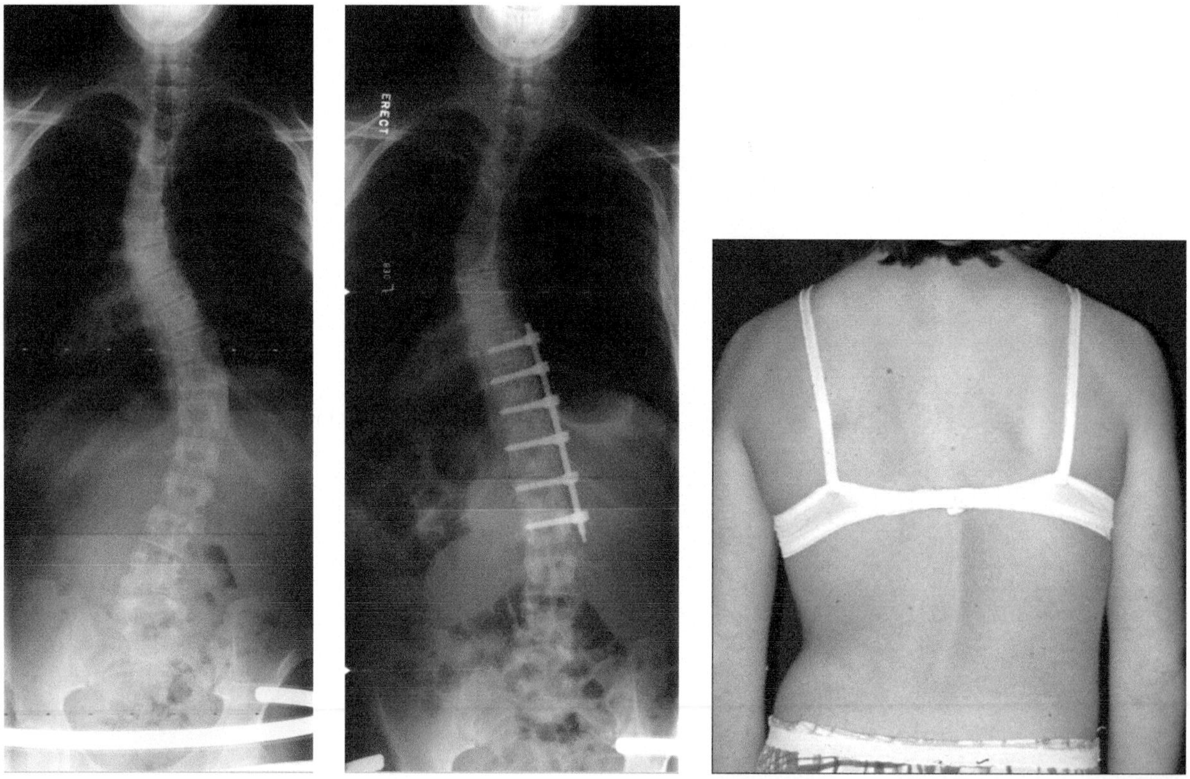


A,B C

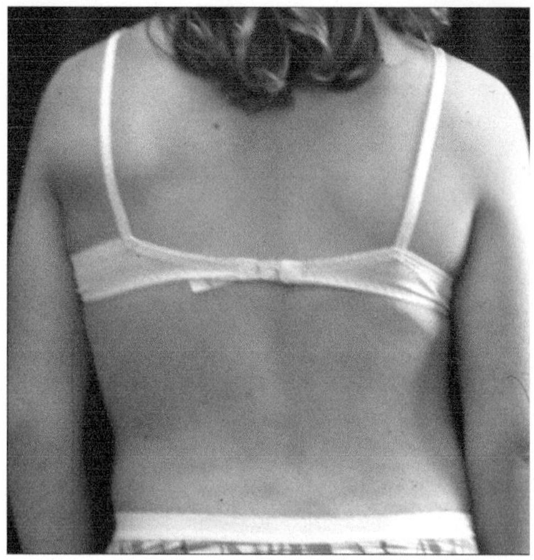

D

**Fig. 18.6** **(A)** Preoperative PA radiograph of 15-year + 1-month-old girl with a progressive Lenke type 2 curve and low apex of the MT curve. The PT curve (T2–T8) measures 42 degrees and reduces to 26 degrees on side-bending. The MT curve extends from T8 to L2 (with its apex at the T11–T12 disc space), measures 49 degrees, and reduces to 10 degrees on side-bending. **(B)** Two-year postoperative radiograph after ASF from T9 to L2 demonstrates decompensation of the unfused PT curve with associated coronal imbalance to the left. **(C)** Preoperative clinical photograph demonstrating waist asymmetry and right truncal shift; however, the shoulders are symmetrical clinically, which is indicative of a structural PT curve. **(D)** Postoperative clinical photograph demonstrating an elevated left shoulder and left truncal shift consistent with decompensation of an unfused PT curve and associated coronal imbalance, as demonstrated on this postoperative radiograph.

relative sizes of the thoracic curves clearly help determine whether or not this occurs.

Choice of approach affected the sagittal contour of the spine, with the anterior approach resulting in more postoperative kyphosis in the T5 to T12 region, whereas the posterior approach resulted in less postoperative kyphosis in this region. The anterior approach caused some reduction of kyphosis from T2 to T5, which is important to the alignment of the cervical spine. The posterior approach caused no kyphosis. The patients in the HSG review were evaluated with the Scoliosis Research Society (SRS)-24 questionnaire. There was no significant difference between the anterior and posterior approaches with respect to outcomes, Patients in both groups had significant improvements in the postoperative general function, health, pain, self-image, and patient satisfaction domains of the questionnaire. Seventy percent of patients with reduced shoulder asymmetry showed an improvement in the self-mage domain. From these data it can be concluded that both anterior and posterior fusions have a role in the management of DT

**Table 18.1 Harms Study Group Pre and Postoperative Radiographic Values Following ASIF or PSIF for Double Thoracic Curve Pattern**

| | ASIF | PSIF | *P-value* |
|---|---|---|---|
| Preoperative PT curve | 34.6° | 42.5° | $P<0.001$ |
| Preoperative MT curve | 58.6° | 60.8° | NS |
| Preoperative lumbar curve | 30.2° | 28.9° | NS |
| Preoperative PT-curve Flexibility | 24.6% | 23.2% | NS |
| Preoperative MT-curve flexibility | 44.0% | 47.3% | NS |
| Preoperative lumbar-curve flexibility | 78.4% | 75.1% | NS |
| Postoperative PT curve | 62% | 47% | $P< 0.001$ |
| Preoperative T1 tilt | 4.0° | 7.5° | $P = 0.002$ |
| Postoperative T1 tilt | 6.2° | 6.9° | NS |
| Change in T2–T5 kyphosis (pre- to postoperative) | −1.5° | +1.1° | |
| Change in T5–T12 kyphosis (pre- to postoperative) | +10.3° | −5.0° | |
| Change in T2–T12 kyphosis (pre- to postoperative) | +8.6° | −4.0° | |

*Abbreviations:* ASIF, anterior instrumented spinal fusion; MT, main thoracic; PSIF, posterior instrumented spinal fusion; PT, proximal thoracic.

**Table 18.2 Harms Study Group Pre and Posteperative T1 Tilt and Shoulder Balance Following ASIF or PSIF for Double Thoracic Curve Pattern**

| | Postoperative T1 Tilt | | T1 Tilt Maintained or Improved Postoperatively |
|---|---|---|---|
| | *Acceptable <5 Degrees* | *Unacceptable ≥5 Degrees* | |
| **ASIF** | | | |
| Preoperatively acceptable $n = 10$ | 7 (70%) | 3 (30%) | 47% |
| Preoperatively unacceptable $n = 15$ | 6 (40%) | 9 (60%) | |
| **PSIF** | | | |
| Preoperatively acceptable $n = 48$ | 32 (67%) | 16 (33%) | 43% |
| Preoperatively unacceptable $n = 29$ | 12 (41%) | 17 (59%) | |

*Abbreviations:* ASIF, anterior instrumented spinal fusion; PSIF, posterior instrumented spinal fusion.

curves. Fusion of the PT curve with the posterior approach provides direct and more powerful correction, but has the drawbacks of being a longer fusion that leaves fewer mobile segments and entails instrumentation in an area prone to implant prominence.

T1 tilt is an approximate radiographic indicator of shoulder asymmetry, and is affected by many factors including the MT-to-PT curve-size ratio and PT-curve flexibility. Postoperative T1 tilt is clearly affected by the extent of fusion and correction, but quantifying this intraoperatively remains difficult, and it is recommended that this be done with a C-arm radiographic image tilted to accommodate the sagittal alignment, resembling a Ferguson view of L5. The HSG prospective database will be invaluable in understanding how to plan the operative treatment of DT curves, as well as in understanding the effect of their correction on long-term function.

## Conclusion

Originally believed to be uncommon, the DT curve pattern in AIS may occur in as many as 20% of cases.[3] Identification of a structural PT curve and routine DT pattern requires routine measurement of the Cobb angles of all of the coronal deformities identified in a PA radiograph routine measurement of all scoliotic curves will prevent distraction by a larger curve. Long-cassette, 36-inch PA and lateral radiographs facilitate accurate evaluation of the curve pattern and associated sagittal profile. Flexibility on side-bending radiographs and focal kyphosis on lateral imaging allow assessment of the structurality of minor curves. The structural characteristics of the PT curve and assessment of shoulder height guide the decision about whether or not to include the PT curve in a fusion. Currently, no formal criteria exist for selecting the UIV in the PT curve, however, inclusion of the curve should be strongly considered if the left shoulder is elevated preoperatively.

## References


1. Cruickshank JL, Koike M, Dickson RA. Curve patterns in idiopathic scoliosis. A clinical and radiographic study. J Bone Joint Surg Br 1989;71:259–263
2. King HA, Moe JH, Bradford DS, Winter RB. The selection of fusion levels in thoracic idiopathic scoliosis. J Bone Joint Surg Am 1983; 65:1302–1313
3. Lenke LG, Betz RR, Clements D, et al. Curve prevalence of a new classification of operative adolescent idiopathic scoliosis: Does classification correlate with treatment? Spine 2002;27: 604–611
4. Moe JH, Kettleson DN. Idiopathic scoliosis. Analysis of curve patterns and the preliminary results of Milwaukee-brace treatment in

one hundred sixty-nine patients. J Bone Joint Surg Am 1970;52: 1509–1533

5. Cummings RJ, Loveless EA, Campbell J, Samelson S, Mazur JM. Interobserver reliability and intraobserver reproducibility of the system of King et al. for the classification of adolescent idiopathic scoliosis. J Bone Joint Surg Am 1998;80:1107–1111
6. Lenke LG, Betz RR, Bridwell KH, et al. Intraobserver and interobserver reliability of the classification of thoracic adolescent idiopathic scoliosis. J Bone Joint Surg Am 1998;80:1097–1106
7. Lenke LG, Betz RR, Harms J, et al. Adolescent idiopathic scoliosis: A new classification to determine extent of spinal arthrodesis. J Bone Joint Surg Am 2001;83A:1169–1181
8. Cheh G, Lenke LG, Lehman RAJ Jr, Kim YJ, Nunley R, Bridwell KH. The reliability of preoperative supine radiographs to predict the amount of curve flexibility in adolescent idiopathic scoliosis. Spine 2007;32:2668–2672
9. Winter RB. The idiopathic double thoracic curve pattern. Its recognition and surgical management. Spine 1989;14:1287–1292
10. Winter RB, Denis F. The King V curve pattern. Its analysis and surgical treatment. Orthop Clin North Am 1994;25:353–362
11. O'Brien MF, Kuklo TR, Blanke K. Spinal Deformity Study Group Radiographic Measurement Manual. Memphis, TN: Medtronic Sofamor Danek, 2004
12. Ginsberg H, Goldstein L, DeVanny J. An evaluation of the upper thoracic curve in idiopathic scoliosis: Guidelines in the selection of the fusion area. 12th Annual Scoliosis Research Society Meeting, Hong Kong, Oct 24–27, 1977
13. Kuklo TR, Lenke LG, Graham EJ, et al. Correlation of radiographic, clinical, and patient assessment of shoulder balance following fusion versus nonfusion of the proximal thoracic curve in adolescent idiopathic scoliosis. Spine 2002;27(18):2013–2020
14. Kuklo TR, Lenke LG, Won DS, et al. Spontaneous proximal thoracic curve correction after isolated fusion of the main thoracic curve in adolescent idiopathic scoliosis. Spine 2001;26:1966–1975
15. Bagó J, Carrera L, March B, Villanueva C. Four radiological measures to estimate shoulder balance in scoliosis. J Pediatr Orthop B 1996; 5:31–34
16. Davids JR, Chamberlin E, Blackhurst DW. Indications for magnetic resonance imaging in presumed adolescent idiopathic scoliosis. J Bone Joint Surg Am 2004;86A:2187–2195
17. Do T, Fras C, Burke S, Widmann RF, Rawlins B, Boachie-Adjei O. Clinical value of routine preoperative magnetic resonance imaging in adolescent idiopathic scoliosis. A prospective study of three hundred and twenty-seven patients. J Bone Joint Surg Am 2001; 83A:577–579
18. Maiocco B, Deeney VF, Coulon R, Parks PF Jr. Adolescent idiopathic scoliosis and the presence of spinal cord abnormalities. Preoperative magnetic resonance imaging analysis. Spine 1997;22:2537–2541
19. Spiegel DA, Flynn JM, Stasikelis PJ, et al. Scoliotic curve patterns in patients with Chiari I malformation and/or syringomyelia. Spine 2003;28:2139–2146
20. Winter RB, Lonstein JE, Heithoff KB, Kirkham JA. Magnetic resonance imaging evaluation of the adolescent patient with idiopathic scoliosis before spinal instrumentation and fusion. A prospective, double-blinded study of 140 patients. Spine 1997; 22:855–858
21. Lonstein JE, Carlson JM. The prediction of curve progression in untreated idiopathic scoliosis during growth. J Bone Joint Surg Am 1984;66:1061–1071
22. Bassett GS, Bunnell WP, MacEwen GD. Treatment of idiopathic scoliosis with the Wilmington brace. Results in patients with a twenty to thirty-nine-degree curve. J Bone Joint Surg Am 1986;68:602–605
23. Clayson D, Luz-Alterman S, Cataletto MM, Levine DB. Long-term psychological sequelae of surgically versus nonsurgically treated scoliosis. Spine 1987;12:983–986
24. Edmonsson AS, Morris JT. Follow-up study of Milwaukee brace treatment in patients with idiopathic scoliosis. Clin Orthop Relat Res 1977; (126):58–61
25. Fällström K, Cochran T, Nachemson A. Long-term effects on personality development in patients with adolescent idiopathic scoliosis. Influence of type of treatment. Spine 1986;11:756–758
26. Lonstein JE, Winter RB. The Milwaukee brace for the treatment of adolescent idiopathic scoliosis. A review of one thousand and twenty patients. J Bone Joint Surg Am 1994;76:1207–1221
27. Lee CK, Denis F, Winter RB, Lonstein JE. Analysis of the upper thoracic curve in surgically treated idiopathic scoliosis. A new concept of the double thoracic curve pattern. Spine 1993;18:1599–1608
28. Lenke LG, Bridwell KH, O'Brien MF, Baldus C, Blanke K. Recognition and treatment of the proximal thoracic curve in adolescent idiopathic scoliosis treated with Cotrel-Dubousset instrumentation. Spine 1994;19:1589–1597
29. Cil A, Pekmezci M, Yazici M, et al. The validity of Lenke criteria for defining structural proximal thoracic curves in patients with adolescent idiopathic scoliosis. Spine 2005;30:2550–2555
30. Kim YJ, Lenke LG, Cho SK, Bridwell KH, Sides B, Blanke K. Comparative analysis of pedicle screw versus hook instrumentation in posterior spinal fusion of adolescent idiopathic scoliosis. Spine 2004;29:2040–2048
31. Suk SI, Lee CK, Kim WJ, Chung YJ, Park YB. Segmental pedicle screw fixation in the treatment of thoracic idiopathic scoliosis. Spine 1995;20:1399–1405
32. Suk SI, Kim WJ, Lee CS, et al. Indications of proximal thoracic curve fusion in thoracic adolescent idiopathic scoliosis: Recognition and treatment of double thoracic curve pattern in adolescent idiopathic scoliosis treated with segmental instrumentation. Spine 2000;25: 2342–2349

# 19 The Surgical Treatment of Lumbar and Thoracolumbar Curve Patterns (Lenke Type 5): Anterior versus Posterior Approach

*Harry L. Shufflebarger, James T. Guille, and Burt Yaszay*

Controversy remains about the best approach to the management of Lenke type 5 or thoracolumbar/lumbar (TL/L) curves. Advocates of anterior instrumentation and fusion report excellent coronal correction, restoration of lumbar lordosis, and derotation of the lumbar spine with the fusion of fewer distal motion segments. Supporters of the posterior approach express concern about the morbidity of the anterior approach and the need for an access surgeon to assist operators who are unfamiliar or uncomfortable with this operative approach. They also discuss the equivalent or greater three-dimensional (3D) curve correction obtained with the multilevel pedicle screws and osteotomies used in the posterior approach relative to the correction achieved with the anterior approach. The following sections describe each technique for the management of the Lenke type 5 curve pattern, with a discussion by the respective advocates of the anterior approach (Dr. Guille) and the posterior approach (Dr. Shufflebarger).

## Anterior Approach

### History

Anterior approaches to the thoracolumbar and lumbar spine were used for decades before their application to the treatment of idiopathic scoliosis. In the mid-1960s, Dwyer and colleagues introduced their system for the anterior correction and stabilization of scoliosis. Large screws were placed across the vertebral bodies and were connected by a flexible titanium cable on the convex side of the curve. Compressive maneuvers were then used to correct scoliosis by shortening the longer, convex side of the curve. Disadvantages of this system were numerous. The instrumentation could not be adjusted after the screw–cable interface had been crimped, nor did it provide rigid internal fixation, which resulted in the poor long-term maintenance of correction and necessitated postoperative immobilization of the spine. The kyphosing effects on the spine of the Dwyer technique, its inability to produce vertebral derotation, and the high pseudarthrosis rates with this technique have lead to its disuse.[1–5]

In 1976, Zielke shared his experience with a modification of the Dwyer system that utilized a solid 3.2-mm threaded rod instead of a flexible cable. This provided more rigid fixation that was able to resist the kyphosing effects of the anterior approach and provided for vertebral derotation. However, postoperative immobilization with a brace was still necessary, and unacceptably high rates of pseudarthrosis were reported in early series using Zielke instrumentation.[6–8]

In the 1980s and1990s, systems utilizing one or two solid rods provided more rigid fixation that obviated postoperative external immobilization, decreased pseudarthrosis rates, and maintained the correction of curvature obtained in both the sagittal and coronal planes.[9–12]

Correction of scoliosis in the coronal plane and hypolordosis in the sagittal plane is achieved by 90-degree rotation of the rod used in the construct for treating scoliosis, with mild compression applied on the convex side of the instrumented curve. Lumbar lordosis is maintained by the stiffness of the treatment construct and the placement of cages around adjacent vertebral bodies at the appropriate levels, or by structural bone grafts. Postoperative immobilization is usually not required.

### Patient Selection

Those patients best suited for anterior instrumentation and fusion of their TL/L curve fit the criteria established by Lenke and colleagues in their description of the surgical treatment of type 5 curves:[13] The proximal thoracic (PT) and main thoracic (MT) curves are nonstructural, whereas the TL/L curve is structural (comprising the major curve in the type 5 category, with the largest Cobb angle). The apex of the thoracolumbar curve is at T12–L1, and that of the lumbar curve is between the L1–L2 disc and L4. All Lenke type 5 curves have a "C" lumbar modifier by definition. A patient who has undergone a prior abdominal operation may not be a candidate for the anterior approach. A dilemma may exist if the last vertebral body to be instrumented is that of L4 or L5, because of the overlying great vessel (aorta) impeding exposure of the anterior lower lumbar spine. A large body habitus should not be a contraindication to anterior instrumentation of the spine.

Sanders and colleagues attempted to set forth criteria for including the thoracic curve in fusion.[14] The preoperative thoracic-curve magnitudes in their study ranged from 30 to 55 degrees. They determined that a patient with a TL/L-to-thoracic-curve Cobb-angle ratio of ≥1.25 and a thoracic curve that bent out to ≤20 degrees, along with closed triradiate cartilages, had the best chance of having a satisfactory result of surgery. A satisfactory result was defined as a thoracic curve ≤40 degrees, "reasonable" balance and sagittal alignment, and no need for additional procedures. The need to treat the thoracic curve is a relative contraindication to anterior fusion, because both the TL/L and thoracic curves cannot be instrumentated through a single thoracoabdominal incision.

Guille and colleagues[15] reviewed the Harms Study Group (HSG) database and found 109 patients with Lenke type 5 curves for whom data had been prospectively collected at the time of fusion. Eighty-four patients (77%) had had a selective fusion of the TL/L curve only, whereas 25 patients (23%) had had fusion of the thoracic curve as well. Preoperatively, the patients' data were statistically similar in terms of sagittal parameters, skeletal maturity, and age at surgery. Surgeons in the HSG broke the rules of the Lenke classification and fused both the TL/L and thoracic curves in patients with larger thoracic curves, larger thoracic rib humps, and greater thoracic apical translations. Scores on the Scoliosis Research Society (SRS)-24 questionnaire were statistically similar in the two study groups at the time of a follow-up review, except that the group with fusion of their thoracic curves reported less function.

## Preoperative Planning

Routine full-length posteroanterior (PA) and lateral radiographs should be made of the patient in the standing position, as well as lateral side-bending films of the patient in the supine position. As outlined earlier in this book, the standard measurements of spinal curvature and shoulder height should be made. Usually, the levels to be fused and instrumented are those within the TL/L Cobb angle. The uppermost level to be instrumented is the proximal vertebra in the measured Cobb angle. Care should be taken if this vertebra is the T12 level. The lower end-vertebra of the measured curve, determined from the standing PA view, is usually the best choice as the last instrumented level. This vertebra usually has minimal rotation, but may have a marked tilt. It is important to view the patient's side-bending films to ensure that this vertebra can be made horizontal (after correction of the scoliosis). The long-term results of residual obliquity at this end-vertebral level, or those of facet incongruity, are unknown.

The vertebral bodies should be evaluated for their ability to accommodate two screws if a dual-rod construct is being considered. The radiographs and operative plan are ideally discussed preoperatively with the access surgeon. The thoracolumbar operative approach will not be discussed in this chapter.

## Operative Technique

The spine should be exposed to reveal all of the vertebrae to be included in the fusion and instrumentation of a Lenke type 5 curve. Postural reduction of the magnitude of the curve is usually obtained by positioning the patient on the operating table, and is even greater after the discectomies are done. Care should be taken to avoid violating disc spaces not to be included in the fusion. Complete discectomies, down to bleeding bone, are done at all intended levels of the fusion procedure. Usually, there is no need to remove the annulus on the concave side of the patient's curve or the posterior longitudinal ligament, but these steps may allow greater correction in larger curves. Soft tissue is removed from the vertebral bodies to allow the accurate placement of instrumentation. It is important to identify the posterior border of the vertebral body to be instrumented so that one of the screws to be inserted in it can be placed as posteriorly as possible, which is especially important with dual-rod constructs. Staples help demarcate screw-insertion sites and aid in avoiding the plowing of screws during corrective maneuvers. Particular care must be taken to accurately measure vertebral screw length and avoid excessive prominence of screws into the distal cortex. With open exposure of the lumbar spine, the surgeon can place an index finger on the contralateral side of the vertebral body during screw placement. Following screw placement, attention is given to the placement of inter-vertebral-body cages or grafts. The cage or graft should be placed on the concave sides of the vertebral bodies to aid in correction of the scoliosis, and in a slightly anterior position to create and maintain lumbar lordosis. The rods in a dual-rod construct are each usually 4.5 mm in diameter, whereas single rods are generally ≥5.0 mm. A mild curve is bent into the rod, which is placed with the apex of the bend facing upward, which aids in insertion of the rod. A 90-degree rod rotation is then done so that the apex of the bend in the rod faces anteriorly, thus creating a lordosis. If a second rod is used, it is inserted in situ, because the correction has already been achieved by the first rod. Mild compression is then done on the convex side of the patient's curve for further correction. Radiographs are then made to ensure that the end instrumented vertebra is horizontal.

## Dual versus Single Rods and Inter-vertebral-body Implants

Discussion of the biomechanical merits of single- versus dual-rod instrumentation abounds in the literature, with proponents of both types of construct.[16-20] There is also debate about optimal rod diameter and the benefits of dual rods.[21,22] Fricka et al have shown in a bovine model that dual-rod constructs are stiffer in torsion and flexion–extension loading.[17] They found that structural support with dual rods helped with lumbar lordosis but did not increase construct stiffness. With single-rod constructs, the addition of structural support added stiffness in flexion. Oda and coworkers demonstrated in a calf-spine model that increased rod diameter did not improve construct stiffness or affect rod–screw strain.[18] Dual-rod constructs had greater construct stiffness and less rod–screw strain. Chang et al showed no statistical difference in range of motion or load sharing when dual rods, each of 6.35 mm or 5.5 mm diameter, were used.[19] Zhang and coworkers described a novel implant for anterior instrumentation.[20] This rod–plate construct was significantly stiffer and provided a more stable bone–screw interface than did a single-rod-with-cages construct, but was comparable in stiffness and stability to dual-rod constructs. If the size of the vertebral body permits, a dual-rod construct should be used, and obviates the need for a brace. Frequently, a brace will be needed when only a single-rod construct is used.

Most studies support anterior inter-vertebral-body grafts and cages as aiding in fusion, sagittal-plane correction, and the maintenance of sagittal-plane correction. Lenke and Bridwell reviewed the use of titanium mesh cages for anterior spine surgery.[21] Described benefits included sagittal-plane correction and the maintenance of lumbar lordosis, as well as a decreased frequency of pseudarthrosis. Lowe et al showed in human cadaver and bovine models that dual rods with structural inter-vertebral-body support were the best combination for increasing stiffness, and that the addition of cross-links did not add to stiffness but to torsional strength.[16] Ouellet and Johnston showed that rib-strut grafting with single-rod constructs decreased the rate of pseudarthrosis, but this particular form of grafting did not affect the maintenance of correction or sagittal alignment.[11,22] They suggested that mesh cages or femoral ring allografts may be better for these functions. The placement of inter-vertebral-body cages or grafts increases anterior column height and stability, but longer follow-up will be needed to ascertain whether they maintain sagittal balance.

## Clinical Results

Guille and colleagues reviewed the HSG database and found 100 patients with Lenke type 5 curves treated with the anterior approach.[23] Thirty-nine of the patients had received single-rod constructs (**Fig. 19.1**) and 61 had received dual-rod constructs (**Fig. 19.2**). Preoperatively,

A–C

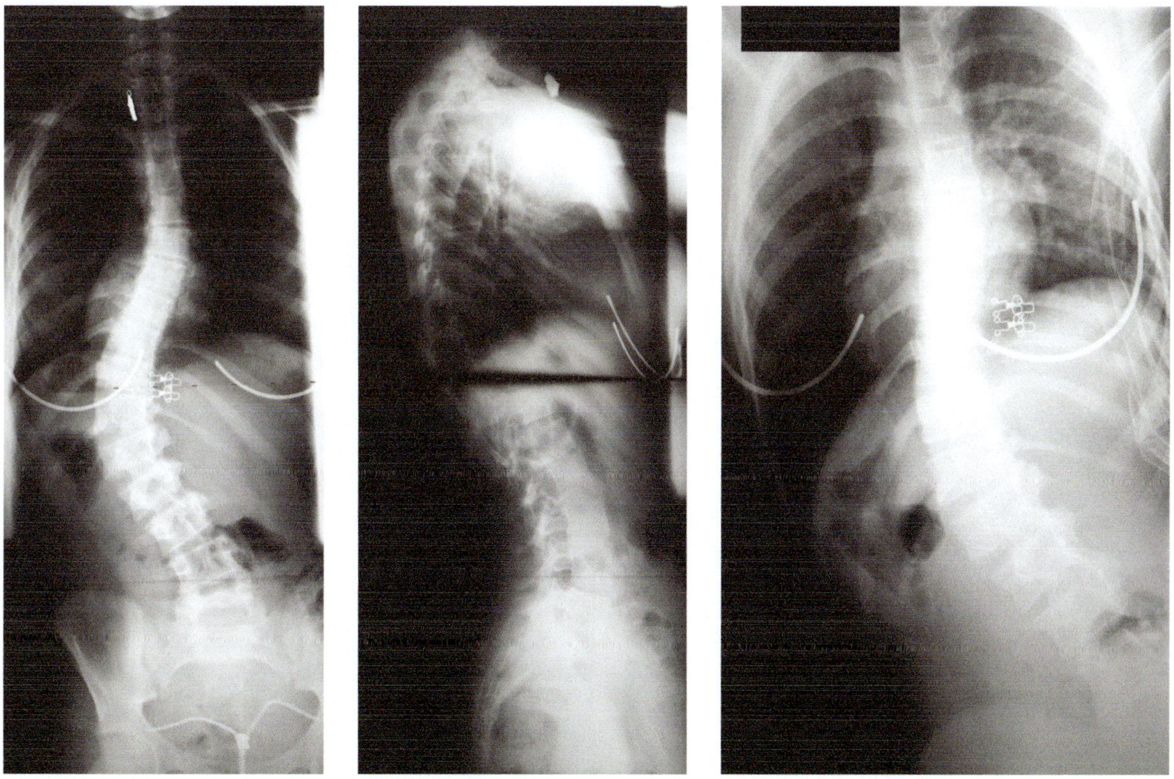

**Fig. 19.1** **(A,B)** Lenke type 5CN curve. The TL/L curve measured 56 degrees. **(C,D)** The TL/L curve bends to 40 degrees.

*(Continued on page 236)*

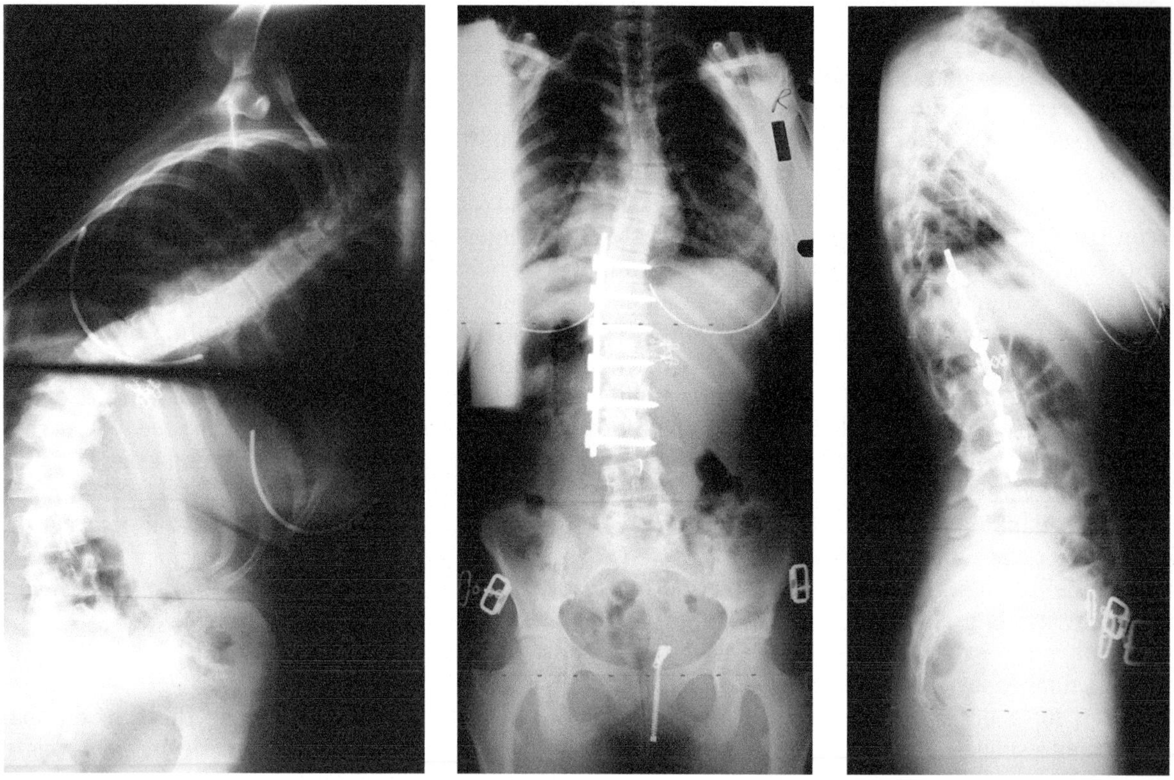

D–F

**Fig. 19.1** (*Continued*) **(C,D)** The TL/L curve bends to 40 degrees. **(E,F)** The patient underwent anterior instrumentation and fusion from T10 to L3 with a single rod, and with interbody cages from T12 to L3. At 2 years postoperatively the patient's TL/L curve was 11 degrees.

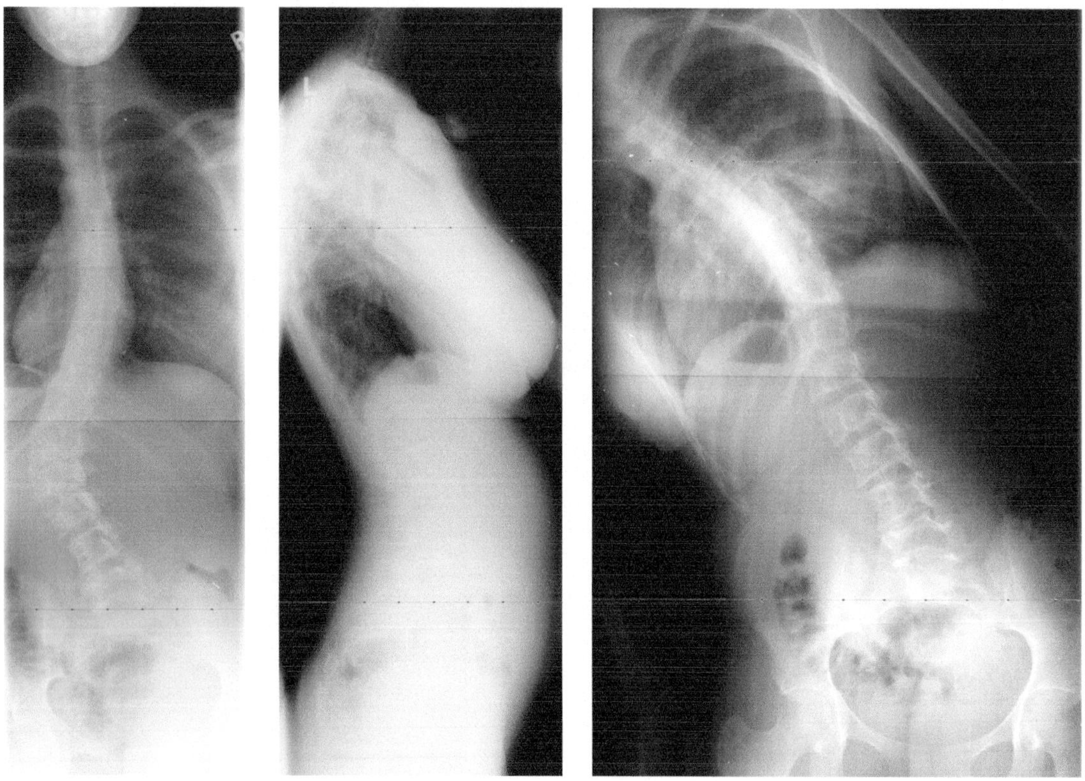

A–C

**Fig. 19.2 (A,B)** Lenke type 5CN curve. The TL/L curve measured 44 degrees. **(C,D)** The TL/L curve bends to 17 degrees.

D–F

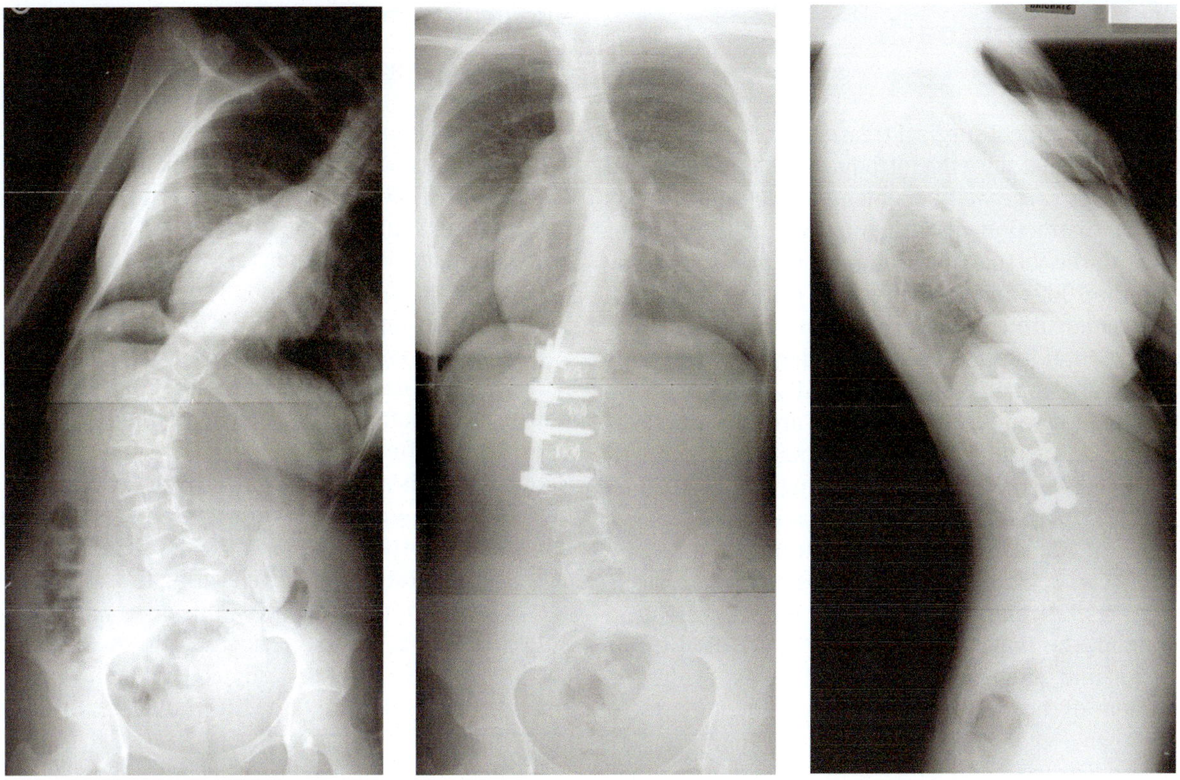

**Fig. 19.2** *(Continued)* **(C,D)** The TL/L curve bends to 17 degrees. **(E,F)** The patient underwent anterior instrumentation and fusion from T12 to L3 with a dual rod, and with interbody cages from T12 to L3. At 2 years postoperatively the patient's TL/L curve was 19 degrees.

the two groups were statistically similar in their radiographic measurements. Intraoperatively, patients with the single-rod constructs had shorter operative times and less blood loss. Average coronal-curve correction was 83% for the single-rod group and 72% for the dual-rod group. Measured values of sagittal alignment were improved and maintained in both groups. At a minimun of 2 years follow-up, the patients treated with single rods had better maintenance of coronal correction, whereas four of the patients treated with dual rods had pseudarthroses.

Turi and coworkers reported their experience with single-rod Texas Scottish Rite Hospital instrumentation in 14 patients.[9] Average coronal-curve correction was 76%, with no pseudarthrosis. There was an average 5-degree loss of correction at follow-up. Sweet and colleagues reviewed 47 patients who had anterior fusions instrumented with 5.0-mm or 5.5-mm single-rods with cages for their TL/L curves. The average correction was 70%. Two patients developed a pseudarthrosis. Kaneda et al reported their experience with 20 patients who had idiopathic TL/L scoliosis treated with dual-rod anterior instrumentation.[12] They showed an 83% coronal-curve correction, maintenance of sagittal alignment, and no pseudarthrosis. Hurford et al reported their experience with 42 patients who underwent dual-rod anterior instrumentation and fusion for idiopathic scoliosis.[24] At follow-up, they found a 67% average correction and no pseudarthrosis. This percent correction compares favorably with the 70% correction seen in a group of patients treated at the same institution with single-rod constructs,[25] also without any cases of pseudarthrosis.

## Hall Concept

Few reports exist of the method of treatment proposed by John Hall.[26,27] Hall suggested that flexible TL/L curves could be treated anteriorly with short fusion (three or four segments) and overcorrection at the apex. Thus, for example, if the apex was at L2, the fusion would extend from L1 to L3. If the apex was a disc space, the fusion would extend two vertebrae above and two vertebrae below the apex. Although good coronal correction can be achieved with this method, the fate of the sagittal alignment is less reliable. Also, the last instrumented vertebra is not rendered horizontal, but is instead overcorrected. The fate of the resulting obliquity and the associated disc-space wedging is unknown.

# Posterior Approach

## History

The search for the ideal surgical treatment of Lenke type 5 curves has continued since the introduction of instrumented fusion for scoliosis. The well-documented deleterious effects of posterior distraction instrumentation on the lumbar spine[28] led to the virtual abandonment of posterior spine surgery in the 1960s and thereafter. The primary goal with this type of idiopathic deformity is to maintain or create normal segmental lumbar lordosis. Inadequate lordosis is probably the single main etiology of late distal degenerative disease. Other goals of posterior surgery are horizontalization of the distal instrumented vertebra, maximum coronal- and axial-plane correction, and balancing of the residual lumbar curve with the compensatory thoracic curve.

Dwyer et al advocated the anterior approach, utilizing vertebral screws connected by a cable to correct idiopathic lumbar curves.[3] Although satisfactory coronal correction was obtained, the universal kyphosing effect of anterior compression and a high rate of pseudarthrosis resulted in abandonment of the Dwyer device.[29] Creation of kyphosis by anterior convex compression is analogous to its creation by posterior distraction. Zielke's use of a 3.2-mm threaded rod in conjunction with anterior vertebral screws was thought to be the solution to the problem of a kyphosing effect.[30] However, the universal kyphosing effect remained with this device, and a high pseudarthrosis rate became evident.[8] The search for the ideal surgical treatment of the Lenke type 5 deformity therefore continued.

The introduction of anterior solid rods with vertebral screws was the natural evolution in this search. Yet despite good coronal correction with their use, the kyphosing effect remained.[25,31] Theoretically, the use of structural intervertebral-body grafts (femoral rings, cages) in conjunction with solid rods should maintain lumbar lordosis, and Harms reported excellent results and normal lordosis with this combination.[32] However, the maximally invasive anterior thoracoabdominal approach is required to achieve 80% correction and normal segmental lordosis.

Posterior alternatives to the anterior thoracoabdominal procedure have also been long sought. Ponte, in the 1980s, introduced the concept of a posterior shortening osteotomy over multiple vertebral levels to achieve purely posterior correction of Scheuerman kyphosis.[33] In this technique, hooks and a threaded 0.24-in. rod were used. A similar procedure has been used since the early 1990s by one of the authors (H.L.S.) to produce or maintain lumbar lordosis in Lenke type 5 scoliosis.[34] Initially, this technique was used with hooks, but with the advent of segmental pedicle screws in idiopathic spinal deformities, consistent and reliable 3D correction is attainable with a relatively simple posterior procedure.[35]

## Surgical Technique of Posterior Fusion

One of the authors (H.L.S.) has used posterior fusion for more than 15 years in correcting scoliotic deformities, initially using hooks. Segmental pedicle screws have been used as the spinal anchors in the technique since the late 1990s. In the patient with a Lenke type 5 curve with normal thoracic kyphosis, the fusion levels are the Cobb-angle levels of the curve. If there is significant thoracic kyphosis (>60 degrees), consideration of the proximal extension of fusion may be appropriate.

The patient is positioned on the Jackson table, and subperiosteal exposure is achieved to the tips of the transverse processes. All soft tissue is removed from the spine. In cases in which the fusion will extend into the thoracic spine, thoracoplasty is accomplished through the original midline incision. Bone grafting from the iliac crest has not been required in posterior fusion for the past 15 years. Thoracoplasty is accomplished by elevating the appropriate subcutaneous flap from the latissimus dorsi and dividing the intercostal muscles and periosteum in the line of the rib. Portions of three ribs are easily accessed with this method, and together with local bone this provides sufficient bone-graft material for the procedure.

The next step in posterior fusion is the excision of all facet joints from the posterior. An osteotome may be used to remove the superior articular process of the inferior vertebra at each level. A 3-mm Leksell rongeur is useful for removing all of the articular cartilage before excision of the articular process. **Figure 19.3** shows the exposed spine with the areas to be excised outlined.

The ligamentum flavum is next excised at each vertebral level. This is best accomplished with a Kerrison rongeur. The excision of the ligamentum flavum must be carried laterally onto the anterior surface of each facet joint, with excision of the extension that constitutes the anterior capsule of the facet joint. The capsule excision is carried into the foramen bilaterally at each vertebral level. **Figure 19.4** shows the TL spine with the osteotomies completed.

Segmental pedicle screws are then inserted. The author's (H.L.S.) preferred technique uses guidance with image intensification, and a hand drill to navigate the pedicle. Polyaxial screws are inserted at the proximal and distal end-vertebrae and at every level on the concave side of the scoliotic curve. Uniplanar pedicle screws are inserted at all other levels on the convex side. These improve the ability to derotate the maximally rotated central portion of the scoliotic deformity.

Rod placement is the next step. The author (H.L.S.) prefers a very stiff stainless-steel rod for instrumentation on both the convex and concave sides of the scoliotic curve. The rod diameter is 5.5 mm. The convex rod must be placed first, because lordosis and correction of the coronal deformity can be accomplished only from this side of the curve. An extensive discussion of the mechanisms of correction of

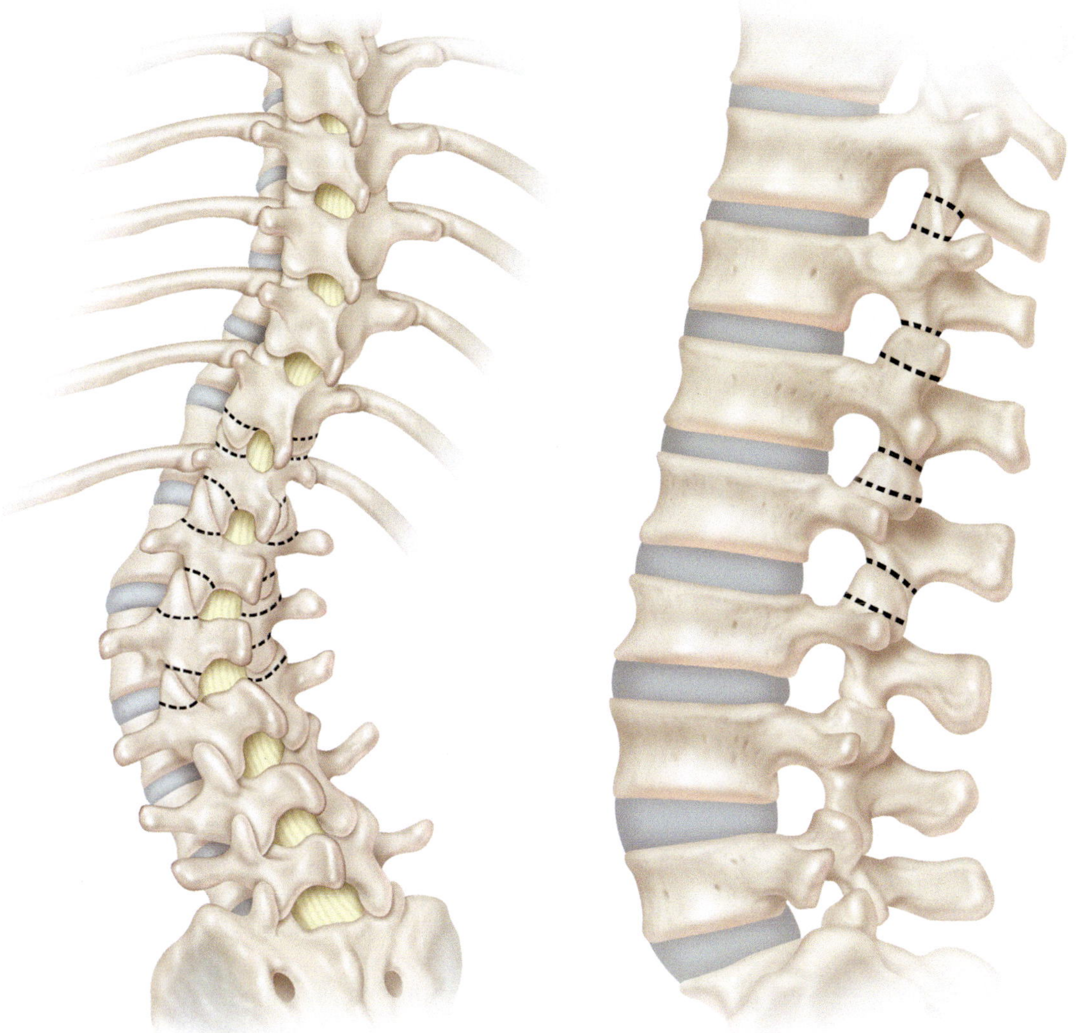

A B

**Fig. 19.3** **(A)** An idiopathic lumbar curve. Wide posterior release would consist of removal of facet joints and ligamentum flavum, and extension of the ligamentum flavum across the anterior portion of the facet joint. The *hatched areas* indicate the portions to be excised to effect a Ponte osteotomy. **(B)** The sagittal view also depicts the portions to be excised to create a Ponte osteotomy across several segments of the lumbar scoliosis.

deformity is provided in Chapter 14.[36] The convex rod is bent to approximate the normal sagittal contours of the spine. Usually, initial insertion of the rod in the distal-most convex implant facilitates rod placement. The rod is fixed distally in the final sagittal position. The rod-rotation maneuver is not used. Sequential entering of successive implants from distal to proximal, using a cantilever maneu ver, accomplishes placement of the first rod.

The concave or second rod is bent to a lesser degree of lordosis than the first rod. This underbending accomplishes an en-bloc derotation as the concave screws are pulled to the rod. Facile placement of this rod is accomplished by placing the rod in both the proximal and distal implants. The central portion of the deformity curve is then pulled posteriorly to the rod.

With both rods in place, direct vertebral derotation is accomplished. Both of the distal implants in the spine are tightened. Several instruments are available to accomplish direct vertebral derotation from the distal to the proximal level. Final tightening of all implants is accomplished in conjunction with stable spinal-cord monitoring. Cross-links are not routinely used. **Figure 19.5** demonstrates the final position of the spine with the two treatment rods in place. Decortication to the tips of the transverse processes, and graft placement followed by closure, completes the procedure.

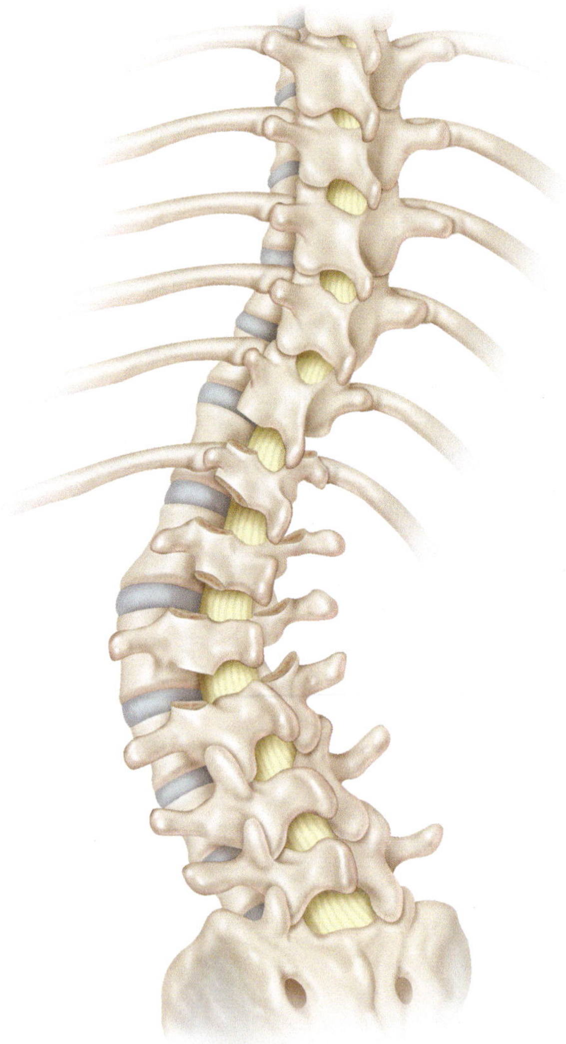

**Fig. 19.4** Ponte osteotomies have been done at every vertebral level to be instrumented and fused in this lumbar scoliosis. Closure of the created spaces permits correction of the coronal deformity and production of lumbar lordosis.

Postoperative care of the patient undergoing posterior fusion includes beginning ambulation on the first day after surgery without bracing or other external immobilization. Sedentary activities are permitted as tolerated. Return to most sporting activities is permitted by 3 to 6 months after surgery.

## Outcomes

Many chapters in this book use the HSG database to report clinical results of scoliosis surgery. The author (H.L.S) was not a participant in the HSG until late 2005. Accordingly, there are a paucity of data on the posterior surgical treatment of Lenke type 5 idiopathic curves. Two groups of patients, both with follow-up of more than 2 years, are discussed to illustrate the efficacy of the posterior approach to such curves. Sixty-one patients with instrumented lumbar curves (51 with Lenke type 5 curves), referred to in the following discussion as 2004 Posterior, have been previously described.[35] An additional 31 patients with Lenke type 5 curves, referred to as 2007 Posterior, have been studied and compared with a matched group of patients, referred to as 2007 Anterior, who were treated with anterior dual-rod constructs.[37] The patients treated with posterior surgery may also be compared with patients with Lenke type 5 curves who had anterior surgery, referred to as HSG Anterior, and described in the section of this chapter on the anterior approach. The two groups of patients treated with posterior surgery were consecutive to one another in their diagnosis and surgery, as were the patients in the 2007 Anterior group. All of the patients having posterior surgery were treated by the author (H.L.S.).

Multiple parameters may be compared in the studies described above. **Table 19.1** lists coronal measurements and sagittal measurements from T12 to the lowest instrumented vertebra (LIV). The correction with the posterior approach is better ($P < 0.01$) and the loss of correction smaller ($P = 0.028$) than in either of the two series in which an anterior approach was used. The change in lordosis between T12 and the LIV is significantly better ($P < 0.001$) in the group treated with a posterior approach. This would indicate the persistent inability of anterior surgery to produce and maintain lordosis over the instrumented segments of the spine.

Multiple other measurements are available in the data described above for the patients treated with an anterior and those treated with a posterior approach. The patients treated with a posterior approach had an average of 4.8 days of hospitalization, as compared with 6.1 days of hospitalization for the group treated with an anterior approach ($P < 0.01$). Blood loss was equivalent with the two approaches. However, in the HSG Anterior group, the operative time was 6 hours as compared with 2.36 hours in the combined posterior groups. Lordosis from T12 to S1 was 53 degrees in both the 2007 Posterior and 2007 Anterior groups. The smaller lordosis with instrumentation in the anterior-treatment group reflects a situation resembling that with the use of posterior Harrington instrumentation in the 2007 Anterior group. There is a straight or relatively kyphotic instrumented segment of the spine, with a distal hyperlordosis below it. Thoracic kyphosis was similar in the posterior-treatment groups (25 degrees) and in the 2007 Anterior group (27 degrees).

The angle of the LIV is one of the more important parameters in the surgical treatment of idiopathic TL/L scoliosis. In both of the posterior-treatment groups in the

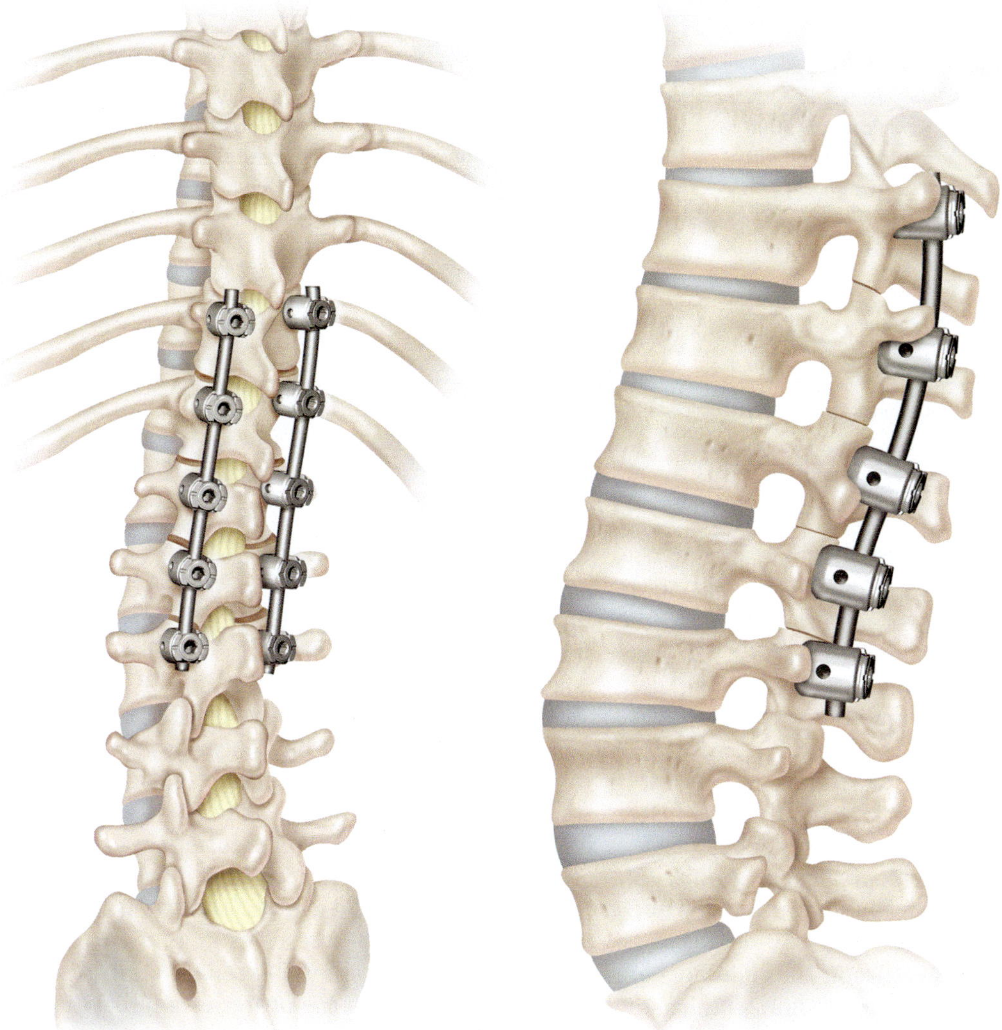

A B

**Fig. 19.5** **(A)** Bilateral pedicle screws have been placed at every vertebral level, and both rods of the corrective instrumentation have been placed, with the convex rod having been placed first. See text for an explanation of the mechanics of correction. Correction of the coronal plane has been achieved. **(B)** In the sagittal plane, a harmonious lumbar lordosis has been produced, as well as a smooth conversion from lumbar lordosis to thoracic kyphosis.

HSG database this was 27 degrees before surgery and 5 degrees at last follow-up. In the 2007 Anterior group, the angle of the LIV was 28 degrees before surgery and 4.5 degrees at last follow-up. Posterior or anterior surgery significantly and equally improved the angle of the LIV.

There were no significant complications in either the two posterior-surgery groups or the 2007 Anterior group. There were no extended hospital stays, no unplanned second surgeries, no infections, and no neurological injuries. In the HSG Anterior group there were two unplanned second surgeries. An L4 screw causing nerve-root irritation required acute revision. One of the four pseudarthroses in this group required a revision.

## Discussion

The foregoing section describes two separate groups of patients treated with wide posterior release and Ponte osteotomy followed by segmental pedicle-screw and rod instrumentation for idiopathic TL/L scoliosis. Both groups were consecutive for diagnosis and surgery. The first group treated with a posterior approach was entered into the HSG database between 1997 and 1999 and the second posterior-treatment group was entered between 2001 and 2004. The total comprises 82 patients treated with the posterior procedure, all of whom had more than 24 months of follow-up. All underwent surgery and instrumentation by the author (H.L.S.).

**Table 19.1 Comparison of Measured Variables with Posterior and Anterior Procedures**

| | AP Cobb Angle (Degrees) | First Postoperative Measurement (Degrees) | Final Postoperative Measurement (Degrees) (Percent Reduction) | T12–LIV Lordosis Preoperative (Degrees) | T12–LIV Lordosis Postoperative (Degrees) |
|---|---|---|---|---|---|
| 2004 Posterior | 52 | 10 | 11 (79%) | | |
| 2007 Posterior | 50 | 6 | 8 (84%) | −10 | −27 |
| 2007 Anterior | 49 | 12 | 16 (68%) | −1 | −0.8 |
| HSG Anterior | 46 | 11.5 | 15 (68%) | | |

*Abbreviations*: AP, anteroposterior; HSG, Harms Study Group; LIV, lowest instrumented vertebra.

Two groups of patients treated with anterior instrumentation for TL/L scoliosis are also discussed. These comprise 99 patients whose entry into the HSG database began in 1995 with the creation of the HSG. Of these patients, 31 had anterior dual-rod instrumentation. There may be some overlap of patients in the two anterior-surgery groups.

Some differences exist in the posterior- and anterior-treatment groups. The correction was significantly better ($P < 0.01$) in the posterior-treatment group, at 84%, than the 67% correction for both anterior-treatment groups. Although this difference is statistically significant, it is difficult to state that the difference between a 10-degree and a 16-degree curve is clinically significant. The ability of both the posterior and anterior approaches to horizontalize the LIV is similar, with both producing excellent distal alignment. This factor is probably critically important in the long term.

Of some concern is the production of a straight segment from T12 to the LIV. This was the specific problem affecting early posterior distraction instrumentation, and it was for this reason that posterior instrumentation of the lumbar spine in scoliosis was abandoned in the 1960s and 1970s. The time is probably approaching when many patients with flatback syndrome from anterior instrumentation for scoliosis will be developing distal degenerative disease. In the 2007 Posterior group identified in the HSG database, measurements for the segment from T12 to the LIV are available, and demonstrate excellent production of lordosis in this segment. This segment, which corresponds to the vertebral levels beginning at T12 and usually ending at L3, had a final lordosis of 27 degrees, with the total lordosis for T12 to S1 of 59 degrees. From the LIV to S1, the lordosis was 32 degrees, as compared with 55 degrees in the 2007 Anterior group. In theory, flatback syndrome is not caused by current posterior-treatment techniques but rather by the compression used in the anterior procedure. Less lordosis is created distal to the LIV in posterior procedures. This, again in theory, should be beneficial in the long term.

Both series of patients treated with posterior surgeries were without complications. This was not true for the HSG Anterior group, in which four pseudarthroses (5%) were reported, although only one patient had a surgical revision (with a posterior instrumented fusion).

Several nonobjective measures favor the posterior approach in treating TL/L curves. The scar is never visible to patients looking at themselves in a mirror. **Figures 19.6** and **19.7** demonstrate the excellent clinical results routinely obtained with the posterior approach. The operative time with this approach is never more than 3 hours, intensive care is never required, and a chest tube is not needed.

The fusion levels in posterior surgery are almost always those involved in the Cobb-angle measurement unless there is significant thoracic hyperkyphosis. The distal level of fusion is always involved in the Cobb-angle measurement, and is frequently one level proximal to this when the distal end-vertebra is L3. **Figures 19.8**, **19.9**, **19.10**, and **19.11** demonstrate the excellent radiographic results shown in the clinical photographs in **Figs 19.6** and **19.7**. The images in **Fig. 19.12** are the clinical photographs of the patient whose radiographs are seen in **Fig. 19.8**, and **Fig. 19.13A** and **B** are the clinical photographs of the patient whose radiographs are seen in **Fig. 19.10**.

In view of the excellent results in the 82 patients treated with posterior surgery for adolescent idiopathic Lenke type 5 curves, it is difficult to envision an instance in which an anterior instrumented procedure would be the procedure of choice.

A B

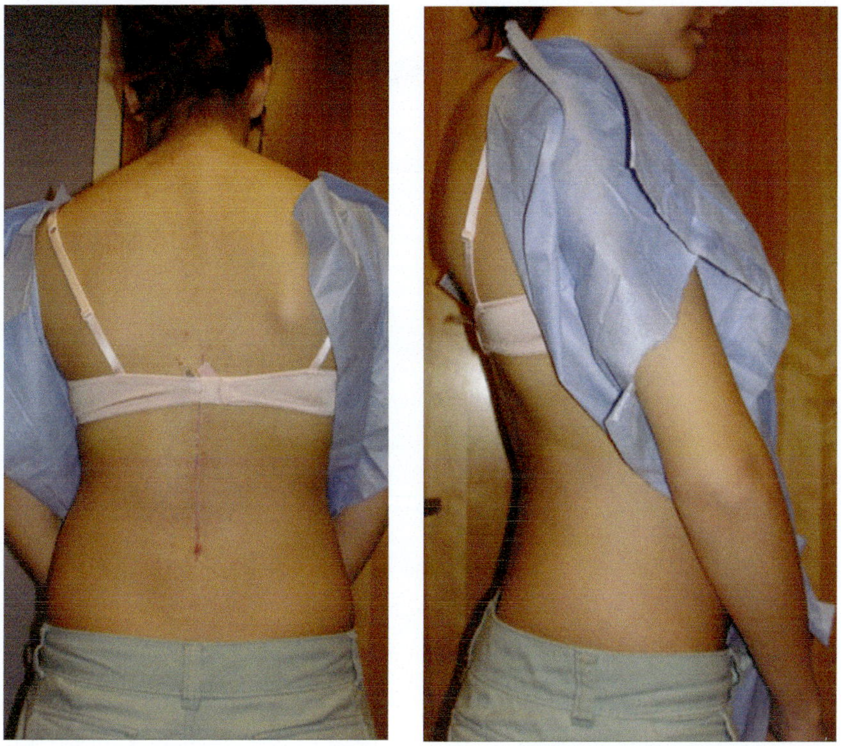

**Fig. 19.6 (A,B)** Excellent clinical appearance in both the coronal and sagittal planes following instrumentation and fusion.

A B

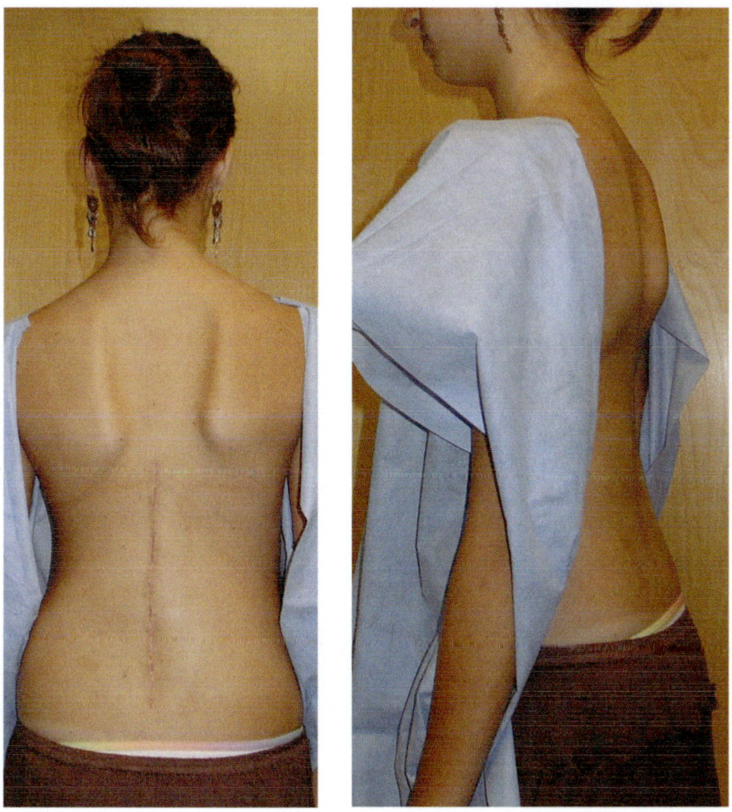

**Fig. 19.7 (A,B)** An excellent clinical result following instrumentation and fusion.

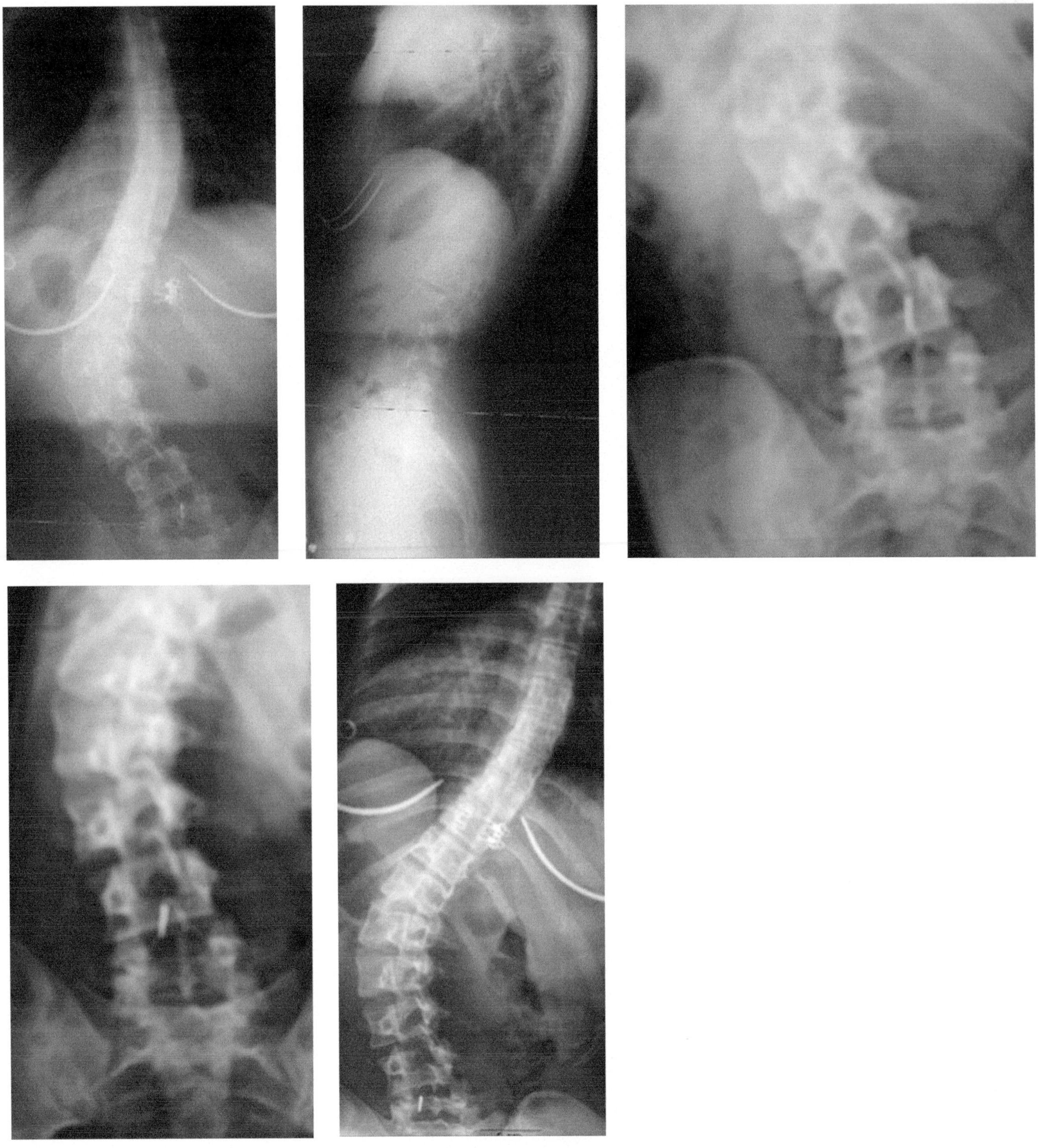

A–C

D,E

**Fig. 19.8** **(A)** Coronal view demonstrating a 55-degree thoracolumbar idiopathic scoliosis. The Cobb-angle measurement is from T10 to L3. **(B)** Sagittal view demonstrates a kyphotic thoracolumbar junction. The total thoracic kyphosis is normal. **(C,D)** The left- and right-bending films at the lumbosacral junction do not demonstrate reduction of L3 on L4 or satisfactory correction of the lumbosacral fractional curve. Some question remains about the advisability of stopping fusion at L3. **(E)** The right-bending film demonstrates correction of the thoracic curve to less than 20 degrees, indicating that the thoracic curve need not be included in the fusion.

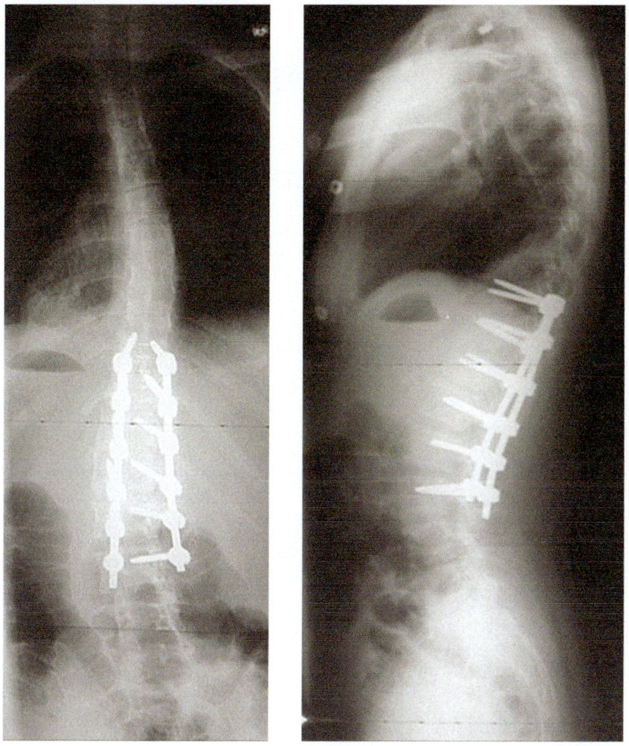

A,B

**Fig. 19.9 (A,B)** Excellent postoperative coronal and sagittal alignment and balance is obtained. Note that the angle of the distal endplate of the LIV is ~5 degrees, and that the disc space is minimally wedged. In the sagittal plane, there is harmonious lumbar lordosis without a distal increase in lordosis.

## Conclusion

Current techniques of either posterior or anterior fusion in Lenke type 5 curves yield excellent results in terms of coronal, sagittal, and rotational correction. The addition of a second rod in the anterior approach has provided stability and rigidity similar to that seen when a posterior approach is used to avoid temporary bracing. The use of an anterior inter-vertebral-body spacer or a posterior-based shortening with an osteotomy gives each approach the ability to maintain lumbar lordosis. The advantages and drawbacks of each of the two techniques have been discussed in this chapter. Historically, the anterior approach has reduced the number of needed fusion levels. It also avoids injury to the paraspinal muscles of the lower back. However, the anterior approach produces greater immediate postoperative morbidity, a scar that is more visible to the patient, and for many spine surgeons a greater dependence on an access surgeon. The posterior approach, on the other hand, is more familiar for the spine surgeon or pediatric orthopedic surgeon. Current techniques allow fusion levels in a posterior approach that are similar to those used in an anterior approach. What is not clear is whether there will be long-term problems (low back pain, etc.) associated with scarring of the paraspinal musculature of the low back. However, it is clear that either an anterior or a posterior technique can be used to effectively manage a Lenke type 5 curve. The choice for the treating surgeon may be related more closely to the surgeon's experience with a particular approach than to other factors.

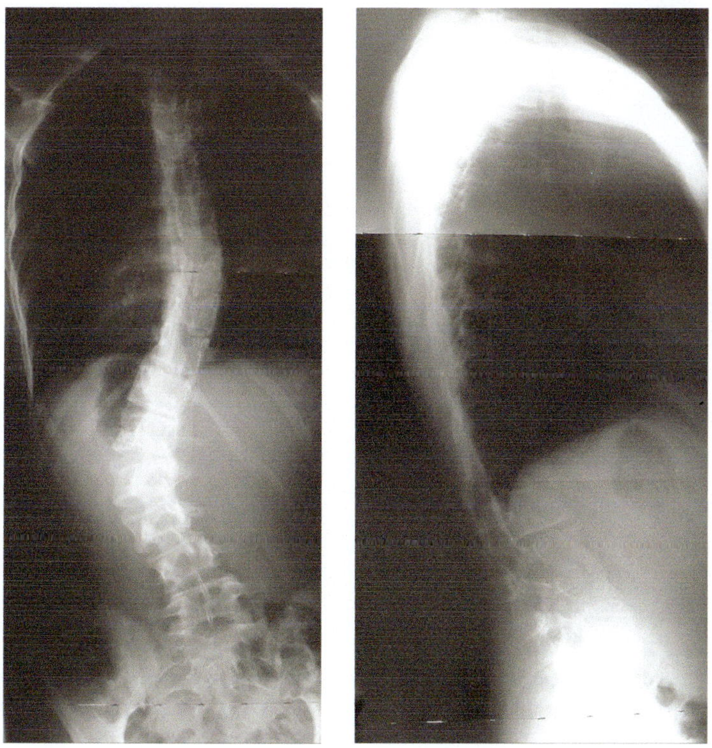

A B

**Fig. 19.10 (A,B)** This idiopathic lumbar curve has an apex at L2 and the ends of its Cobb angle at T11 and L4. The lateral film demonstrates a kyphotic upper lumbar spine and distal lumbar increased lordosis.

*(Continued on page 246)*

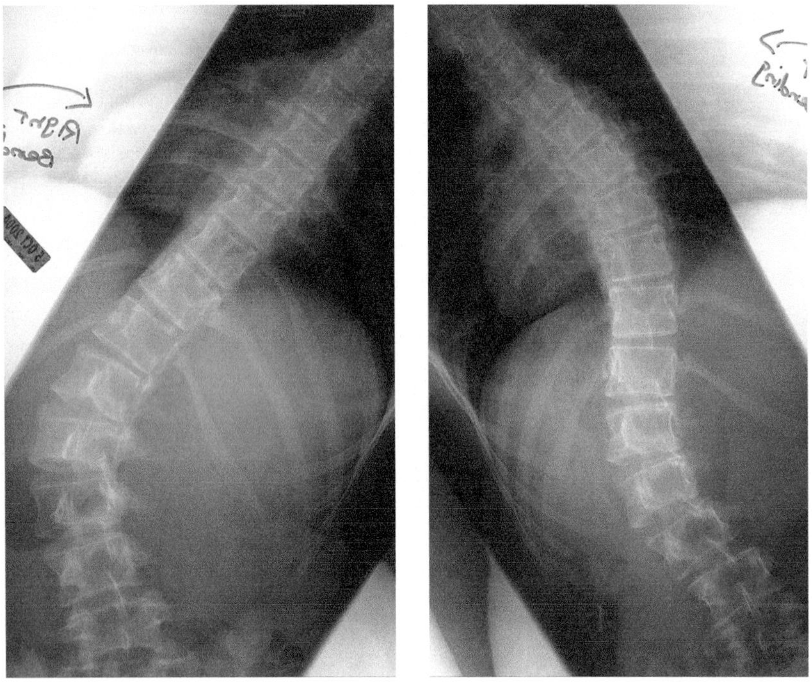

C D

**Fig. 19.10** (*Continued*) **(C,D)** The right-bending film shows that L4 is nearly horizontal over the sacrum, with nearly complete correction of the thoracic curve. The left- bending film shows the main lumbar curve is relatively rigid.

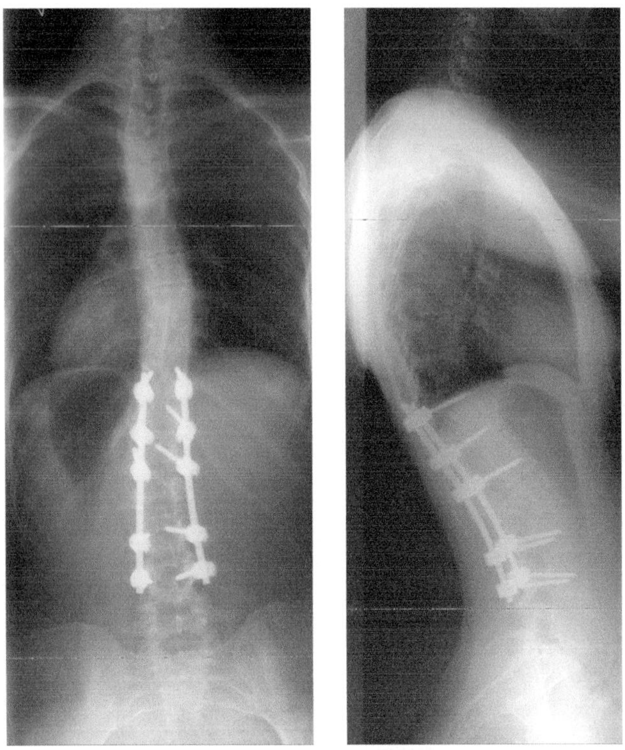

A B

**Fig. 19.11** **(A,B)** At 2 years after surgery, this patient's coronal and sagittal balance are excellent. The coronal correction is nearly complete, L4 is parallel, and the L4–L5 disc is not wedged. In the sagittal plane there is harmonious lumbar lordosis, and the distal hyperlordosis has been alleviated.

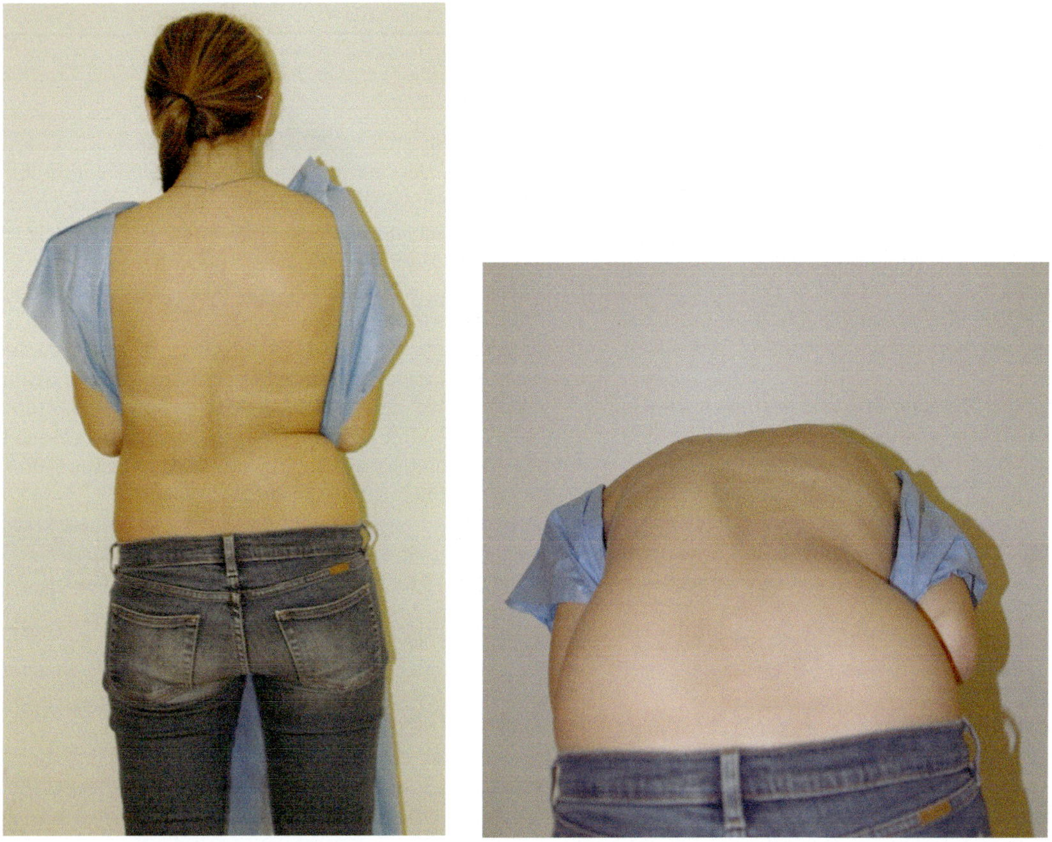

A B

**Fig. 19.12 (A,B)** Clinical photographs of the patient whose radiographs are shown in Fig. 19.8 illustrate marked waist asymmetry and a significant lumbar rotational prominence.

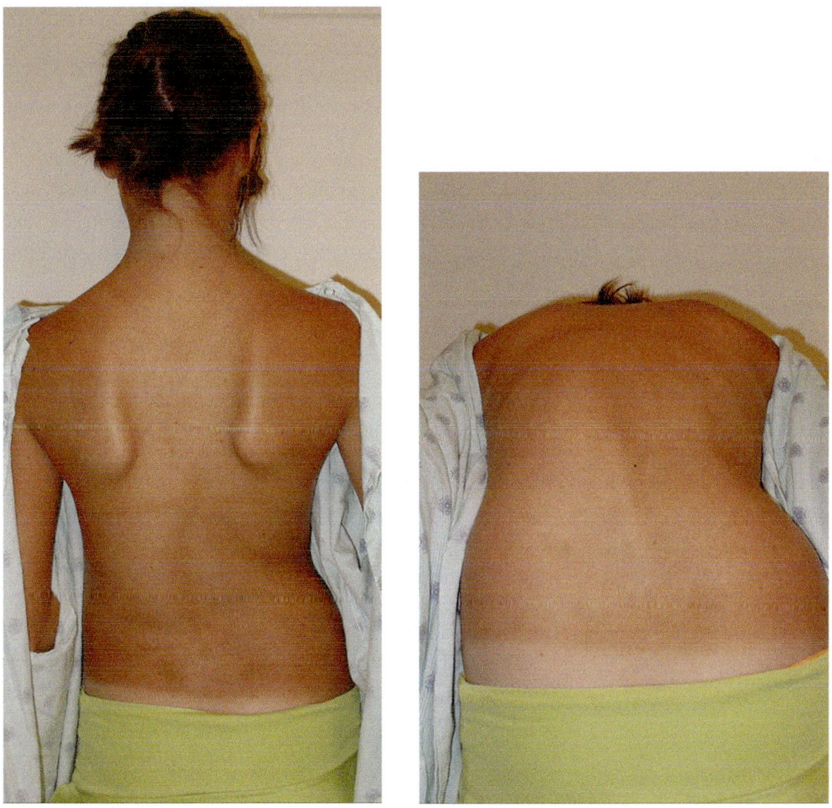

A,B

**Fig. 19.13 (A,B)** The clinical deformity in this case is quite significant.

## References


1. Dwyer AF, Newton NC, Sherwood AA. An anterior approach to scoliosis. A preliminary report. Clin Orthop Relat Res 1969;62:192–202
2. Dwyer AF. Experience of anterior correction of scoliosis. Clin Orthop Relat Res 1973;93:191–214
3. Dwyer AF, Schafer MF. Anterior approach to scoliosis. Results of treatment in fifty-one cases. J Bone Joint Surg Br 1974;56:218–224
4. Dwyer AF, O'Brien JP, Seal PP. The late complications after the Dwyer anterior spinal instrumentation for scoliosis. J Bone Joint Surg Br 1977;59:117
5. Hsu LC, Zucherman J, Tang SC, Leong JC. Dwyer instrumentation in the treatment of adolescent idiopathic scoliosis. J Bone Joint Surg Br 1982;64:536–541
6. Hammerberg KW, Rodts MF, DeWald RL. Zielke instrumentation. Orthopedics 1988;11:1365–1371
7. Trammell TR, Benedict F, Reed D. Anterior spine fusion using Zielke instrumentation for adult thoracolumbar and lumbar scoliosis. Spine 1991;16:307–316
8. Kaneda K, Fujiya N, Satoh S. Results with Zielke instrumentation for idiopathic thoracolumbar and lumbar scoliosis. Clin Orthop Relat Res 1986;205:195–203
9. Turi M, Johnston CE II, Richards BS. Anterior correction of idiopathic scoliosis using TSRH instrumentation. Spine 1993;18: 417–422
10. Hopf CG, Eysel P, Dubousset J. Operative treatment of scoliosis with Cotrel-Dubousset-Hopf instrumentation. New anterior spinal device. Spine 1997;22:618–627, discussion 627–628
11. Johnston CE II. Anterior correction of thoracolumbar and lumbar idiopathic scoliosis. Semin Spine Surg 1997;9:150
12. Kaneda K, Shono Y, Satoh S, Abumi K. New anterior instrumentation for the management of thoracolumbar and lumbar scoliosis. Application of the Kaneda two-rod system. Spine 1996;21:1250–1261, discussion 1261–1262
13. Lenke LG, Betz RR, Harms J, et al. Adolescent idiopathic scoliosis: A new classification to determine extent of spinal arthrodesis. J Bone Joint Surg Am 2001;83A:1169–1181
14. Sanders AE, Baumann R, Brown H, Johnston CE II, Lenke LG, Sink E. Selective anterior fusion of thoracolumbar/lumbar curves in adolescents: When can the associated thoracic curve be left unfused? Spine 2003;28:706–713, discussion 714
15. Newton PO, Faro FD, Lenke LG, et al. Factors involved in the decision to perform a selective versus nonselective fusion of Lenke 1B and 1C (King-Moe II) curves in adolescent idiopathic scoliosis. Spine 2003;28:S217–S223
16. Lowe TG, Enguidanos ST, Smith DA, et al. Single-rod versus dual-rod anterior instrumentation for idiopathic scoliosis: A biomechanical study. Spine 2005;30:311–317
17. Fricka KB, Mahar AT, Newton PO. Biomechanical analysis of anterior scoliosis instrumentation: Differences between single and dual rod systems with and without interbody structural support. Spine 2002;27:702–706
18. Oda I, Cunningham BW, Lee GA, Abumi K, Kaneda K, McAfee PC. Biomechanical properties of anterior thoracolumbar multisegmental fixation: An analysis of construct stiffness and screw-rod strain. Spine 2000;25:2303–2311
19. Chang UK, Lim J, Kim DH. Biomechanical study of thoracolumbar junction fixation devices with different diameter dual-rod systems. J Neurosurg Spine 2006;4:206–212
20. Zhang H, Johnston CE II, Pierce WA, Ashman RB, Bronson DG, Haideri NF. New rod-plate anterior instrumentation for thoracolumbar/lumbar scoliosis: biomechanical evaluation compared with dual-rod and single-rod with structural interbody support. Spine 2006;31:E934–E940
21. Lenke LG, Bridwell KH. Mesh cages in idiopathic scoliosis in adolescents. Clin Orthop Relat Res 2002;394:98–108
22. Ouellet JA, Johnston CE II. Effect of grafting technique on the maintenance of coronal and sagittal correction in anterior treatment of scoliosis. Spine 2002;27:2129–2135, discussion 2135–2136
23. Guille JT, D'Andrea LP, Lonner BS, et al. Anterior treatment of structural thoracolumbar and lumbar curves: a comparison of dual vs single rod constructs in 100 patients. In preparation
24. Hurford RK Jr, Lenke LG, Lee SS, Cheng I, Sides B, Bridwell KH. Prospective radiographic and clinical outcomes of dual-rod instrumented anterior spinal fusion in adolescent idiopathic scoliosis: comparison with single-rod constructs. Spine 2006;31:2322–2328
25. Sweet FA, Lenke LG, Bridwell KH, Blanke KM, Whorton J. Prospective radiographic and clinical outcomes and complications of single solid rod instrumented anterior spinal fusion in adolescent idiopathic scoliosis. Spine 2001;26:1956–1965
26. Bernstein RM, Hall JE. Solid rod short segment anterior fusion in thoracolumbar scoliosis. J Pediatr Orthop B 1998;7:124–131
27. Hall JE. Short segment anterior instrumentation for thoracolumbar scoliosis. In: Bridwell KH, DeWald RL, eds. The Textbook of Spinal Surgery, ed. 2. Philadelphia: Lippincott-Raven, 1997:665–670
28. Lagrone MO, Bradford DS, Moe JH, Lonstein JE, Winter RB, Ogilvie JW. Treatment of symptomatic flatback after spinal fusion. J Bone Joint Surg Am 1988;70:569–580
29. Kohler R, Galland O, Mechin H, Michel CR, Onimus M. The Dwyer procedure in the treatment of idiopathic scoliosis. A 10-year follow-up review of 21 patients. Spine 1990;15:75–80
30. Lowe TG, Peters JD. Anterior spinal fusion with Zielke instrumentation for idiopathic scoliosis. A frontal and sagittal curve analysis in 36 patients. Spine 1993;18:423–426
31. Sweet FA, Lenke LG, Bridwell KH, Blanke KM. Maintaining lumbar lordosis with anterior single solid-rod instrumentation in thoracolumbar and lumbar adolescent idiopathic scoliosis. Spine 1999; 24:1655–1662
32. Harms JG. personal communication
33. Ponte A, Sicardi G. Progress in spinal deformity: Kyphosis. In: Goggi A, ed. Bologna, 1988:75–88
34. Shufflebarger HL, Clark CE. Effect of wide posterior release on correction in adolescent idiopathic scoliosis. J Pediatr Orthop B 1998; 7:117–123
35. Shufflebarger HL, Geck MJ, Clark CE. The posterior approach for lumbar and thoracolumbar adolescent idiopathic scoliosis: Posterior shortening and pedicle screws. Spine 2004;29:269–276, discussion 276
36. Shufflebarger HL. Posterior Hook/Screw/Rod Constructsed. Philadelphia: Hanley & Belfus, 2000
37. Geck MJ, Rinella A, Kim YJ. Comparison of surgical treatment in Lenke 5C adolescent idiopathic scoliosis: Anterior dual rod versus posterior pedicle fixation surgery: A comparison of two practices. Paper presented at: Annual Meeting for the Scoliosis Research Society, Edinburgh, Scotland, 2007

# 20 The Surgical Treatment of Double and Triple Curves (Lenke Types 3, 4, and 6)

*Burt Yaszay, William F. Lavelle, and Baron S. Lonner*

In 2001, Lenke and colleagues reported a new classification system for adolescent idiopathic scoliosis (AIS).[1] The intended goal was that the system be inclusive of all types of scoliotic curves, have good-to-excellent inter- and intraobserver reliability, include an assessment of sagittal alignment, and help in comparing treatment modalities and outcomes. The new classification is described in further detail in Chapter 9.

Before the Lenke classification, the King classification had been considered the gold standard for classifying AIS.[2] However, the King classification described five types of curves relative to each other, and was therefore not inclusive of all types of curves. Except for the King type I curve, which some consider a true double major curve, the King system did not specifically describe patterns with multiple structural curves.[3,4] In contrast, the Lenke classification provides an independent evaluation of each of the scoliotic curves (proximal thoracic [PT], main thoracic [MT], and thoracolumbar [TL]) for structurality. Once a curve is defined as structural, the recommendation is to treat the curve. Cases in which there was more than one structural curve created the need for defined types of double and triple major curves.

## Curve Definitions

The Lenke type 3 or double major curve is defined by both a structural MT (major) and a structural but minor thoracolumbar/lumbar (TL/L) curve (**Fig. 20.1A**). In the Lenke system, these curves typically have a lumbar "C" modifier but may also have a lumbar "B" or even an "A" modifier.[5] There may be varying degrees of TL kyphosis between the two curves that can affect treatment decisions. As discussed earlier, TL kyphosis >20 degrees from T10 through L2 also defines a curve as structural, even when the side-bending Cobb-angle measurement is <25 degrees. A multicenter study of 606 patients demonstrated a prevalence of 11% for Lenke type 3 double major curves.[6]

The Lenke type 4 or triple major curve pattern has a structural curve in all three regions of the spine, consisting of a PT (minor), MT (major), and TL/L (minor) curve (**Fig. 20.1B**). The lumbar apical vertebrae will typically lie lateral to the center sacral vertical line (CSVL) (lumbar modifier C) for curves of this type; however, this is not always the case.[6] The type 4 curve is also considered the least common of the curves in idiopathic, with a reported frequency in the literature of 1.4 to 3%.[6–8]

The Lenke type 6 curve is also a structural double curve (**Fig. 20.1C**). In contrast to a Lenke type 3, the type 6 curve pattern resembles the King type I curve pattern, with the TL/L curve being the larger or major curve. All Lenke type 6 curves have a lumbar "C" modifier.[1] Lenke type 6 curves are also rare, with a prevalence just above 3%.[6]

## Treatment Principles

The surgical management of Lenke type 3, 4, and 6 curves follows the same set of basic principles that apply to all AIS curves. The primary goal is to prevent progression while achieving maximal correction of deformity. This objective must not be achieved at the expense of maintaining or achieving optimal coronal and sagittal balance. Axial derotation to a neutral position should be attempted. Most thoracic deformities in AIS are accompanied by thoracic hypokyphosis or even thoracic lordosis. Correction of these sagittal deformities should also be attempted.

Improvement in the cosmetic appearance of the patient also plays an important role in the treatment of AIS. Although it is difficult to evaluate, cosmetic deformity can have profound psychosocial effects and drive patients to seek surgery.[9–13] Rib prominence, shoulder balance, flank symmetry, and a postoperative scar have all been shown to have an impact on patient satisfaction following the surgical treatment of AIS.[14] By achieving physiological coronal-, sagittal-, and axial-plane correction, the surgeon will optimize body symmetry and the patient's self-image.

Minimizing the number of fusion levels remains a fundamental principle of surgery for AIS. With the introduction of instrumentation by Harrington in the late 1950s, fusions were long and typically extended into the lower lumbar region.[15,16] Long-term follow-up studies of patients who had such fusions have found that they have greater than average back pain and risk of lumbar degeneration below the end-instrumented vertebra (EIV).[17–22] Reducing

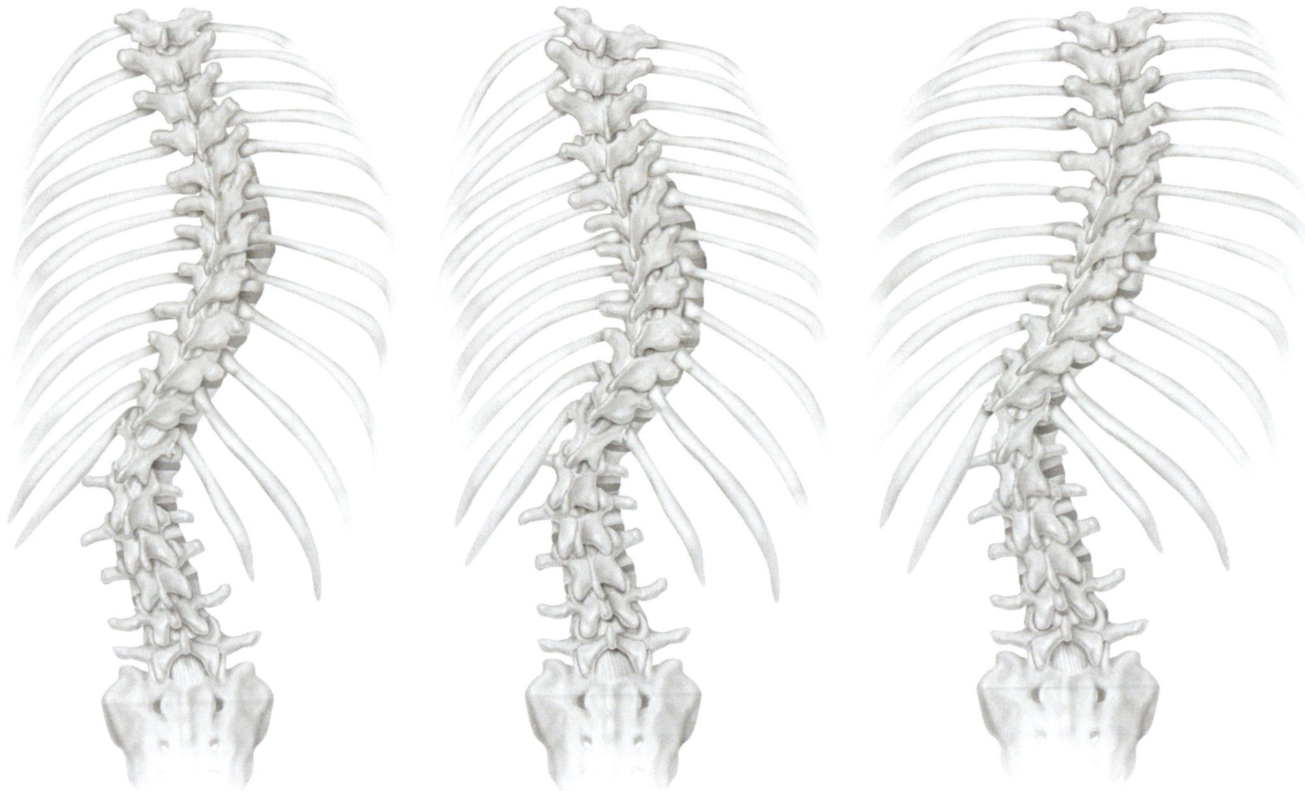


**Fig. 20.1** Drawings representing **(A)** Lenke type 3, **(B)** type 4, and **(C)** type 6 curves.

the number of fused vertebral levels maximizes spinal flexibility and distributes stress across a larger number of remaining distal lumbar motion segments.[23] Theoretically, this may diminish the long-term risk of disc degeneration at adjacent distal levels.

Beyond these basic principles, little has been written to guide the surgeon in treating double and triple major curves. Because these curves are less common than others, they have typically been discussed as part of larger, more comprehensive series of AIS patients. The traditional treatment for double and triple major curves has been arthrodesis of all curves.[3,4,24–29] In the Lenke classification, the recommendation is fusion of all the structural curves to prevent coronal decompensation through the uninstrumented curve.[1] In addition, the literature contains information on the treatment of these curves with third-generation hook-and-rod implants. To our knowledge, there is no analysis of double and triple major curves treated with current pedicle screw–rod implant technology. Barr et al reported that lumbar pedicle screws provided greater lumbar curve correction as well as maintenance of the correction in double major curves treated with hybrid constructs.[28] Some authors believe that all-pedicle-screw instrumentation provides better curve correction than all-hook or hybrid constructs.[30,31] Other studies challenge this, reporting similar curve correction without the expense of pedicle screws.[32–34] Regardless of whether or not pedicle screws improve coronal or sagittal curve correction, their true benefits may not be appreciated until the three-dimensional (3D) deformity of scoliosis can be adequately analyzed. By engaging both the posterior and anterior column of a vertebra, pedicle screws may improve axial rotation to a greater extent than do hooks or wires. However, it is unreasonable to subject young pediatric patients to preoperative and postoperative computed tomography (CT) to determine their axial deformity. New methods are currently being investigated for better analyzing the 3D deformity associated with scoliosis. Once a reliable and viable method is developed to fully quantify 3D spinal deformity, the effectiveness of pedicle-screw instrumentation can be compared with that of hybrid and other constructs.

## Selective Fusion

In keeping with the principle of minimizing fusion levels, the concept of selective fusion was introduced. Selective fusion is defined as fusion of the major curve when the apices of both the thoracic and TL curves deviate from the C7 plumbline or CSVL, respectively. King et al discussed the concept when they recommended selective thoracic fusion for their type II curves.[2] Lenke et al further refined this recommendation by listing parameters that would maximize success with selective thoracic fusions.[27] The purpose of these parameters was to differentiate true double major curves from MT curves in which the thoracic curvature was greater or more rigid than that of the TL curve, or both. At 10 years postoperatively, Large and colleagues found that patients who had a successful selective fusion of a double major curve had significantly less back pain and stiffness than those who had both curves fused.[35] Because their study predated the current Lenke classification, it is unclear whether all of the lumbar curves in Large and colleagues' patients were structural and would have required fusion under the current guidelines. The criteria for selective thoracic fusion under the current Lenke classification requires that a structural lumbar curve remain mobile and unfused. If, however, Large and coworkers' patients had true double major curves, this would call into question the definition of a structural TL curve as defined by the Lenke classification. Persistent lumbar motion may be a more important postoperative goal than a residual lumbar curve. If selective thoracic fusion is chosen, the surgeon will have to temper the degree of thoracic-curve correction to maintain coronal balance with the uninstrumented lumbar curve.

When considering fusion of the PT curve in a Lenke type 4 curve pattern, indications for arthrodesis can be extrapolated from data for double thoracic or King type V curves. Although spontaneous correction of the upper thoracic region can occur, both proximal extension of the instrumentation used in treating these curves, and failure to correct a PT curve, can have significant effects on shoulder balance.[36–38] Before the development of the Lenke classification, the criteria for recommending instrumentation and fusion of the PT curve included a Cobb angle >20 degrees on bending films, >1 cm of translation at the apex of the curve, elevation of the left shoulder, 5 degrees or more of T1 tilt into the concavity of the curve, or transition between the two curves at T6 or below.[39] One may consider making the proximal instrumented vertebra the vertebra at the apex of the PT curve if the T1 tilt is less than 5 degrees. Other literature has suggested that the best predictor of postoperative shoulder balance is the clavicle angle rather than the absolute or bending Cobb angle or the T1 tilt.[37] The clavicle line is defined by the intersection of a tangential line connecting the two highest points of each clavicle with a horizontal reference line. If the clavicle angle is positive (left clavicle higher than right clavicle), then fusion of the PT curve is likely to result in improved shoulder symmetry. The criteria for fusion in the Lenke classification include a side-bending Cobb angle >25 degrees or T2 to T5 kyphosis >20 degrees, or both. Cil and coworkers attempted to evaluate these criteria by retrospectively evaluating patients who had undergone fusion before the development of the Lenke classification.[40] They divided patients who had nonstructural PT curves into two groups: group 1 had a proximal fusion to T3 or above and group 2 had an upper instrumented vertebra at T4 or below. They then compared postoperative bilateral coracoid heights, clavicle angles, and T1 tilt in the two groups and found similar outcomes. This suggested that the Lenke criteria for leaving a PT curve unfused were safe. Unfortunately, Cil and coworkers did not comment on patient satisfaction or actual clinical assessments of shoulder heights. These data did not comment on whether structural PT curves absolutely required fusion, especially with a large MT curve and a low left shoulder. When considering fusion of a PT curve, we use the bending Cobb angle, but also evaluate the patient's radiographic clavicle angle and clinical shoulder height. A patient with either a level or slightly lower left shoulder height may need instrumentation of the upper thoracic curve if correction of a large MT curve is anticipated. It is important to include the curve flexibility with the radiographic and clinical shoulder-height measurements when determining the need to instrument an upper thoracic curve.

Selective TL/L fusion is also a consideration in attempting to minimize fusion levels. In a study of 49 patients with major TL/L and "partially structural" thoracic curves, Sanders et al assessed compensatory thoracic-curve correction when anterior fusion was done only on the TL/Lscoliosis.[41] They determined that a lumbar-to-thoracic Cobb-angle ratio >1.25 and a thoracic curve of <20 degrees on bending films, as well as a closed triradiate cartilage, were the best predictors of successful selective fusion. Lenke et al expanded on this, utilizing the specific curve patterns of the Lenke classification as a template.[42] Their radiographic criteria for selective fusion of type 6C curves included a ratio >1.25 for lumbar-to-thoracic curve Cobb-angle, apical vertebral translation and apical vertebral rotation, a flexible thoracic curve (ideally <25 degrees), and TL junctional kyphosis of <10 degrees. Their clinical criteria for selective fusion included a level or high left shoulder (for a right thoracic and left TL curve pattern), a lumbar truncal shift exceeding the thoracic truncal shift, a lumbar-to-thoracic curve ratio >1.2 by scoliometric measurement, and an acceptable rib prominence.

In the same article, Lenke and colleagues also suggested a more comprehensive list of parameters for selective thoracic fusion. Their radiographic criteria for selective thoracic fusion included a ratio >1.2 for thoracic-to-lumbar Cobb angle, apical vertebral translation and apical vertebral rotation, a flexible TL/L curve (ideally <25 degrees on side-bending), and TL kyphosis of <10 degrees. Clinical criteria for selective thoracic fusion included a level or high right shoulder, thoracic truncal shift exceeding lumbar waistline asymmetry, and a thoracic-to-lumbar curve ratio >1.2 by scoliometric measurement. Although not specifically assessed in the article, some Lenke type 3 curves may qualify for selective fusion.[43]

For both selective thoracic and selective TL fusion, these expanded radiographic and clinical criteria suggest that fusing curves simply on the basis of the Lenke classification is not absolutely adequate. Either the definitions for structural curves as delineated by the new classification system simply constitute an expandable template, or some structural curves do not need to be fused. Unfortunately, there have not been enough data about such fusion to fully resolve these issues.

## Surgical Approaches

The traditional approach to the treatment of double and triple major curves is posterior instrumentation and fusion.[28,44–46] Whether using pedicle screws, hooks, wires, or hybrid constructs, a posterior approach allows access to all curves through a single incision. Sagittal deformities can be addressed with multilevel posterior osteotomies.[47]

Anterior approaches, on the other hand, can be used in combination with a posterior approach for rigid curves, prevention of the crankshaft phenomenon, and the treatment of severe sagittal deformities.[48–50] We consider anterior release for curves >90 degrees or particularly stiff curves that do not bend below 50 degrees. However, with pedicle-screw instrumentation and wide posterior osteotomies, the role of anterior release is less clear. Historically, as compared with posterior instrumentation, anterior instrumentation has been shown to save fusion levels and result in better correction of the uninstrumented lumbar curve.[43,51–53] However, as new surgical instrumentation and techniques continue to be evaluated, this may not remain the case. When instrumentation is used in compression, anterior surgery of the thoracic curvature has more reliably resulted in the restoration of kyphosis than has posterior surgery.[51,54] Anterior arthrodesis of both double major curves through a single incision has not been previously discussed in the literature. However, it has been done and will be discussed later in this chapter.

When considering anterior approaches, one must understand the associated morbidity. An anterior fusion through an open thoractomy has been shown to adversely affect pulmonary function.[55–57] More recently, video-assisted thorascopic surgery (VATS) has become a popular alternative to open thoracotomy.[54,58–60] Studies have demonstrated a reduced effect of VATS on pulmonary function testing.[61–63] Whether this translates into improved clinical outcomes remains unclear. Interestingly, no significant diminution in pulmonary function was found for the thoracoabdominal approach despite the associated disruption of the diaphragm.[64] In patients with severe pulmonary compromise, anterior thoracic surgery should be avoided because of a possibly significant risk of further deterioration.

## The Harms Study Group Experience

### Lenke Type 3 Curves

Of the 1285 patients in the Harms Study Group (HSG) prospective AIS database, 57 (4.4%) were classified as having Lenke type 3 curves. Complete 2-year follow-up was reached in 22 of the patients. Most of the 57 patients with type 3 curves were female (86.4%), with a mean age of 14.4 years at the time of treatment. The magnitudes of their MT and TL/L curves were 66 degrees and 52 degrees, respectively. Thirteen lumbar curves had a "C" modifier, with the remaining curves having a "B" modifier. The sagittal modifier was "N" (normal [10 to 40 degrees]) for 14 patients, positive (>40 degrees) for 4 patients, and negative (<10 degrees) for 4 patients.

Of the 22 patients with 2-year follow-up, 13 patients underwent nonselective arthrodesis of both their MT and TL/L curves, with an average of 13.5 fused levels (**Fig. 20.2**). The other 9 patients had selective fusion of their MT curve, as discussed below. All 13 patients with nonselective fusions underwent instrumentation and fusion through a posterior exposure. One patient who was of Risser grade 0 underwent an additional thoracoscopic release and fusion from T6 to T10. The postoperative magnitude of the patient's MT curve was 23 degrees and that of the TL/L curve was 22 degrees, representing corrections of 61% and 60%, respectively. There was no significant difference in the patient's pre- and postoperative coronal balance as measured by the difference between the C7 plumbline and the CSVL. Overall, there was an improvement in clinical outcomes as measured with the Scoliosis Research Society (SRS)-24 questionnaire in all domains except that of activity, which remained the same from before to after surgery.

Depending on curve apex and shoulder symmetry for the 13 patients who underwent nonselective fusion, proximal instrumentation began between T2 and T5. The lowest instrumented vertebra (LIV) was L3 in eight patients and L4 in five patients. This was typically the most caudal vertebra touched by the CSVL.

### Lenke Type 4 Curves

Forty-two of the 1285 patients (3.3%) were classified as having Lenke type 4 curves. Seventeen of these patients had a 2-year follow-up. In semblance to the corresponding percentage in the group of patients with Lenke type 3 curves, 82% of those with type 4 curves were female. The average age of the patients at the time of arthrodesis was 14.5 years. The mean Cobb angles of their PT, MT, and TL/L curves were 38 degrees, 80 degrees, and 60 degrees, respectively. The majority had a lumbar "C" modifier (71%) and a neutral sagittal modifier (82%).

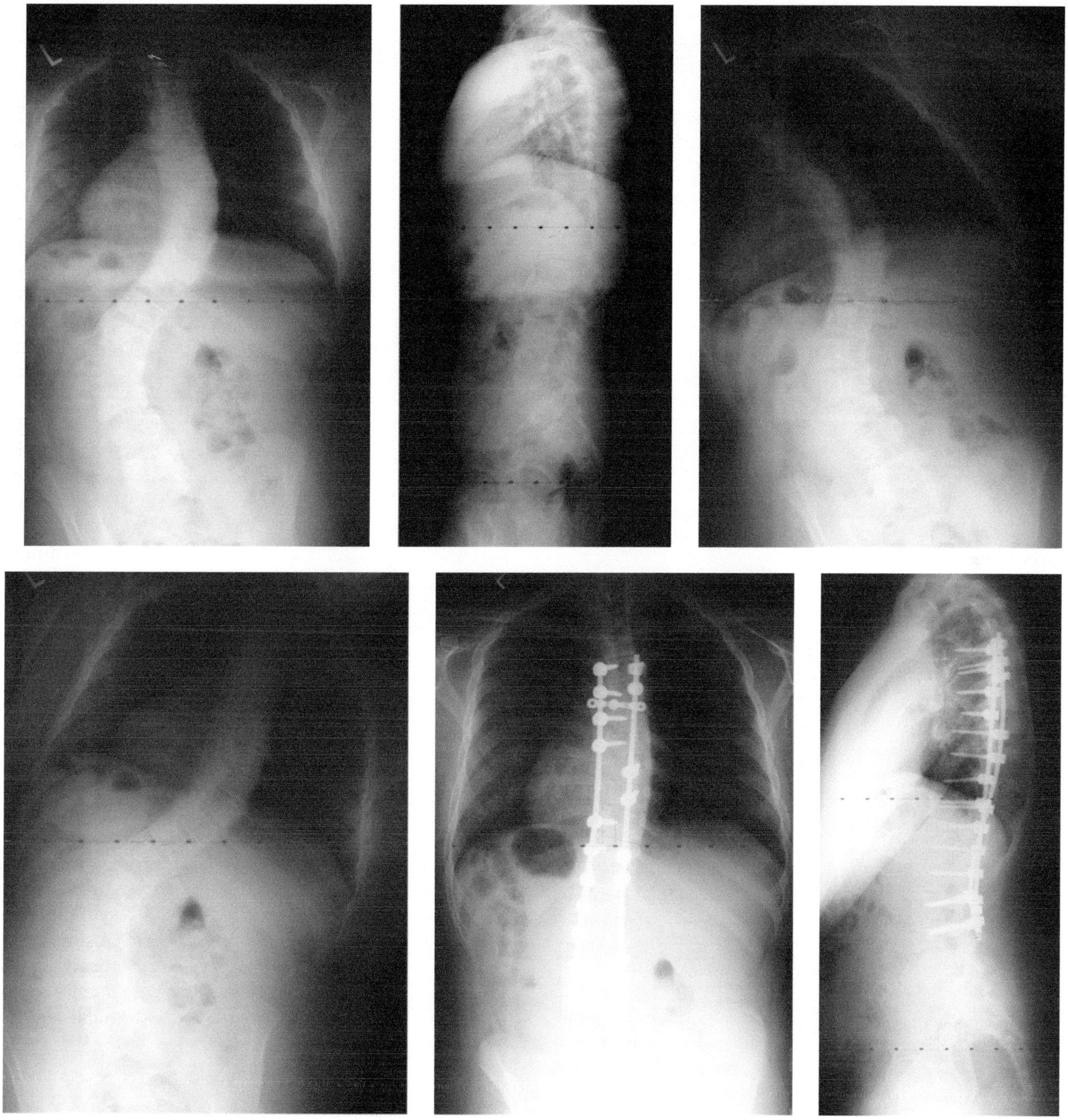


**Fig. 20.2** **(A,B)** Lenke type 3CN curve. The MT and TL/L curves measured 63 degrees and 61 degrees, respectively. **(C,D)** The MT and TL/L curves bend to 45 degrees and 47 degrees, respectively. **(E,F)** The patient underwent posterior instrumentation and fusion from T4 to L4. At 2 years postoperatively the patient's MT curve was 19 degrees and the TL/L curve was 21 degrees.

Fourteen of the patients had nonselective fusion of all of their structural curves through a posterior approach (**Fig. 20.3**). Selective fusion was performed in three patients as discussed below. Excluding those patients who had selective fusion, the average number of fused segments was 14. Final magnitudes of the patients' PT, MT, and TL/L curves were 16 degrees, 23 degrees, and 22 degrees, respectively. This resulted in 54%, 67%, and 65% corrections of the respective curves. Coronal balance improved from –0.34 cm to –0.05 cm. Outcomes as measured with the SRS-24 questionnaire included significant improvements in self-image and general function. The

A–C

D–F

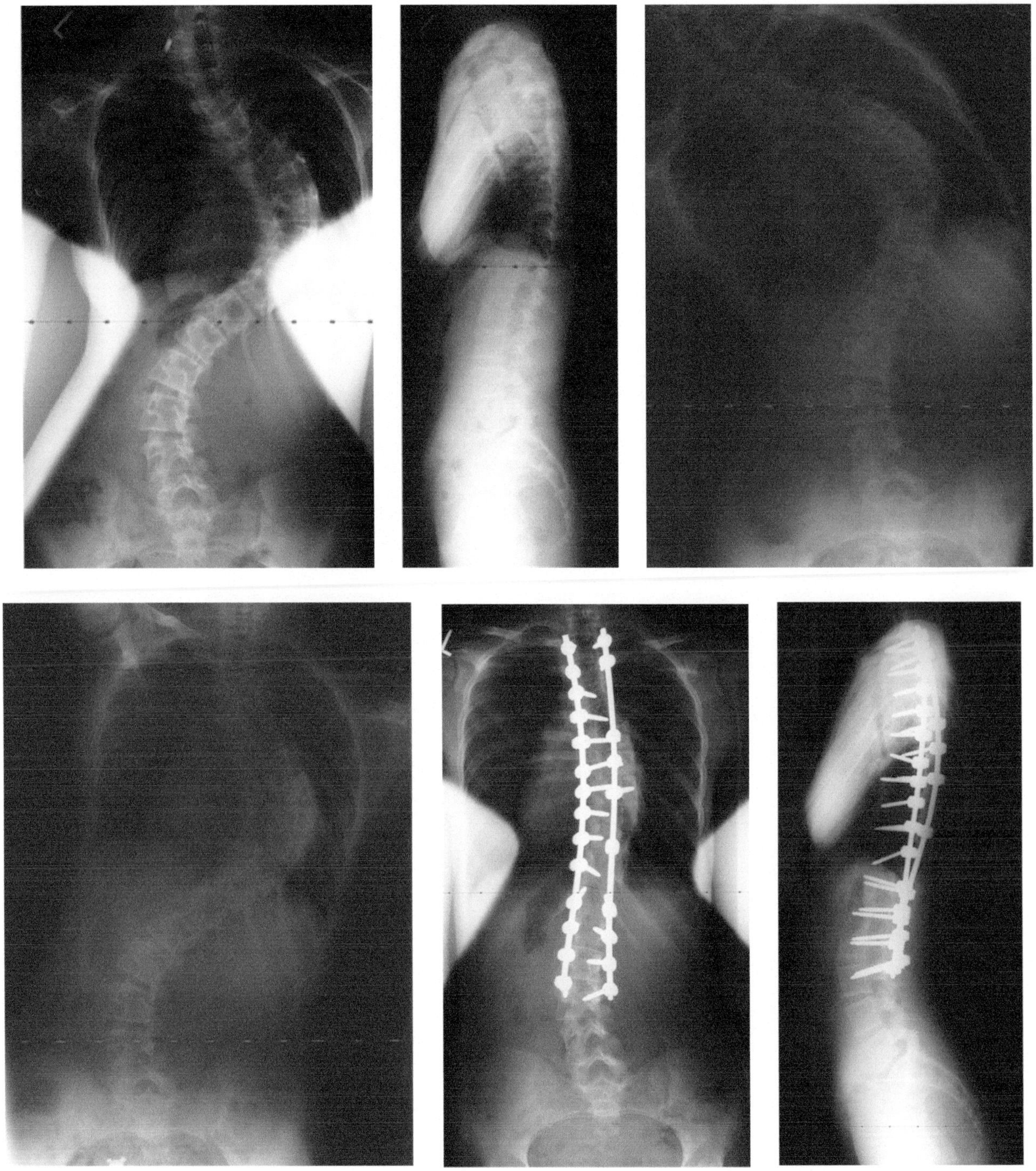

**Fig. 20.3 (A,B)** Lenke type 4CN curve. The PT, MT, and TL/L curves measured 49 degrees, 100 degrees, and 60 degrees, respectively. **(C,D)** The PT, MT, and TL/L curves bend to 40 degrees, 82 degrees and 33 degrees, respectively. **(E,F)** The patient underwent anterior release of the thoracic curve followed by posterior instrumentation and fusion from T2 to L3. At 6 months postoperatively the patient's PT, MT, and TL/L curves measured 33 degrees, 31 degrees, and 21 degrees, respectively.

overall score on the SRS-24, as well as the pain and activity measures, were improved but not statistically significantly at 2 years of follow-up. Proximal instrumentation began at T2 in six patients, T3 in six patients, and T4 in two patients. As recommended, patients with a preoperatively high left shoulder typically had instrumentation and fusion extended to T2.[29] Patients with a preoperatively high right shoulder often had an arthrodesis beginning at T3 or T4. The LIV was L3 in 4 patients and L4 in 10 patients.

## Lenke Type 6 Curves

Seventy-one (5.5%) of the 1285 patients in the HSG prospective AIS database had Lenke type 6 curves. Two-year follow-up was available for 26 of these patients. The majority of the 71 patients were female (85%), and the average age of the patients was 14.8 years at the time of surgery. All patients had a lumbar "C" modifier by definition. The sagittal modifier was "N" for 17 patients, and was positive for 4 patients and negative for 5 patients.

Twenty-five of the patients underwent instrumentation and fusion of both the MT and TL/L curves (**Fig. 20.4**). One

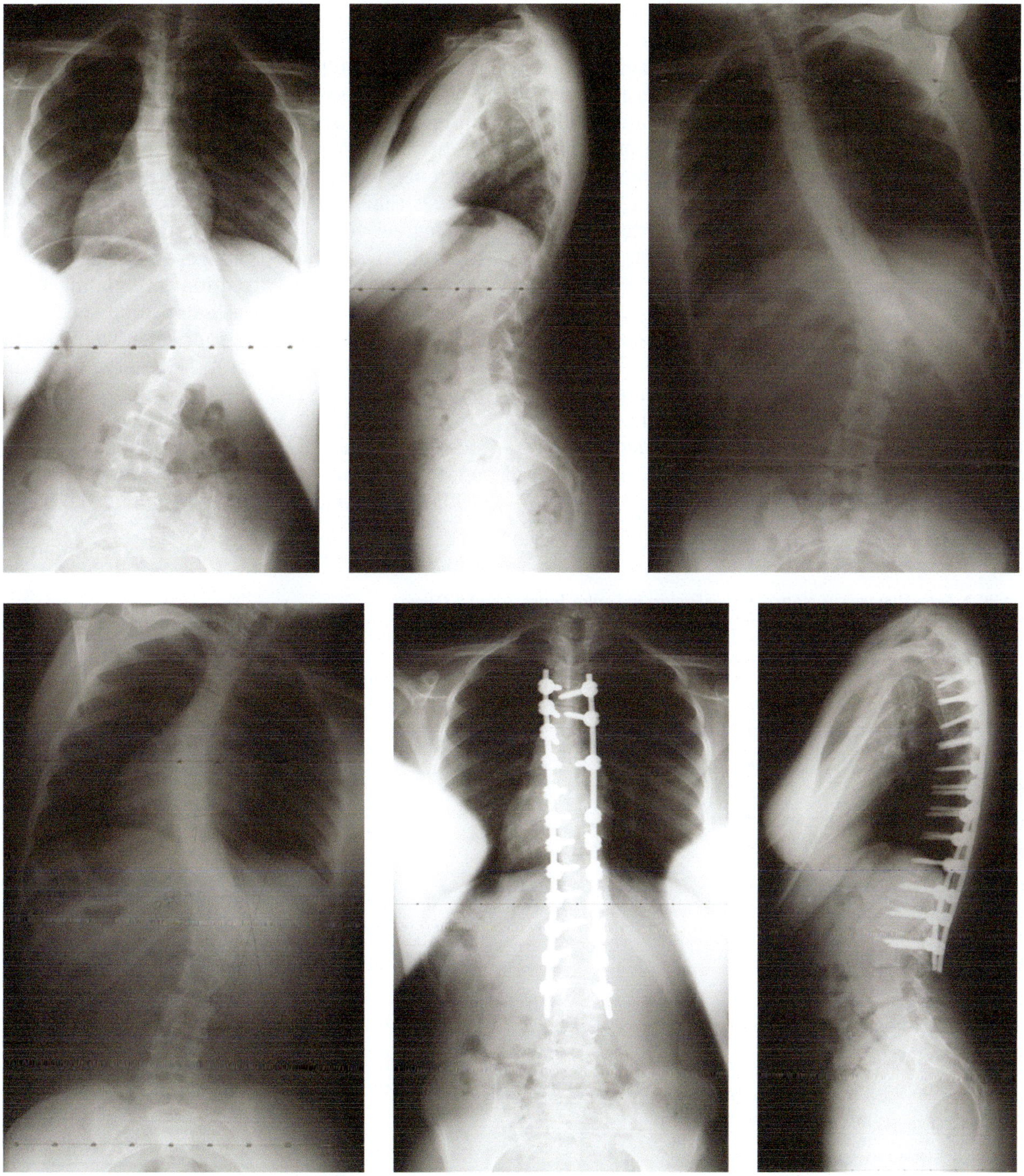

A–C

D–F

**Figs. 20.4 (A,B)** Lenke type 6CN curve. The MT and TL/L curves measured 35 degrees and 51 degrees, respectively. **(C,D)** The MT and TL/L curves bend to 25 degrees and 27 degrees, respectively. **(E,F)** The patient underwent posterior instrumentation and fusion from T4 to L3. At 6 months postoperatively the patient's MT and TL/L curves measured 17 degrees and 10 degrees, respectively.

patient underwent selective fusion. Seven of the patients who had nonselective fusion underwent a concomitant anterior release, four other patients had an open release of their TL curve, and three patients had thoracoscopic release of their thoracic curve. The TL/L curve improved from 63 degrees preoperatively to 17 degrees postoperatively (a 66% correction). The main thoracic curve decreased from 55 degrees to 17 degrees (68% correction). A mean of 13.1 vertebral levels were fused. Coronal balance improved from –2.5 cm to –0.8 cm. Evaluation with the SRS-24 questionnaire demonstrated improvement in pain at 2 years. Otherwise the patients' overall SRS-24 scores and their self-image, general function, and activity measures did not change significantly. In semblance to the case for the patients with Lenke type 3 curves, the upper instrumented level in those with type 6 curves was T2 (2 patients), T3 (8 patients), T4 (13 patients), and T5 (1 patient), and the LIV was L3 (9 patients), L4 (14 patients), and L5 (1 patient).

## Selective Fusion

In those patients with 2-year follow-ups, selective fusion of a structural curvature was done in 13 patients (9 with Lenke type 3, 3 with Lenke type 4, and 1 with Lenke type 6 curves) (**Table 20.1**). No differences in gender or age were found in the patients who had selective and those who had nonselective fusions for any curve type.

Selective fusion of Lenke type 3 curves was done on an average of 9.2 vertebral levels, as compared with 13.5 levels in nonselective fusions (**Fig. 20.5**). Anterior instrumentation and fusion of the thoracic curve was done in five of the patients who had selective fusion, with the other patients having selective posterior fusions. This saved an additional one or two caudal levels as compared with selective posterior fusions. Patients in the two treatment groups had MT curves of similar pre- and postoperative magnitudes. They also had similar postoperative Cobb-angle measurements for their TL/L curves, of 22 degrees and 21 degrees, respectively. At 2 years there was no difference in the anterior and posterior fusion groups' outcomes on the SRS-24 questionnaire.

In a comparison of radiographic parameters, the patients who had selective fusion had smaller TL/L curves than did those who had nonselective fusion, at 47 degrees versus 55 degrees, respectively. The curves in the selective-fusion group were also more flexible, with an average of 46% correction on bending films,versus 32% in the nonselective-fusion group. In accord with Lenke's recommendations for selective fusion, patients who had such fusion had a TL/L-curve Cobb-angle and apical translation ratio >1.2.[42]

Among patients with Lenke type 4 curves, selective fusion saved an average of 3.3 vertebral levels (11.7 levels, vs. 14 levels for patients who had nonselective fusion). The PT curve was included in the fusion in all of the patients.

**Table 20.1 Selective versus Nonselective Fusion in Lenke Types 3 and 4 Curves**

| | Lenke Type 3 | | Lenke Type 4 | |
|---|---|---|---|---|
| | Nonselective Fusion | Selective Fusion | Nonselective Fusion | Selective Fusion |
| *n* | 13 | 9 | 14 | 3 |
| Age (years) | 14.4 | 14.3 | 14.4 | 14.3 |
| Preoperative UT Cobb angle (degrees) | 22 | 35 | 38 | 41 |
| Preoperative MT Cobb angle (degrees) | 66 | 66 | 80 | 80 |
| Preoperative TL/L Cobb angle (degrees) | 55 | 47 | 62 | 51 |
| 2-Year UT Cobb angle (degrees) | 11 | 17 | 17 | 11 |
| 2-Year MT Cobb angle (degrees) | 25 | 28 | 26 | 8 |
| 2 Year TL/L Cobb angle (degrees) | 21 | 22 | 23 | 21 |
| 2-Year C7–CSVL distance (cm) | −0.04 | −0.38 | −0.14 | 0.90 |
| 2-Year SRS score | 4.26 | 4.26 | | |
| 2-Year activity score | 4.38 | 4.42 | | |
| 2-Year self-image score | 4.52 | 4.75 | | |
| 2-Year general function score | 4.29 | 4.75 | | |
| 2-Year pain score | 4.48 | 4.00 | | |

*Abbreviations*: CSVL, center sacral vertical line; UT, upper thoracic; MT, main thoracic; TL/L, thoracolumbar/lumbar.

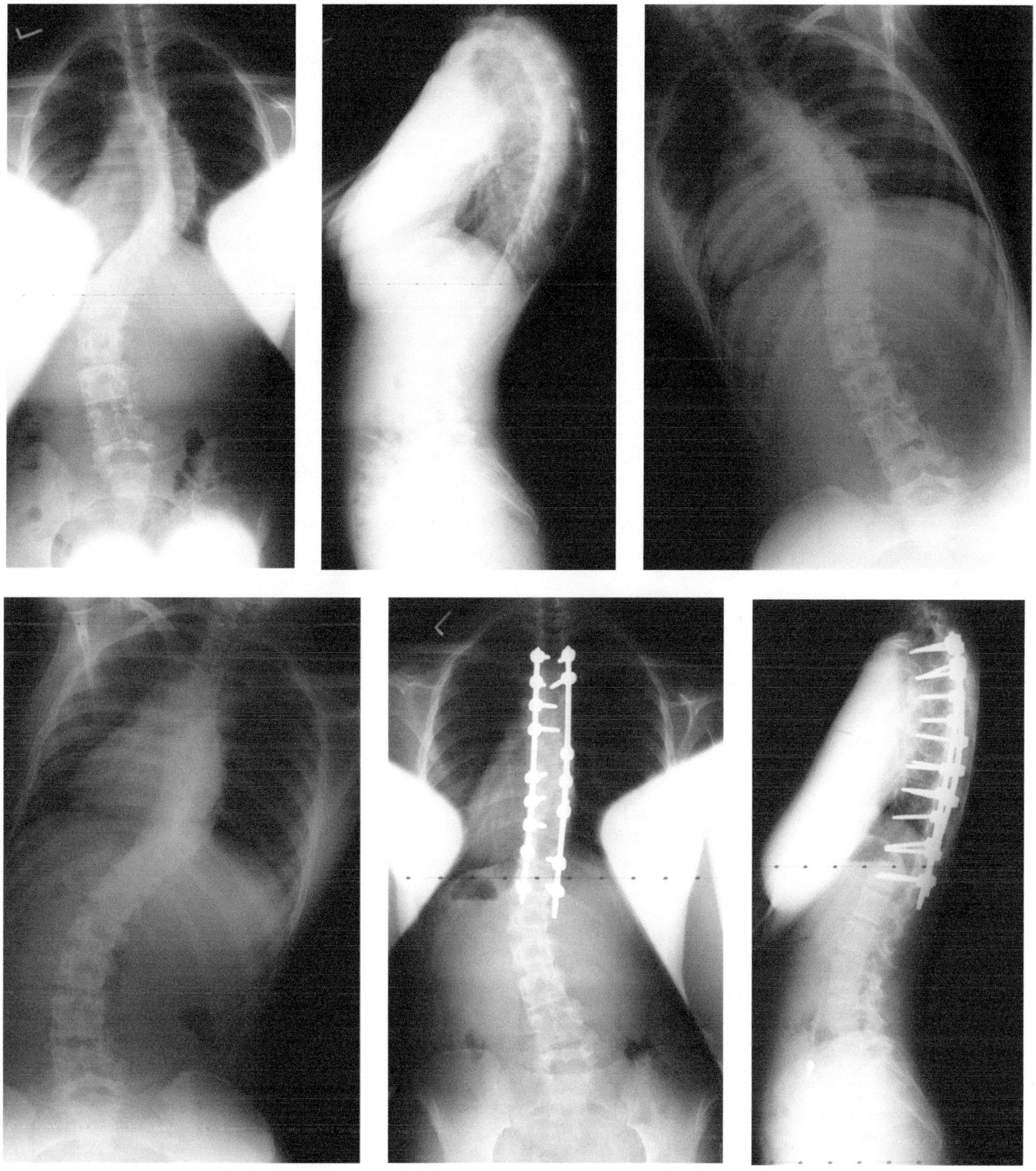

A–C

D–F

**Fig. 20.5** **(A,B)** Selective fusion of a Lenke type 3CN curve. The MT and TL/L curves measured 68 degrees and 55 degrees, respectively. **(C,D)** Preoperative bending films demonstrate greater flexibility of the TL/L curve than of the MT curve (28 degrees vs. 48 degrees, respectively). **(E,F)** The patient underwent selective posterior instrumentation and fusion of the MT curve from T3 to T12. At 1 year postoperatively the patient's MT curve was 28 degrees and the TL/L curve was 27 degrees.

No differences were seen in the selective- and nonselective-fusion groups in pre- or postoperative PT and MT curve magnitudes. In resemblance to what was found for the patients with Lenke type 3 curves, all the radiographic criteria for selective thoracic fusion were followed in the patients who had Lenke type 4 curves.

Selective fusion was done in one patient with a Lenke type 6 curve. Interestingly, this patient had a selective thoracic

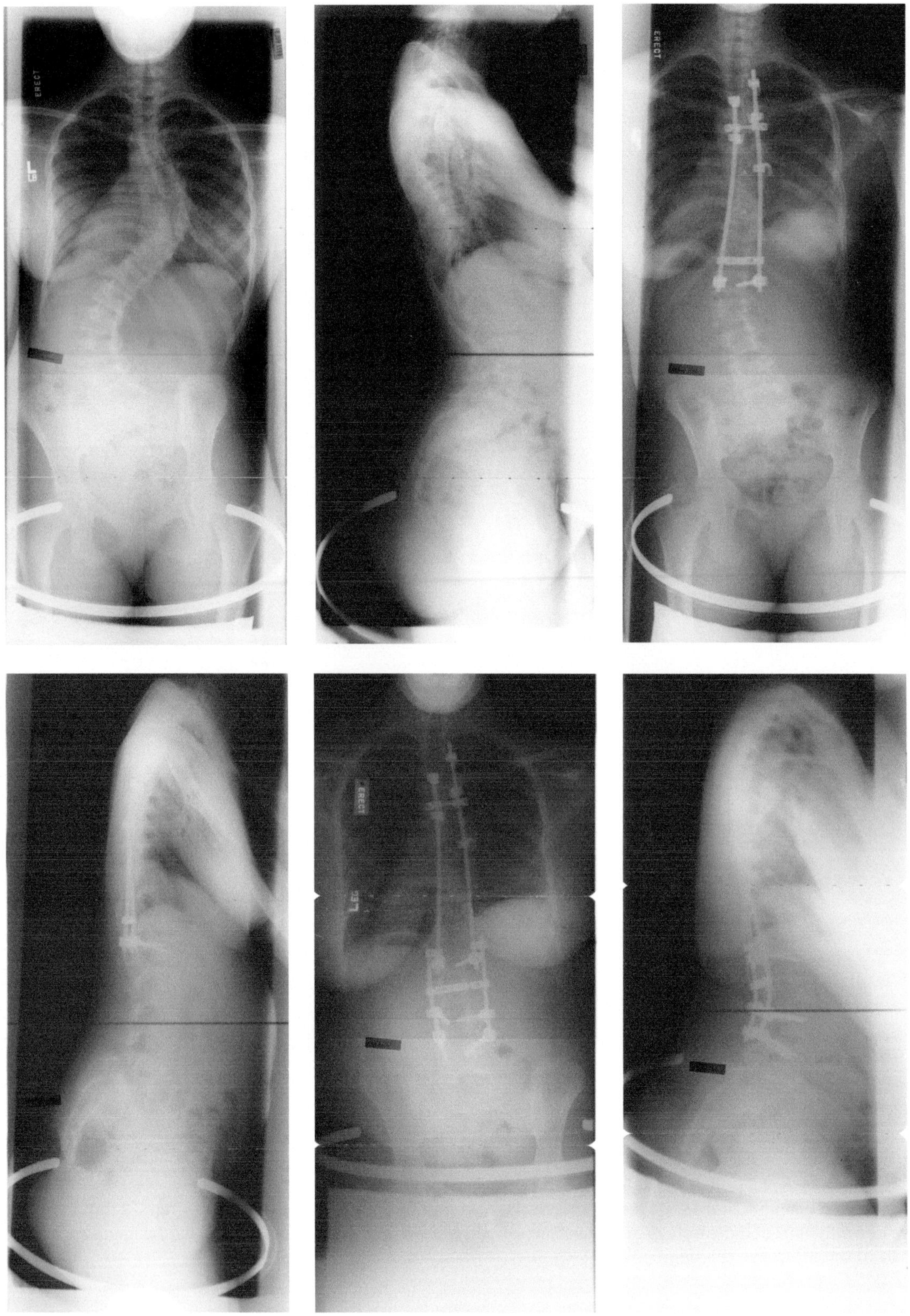

A–C

D–F

**Fig. 20.6 (A,B)** Lenke type 3CN curve. The PT, MT, and TL/L curves measured 33 degrees, 70 degrees, and 54 degrees, respectively. The PT, MT, and TL/L curves bend to 16 degrees, 50 degrees, and 31 degrees, respectively. **(C,D)** The patient underwent open anterior release from T5 to T12 followed by selective posterior instrumentation and fusion from T2 to L1. Postoperatively the patient showed residual lumbar curvature with a significant truncal shift. **(E,F)** Extension of the fusion from L1 to L4 was subsequently undertaken. At 2 years postoperatively the patient's PT, MT, and TL/L curves measured 9 degrees, 20 degrees, and 10 degrees, respectively.

fusion or arthrodesis of the minor structural curve. In the patients with type 6 curves, the TL curve was similar in magnitude to the MT curve (41 degrees vs. 40 degrees, respectively) but was defined as the major curve because it was less flexible on bending films. The postoperative Cobb angles of the MT and TL curves in the patients with type 6 curves were 27 degrees and 35 degrees, respectively.

Revision to extend a fusion to include both structural curves was done in one patient with a Lenke type 3 curve that was initially treated with a selective fusion (**Fig. 20.6**). This patient had an unacceptable residual lumbar curve as well as mechanical lumbar pain. The fusion was extended from L1 to L4. The guidelines of the Lenke classification system would have recommended arthrodesis of both of this patient's curves.

## Complications

A detailed analysis of complications of the surgical treatment of the patients in the HSG prospective AIS database is presented in Chapter 22. No deaths or neurological injuries occurred among the patients with Lenke type 3, 4, and 6 curves. Otherwise, the rates of pulmonary complications, wound infection, hardware failure, urinary tract infection, gastric complications, and excessive pain were similar to those seen in other patients with AIS.[29]

At 2-year follow-up, revision surgery was required in four patients. One patient with a Lenke type 3 curve who underwent selective thoracic fusion required extension of the fusion to L4 for coronal decompensation. Sagittal decompensation was not seen in any patients. At 2 years no patient showed evidence of proximal or distal junctional kyphosis. Two patients required revision fusion for implant failure and pseudarthrosis. One case of pseudarthosis occurred in a patient who underwent selective open anterior instrumentation and fusion for a Lenke type 3 curve. This was treated with supplemental posterior instrumentation and fusion. The other pseudoarthrosis occurred at the distal end of a nonselective posterior fusion of a Lenke type 6 curve. This patient underwent revision with posterior instrumentation as well as supplemental anterior cage placement at L3–L4. The last patient underwent scar revision as well as thoracoplasty for unacceptable rib prominence and a surgical scar.

## Conclusion

The combined frequency of Lenke type 3, 4, and 6 curves is between 10 and 15%. The standard treatment for these curves is posterior fusion and instrumentation of all structural curves. This is the optimal method for preventing progression and correcting deformity while maintaining coronal and sagittal balance and axial correction. Proper spinal alignment should ensure favorable cosmesis and preserve physiological function. Techniques that minimize fusion levels are also critical in potentially reducing the pain and disc degeneration associated with long fusions.

Better understanding of the long-term effects of long instrumentation and fusion has increased interest in decreasing the morbidity associated with the surgical treatment of double and triple major scoliotic curves. Initially applied to thoracic scoliosis with compensatory lumbar curves, the concept of selective fusion has now been applied to double and triple major curves. Ideally, refining the criteria for selective fusion of a major curve will maximize the benefits of maintaining spinal flexibility and motion segments and minimize the risk of decompensation through uninstrumented curves. With 2 years of postoperative follow-up, outcome scores on the SRS-24 instrument have not demonstrated any benefit for selective fusion. Only long-term follow-up will delineate the benefit of maintaining motion segments.

Among the 13 patients who underwent selective fusion in the HSG prospective AIS database, only 1 experienced failure and required extension of the fusion. As recommended in the Lenke classification, this patient should have undergone fusion of both structural curves. Eleven of the 12 patients who had successful selective fusions did not have any decompensation through their uninstrumented curves at 2 years. This suggests that the definition of a structural curve in the Lenke classification is not absolute. Other criteria, whether radiographic, clinical, or both must be considered when determining whether a structural curve should be fused. However, additional studies are needed to determine the parameters for performing these selective fusions.

## References

1. Lenke LG, Betz RR, Harms J, et al. Adolescent idiopathic scoliosis: A new classification to determine extent of spinal arthrodesis. J Bone Joint Surg Am 2001;83A:1169–1181
2. King HA, Moe JH, Bradford DS, Winter RB. The selection of fusion levels in thoracic idiopathic scoliosis. J Bone Joint Surg Am 1983; 65:1302–1313
3. Bridwell KH, The RLD. Textbook of Spinal Surgery, ed. 2. Philadelphia: Lippincott-Raven; 1997
4. Morrissy RT, Weinstein SL. Lovell and Winter's Pediatric Orthopaedics, ed. 5. Philadelphia: Lippincott, Williams & Wilkins; 2001
5. Lenke LG. Lenke classification system of adolescent idiopathic scoliosis: Treatment recommendations. Instr Course Lect 2005;54: 537–542
6. Lenke LG, Betz RR, Clements D, et al. Curve prevalence of a new classification of operative adolescent idiopathic scoliosis: Does classification correlate with treatment? Spine 2002;27:604–611

7. Stokes IA, Armstrong JG, Moreland MS. Spinal deformity and back surface asymmetry in idiopathic scoliosis. J Orthop Res 1988;6: 129–137
8. Coonrad RW, Murrell GA, Motley G, Lytle E, Hey LA. A logical coronal pattern classification of 2,000 consecutive idiopathic scoliosis cases based on the scoliosis research society-defined apical vertebra. Spine 1998;23:1380–1391
9. Iwahara T, Imai M, Atsuta Y. Quantification of cosmesis for patients affected by adolescent idiopathic scoliosis. Eur Spine J 1998;7:12–15
10. Theologis TN, Jefferson RJ, Simpson AH, Turner-Smith AR, Fairbank JC. Quantifying the cosmetic defect of adolescent idiopathic scoliosis. Spine 1993;18:909–912
11. Goldberg MS, Mayo NE, Poitras B, Scott S, Hanley J. The Ste-Justine Adolescent Idiopathic Scoliosis Cohort Study. Part II: Perception of health, self and body image, and participation in physical activities. Spine 1994;19:1562–1572
12. Lonstein JE. Scoliosis: surgical versus nonsurgical treatment. Clin Orthop Relat Res 2006;443:248–259
13. Danielsson AJ, Wiklund I, Pehrsson K, Nachemson AL. Health-related quality of life in patients with adolescent idiopathic scoliosis: A matched follow-up at least 20 years after treatment with brace or surgery. Eur Spine J 2001;10:278–288
14. Koch KD, Buchanan R, Birch JG, Morton AA, Gatchel RJ, Browne RH. Adolescents undergoing surgery for idiopathic scoliosis: How physical and psychological characteristics relate to patient satisfaction with the cosmetic result. Spine 2001;26:2119–2124
15. Harrington PR. Treatment of scoliosis. Correction and internal fixation by spine instrumentation. J Bone Joint Surg Am 1962;44A: 591–610
16. La Grone MO. Loss of lumbar lordosis. A complication of spinal fusion for scoliosis. Orthop Clin North Am 1988;19:383–393
17. Danielsson AJ, Cederlund CG, Ekholm S, Nachemson AL. The prevalence of disc aging and back pain after fusion extending into the lower lumbar spine. A matched MR study twenty-five years after surgery for adolescent idiopathic scoliosis. Acta Radiol 2001; 42:187–197
18. Cochran T, Irstam L, Nachemson A. Long-term anatomic and functional changes in patients with adolescent idiopathic scoliosis treated by Harrington rod fusion. Spine 1983;8:576–584
19. Danielsson AJ, Nachemson AL. Back pain and function 23 years after fusion for adolescent idiopathic scoliosis: A case-control study-part II. Spine 2003;28:E373–E383
20. Hayes MA, Tompkins SF, Herndon WA, Gruel CR, Kopta JA, Howard TC. Clinical and radiological evaluation of lumbosacral motion below fusion levels in idiopathic scoliosis. Spine 1988;13:1161–1167
21. Connolly PJ, Von Schroeder HP, Johnson GE, Kostuik JP. Adolescent idiopathic scoliosis. Long-term effect of instrumentation extending to the lumbar spine. J Bone Joint Surg Am 1995;77:1210–1216
22. Paonessa KJ, Engler GL. Back pain and disability after Harrington rod fusion to the lumbar spine for scoliosis. Spine 1992;17(8, suppl): S249–S253
23. Wilk B, Karol LA, Johnston CE II, Colby S, Haideri N. The effect of scoliosis fusion on spinal motion: A comparison of fused and non-fused patients with idiopathic scoliosis. Spine 2006;31:309–314
24. Puno RM, An KC, Puno RL, Jacob A, Chung SS. Treatment recommendations for idiopathic scoliosis: An assessment of the Lenke classification. Spine 2003;28:2102–2114, discussion: 2114–2115
25. Davidson D, Letts M, Jarvis J. Triple major curves in children. Can J Surg 2003;46(3):193–198
26. Hamill CL, Lenke LG, Bridwell KH, Chapman MP, Blanke K, Baldus C. The use of pedicle screw fixation to improve correction in the lumbar spine of patients with idiopathic scoliosis. Is it warranted? Spine 1996;21:1241–1249
27. Lenke LG, Bridwell KH, Baldus C, Blanke K. Preventing decompensation in King type II curves treated with Cotrel-Dubousset instrumentation. Strict guidelines for selective thoracic fusion. Spine 1992;17(8, suppl):S274–S281
28. Barr SJ, Schuette AM, Emans JB. Lumbar pedicle screws versus hooks. Results in double major curves in adolescent idiopathic scoliosis. Spine 1997;22:1369–1379
29. Frymoyer JW, Wiesel SW. The Adult and Pediatric Spine, ed. 3. Philadelphia: Lippincott, Williams & Wilkins; 2004
30. Kim YJ, Lenke LG, Kim J, et al. Comparative analysis of pedicle screw versus hybrid instrumentation in posterior spinal fusion of adolescent idiopathic scoliosis. Spine 2006;31:291–298
31. Dobbs MB, Lenke LG, Kim YJ, Kamath G, Peelle MW, Bridwell KH. Selective posterior thoracic fusions for adolescent idiopathic scoliosis: comparison of hooks versus pedicle screws. Spine 2006;31: 2400–2404
32. Cheng I, Kim Y, Gupta MC, et al. Apical sublaminar wires versus pedicle screws—which provides better results for surgical correction of adolescent idiopathic scoliosis? Spine 2005;30:2104–2112
33. Lowenstein JE, Matsumoto H, Vitale MG, et al. Coronal and sagittal plane correction in adolescent idiopathic scoliosis: A comparison between all pedicle screw versus hybrid thoracic hook lumbar screw constructs. Spine 2007;32:448–452
34. Vora V, Crawford A, Babekhir N, et al. A pedicle screw construct gives an enhanced posterior correction of adolescent idiopathic scoliosis when compared with other constructs: Myth or reality. Spine 2007;32:1869–1874
35. Large DF, Doig WG, Dickens DR, Torode IP, Cole WG. Surgical treatment of double major scoliosis. Improvement of the lumbar curve after fusion of the thoracic curve. J Bone Joint Surg Br 1991;73: 121–124
36. Kuklo TR, Lenke LG, Won DS, et al. Spontaneous proximal thoracic curve correction after isolated fusion of the main thoracic curve in adolescent idiopathic scoliosis. Spine 2001;26:1966–1975
37. Kuklo TR, Lenke LG, Graham EJ, et al. Correlation of radiographic, clinical, and patient assessment of shoulder balance following fusion versus nonfusion of the proximal thoracic curve in adolescent idiopathic scoliosis. Spine 2002;27:2013–2020
38. Winter RB. The idiopathic double thoracic curve pattern. Its recognition and surgical management. Spine 1989;14:1287–1292
39. Lenke LG, Bridwell KH, O'Brien MF, Baldus C, Blanke K. Recognition and treatment of the proximal thoracic curve in adolescent idiopathic scoliosis treated with Cotrel-Dubousset instrumentation. Spine 1994;19:1589–1597
40. Cil A, Pekmezci M, Yazici M, et al. The validity of Lenke criteria for defining structural proximal thoracic curves in patients with adolescent idiopathic scoliosis. Spine 2005;30:2550–2555
41. Sanders AE, Baumann R, Brown H, Johnston CE II, Lenke LG, Sink E. Selective anterior fusion of thoracolumbar/lumbar curves in adolescents: When can the associated thoracic curve be left unfused? Spine 2003;28:706–713, discussion 714
42. Lenke LG, Edwards CC II, Bridwell KH. The Lenke classification of adolescent idiopathic scoliosis: How it organizes curve patterns as a template to perform selective fusions of the spine. Spine 2003; 28:S199–S207

43. Lowe TG, Betz R, Lenke L, et al. Anterior single-rod instrumentation of the thoracic and lumbar spine: saving levels. Spine 2003;28: S208–S216
44. Lenke LG, Betz RR, Haher TR, et al. Multisurgeon assessment of surgical decision-making in adolescent idiopathic scoliosis: Curve classification, operative approach, and fusion levels. Spine 2001; 26:2347–2353
45. Lenke LG, Betz RR, Harms J. Modern Anterior Scoliosis Surgery, ed. 1. St. Louis: Quality Medical Publishing; 2004
46. Moe JH, Winter RB, Bradford DS, et al. Scoliosis and Other Spinal Deformities. Philadelphia: W.B Saunders, 1978
47. Shufflebarger HL, Geck MJ, Clark CE. The posterior approach for lumbar and thoracolumbar adolescent idiopathic scoliosis: Posterior shortening and pedicle screws. Spine 2004;29:269–276, discussion 276
48. Floman Y, Micheli LJ, Penny JN, Riseborough EJ, Hall JE. Combined anterior and posterior fusion in seventy-three spinally deformed patients: Indications, results and complications. Clin Orthop Relat Res 1982;(164):110–122
49. Lapinksy AS, Richards BS. Preventing the crankshaft phenomenon by combining anterior fusion with posterior instrumentation. Does it work? Spine 1995;20:1392–1398
50. Shufflebarger HL, Clark CE. Prevention of the crankshaft phenomenon. Spine 1991;16(8, suppl):S409–S411
51. Betz RR, Harms J, Clements DH III, et al. Comparison of anterior and posterior instrumentation for correction of adolescent thoracic idiopathic scoliosis. Spine 1999;24:225–239
52. Lenke LG, Betz RR, Bridwell KH, Harms J, Clements DH, Lowe TG. Spontaneous lumbar curve coronal correction after selective anterior or posterior thoracic fusion in adolescent idiopathic scoliosis. Spine 1999;24:1663–1671, discussion 1672
53. Kuklo TR, O'Brien MF, Lenke LG, et al; Spinal Deformity Study Group: AIS Section. Comparison of the lowest instrumented, stable, and lower end vertebrae in "single overhang" thoracic adolescent idiopathic scoliosis: Anterior versus posterior spinal fusion. Spine 2006;31:2232–2236
54. Lonner BS, Kondrachov D, Siddiqi F, Hayes V, Scharf C. Thoracoscopic spinal fusion compared with posterior spinal fusion for the treatment of thoracic adolescent idiopathic scoliosis. Surgical technique. J Bone Joint Surg Am 2007;89(suppl 2 Pt.1): 142–156
55. Graham EJ, Lenke LG, Lowe TG, et al. Prospective pulmonary function evaluation following open thoracotomy for anterior spinal fusion in adolescent idiopathic scoliosis. Spine 2000;25:2319–2325
56. Vedantam R, Lenke LG, Bridwell KH, Haas J, Linville DA. A prospective evaluation of pulmonary function in patients with adolescent idiopathic scoliosis relative to the surgical approach used for spinal arthrodesis. Spine 2000;25:82–90
57. Wong CA, Cole AA, Watson L, Webb JK, Johnston ID, Kinnear WJ. Pulmonary function before and after anterior spinal surgery in adult idiopathic scoliosis. Thorax 1996;51:534–536
58. Levin R, Matusz D, Hasharoni A, Scharf C, Lonner B, Errico T. Mini-open thoracoscopically assisted thoracotomy versus video-assisted thoracoscopic surgery for anterior release in thoracic scoliosis and kyphosis: A comparison of operative and radiographic results. Spine J 2005;5:632–638
59. Newton PO, Parent S, Marks M, Pawelek J. Prospective evaluation of 50 consecutive scoliosis patients surgically treated with thoracoscopic anterior instrumentation. Spine 2005;30(17, suppl): S100–S109
60. Newton PO. The use of video-assisted thoracoscopic surgery in the treatment of adolescent idiopathic scoliosis. Instr Course Lect 2005;54:551–558
61. Newton PO, Marks M, Faro F, et al. Use of video-assisted thoracoscopic surgery to reduce perioperative morbidity in scoliosis surgery. Spine 2003;28:S249–S254
62. Faro FD, Marks MC, Newton PO, Blanke K, Lenke LG. Perioperative changes in pulmonary function after anterior scoliosis instrumentation: Thoracoscopic versus open approaches. Spine 2005;30: 1058–1063
63. Kishan S, Bastrom T, Betz RR, et al. Thoracoscopic scoliosis surgery affects pulmonary function less than thoracotomy at 2 years postsurgery. Spine 2007;32:453–458
64. Yaszay B, Jazayeri R, Lonner B. The effect of surgical approaches on pulmonary function in adolescent idiopathic scoliosis. J Spinal Disord Tech 2009;22:278–283

# 21 Outcomes of Treatment of Adolescent Idiopathic Scoliosis

*Michelle C. Marks, Tracey Bastrom, William F. Lavelle, and Peter O. Newton*

With any medical treatment or intervention, knowledge of the treatment outcome is invaluable for ensuring patient safety and quality of life, in addition to providing valuable information for the advancement of care. The need to demonstrate that a treatment has an effect on health is becoming increasingly important in the face of rapidly rising healthcare costs, growing consumer involvement in healthcare decision-making, and third-party demands to increase the efficiency and control the costs of healthcare.[1]

Outcomes research evaluates both a treatment process and the response of the patient's condition to the treatment process. It is a rapidly evolving field that incorporates epidemiology, health economics, psychometrics, and health-services research. This field has expanded dramatically in recent years as a result of rising interest in improving outcomes while controlling healthcare costs.[1] During the 1990s the number of publications on the development and validation of outcome tools more than doubled, with 46% of these tools being disease specific.[2]

The term *outcome* is linked to many different measures extending from subjective clinical measures to well-designed and validated patient-based quality-of-life assessment tools.[1] The physician is routinely interested in one or two specific outcomes, whereas the patient may be more interested in an entirely different set of outcomes. The "success" of a treatment is measured by a combination of these variables. With that being the case, the accurate measurement of these variables is essential in guiding treatment.

Defining the success of treatment for adolescent idiopathic scoliosis (AIS) can be a challenge, despite a multitude of potential outcome measures. This challenge is primarily related to the difficulty of interpreting change as reflected by a given specific outcome tool. What, for example, is the meaning of a 20-degree improvement in a 40-degree scoliotic curve? Or what is the meaning of a 10-point change on a 125-point health-related quality-of-life (HRQOL) scale? Researchers are just beginning to critically assess and define what in fact is a clinically significant change as reflected in an outcome tool after a treatment. The science of relating changes in outcome-tool results to one another, such as relating an objective measurement like the Cobb angle to a subjective measurement such as an outcome survey score, is also in its infancy, and this has been an area of interest in adult spine surgery as well as in AIS. Recently, some authors have critically examined the concept known as the minimum clinically important difference (MCID). This is defined as a threshold value used to measure the effect of a clinical treatment. Variable threshold values have been proposed as MCIDs for different outcome-assessment instruments, despite a lack of agreement about the optimal method for calculating an MCID.[3]

This method has encountered some challenges. In some cases outcome assessments may be completely unrelated, leaving the investigator without any conclusions about the overall outcome of a treatment. For example, in a multicenter study of the impact of a standardized radiographic score on the Scoliosis Research Society (SRS)-24 outcomes instrument, the radiographic measure (specifically, the size of a spinal curve) explained from 3 to 7% of the variability in the overall score provided by the SRS-24 instrument.[4] Considerable additional research on the meaning and application of outcomes is required.

In AIS, a condition that some may consider largely a cosmetic problem; there is a strong need for methodological studies. Efforts toward improving the methodology of AIS research need to be multifaceted, with emphasis on developing better outcome tools (measures of clinical status, functional status, health perceptions, severity of illness, and standardized measures of costs), better methods for data collection and analysis, and a better understanding of research findings (e.g., what does a change of 1 point mean on a 5-point scale?).

This chapter will focus on the components of outcomes research in AIS. Specifically, it will describe the elements of sound research design and analysis. The currently available outcome-measurement "tools" in the area of AIS research will be defined, and their shortcomings will be discussed. Suggestions will also be made for developing and improving those tools. This chapter will highlight research done by the Harms Study Group (HSG), a large, multicenter AIS research study group. As a concluding element, predictions and recommendations will be given for the future of outcomes research in the AIS patient population.

## Radiographic Outcomes

Outcomes research in AIS began as an attempt to document the radiographic outcomes of its surgical treatment with the earliest form of posterior instrumentation, which was developed by Harrington in the 1960s.[5,6] Advances in the treatment of AIS led to the development of techniques for anterior spinal fusion (ASF) for the correction of scoliosis, which was popularized by Zielke in the mid-1970s.[7] Research on the anterior approach in this patient population was expanded to the assessment of outcomes with various treatment techniques.[8–11] However, because the correction achieved with ASF did not justify its morbidity and difficulty, posterior spinal fusion (PSF) had remained the standard of care for AIS. In the 1980s, Dr. Jürgen Harms began repopularizing the idea of anterior instrumentation for the correction of idiopathic scoliosis. However, although excellent clinical results were obtained with ASF, the procedure had not become the standard of care for AIS. The members of the HSG began using an improved anterior system for the correction of scoliosis. The HSG then began to report the outcomes associated with this new procedure, and for perhaps the first time, serious comparisons were made of the anterior and posterior approaches.

In a prospective study comparing the results of anterior instrumentation and posterior instrumentation, Betz reported equivalent coronal correction and balance on the basis of the outcomes of 78 patients in the anterior-instrumentation group and 100 patients in the posterior-instrumentation group. The most significant benefits of ASF over PSF in this study included improvement in the sagittal alignment of the spine when patients were hypokyphotic preoperatively, and the saving of distal fusion levels, averaging 2.5 more levels saved per patient with the anterior than with the posterior approach.[12] Despite posterior instrumentation remaining the gold standard for scoliosis surgery, anterior instrumentation had become and remains a viable option.[13]

Lenke and colleagures evaluated correction of the instrumented thoracic curve as well as the uninstrumented compensatory lumbar curve in primary thoracic scoliosis treated with either anterior or posterior selective thoracic fusion. They compared 70 cases of an anterior with 53 cases of a posterior single approach. At 2-year follow-up, the percentage of thoracic-curve correction was greater with the anterior (58%) than with the posterior (38%) approach ($P < 0.05$); the spontaneous lumbar-curve correction was also greater with the anterior (56%) than with the posterior (37%) approach ($P < 0.05$).[14]

Analysis of the radiographic parameters assessed in sagittal-plane films began to hold a more important place in treatment outcomes in AIS. An analysis of patients who had undergone anterior instrumentation for thoracic idiopathic scoliosis revealed that sagittal curve progression, defined as an increase in kyphosis of >10 degrees between T5 and T12, occurred in 6 of 10 patients (60%) who were of Risser grade 0 at the time of fusion. In contrast, sagittal curve progression occurred in only 10 of 37 patients (27%) who were of Risser grades 1 to 5. The investigators who performed the analysis concluded that skeletally immature patients with adolescent idiopathic thoracic scoliosis treated with anterior instrumentation may be at risk for progressive sagittal kyphosis as a result of growth.[15]

Evaluating the radiographic parameters in both the coronal and sagittal planes led to critical analysis of the standard scoliosis classification system[16] and to the development of a new classification system for scoliosis.[17] The selection of operative approaches and both proximal and distal fusion levels was investigated,[18] and correlation of the curve classification with selected treatments was evaluated.[19]

Critical evaluation of radiographic parameters other than the standard Cobb angles has improved the understanding of factors involved in the choice of selective over nonselective fusion in primary thoracic scoliosis. However, substantial variation in the frequency of fusing the lumbar curve confirms the persistence of controversy about when surgeons feel the lumbar curve can be spared in Lenke type 1B and 1C curves.[20]

## Pulmonary Function Testing

Patients with AIS may have significant pulmonary morbidity. The deformation of the rib cage caused by the scoliotic deformity of the spine can adversely affect lung function. Pulmonary function test (PFT) data are important in this patient population because of the potential for increased morbidity and even early mortality from pulmonary deficiency as a result of untreated, progressive scoliosis.[21] Postoperatively, pulmonary function is an important outcome variable in scoliosis surgery for two reasons: (1) to quantify the effect of various treatment approaches on the change in perioperative pulmonary function; and (2) to understand the long-term effects of both the spinal deformity and the surgical intervention on pulmonary function in this patient population.

Standard pulmonary function testing includes plethysmography and spirometry to measure total lung capacity (TLC), forced vital capacity (FVC: the total amount of air that can be forcibly blown out after full inspiration, measured in liters), and forced expiratory volume in 1 second (FEV1: the amount of air that can be forcibly blown out in 1 second, measured in liters). Plethysmography measures variations in the size of the lungs, and is represented as

TLC. In traditional plethysmography, the test subject is placed inside a sealed chamber the size of a small telephone booth. At the end of normal expiration, the breathing mouthpiece used for testing is closed while the patient makes an inspiratory effort. The increase in the pressure within the box as the patient's chest expands is used to calculate the volume within the lungs. Spirometry measures the volumes of gas that can be moved in or out of the lungs. Volume changes can also be determined from measurements of flow or the rate of volume change that can be sensed and recorded continuously by a transducer. The flow signal can be continuously integrated to yield a volume trace.[22] Plethysmographic pulmonary testing of this type should be performed in a pulmonary laboratory and should follow the guidelines of the American Thoracic Society/European Respiratory Society (ATS/ERS) Standardization of Lung Function Testing.[23] If spirometry is performed in a clinical setting (rather than in the pulmonary laboratory), the results obtained from a portable spirometer should be validated with the pulmonary laboratory.

Because research had suggested a correlation between pulmonary impairment and thoracic spinal deformity,[21,24] the HSG conducted a prospective study of pulmonary function in patients with AIS to test the hypothesis that increasing thoracic deformity was associated with decreasing pulmonary function and to determine which, if any, radiographic measurements of deformity predicted moderate or severe pulmonary impairment. Analysis of PFT data for 631 patients with AIS revealed that thoracic-curve magnitude, thoracic-curve length, and thoracic hypokyphosis had a minimal but significant effect on pulmonary function. It was found that clinically significant decreases in pulmonary function occurred with much smaller scoliotic curves than had previously been described (**Fig. 21.1**). The HSG investigators concluded that some patients may have clinically significant pulmonary impairment disproportionate to the apparent severity of their scoliosis. Investigating pulmonary function in each individual scoliosis patient preoperatively may facilitate decision-making about the timing of and approach to correction of the patient's spinal deformity.[25]

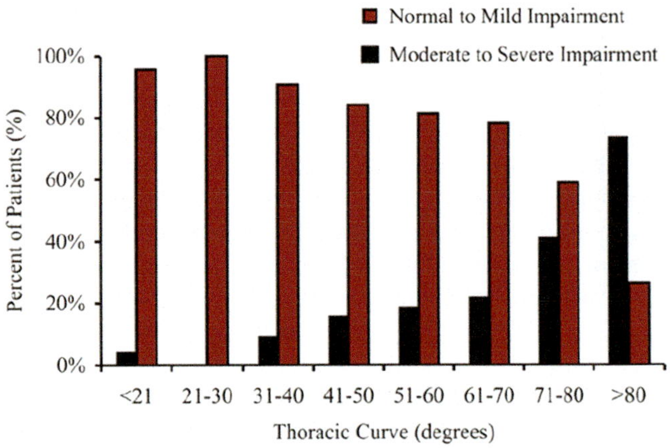


**Fig. 21.1** Bar graph illustrating association of increased coronal deformity with increased pulmonary impairment. (From Results of pre-operative pulmonary function testing of adolescent with idiopathic scoliosis, Newton et al. 2005. Reprinted with permission.)

The HSG has also made a comparison of the effects of treatment approaches on pulmonary function. In an attempt to determine whether the minimally invasive thoracoscopic approach impaired postoperative pulmonary function to a lesser extent than did open anterior instrumentation, the HSG evaluated 54 patients before surgery, as well as 3 months and 1 year after surgery. The results showed that for the instrumented anterior correction of AIS, the thoracoscopic approach causes a smaller decline in pulmonary function at 3 months and 1 year after surgery than does the more invasive technique of open thoracotomy (**Figs. 21.2**, **21.3**).[26] A follow-up to this HSG study investigated PFT outcomes in patients undergoing thoracoscopic instrumentation, thoracotomy, or thoracotomy with thoracoplasty at 2 years. Results showed that thoracoscopic instrumentation only minimally affected pulmonary function at 2 years postoperatively, with improvements noted in

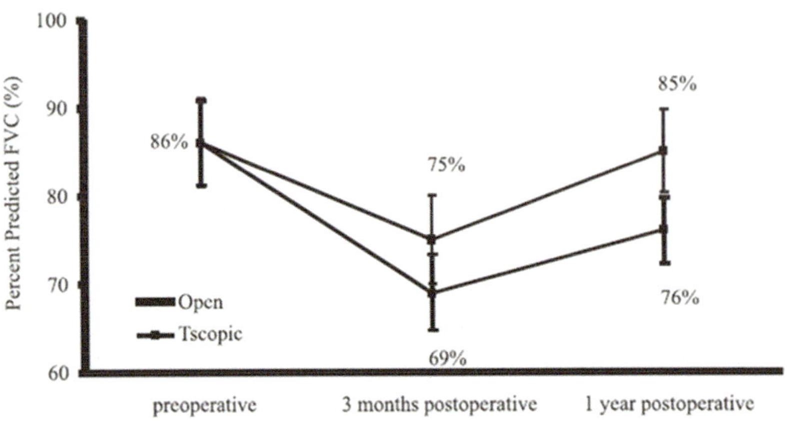


**Fig. 21.2** The changes in percent predicted FVC for thoracoscopic (Tscopic) and open anterior instrumentation groups. (From Results of perioperative changes in pulmonary function after anterior scoliosis instrumentation: thorascopic versus anterior approaches, Faro et al. 2005. Reprinted with permission.)

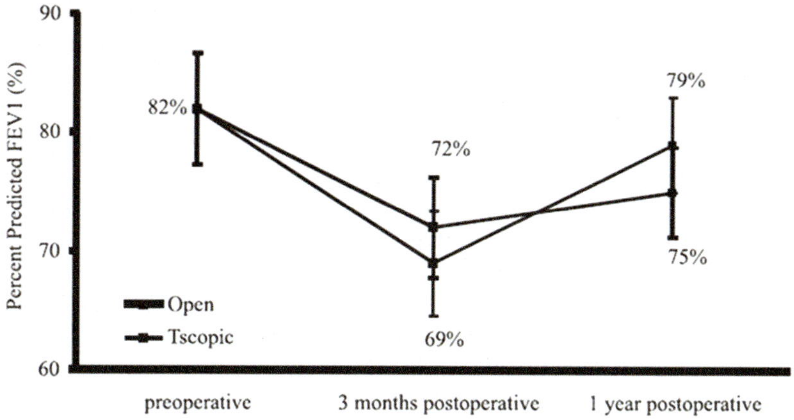


**Fig. 21.3** The changes in percent predicted FEV1 for thoracoscopic (Tscopic) and open anterior instrumentation groups. (From Results of perioperative changes in pulmonary function after anterior scoliosis instrumentation: thorascopic versus anterior approaches, Faro et al. 2005. Reprinted with permission.)

absolute FVC, FEV1, TLC, and percent-predicted TLC. Patients who underwent thoracotomy had a persistent reduction in FEV1 and FVC at 2 years, although their TLC had returned to its preoperative value. Thoracoplasty added to thoracotomy predictably, caused even greater pulmonary morbidity, with significant deficits in all measured PFTs at 2 years (**Figs. 21.4, 21.5**).[27]

The HSG also explored pulmonary function in patients undergoing endoscopic versus open anterior fusion (without instrumentation) together with posterior segmental fixation and fusion. Twenty-one patients with AIS who underwent a video-assisted thoracoscopic release followed by a PSF and segmental spinal fixation were compared with 16 patients who underwent a release through an open thoracotomy followed by a PSF. Results showed that although both groups had statistically significant improvement in postoperative versus preoperative PFT parameters, there were no significant differences between the endoscopic and the thoracotomy groups in any specific parameter.[28]

Most recently, the HSG has sought to determine factors relating to outcomes in pulmonary function after surgery for AIS. They conducted a study to: (1) identify the factors that determine pulmonary function beyond 2 years after surgery for AIS; and (2) determine what factors, if any, can predict an increase or decrease in percent-predicted 2-year pulmonary function. To accomplish this, the HSG conducted a study of demographic data and performed a correlation analysis and subsequent stepwise multiple regression analysis of associations between radiographic measurements of spinal deformity and the results of spirometry in a series of 254 patients with AIS. The variables found to be significant predictors of

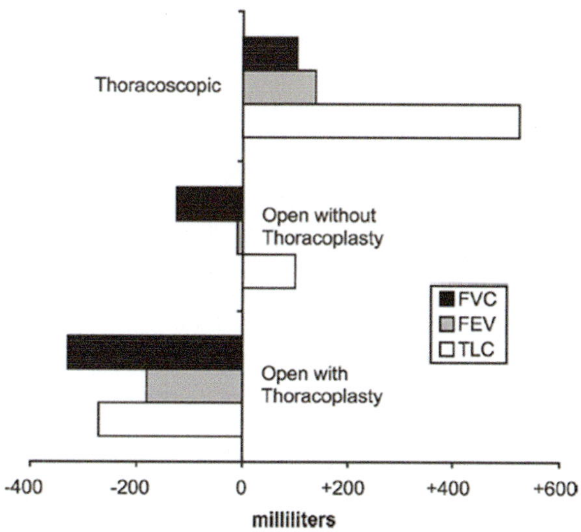


**Fig. 21.4** Change in absolute values (preoperative to 2-year postoperative) of all PFT parameters. (From Thorascopic scoliosis surgery affects pulmonary function less than thoracotomy at 2-years post surgery, Kishan et al. 2007. Reprinted with permission.)

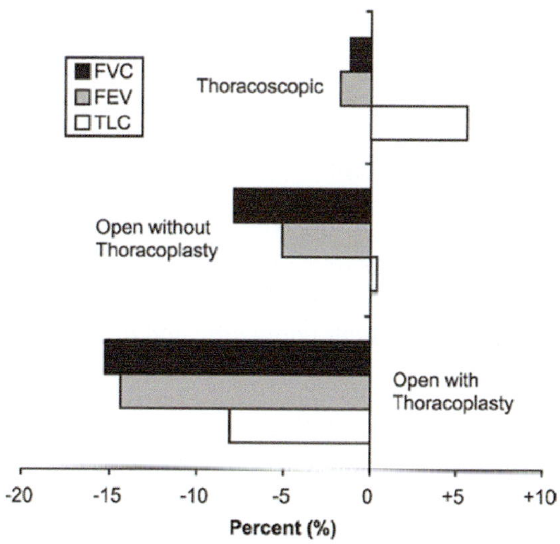


**Fig. 21.5** Change in percent predicted values (preoperative to 2-year postoperative) for all PFT parameters. (From Thorascopic scoliosis surgery affects pulmonary function less than thoracotomy at 2-years post surgery, Kishan et al. 2007. Reprinted with permission.)

2-year pulmonary function included: preoperative PFT scores in patients having open thoracotomy (as opposed to a thoracoscopic or posterior approach), surgical time, and use of thoracoplasty. These variables explained 40 to 51% of the variance in 2-year PFT data.[29] Pulmonary function is one of many outcome variables important in assessing the results of surgical correction of AIS.

## Health-Related Quality-of-Life Assessments

Because assessing HRQOL outcomes has become widely expected and accepted, appropriate research into the development of disease-specific tools for this purpose is increasingly essential. Extensive psychometric testing needs to go into the development of such tools to determine their validity and reliability in assessing HRQOL outcomes.[30]

For a surgical outcome to be considered successful, patient satisfaction must be taken into account. The tools and methods used to assess patient satisfaction are complicated because the relevant outcome measures must stratify the various aspects of daily living, personal perception, and overall well-being. Assessment with HRQOL tools allows physicians to determine the efficacy of an intervention in improving a patient's daily life. Because this yields data based on patient perception, the interpretation and analysis of these data can prove challenging in that the variability within a group can be largely based on nonmedical factors. This is particularly true with the population of patients with AIS. The surgeon is often left wondering whether it was truly the treatment that changed a patient's happiness, or an issue related to normal adolescence. Nonetheless, patient expectations and satisfaction should be of prime importance and should be addressed in any treatment-outcome study.[31]

The appropriate timepoint for assessing this, and the infrastructure for acquisition of the assessment data, can make the measurement of HRQOL outcomes a challenging goal for use in the care of spinal disorders.[32] This can be taxing' to the infrastructure of a busy clinic, and the management and analysis of the necessary data can be a burden to the staff members responsible for it. However, identification of the appropriate patient population and intervals for data acquisition is vital.

The HRQOL questionnaire of the SRS-24 was developed to evaluate patient satisfaction and performance, and to differentiate subgroups of patients with AIS from one another. The instrument consists of 24 questions divided into 7 equally weighted domains as determined by factor analysis. The domains are: (1) pain, (2) general self-image, (3) postoperative self-image, (4) general function, (5) overall level of activity, (6) postoperative function, and (7) satisfaction. The reliability and validity of the questionnaire were evaluated in 244 patients. The initial validation study concluded that the questionnaire allows the dynamic monitoring of scoliosis patients as they become adults, and is a validated instrument with good reliability.[33]

The SRS-24 questionnaire was used to demonstrate the ability of surgery to improve the outcome of patients with AIS. In a multicenter study of 242 patients, statistically significant improvements were seen in the pain, general self-image, function from back condition, and level of activity domains of the SRS-24 questionnaire at 2-year postoperative follow-up. The study also found that preoperative pain exists in the AIS population.[34]

It is often necessary for an HRQOL tool to be refined. This is beneficial for continued improvement of outcomes assessment with HRQOL tools, but presents a challenge to long-term data collection if one version of a tool is used preoperatively and a new version is administered postoperatively, because a pre- to postoperative analysis cannot then be done. The SRS-24 questionnaire has been revised from its original version with 24 questions to a version with 22 questions,[35–37] and more recently to version 22-R. During validation of the English version of the questionnaire, as well as in Spanish and Turkish transcultural adaptation studies, low internal consistency was discovered in the function domain of the questionnaire, and the problem was traced to questions 15 (relating to financial considerations) and 18 (relating to going out with friends). A minor revision was made to question 18, and question 15 was removed from the questionnaire, after which the internal consistency of the function domain improved. **Figure 21.6** summarizes the questions and domains that make up each validated version of the SRS questionnaire.

The HSG has conducted studies directed at understanding the correlation between HRQOL outcomes and other outcome measures in AIS research. These studies included the use of a radiographic outcomes assessment and the SRS-24 questionnaire. However, in a series of 78 patients, little correlation was found between the results of the radiographic assessment and the scores on the questionnaire,[38] and in a larger follow-up study, radiographic measures in the AIS population were only weak predictors of scores on the postoperative domain of the SRS-24 outcomes questionnaire.[4] This lack of correlation is troublesome, in that the "gold standard" for the outcome of surgery for AIS has been based on radiographic parameters, yet the patient's quality-of-life measures represent a highly valuable assessment, particularly in a relatively healthy teenage population with a diagnosis that creates little disability early in life. However, the observed lack of correlation may be a consequence of the inaccurate capture of radiographic factors that underlie patient satisfaction. As an example of this, a rib hump would be more of a rotational deformity than a pure coronal or sagittal deformity, but the means for measuring the rotation that causes a rib hump are very inaccurate.

| | | | | | | | |
|---|---|---|---|---|---|---|---|
| | | | 5 Domains: Pain (5), Self Image (5), Function/Activity (5), Mental Health (5), Satisfaction (5) | | 5 Domains: Pain (5), Self Image (5), Function/Activity (5), Mental Health (5), Satisfaction (5) | | 7 Domains: Pain (7), Self Image (3), General Function (3), Function/Activity (3), Self Image After Surgery (3), Function After Surgery (2), Satisfaction with Surgery (3) |
| Combined SRS 22 & 24 | | | | | | | |
| Question | | SRS 22 | | SRS 22R | | SRS 24 | |
| Which of the following best describes the amount of pain you have experienced during the past 6 months? | 1 | 1 | Pain | 1 | Pain | 1 | Pain |
| Which one of the following best describes the amount of pain you have experienced over the last month? | 2 | 2 | Pain | 2 | Pain | 2 | Pain |
| During the past 6 months have you been a very nervous person? | 3 | 3 | Mental Health | 3 | Mental Health | N/A | N/A |
| If you had to spend the rest of your life with your back shape as it is right now, how would you feel about it? | 4 | 4 | Self Image | 4 | Self Image | 3 | Pain |
| What is your current level of activity? | 5 | 5 | Function/Activity | 5 | Function/Activity | 4 | Function/Activity |
| How do you look in clothes? | 6 | 6 | Self Image | 6 | Self Image | 5 | Self Image |
| In the past 6 months have you felt so down in the dumps that nothing could cheer you up? | 7 | 7 | Mental Health | 7 | Mental Health | N/A | N/A |
| Do you experience back pain when at rest? | 8 | 8 | Pain | 8 | Pain | 6 | Pain |
| What is your current level of work/school activity? | 9 | 9 | Function/Activity | 9 | Function/Activity | 7 | General Function |
| Which of the following best describes the appearance of your trunk; defined as the human body except for the head and extremities? | 10 | 10 | Self Image | 10 | Self Image | N/A | N/A |
| Which one of the following best describes your medication usage for your back? | 11 | 11 | Pain | 11 | Pain | 8 | Pain |
| Does your back limit your ability to do things around the house? | 12 | 12 | Function/Activity | 12 | Function/Activity | 9 | Function/Activity |
| Have you felt calm and peaceful during the past 6 months? | 13 | 13 | Mental Health | 13 | Mental Health | N/A | N/A |
| Do you feel that your back condition affects your personal relationships? | 14 | 14 | Self Image | 14 | Self Image | 11 | Pain |
| Are you and/or your family experiencing financial difficulties because of your back? | 15 | 15 | Function/Activity | 15 | Function/Activity | 12 | General Function |
| In the past 6 months have you felt down hearted and blue? | 16 | 16 | Mental Health | 16 | Mental Health | N/A | N/A |
| In the last 3 months have you taken any sick days from work/school due to back pain, and if so, how many? | 17 | 17 | Pain | 17 | Pain | 10 | Function/Activity |
| Do you go out more or less than your friends? | 18 | 18 | Function/Activity | Reworded 18 | Function/Activity | 13 | General Function |
| Do you feel attractive with your current back condition? | 19 | 19 | Self Image | 19 | Self Image | 14 | Self Image |
| Have you been a happy person during the past 6 months? | 20 | 20 | Mental Health | 20 | Mental Health | N/A | N/A |
| Are you satisfied with the results of your back management? | 21 | 21 | Satisfaction | 21 | Satisfaction | 22 | Satisfaction |
| Would you have the same management again if you had the same condition? | 22 | 22 | Satisfaction | 22 | Satisfaction | 24 | Satisfaction |
| On a scale of 1 to 9, with 1 being very low and 9 being extremely high, how would you rate your self image? | 23 | N/A | N/A | N/A | N/A | 15 | Self Image |
| Compared with before treatment, how do you feel you look now? | 24 | N/A | N/A | N/A | N/A | 23 | Satisfaction |
| Has your back treatment changed your function and daily activity? | 25 | N/A | N/A | N/A | N/A | 16 | Function After Surgery |
| Has your back treatment changed your ability to enjoy sports/hobbies? | 26 | N/A | N/A | N/A | N/A | 17 | Function After Surgery |
| Has your back treatment your back pain? | 27 | N/A | N/A | N/A | N/A | 18 | Pain |
| Has your treatment changed your confidence in personal relationships with others? | 28 | N/A | N/A | N/A | N/A | 19 | Self Image After Surgery |
| Has your treatment changed the way others view you? | 29 | N/A | N/A | N/A | N/A | 20 | Self Image After Surgery |
| Has your treatment changed your self image? | 30 | N/A | N/A | N/A | N/A | 21 | Self Image After Surgery |

**Fig. 21.6** Breakdown of the different versions of the SRS questionnaire.

Other research groups have also evaluated postoperative residual spinal deformity and patient quality-of-life outcomes and have found that patients with a greater Cobb angle or rotational deformity in their thoracic curve had a more negative self-image preoperatively and had their self-image improved after surgery. This score bore a direct relationship to the magnitude of correction of the thoracic Cobb angle.[39] However, as with the findings of the HSG, the presence of low $R^2$ values in both studies (0.03 to 0.07) for the correlation of the change in self-image score with the change in Cobb angle indicates that variables other than the radiographic appearance of a deformity must also be affecting such scores (e.g., psychosocial, functional variables).[4]

The limitation of the currently available outcome instruments may be a lack of adquate sensitivity, with all healthy adolescents falling within a relatively narrow outcome range regardless of the severity of their scoliosis. Or it may be that the radiographic measurements of scoliosis now being compared with outcome-instrument measures instruments do not account for factors that explain most of the variability in these measures, such as rotational deformity. Further research is required in this area.

## Functional Assessments

Assessment of the scoliotic spine is routinely limited to radiographic examinations that provide individual measures of global and regional spinal alignment in the coronal and sagittal planes. These routine procedures provide a static assessment of spinal alignment while the patient is standing, and do not represent functional movement of the spine. Thus, most current knowledge of preoperative AIS and its response to treatment is limited to nonfunctional, uniplanar measurements.

Until recently, the postoperative function of the patient with AIS was rarely considered. The shift in surgical treatment to fusion only of selected regions of the spine, with the thought of sparing a greater number of vertebral segments, initiated the need to document a patient's functional status as a means of proving the benefit of leaving regions of the spine unfused. The hypothesis underlying this is that preserving mobile segments of a patient's spine (rather that fusing them) should increase function over what it would be with a longer spinal fusions. Surprisingly, proving this has remained challenging.

The functional consequences of a longer fusion are unknown. Alhough improvements in function are of concern in treating patients with AIS, there is little understanding of how the deformity and its treatment affect the magnitude and quality of functional, dynamic spinal motion. An improved understanding of the connection between AIS and potential functional deficiencies may improve both the evaluationof AIS and decision-making for its correction.

Numerous studies have documented improvements in standing spinal alignment and trunk shape after corrective surgery for AIS.[40–42] However, there is a paucity of research on postoperative changes in the capabilities of the spine for functional movement. Engsberg et al[41] examined lower-extremity kinematics and parameters of spinopelvic balance during gait in patients with AIS before and at 1 year after fusion surgery. They observed improvements in head-over-neck positioning and shoulder–pelvis symmetry. Interestingly, surgery did not significantly alter the patients' lower-extremity kinematics, although a significant decrease in walking speed was observed. However, the dynamic functional limits of axial spinal rotation in patients with AIS have not been established pre- or postoperatively.

Engsberg and colleagues[40] compared the pre- and postoperative range of motion (ROM) of the spine in patients with AIS during uniplanar movements of the trunk. They measured global and regional spinal motion with a camera system and reflective markers attached to the skin overlying the spinous processes. They observed a significant decrease in postoperative global spinal ROM during lateral and forward-bending movements of the trunk. Decreased ROM above and below the fused region of the spine was also reported. Although subjects were instructed to perform uniplanar bending movements, it is likely that the complex nature of the deformity in scoliosis will still produce three-dimensional (3D) rotations that may be undetectable with two-dimensional (2D) means of assessment.

Challenges exist in the ability to accurately and noninvasively measure motion of the spine. Because most clinicians do not have access to a motion-analysis laboratory, and repeated functional testing in the laboratory setting is prohibitive in terms of both cost and time, the assessment of AIS patients' function has been limited. The HSG has adopted a noninvasive method for measuring spinal mobility in the AIS patient population. This method incorporates three measures of trunk flexibility, which are acquired both pre- and postoperatively from patients with AIS. Truncal flexion motion is assessed with a modified version of Shoberg's method.[43] This involves a noninvasive measurement of the length of the spine as the distance between the C7 and S1 spinous processes (**Fig. 21.7**). Lateral flexion of the trunk is measured by having patients touch their fingertips to the floor (**Fig. 21.8**). In an initial evaluation of this method, Marks et al[44] grouped patients according to the location of their spinal fusion as having been in the thoracic region only, in the lumbar region only, or in both the thoracic and lumbar regions. Data for 68 patients with pre- and postoperative mreasures of trunk flexibility were included in this evaluation. This simple noninvasive clinical measure of trunk motion identified reductions in trunk flexibility following scoliosis surgery.

**Trunk Flexibility Evaluation**

**1. Thoracic & Lumbar Flexion**

To Measure: Subject stands with trunk erect while tape is placed proximally on the spinous process of C7 and distally to S1. Following flexion of the vertebrae, using the same bony landmarks, calculate the difference in distance between the starting and ending positions.

Example Case (normal teenager):
Distance Standing = 45 cm
Distance @ Bend = 58 cm
Amount of Flexion = 13 cm

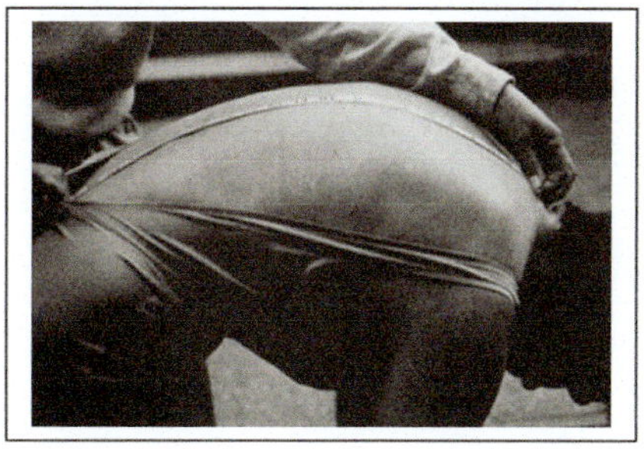

| PT Eval-Scoliosis | Pre-Op | 1 year post-op | 2 year post-op |
|---|---|---|---|
| AROM | Date: | Date: | Date: |
| 1.Thoracic & Lumbar Flexion | | | |

**Fig. 21.7** Truncal flexibility measurement method used by the HSG (part 1).

As expected, longer fusions resulted in greater reductions in motion, but these reductions were modest, ranging from 5 to 36%. The spinal motion affected to the greatest degree was lateral bending, with very little change being observed in axial rotation (**Figs. 21.9, 21.10**). In a recent study, Marks et al[45] measured intervertebral motion of the unfused distal segments of the spine in patients with AIS who underwent PSF and instrumentation. Motion was assessed with standardized radiographs acquired in the maximum right-, left-, and forwarding-bending positions. The intervertebral angles were measured with digital radiographic software at each vertebral level from T12 to S1. The relationship of the vertebral segmental motion for the region from each interspace to the LIV was evaluated. As the LIV progressed distally, motion at the L4–L5 level increased significantly in lateral bending, raising concern about potential early degeneration. A relationship between the increased lateral motion L4–L5 and subsequent disc degeneration with more distal fusion is unknown but considered at potential risk.

The implications of hyper- or hypomobility in unfused segments of the spine after instrumentation for scoliosis is poorly understood, and further research in this area is required.

**3. Thoracic and Lumbar Lateral Flexion**

To Measure: Subject stands erect with the feet flat on the floor. Place one end of a measuring tape on the tip of the middle finger and the other on the floor on a point directly beneath the middle finger. Measure the difference in inches following the lateral flexion motion.

Example Case (normal teenager):
Distance Standing = 77 cm
Distance @ max lateral bend = 48 cm
Amount of lateral bend = 29 cm

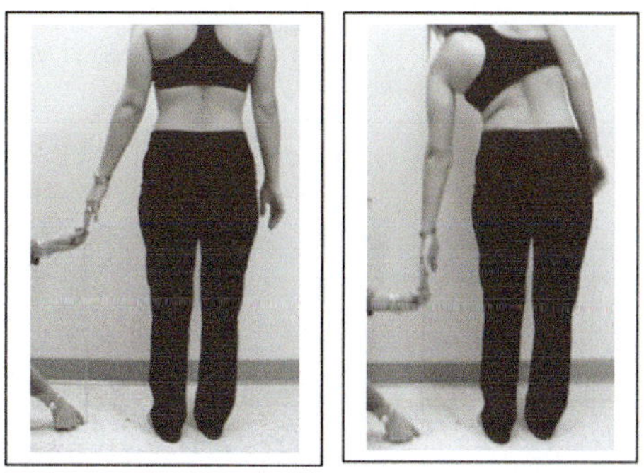

| PT Eval-Scoliosis | Pre-Op | 1 year post-op | 2 year post-op |
|---|---|---|---|
| AROM | Date: | Date: | Date: |
| 3.Right Thoracic & Lumbar Lateral Flexion | | | |
| 4.Left Thoracic & Lumbar Lateral Flexion | | | |

**Fig. 21.8** Trunkal flexibility measurement method utilized by the HSG (part 2).

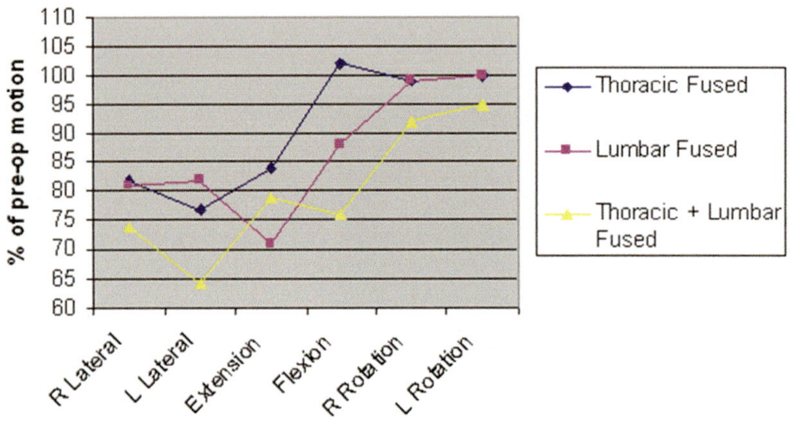


**Fig. 21.9** Percent of preoperative motion in each type of movement for various regions of spinal fusion in AIS.

## Clinical Appearance/Trunk Shape Assessments

According to patients, clinical appearance may be the most important component of AIS outcomes research. The age range in which AIS is most often diagnosed can be a phase of life in which a patient's physical appearance is very important. The asymmetrical trunk shape and altered appearance resulting from spinal deformity are components of AIS that the patient experiences most acutely. They can become manifest as a posterior scapular or rib deformity, an anterior rib deformity, breast asymmetry, shoulder-height asymmetry, or an asymmetrical waistline. Any one or a multitude of these components can have a marked effect on a patient's psychological status. It has been shown that the appearance of the back and shoulders is critically important to the adolescent with idiopathic scoliosis.[46] With respect to postoperative expectations and patients' own ratings of their physical appearance, surgeons and patients are clearly not on the same page. In a study of orthopedists' ratings of outcome in relation to patient satisfaction with postoperative results, the two sets of ratings were not significantly correlated.[47] It is apparent that this area of outcomes research in AIS needs significant attention.

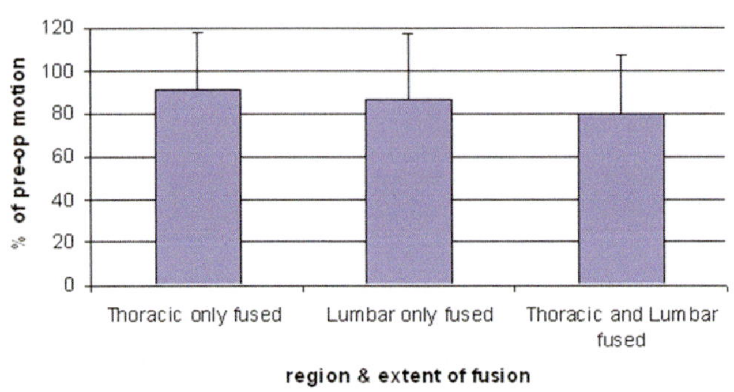


**Fig. 21.10** Percent of preoperative motion in each type of movement for various regions of spinal fusion in AIS.

However, the quantification of cosmesis and its integration into the surgical outcomes of AIS have been challenging. Studies in surface topography have shown that the relationship between spinal curvature and cosmetic effect is not simple. Unfortunately, the equipment for making topographic measurements can be costly and is not practical for routine clinical care.[48] Radiographic and physical measurements of trunk shape and alignment may not correlate well with patients' and parents' perceptions of appearance and patients' assessments of their deformity.[49] In a study of outcome in terms of physical appearance, 73% of patients reported satisfaction with the cosmetic result of surgical correction of their AIS. Dissatisfied patients and those with neutral opinions shared preoperative physical characteristics such as specific curve types and lower body-mass indices, as well as preoperative psychological difficulties and unrealistic expectations.[50]

In a study to determine whether spinal- or truncal-deformity measurements correlated with patients' responses on a quality-of-life questionnaire, Asher and coworkers found that the magnitude of spinal deformity correlated well with such responses, whereas truncal deformity did not. In this study, spinal deformity was defined as the measured curvature of the spine, and truncal deformity was defined as the external deformity in the trunk as a result of the underlying spinal deformity. Asher and coworkers concluded that this was somewhat surprising because it is the truncal deformity that is typically considered the most apparent component of the deformity to the patient with scoliosis, and cautioned that these findings illustrate the pitfalls of assuming what is important to the patient on the basis of current clinical measurements.[51]

The HSG has evaluated truncal-shape correction and its relationship to patient satisfaction in AIS. In a prospective multicenter study, patients who had a diagnosis of AIS with a structural primary thoracic curve (Lenke type 1) were evaluated with preoperative radiographs, 2-year postoperative radiographs, truncal-shape measures, and results on SRS-24 questionnaires. Patients showed a significant

**Table 21.1 Mean Preoperative Trunk Shape Measures for 909 Patients with AIS Categorized by Lenke Classification**

| Lenke Curve Type | *n* | UT curve | TH curve | L/ThL curve | Coronal Decompensation | Rib Humps Thoracic | Rib Humps Left | Shoulder Height | Truncal Shift |
|---|---|---|---|---|---|---|---|---|---|
| 1 | 472 | 25 | 52 | 33 | 1.2 | 14.1 | 6.1 | 1.5 | 1.8 |
| 2 | 136 | 40 | 62 | 33 | 1.4 | 15.4 | 6.2 | 1.5 | 1.9 |
| 3 | 50 | 28 | 67 | 55 | 1.2 | 14.3 | 10.1 | 1.9 | 1.6 |
| 4 | 33 | 39 | 82 | 57 | 1.4 | 17.5 | 8.5 | 1.9 | 2.2 |
| 5 | 159 | 9 | 29 | 47 | 2.1 | 7.0 | 11.2 | 1.5 | 1.9 |
| 6 | 59 | 17 | 52 | 63 | 2.0 | 9.9 | 11.9 | 1.8 | 1.5 |

*Abbreviations:* L/ThL, lumbar/thoracolumbar; TH, Thoracic; UT, upper thoracic

($P < 0.001$) improvement in all measures at follow-up. Although there was no statistically significant difference between the patients treated with ASF or PSF in either radiographic or truncal-shape correction, patient satisfaction and self-image improved significantly after ASF but not after PSF.[52]

Currently, there are 909 AIS patients with preoperative truncal-shape measurements in the HSG database. The preoperative characteristics of patients' truncal deformities stratified according to the Lenke classification are found in **Table 21.1.** In a comparison of the cosmetic deformity in different Lenke curve classifications, Lenke type 5 and type 6 curves show the greatest coronal decompensation ($P < 0.05$). Rib humps are larger in Lenke types 1, 2, 3, and 4 curves, and lumbar humps are larger in the Lenke types 3, 5, and 6 curves ($P < 0.05$). There are no differences in shoulder height or truncal shift among the various Lenke types of curve. The patient population in the study was also assessed to evaluate the correlation between radiographic change from before to after surgery and the corresponding change in trunk shape. It was found that the greater the percent correction in curvature of the thoracic and upper thoracic spine, the greater the reduction in the thoracic rib hump (**Fig. 21.11**). Truncal deformity in the group as a whole (not stratified according to the Lenke classification) showed moderate correlations with thoracic or upper thoracic curve size or both, and with rib-hump deformity ($r = 0.52$ and $r = 0.41$, respectively; $P = 0.00$) (**Table 21.2**). Similarly, a significant correlation was found between lumbar curve size and lumbar-hump deformity ($r = 0.41$; $P = 0.00$).

Measurements of trunk shape are best acquired from the patient as opposed to the patient's radiograph, because doing this includes the soft-tissue component of the underlying bony deformity in the measurements. The HSG had developed a system for acquiring measurements of trunk shape that were made directly from the patient and recorded on a white board or paper against which the patient stood. All attempts were made to have the patient stand in a relaxed, reproducible position to reduce error. However, this methodology introduced unavoidable error as a result of patient movement, and measures of trunk shape are now made on radiographs. Measures of coronal decompensation, shoulder height, and truncal shift are all now acquired from radiographs (**Fig. 21.12**).

Further work in the area of trunk shape assessment in AIS is underway in the HSG, specifically on the relationship between the preoperative truncal deformities of AIS patients and HRQOL measurements. In addition, an attempt is being made to correlate the impact of postoperative cosmetic change in AIS and the reflection of that change as assessed with HRQOL tools.

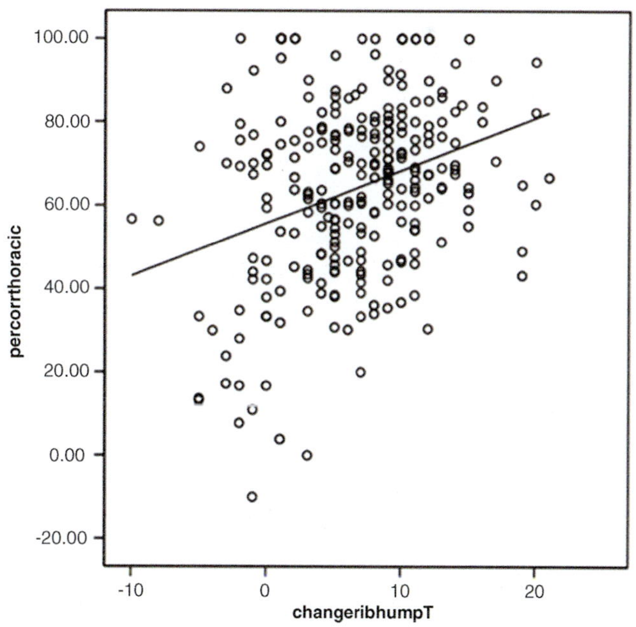


**Fig. 21.11** Scatterplot demonstrating correlation between postoperative Cobb angle correction and subsequent change in trunk shape: The greater percent correction in the thoracic and upper thoracic spine, the greater the change (decrease) in the thoracic rib hump.

**Table 21.2 Correlations of Curve Size with Cosmetic Deformity for 909 Patients**

| Correlations | | Coronal Decompensation | Rib Humps: Thoracic | Rib Humps: Lumbar | Shoulder Height Side | Truncal Shift Side |
|---|---|---|---|---|---|---|
| Thoracic curve | *r* | −0.07 | 0.52 | −0.11 | 0.15 | 0.11 |
| | Sig. (2-tailed) | 0.05 | 0.00 | 0.00 | 0.00 | 0.00 |
| Upper thoracic curve | *r* | −0.13 | 0.41 | −0.24 | 0.01 | 0.03 |
| | Sig. (2-tailed) | 0.00 | 0.00 | 0.00 | 0.77 | 0.34 |
| Lumbar curve | *r* | 0.17 | −0.13 | 0.41 | 0.11 | −0.01 |
| | Sig. (2-tailed) | 0.00 | 0.00 | 0.00 | 0.00 | 0.79 |

## The Development of Scientific Research Design

### Starting with a Hypothesis

To develop a useful research hypothesis for a relevant clinical question, the researcher must be exposed to challenges or problems in current treatment techniques. Sometimes this comes through the systematic prospective collection of data that are then "mined" retrospectively to answer specific clinical questions. In the best-case scenario; a clinical question arises, a null hypothesis is formulated as its answer, and a prospective study is designed to test the hypothesis in the most scientific way possible.

### Study Design

The process of research is an application of the scientific method.[53] Ensuring that the five phases of the research process are completed helps to guarantee that a specific

A

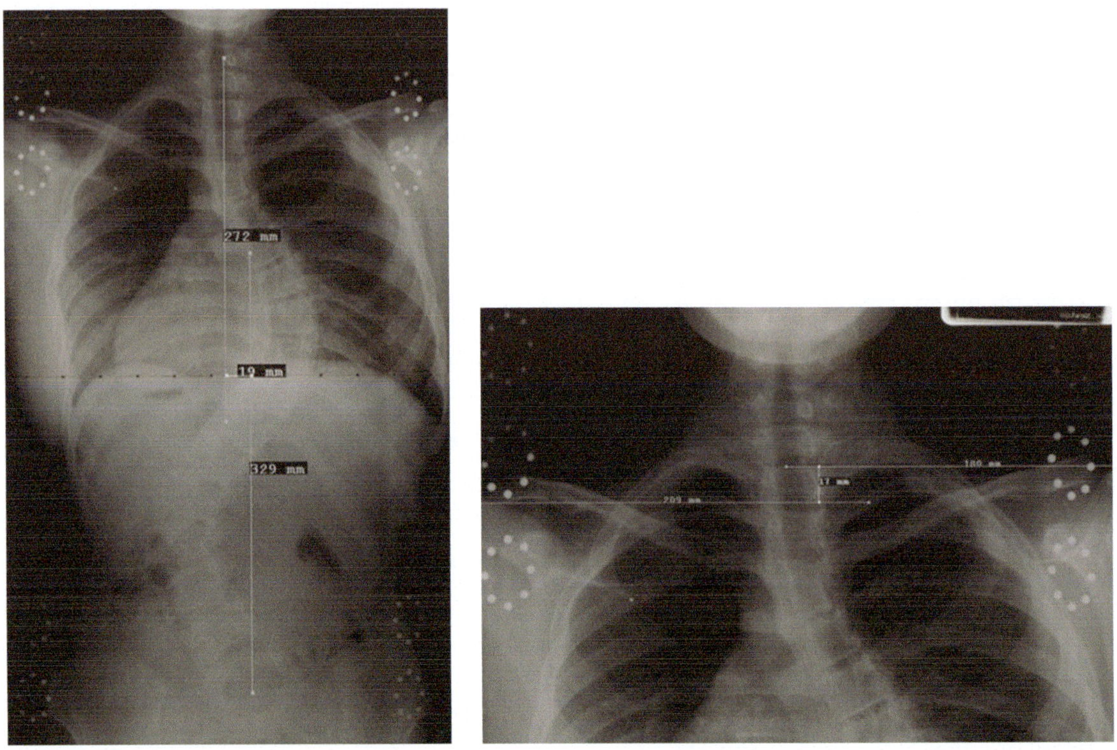


B

**Fig. 21.12 (A)** Trunk-shape measure of coronal decompensation acquired via radiographs. **(B)** Trunk-shape measure of shoulder height acquired via radiographs.

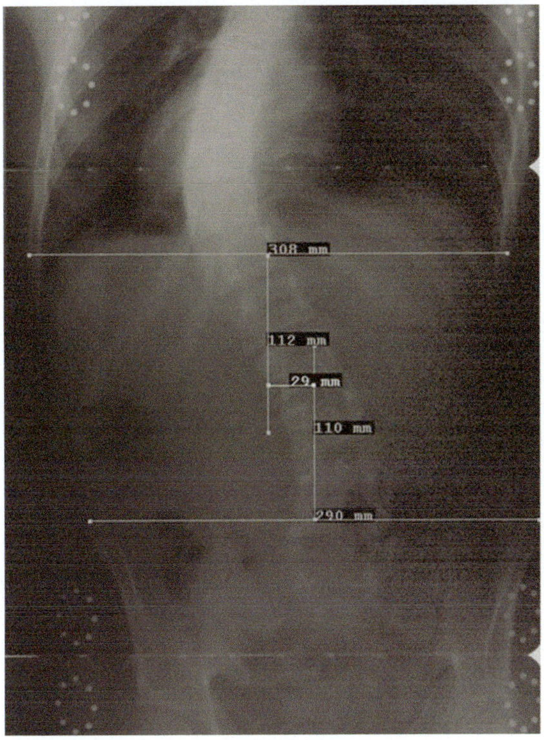


**Fig. 21.12** *(Continued)* **(C)** Trunk-shape measure of shoulder height acquired via radiographs.

research endeavor will be systematic, empirical, controlled, and critical (**Fig. 21.13**). The most reliable design for a research study design is a blinded, randomized controlled trial (RCT). This type of study may be very difficult to conduct in AIS, particularly through research on surgical outcomes. As medicine has become increasingly scientific and less accepting of unsupported opinion or proof by anecdote, the RCT has become the standard technique for changing diagnostic or therapeutic methods. Many journals require that authors designate a "level of evidence" for any study (**Fig. 21.14**). Level-1 studies (blinded, randomized trials) are given priority during manuscript review.

The use of the RCT as a research design can be problematic in that it is often impossible to blind participants to their treatment. This also creates an ethical dilemma related to the issue of randomization for a surgical treatment.[54] Such randomization was attempted by the HSG in a prospective study aimed at comparing three treatment approaches (anterior open, anterior thoracoscopic, and posterior fusion) for the treatment of primary right-thoracic (Lenke type 1) curves. The treatment approach for each patient was to be randomized at the time of enrollment in the study, but this proved impossible to do. The surgeons felt the need to do what was best for the patient, and not allow "chance" to deny what seemed to be the correct treatment for the patient. Even though the "best" treatment approach to Lenke type 1 curves had not been proven scientifically, the investigators allowed empirical clinical judgment to guide their decision-making. The RCT requires physicians to act also and simultaneously as scientists. This puts them in a difficult and sometimes untenable ethical position.[54] Besides the difficulty it presented to the surgeon members of the HSG, the RCT of the three surgical approaches to Lenke type 1 curves was also challenged by a lack of willing participants. When a subgroup of 10 patients was polled during the informed consent process and was asked whether they would be willing to participate if the study was an RCT, all 10 of the patients answered "no." Although the objective clinical data supplied by RCTs is desirable, neither physicians nor patients seem willing to yield their freedom of choice and clinical decision-making to a randomization process.

The primary purpose of the RCT is to ensure that the study sample is representative of the general population and to give each participant an equal chance of being assigned to the treatment being studied. The randomization technique was devised by statisticians in an attempt to prevent bias by eliminating the influence of an investigator's opinions or preferences on patient selection.[55] However, the ethical dilemmas associated with randomization may put its use at variance with primary obligations of the physicians.[54] If there are no data, either anecdotal or more concrete, to support one treatment over another, randomization may be easier, but if data are beginning to support one treatment as superior to another in a physician's opinion, the physician may feel ethically obligated to choose the

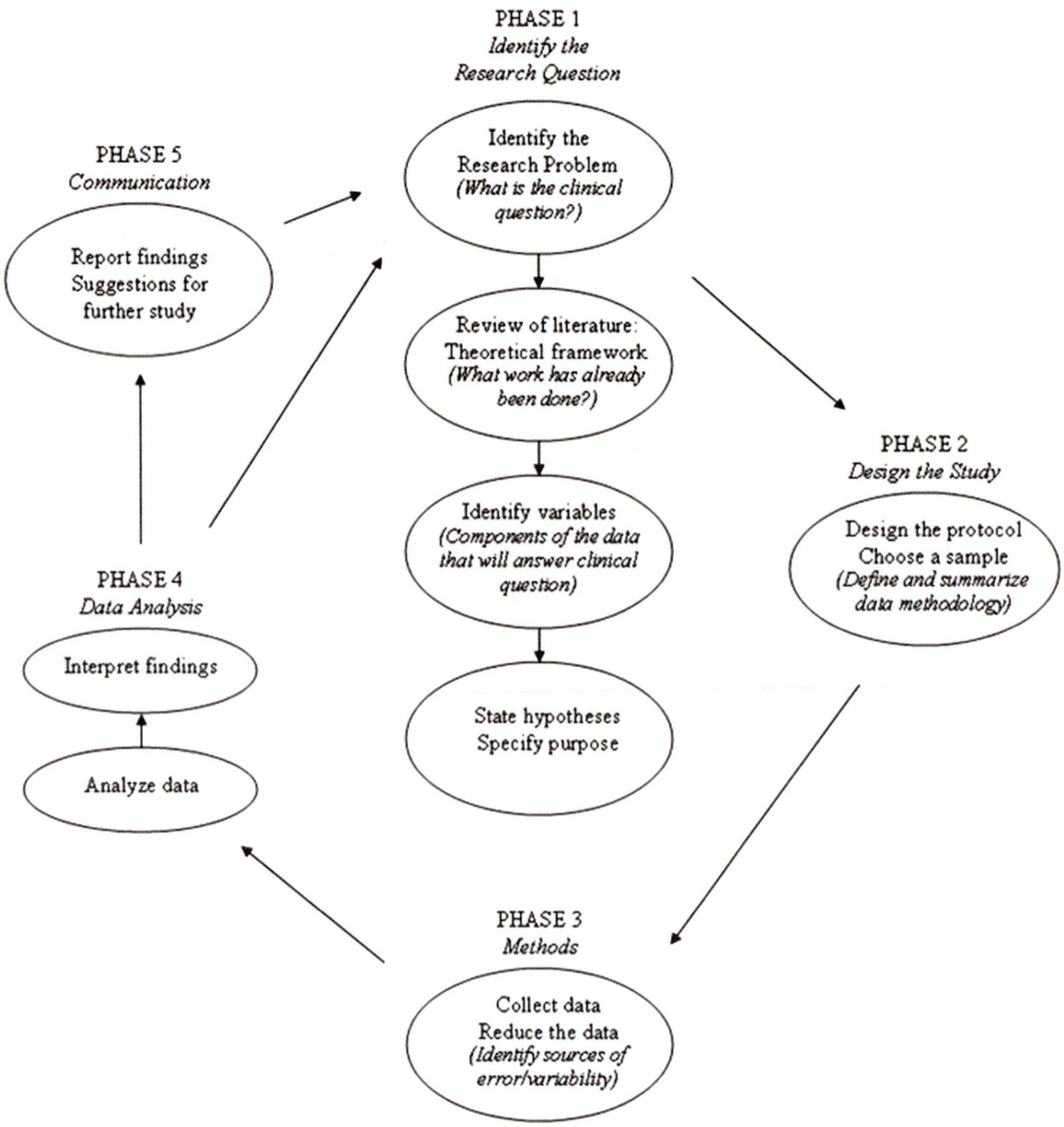


**Fig. 21.13** A model of the research process. (From Foundations of Clinical Research–Applications to Practice. Portney Watkins, 1993. Adapted with permission.)

seemingly superior treatment rather than leaving the decision to chance. This makes for good care, but not good research. The recourse is to conduct a good level-2 study that is prospective and comparative but not necessarily blinded and randomized.

## Good Clinical Research Practices

Research involving the AIS patient population is routinely based on data collected as a component of routine clinical care. In a busy clinical setting, the reliability and consistency of these data can sometimes be compromised by the very busyness and crowding of the clinical setting. It is a reality that clinical data are not collected in a sterile, quiet laboratory setting but in a busy patient-centered setting. These environmental constraints can often jeopardize the quality of the data.

All attempts should be made to follow good clinical research practices when acquiring data for a research protocol. FDA regulations governing clinical research, state and local laws, and institutional standard operating procedures as mandated by the institutional review board (IRB) should all be followed. Sources of error should be minimized and consistency and reliability of measurements should be the goal. Some mechanisms to help achieve this include instituting protocol-specific procedures that are understood by trained clinical staff members. The number of staff members collecting the data for a research protocol should be limited, to reduce inter-rater inconsistency. The procedures for data collection should thoroughly describe the measurement

| Level | Therapy/Prevention, Aetiology/Harm | Prognosis | Diagnosis |
|---|---|---|---|
| 1a | SR (with homogeneity*) of RCTs | SR (with homogeneity*) of inception cohort studies; CDR† validated in different populations | SR (with homogeneity*) of Level 1 diagnostic studies; CDR† with 1b studies from different clinical centres |
| 1b | Individual RCT (with narrow Confidence Interval‡) | Individual inception cohort study with > 80% follow-up; CDR† validated in a single population | Validating** cohort study with good††† reference standards; or CDR† tested within one clinical centre |
| 1c | All or none§ | All or none case-series | Absolute SpPins and SnNouts†† |
| 2a | SR (with homogeneity*) of cohort studies | SR (with homogeneity*) of either retrospective cohort studies or untreated control groups in RCTs | SR (with homogeneity*) of Level >2 diagnostic studies |
| 2b | Individual cohort study (including low quality RCT; e.g., <80% follow-up) | Retrospective cohort study or follow-up of untreated control patients in an RCT; Derivation of CDR† or validated on split-sample§§§ only | Exploratory** cohort study with good††† reference standards; CDR† after derivation, or validated only on split-sample§§§ or databases |
| 2c | "Outcomes" Research; Ecological studies | "Outcomes" Research | |
| 3a | SR (with homogeneity*) of case-control studies | | SR (with homogeneity*) of 3b and better studies |
| 3b | Individual Case-Control Study | | Non-consecutive study; or without consistently applied reference standards |
| 4 | Case-series (and poor quality cohort and case-control studies§§) | Case-series (and poor quality prognostic cohort studies***) | Case-control study, poor or non-independent reference standard |
| 5 | Expert opinion without explicit critical appraisal, or based on physiology, bench research or "first principles" | Expert opinion without explicit critical appraisal, or based on physiology, bench research or "first principles" | Expert opinion without explicit critical appraisal, or based on physiology, bench research or "first principles" |

A

### Notes

Users can add a minus-sign "-" to denote the level of that fails to provide a conclusive answer because of:

- EITHER a single result with a wide Confidence Interval (such that, for example, an ARR in an RCT is not statistically significant but whose confidence intervals fail to exclude clinically important benefit or harm)
- OR a Systematic Review with troublesome (and statistically significant) heterogeneity.
- Such evidence is inconclusive, and therefore can only generate Grade D recommendations.

| | |
|---|---|
| * | By homogeneity we mean a systematic review that is free of worrisome variations (heterogeneity) in the directions and degrees of results between individual studies. Not all systematic reviews with statistically significant heterogeneity need be worrisome, and not all worrisome heterogeneity need be statistically significant. As noted above, studies displaying worrisome heterogeneity should be tagged with a "-" at the end of their designated level. |
| † | Clinical Decision Rule. (These are algorithms or scoring systems which lead to a prognostic estimation or a diagnostic category.) |
| ‡ | See note #2 for advice on how to understand, rate and use trials or other studies with wide confidence intervals. |
| § | Met when all patients died before the Rx became available, but some now survive on it; or when some patients died before the Rx became available, but none now die on it. |
| §§ | By poor quality cohort study we mean one that failed to clearly define comparison groups and/or failed to measure exposures and outcomes in the same (preferably blinded), objective way in both exposed and non-exposed individuals and/or failed to identify or appropriately control known confounders and/or failed to carry out a sufficiently long and complete follow-up of patients. By poor quality case-control study we mean one that failed to clearly define comparison groups and/or failed to measure exposures and outcomes in the same (preferably blinded), objective way in both cases and controls and/or failed to identify or appropriately control known confounders. |
| §§§ | Split-sample validation is achieved by collecting all the information in a single tranche, then artificially dividing this into "derivation" and "validation" samples. |
| †† | An "Absolute SpPin" is a diagnostic finding whose Specificity is so high that a Positive result rules-in the diagnosis. An "Absolute SnNout" is a diagnostic finding whose Sensitivity is so high that a Negative result rules-out the diagnosis. |
| ‡‡ | Good, better, bad and worse refer to the comparisons between treatments in terms of their clinical risks and benefits. |
| ††† | Good reference standards are independent of the test, and applied blindly or objectively to applied to all patients. Poor reference standards are haphazardly applied, but still independent of the test. Use of a non-independent reference standard (where the 'test' is included in the 'reference', or where the 'testing' affects the 'reference') implies a level 4 study. |
| †††† | Better-value treatments are clearly as good but cheaper, or better at the same or reduced cost. Worse-value treatments are as good and more expensive, or worse and the equally or more expensive. |
| ** | Validating studies test the quality of a specific diagnostic test, based on prior evidence. An exploratory study collects information and trawls the data (e.g. using a regression analysis) to find which factors are 'significant'. |
| *** | By poor quality prognostic cohort study we mean one in which sampling was biased in favour of patients who already had the target outcome, or the measurement of outcomes was accomplished in <80% of study patients, or outcomes were determined in an unblinded, non-objective way, or there was no correction for confounding factors. |
| **** | Good follow-up in a differential diagnosis study is >80%, with adequate time for alternative diagnoses to emerge (eg 1-6 months acute, 1 - 5 years chronic) |

### Grades of Recommendation

| | |
|---|---|
| A | consistent level 1 studies |
| B | consistent level 2 or 3 studies *or* extrapolations from level 1 studies |
| C | level 4 studies *or* extrapolations from level 2 or 3 studies |
| D | level 5 evidence *or* troublingly inconsistent or inconclusive studies of any level |

B *"Extrapolations" are where data is used in a situation which has potentially clinically important differences than the original study situation.*

**Fig. 21.14 (A,B)** Oxford Centre for Evidence-based Medicine Levels of Evidence (May 2001) for research studies. (From the Centre for Evidence-based Medicine website: http://www.cebm.net/index.aspx?o=1116.)

method to be used in the research protocol, to reduce inconsistencies stemming from individual biases in data acquisition and measurement (**Fig. 21.15**). Radiographic measurements should be made by one individual, and if a study is multicentered, all attempts should be made to centralize X-ray measurements. The radiographic measures to be used in a research protocol should be standardized and described thoroughly in an instruction manual with a

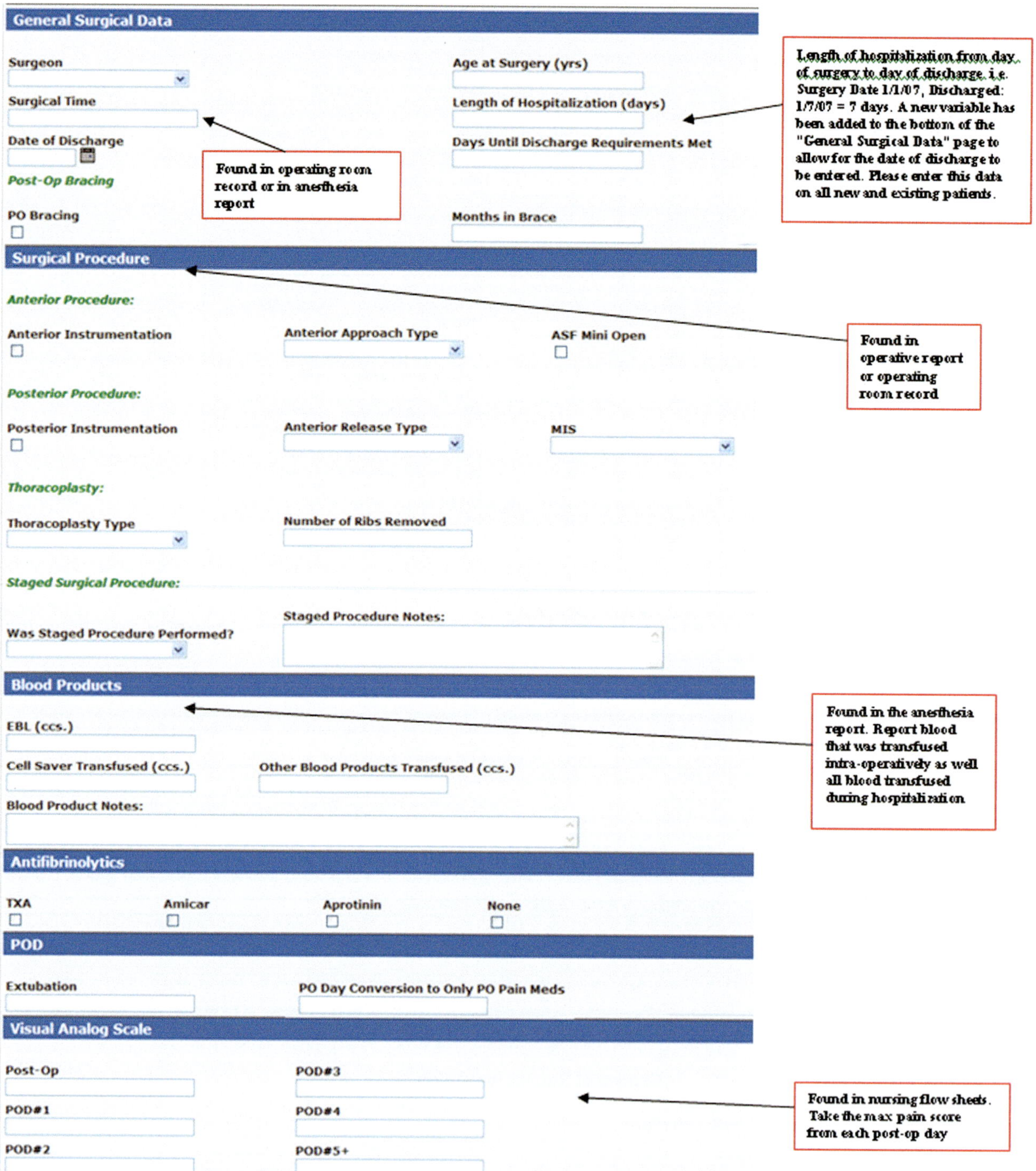


**Fig. 21.15** Example of guidelines and manual for data acquisition, for standardizing methods used for data collection.

textual and pictorial description of each measure (**Fig. 21.16**). The standardization of radiographic data acquisition[56,57] and measurement techniques[58] is vital to the accuracy and validity of radiographic outcomes reporting. Despite attempts to minimize error by standardization, error can be introduced by multiple measurers. Having a single individual make the measurements based directly on digital images (to enhance the visualization of landmarks) is optimal (**Fig. 21.17**). Measurements made directly on the patient should minimize patient-induced error by standardizing positioning and

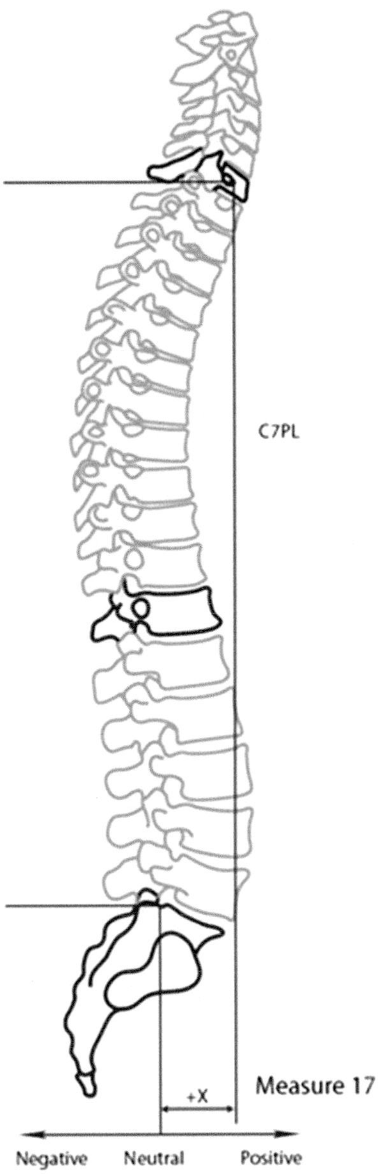


Fig. 21.16 Example of radiographic measurement manual for standardizing methods used for radiographic measurements.

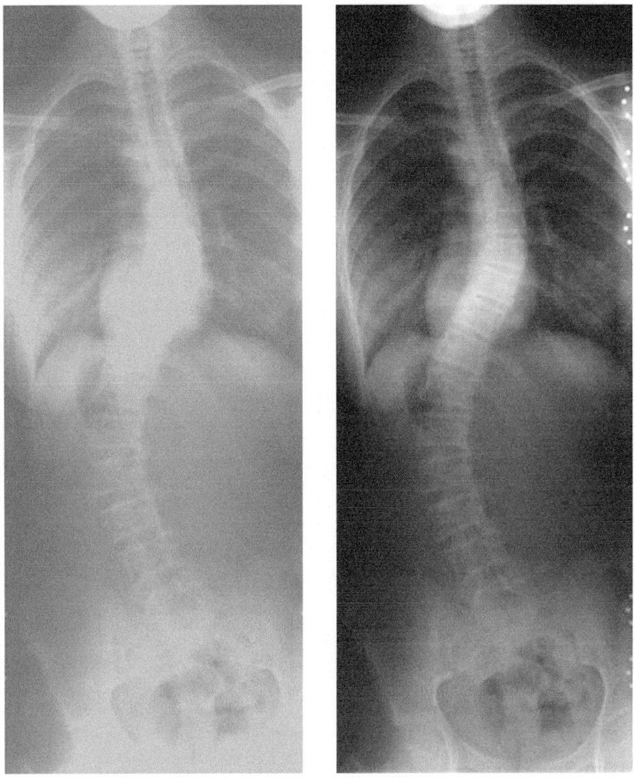

A,B

Fig. 21.17 (A) Examples of visualization on a standard hard-copy film, and (B) a Digital Imaging and Communications in Medicine (DICOM) image that has been enhanced with measuring software.

clear instructions to the patient (Fig. 21.18). Guidelines for administering standardized HRQOL instruments should be followed and the forms should be checked for completeness at the time patients submit them, to avoid data loss from unanswered questions or incomplete forms. Internal measures for quality assurance should be taken for every aspect of data acquisition. These may include two-person data acquisition teams, in which the first member collects the data and the second member checks the data for accuracy. Internal quality-assurance measures may also include random checks for errors in data entry or data comparisons by two individuals, to ensure acceptable interrater reliability.

The HSG adheres to the following standards for quality assurance in data collection:

1. The study group utilizes trained site coordinators who collect the data for the study according to standardized data collection methods, utilizing standardized data-collection forms.
2. Data are collected and managed in compliance with good clinical research practices, and institutional review board approval is required at every site.
3. The data are entered into a central web-based database and new data that are entered remain unverified and are not used in any analyses until the data QA process is complete.
4. The data QA process involves an experienced central individual who reviews each patient file. Every variable in the patient file is evaluated. Any questionable data are sent back to the site at which they were collected for evaluation and rechecking.
5. Radiographic images and clinical photographs are evaluated and used to check the accuracy of radiographic and trunk-shape measures.

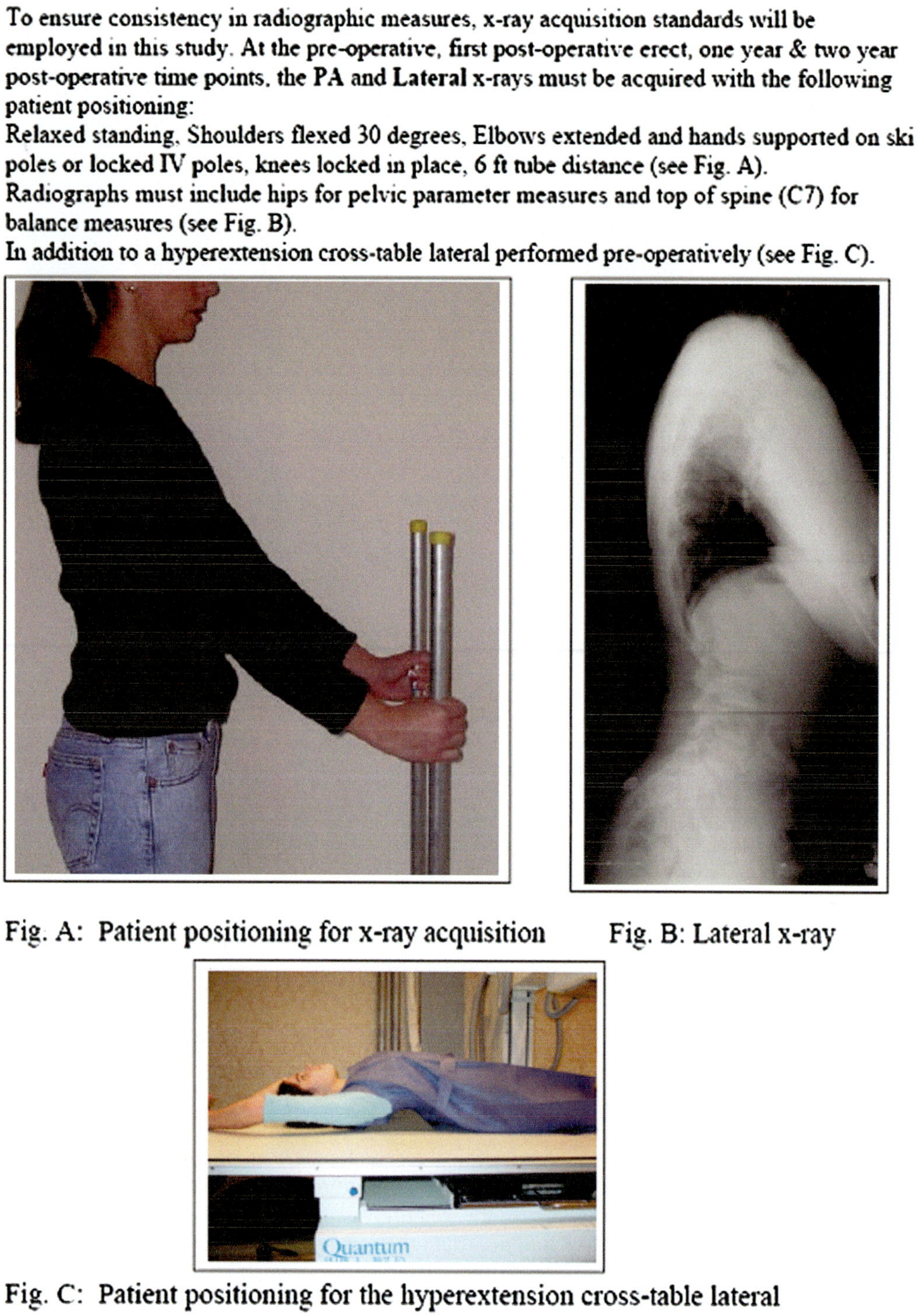
**To ensure consistency in radiographic measures, x-ray acquisition standards will be employed in this study. At the pre-operative, first post-operative erect, one year & two year post-operative time points, the PA and Lateral x-rays must be acquired with the following patient positioning:**

**Relaxed standing, Shoulders flexed 30 degrees, Elbows extended and hands supported on ski poles or locked IV poles, knees locked in place, 6 ft tube distance (see Fig. A).**

**Radiographs must include hips for pelvic parameter measures and top of spine (C7) for balance measures (see Fig. B).**

**In addition to a hyperextension cross-table lateral performed pre-operatively (see Fig. C).**

**Fig. A: Patient positioning for x-ray acquisition**

**Fig. B: Lateral x-ray**



**Fig. C: Patient positioning for the hyperextension cross-table lateral**

**Fig. 21.18** Example of standarization of patient positioning.

6. The study group database is built with internal data checks to ensure data completeness and accuracy.
7. Patient files are not verified for use in analyses until all data-related questions are resolved.
8. A second phase of data QA occurs when study data are analyzed. The HSG database is queried centrally for specific study variables, and a central statistician analyzes the data set. If any outliers are identified in a specific data set, the questionable data are again sent back to the collection site to assess their accuracy.

The methods used by the HSG are as good as can be expected short of sending a site monitor to each site to

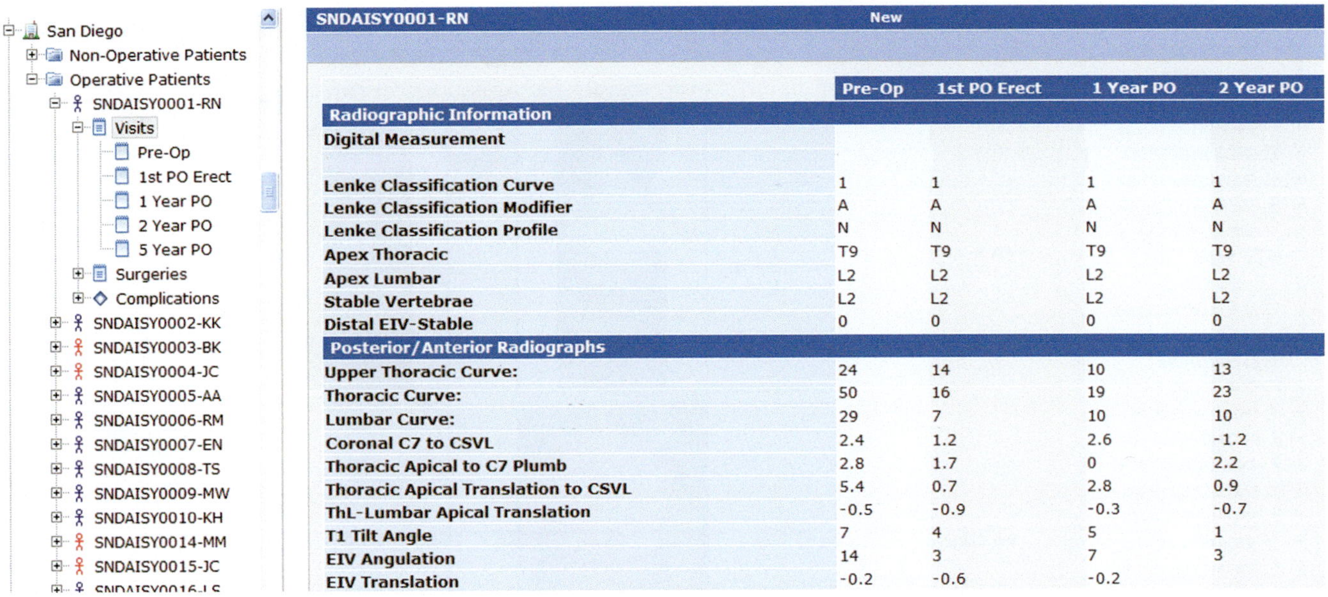


| | Pre-Op | 1st PO Erect | 1 Year PO | 2 Year PO |
|---|---|---|---|---|
| **Radiographic Information** | | | | |
| **Digital Measurement** | | | | |
| **Lenke Classification Curve** | 1 | 1 | 1 | 1 |
| **Lenke Classification Modifier** | A | A | A | A |
| **Lenke Classification Profile** | N | N | N | N |
| **Apex Thoracic** | T9 | T9 | T9 | T9 |
| **Apex Lumbar** | L2 | L2 | L2 | L2 |
| **Stable Vertebrae** | L2 | L2 | L2 | L2 |
| **Distal EIV-Stable** | 0 | 0 | 0 | 0 |
| **Posterior/Anterior Radiographs** | | | | |
| **Upper Thoracic Curve:** | 24 | 14 | 10 | 13 |
| **Thoracic Curve:** | 50 | 16 | 19 | 23 |
| **Lumbar Curve:** | 29 | 7 | 10 | 10 |
| **Coronal C7 to CSVL** | 2.4 | 1.2 | 2.6 | -1.2 |
| **Thoracic Apical to C7 Plumb** | 2.8 | 1.7 | 0 | 2.2 |
| **Thoracic Apical Translation to CSVL** | 5.4 | 0.7 | 2.8 | 0.9 |
| **ThL-Lumbar Apical Translation** | -0.5 | -0.9 | -0.3 | -0.7 |
| **T1 Tilt Angle** | 7 | 4 | 5 | 1 |
| **EIV Angulation** | 14 | 3 | 7 | 3 |
| **EIV Translation** | -0.2 | -0.6 | -0.2 | |

**Fig. 21.19** Example of database design enabling easy QA of radiographic measures over time.

check source documents, which entails logistic, personnel, and financial requirements not entailed by the currently available resources of the HSG.[59]

The common phrase "garbage in, garbage out" holds true in outcomes research and the acquisition of outcomes data; complete and accurate data entry and QA measures are of utmost importance.

## Building a Database

Having an efficient method for data entry and storage in AIS outcomes research is vitally important. A well-designed database can greatly ease the process of data entry, QA, analysis and reporting. The design of the database should be consistent with the specific aims and hypothesis of the study in which the data will be collected, but should allow new areas of study in the patient population from which the study sample is drawn. The database should allow "user-friendly" data entry and the comprehensive viewing of data for QA purposes (**Fig. 21.19**). Optimally, the database should have the ability to house text data as well as image data (**Fig. 21.20**), which not only augments the QA process (i.e., clinical trunk-shape measures can be verified with clinical photographs), but provides for easy retrieval of case examples during manuscript preparation. Ultimately, the most important aspect of a database is the ability to query and extract the data. New questions sometimes arise during the collection of study data (other than the original questions defined by the specific aims of the study), and the ability to answer those questions by querying the appropriate data gathered at the specific time points at which they were entered into the database is crucial. A well-designed query tool makes this possible. The query tool designed for the HSG database allows all variables in the database to be queried and "filtered." The filters used for this define criteria for which specific data are pulled from the database. For example, variables can be filtered by attributes such as curve type or gender, and can be filtered over time, such as for 70-degree curves that are corrected to 20 degrees. This filtering allows efficient data querying, data organization, and preparation of data for analysis.

Data archiving is also an important issue. For example, a backup of the HSG database is created nightly, with the new database replacing the previous night's backup version. Only one daily backup version is saved. Once a week, the daily backup is written to a tape archive. This provides secondary protection of the database. The data are also backed up at an offsite location. Therefore, in the case of a disaster, a database that is no more than 48 hours older than the time of occurrence of the disaster is available.

If funding or time is limited during a study, and a custom-made database cannot be created, a common spread sheet file can be used. However, it is important to design the spreadsheet with the database qualities noted earlier, of user-friendly data entry, easy QA, and good organization for efficient data analysis.

## Statistical Analysis

Statistical analysis is an important component of scientific research. In a well-designed study, statistics enters the picture before any data are collected. The statistical plan should be formulated in conjunction with the development of the

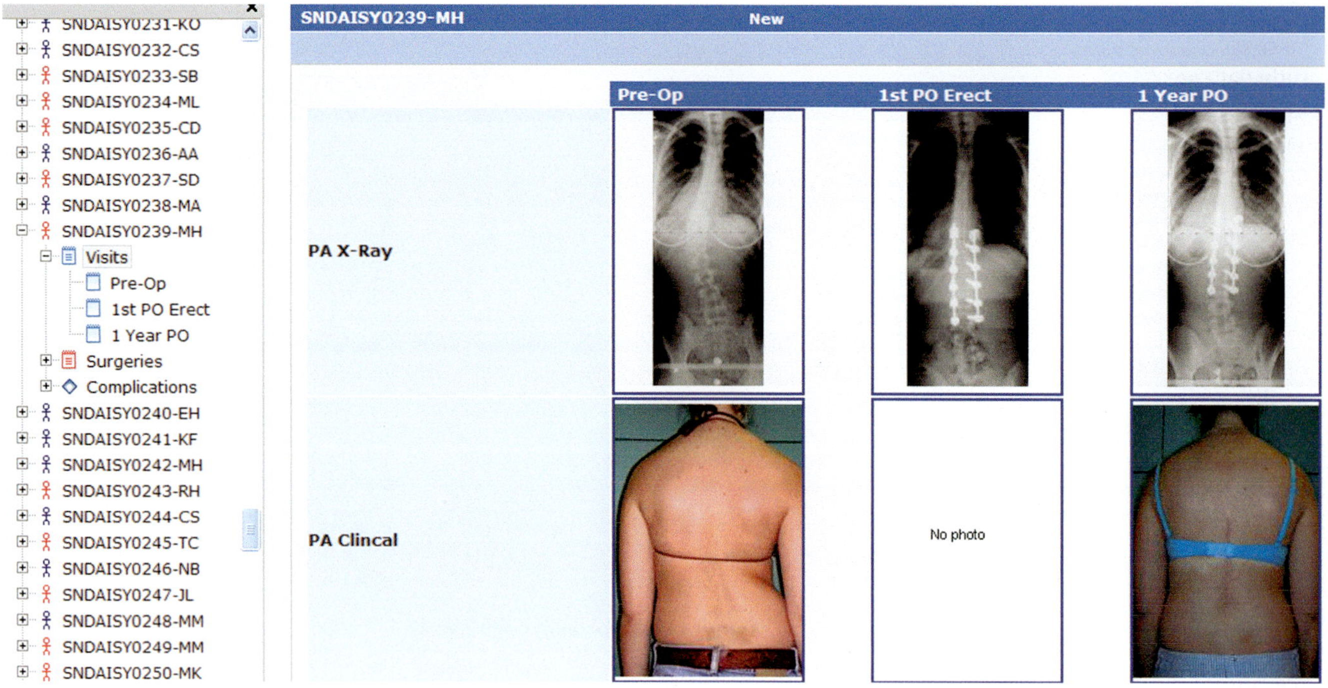


**Fig. 21.20** Example of database design encompassing clinical photographs and radiographic images.

study protocol. A statistician should review the hypothesis underlying the study and determine the best statistical tests for adequately testing the null hypothesis. If the study is prospective in design, a power analysis can be done to determine the sample size needed for the study to have statistical power sufficient to validate its results. Even an RCT does not meet level-1 criteria (Centre for Evidence- based Medicine website: http://www.cebm.net/index. aspx?o=1116) if it has insufficient statistical power. Before being analyzed, the data should undergo a secondary QA process to ensure the accuracy of data collection and entry. The statistician can apply descriptive statistics to all of the outcome variables to seek outliers and illogical data. Alpha (*P*-value) levels are typically set at 0.05 to protect against type 1 error. If multiple outcome variables are being analyzed in a single study, the study $\alpha$ level should be adjusted with the Bonferroni correction to ensure that the chance of type 1 error for the entire study remains at 0.05 (or 5%).

Descriptive, relational, and quasiexperimental (nonrandomized) research have all been done within the AIS population. Despite the difficulty in conducting the RCTs that are the gold standards of surgical studies, statistical analyses can be used in an appropriate and effective manner in designing these alternate kinds of studies. An example of this is the description in the literature of the results of thoracoscopically treatment in a series of patients with AIS.[60] Such analysis is typical of descriptions of the effects of treatment over time.

Relational research and analysis is exemplified in Newton and colleagues'[25] examination of the relationship between preoperative PFT and preoperative radiographic characteristics of scoliotic spines. Although the variables examined in their study did not explain a large percentage of the variance in preoperative PFT, it was found that four radiographic characteristics (thoracic-curve size, number of vertebrae in the curve, thoracic kyphosis, and coronal imbalance) significantly predicted a patient's preoperative PFT values. Although prospective studies are not RCTs, well-collected prospective data, on which responsible statistical analyses have been done, can provide important clinical information.

Quasiexperimental projects involve comparing characteristics of nonrandomized groups to evaluate the effects of a treatment. One such study evaluated the effect of surgical approach on PFT data.[27] The statistical analysis done in this study allowed the investigators to quantify the estimated effect of each surgical approach on 2-year postoperative pulmonary function. Although bias cannot be eliminated in quasiexperimental studies, and the cause–effect relationship is not as definitive as with an RCT, the information gained from the research can still be of benefit in clinical practice.

## Abstract and Manuscript Preparation

A research study is not worth performing if its results are not going to be shared. Unfortunately, writing the manuscript that describes a study is often the most difficult part of the study. Devoting adequate time, thought, and expert collaboration to the refinement of one's research question, the design of the study for answering the question (including appropriate outcome measures), the careful performance of the study, and the correct analysis and interpretation of the study data are the most important components of writing a research article. No amount of analytical or writing skill can make a good article from poor data.[61] The effort of manuscript preparation can be eased by documenting the study from its initiation. If this is done, the manuscript is practically written by the time the study is completed.

For example, when a study proposal is initially written, it clearly defines the purpose of the study and the scope of the work to be done in it. This in turn should be the basis for the "introduction" section of the manuscript. In addition, when the literature review is done in developing the protocol for the study, it can be updated at the completion of the study and the background and significance sections of the manuscript will be complete. It helps to use a program (e.g., Endnote) to save references in a "library," so that they are easily retrievable and help in formatting of the manuscript. Because the methods to be used in a study are clearly defined during development of the study protocol, the "methods" section of the manuscript is essentially written and requires only fine-tuning for the final manuscript. The "results" section of the manuscript is filled in with data reported by a statistician or a surgeon experienced in statistical analysis, as described above. The "conclusion" section of the manuscript should be thought out and described only after the results have been interpreted. The conclusions and clinical recommendations should match the quantitative findings in the "results" section of the manuscript. If all the above are followed during the study, generating a manuscript to submit for publication is straight-forward.

## Areas for Growth and Progress in Outcomes Research in Adolescent Idiopathic Scoliosis

Although a plethora of research exists in AIS (a Pubmed search of the keywords "adolescent idiopathic scoliosis" currently retrieves 2262 records), there are just as many questions that remain unanswered. Within the realm of outcomes of treatment in AIS, the opportunity for research lies within the current limitations discussed throughout this chapter. Many of these limitations revolve around the lack of uniform measures for outcomes in AIS. Clinicians' and researchers' questions will remain unanswered until each outcome measure is standardized and the results of published works can be compared across studies. A perfect example of this exists in the area of radiographic data acquisition and radiographic measurement. Furthermore, a standardized method of measuring and quantifying the external appearance of the body is needed to understand the effect of treatment of AIS on patients' appearances.

The use of the SRS outcomes instrument has allowed the standardization of HRQOL assessment in AIS. However, gaps remain in understanding the effect of treatment on patients' quality of life. Why does what the surgeon sees (curve magnitude) not predict a larger proportion of the variation in what the patient reports on the quality-of-life assessment instrument? Why is there a gap between the orthopedists' ratings of appearance and outcome and patients' views of their own cosmesis?

Technology is constantly expanding and affecting medical care. This expansion translates into fertile areas of research. Newer technologies are providing rapid, low-dose radiation methods of obtaining 3D images of the spine. The current system of classifying scoliotic curves does not take into account the three dimensions in which these deformities exist. The new technologies will allow the development of a new classification system, which will ultimately require research to validate and translate existing findings into categories of scoliosis. Technological advances may also help to create noninvasive methods for understanding the effect of scoliotic deformity and associated surgery on truncal mobility.

Perhaps the most critical component of outcomes research in AIS will be answered not with standardization or technology, but simply with time. The long-term effects of treatments for AIS are very poorly understood. Bridging the gap between the pediatric spine surgeon who may initially operate on the adolescent patient with scoliosis and the adult spine surgeon who cares for the same patient in late adulthood is desperately needed.

## Conclusion

No single variable can accurately assess outcome in the surgical treatment of AIS. It is the integration of multiple variables, always to include the patient's perception, that will lead to a greater understanding of effective and successful treatment strategies.

The spine surgeons who dedicate their efforts to developing research infrastructures and devote their time to answering important clinical questions in AIS must be applauded. They are the key components in advancing the science of the surgical treatment of AIS, because of their position in the "trenches." They are the ones who will apply the proven methodologies for treating AIS in their clinical practice, and who will benefit the patient in an almost immediate way.

However, the most important aspect of research in AIS is that in reality, conducting a true RCT of treatment for this condition is virtually impossible. Therefore, the professionals associated with scoliosis research must be committed to performing excellent prospective studies in the clinical setting, with consistent processes of measurement, data collection, and data analysis.

## References


1. Epstein RS, Sherwood LM. From outcomes research to disease management: A guide for the perplexed. Ann Intern Med 1996;124:832–837
2. Garratt A, Schmidt L, Mackintosh A, Fitzpatrick R. Quality of life measurement: Bibliographic study of patient assessed health outcome measures. BMJ 2002;324:1417–1419
3. Copay AG, Glassman SD, Subach BR, Berven S, Schuler TC, Carreon LY. Minimum clinically important difference in lumbar spine surgery patients: A choice of methods using the Oswestry Disability Index, Medical Outcomes Study questionnaire Short Form 36, and pain scales. Spine J 2008;8:968–974
4. Wilson PL, Newton PO, Wenger DR, et al. A multicenter study analyzing the relationship of a standardized radiographic scoring system of adolescent idiopathic scoliosis and the Scoliosis Research Society outcomes instrument. Spine 2002;27: 2036–2040
5. Harrington PR. Spinal fusion in the treatment of idiopathic adolescent scoliosis. J Tenn Med Assoc 1963;56:470–479
6. Savastano AA, Thayer JB, Gibson TK. Experiences with the Harrington instrumentation method in the treatment of idiopathic scoliosis: A preliminary report. J Int Coll Surg 1964;42:421–428
7. Zielke K, Berthet A. [VDS—ventral derotation spondylodesis: A preliminary report on 58 cases]. Beitr Orthop Traumatol 1978;25: 85–103
8. Dwyer AF, Schafer MF. Anterior approach to scoliosis. Results of treatment in fifty-one cases. J Bone Joint Surg Br 1974;56:218–224
9. Giehl JP, Völpel J, Heinrich E, Zielke K. Correction of the sagittal plane in idiopathic scoliosis using the Zielke procedure (VDS). Int Orthop 1992;16:213–218 (SICOT)
10. Lowe TG, Peters JD. Anterior spinal fusion with Zielke instrumentation for idiopathic scoliosis. A frontal and sagittal curve analysis in 36 patients. Spine 1993;18:423–426
11. Turi M, Johnston CE II, Richards BS. Anterior correction of idiopathic scoliosis using TSRH instrumentation. Spine 1993;18:417–422
12. Betz RR, Harms J, Clements DH III, et al. Comparison of anterior and posterior instrumentation for correction of adolescent thoracic idiopathic scoliosis. Spine 1999;24:225–239
13. Betz RR, Shufflebarger H. Anterior versus posterior instrumentation for the correction of thoracic idiopathic scoliosis. Spine 2001; 26:1095–1100
14. Lenke LG, Betz RR, Bridwell KH, Harms J, Clements DH, Lowe TG. Spontaneous lumbar curve coronal correction after selective anterior or posterior thoracic fusion in adolescent idiopathic scoliosis. Spine 1999;24:1663–1671, discussion 1672
15. D'Andrea LP, Betz RR, Lenke LG, Harms J, Clements DH, Lowe TG. The effect of continued posterior spinal growth on sagittal contour in patients treated by anterior instrumentation for idiopathic scoliosis. Spine 2000;25:813–818
16. Lenke LG, Betz RR, Bridwell KH, et al. Intraobserver and interobserver reliability of the classification of thoracic adolescent idiopathic scoliosis. J Bone Joint Surg Am 1998;80:1097–1106
17. Lenke LG, Betz RR, Harms J, et al. Adolescent idiopathic scoliosis: A new classification to determine extent of spinal arthrodesis. J Bone Joint Surg Am 2001;83A:1169–1181
18. Lenke LG, Betz RR, Haher TR, et al. Multisurgeon assessment of surgical decision-making in adolescent idiopathic scoliosis: Curve classification, operative approach, and fusion levels. Spine 2001; 26:2347–2353
19. Lenke LG, Betz RR, Clements D, et al. Curve prevalence of a new classification of operative adolescent idiopathic scoliosis: Does classification correlate with treatment? Spine 2002;27:604–611
20. Newton PO, Faro FD, Lenke LG, et al. Factors involved in the decision to perform a selective versus nonselective fusion of Lenke 1B and 1C (King-Moe II) curves in adolescent idiopathic scoliosis. Spine 2003;28:S217–S223
21. Weinstein SL, Zavala DC, Ponseti IV. Idiopathic scoliosis: Long-term follow-up and prognosis in untreated patients. J Bone Joint Surg Am 1981;63:702–712
22. Crapo RO. Pulmonary-function testing. N Engl J Med 1994; 331:25–30
23. Miller MR, Crapo R, Hankinson J, et al; ATS/ERS Task Force. General considerations for lung function testing. Eur Respir J 2005;26: 153–161
24. Aaro S, Ohlund C. Scoliosis and pulmonary function. Spine 1984;9: 220–222
25. Newton PO, Faro FD, Gollogly S, Betz RR, Lenke LG, Lowe TG. Results of preoperative pulmonary function testing of adolescents with idiopathic scoliosis. A study of six hundred and thirty-one patients. J Bone Joint Surg Am 2005;87:1937–1946
26. Faro FD, Marks MC, Newton PO, Blanke K, Lenke LG. Perioperative changes in pulmonary function after anterior scoliosis instrumentation: Thoracoscopic versus open approaches. Spine 2005;30: 1058–1063
27. Kishan SBT, Bastrom T, Betz RR, et al. Thoracoscopic scoliosis surgery affects pulmonary function less than thoracotomy at 2 years postsurgery. Spine 2007;32:453–458
28. Lenke LG, Newton PO, Marks MC, et al. Prospective pulmonary function comparison of open versus endoscopic anterior fusion combined with posterior fusion in adolescent idiopathic scoliosis. Spine 2004;29:2055–2060
29. Newton PO, Perry A, Bastrom TP, et al. Predictors of change in postoperative pulmonary function in adolescent idiopathic scoliosis: A prospective study of 254 patients. Spine 2007;32:1875–1882
30. Murphy KR, Davidshofer CO. Psychological Testing: Principles and Applications ed. Englewood Cliffs, NJ: Prentice-Hall; 1994
31. Haher TR, Valdevit A. The use of outcomes instruments in the assessment of patients with idiopathic scoliosis. Instr Course Lect 2005;54:543–550
32. Berven S, Smith A, Bozic K, Bradford DS. Pay-for-performance: considerations in application to the management of spinal disorders. Spine 2007;32(11, suppl):S33–S38
33. Haher TR, Gorup JM, Shin TM, et al. Results of the Scoliosis Research Society instrument for evaluation of surgical outcome in adolescent idiopathic scoliosis. A multicenter study of 244 patients. Spine 1999;24:1435–1440
34. Merola AA, Haher TR, Brkaric M, et al. A multicenter study of the outcomes of the surgical treatment of adolescent idiopathic scoliosis using the Scoliosis Research Society (SRS) outcome instrument. Spine 2002;27:2046–2051
35. Asher M, Min Lai S, Burton D, Manna B. The reliability and concurrent validity of the scoliosis research society-22 patient questionnaire for idiopathic scoliosis. Spine 2003;28:63–69
36. Asher M, Min Lai S, Burton D, Manna B. Scoliosis research society-22 patient questionnaire: responsiveness to change associated with surgical treatment. Spine 2003;28:70–73

37. Asher M, Min Lai S, Burton D, Manna B. Discrimination validity of the scoliosis research society-22 patient questionnaire: Relationship to idiopathic scoliosis curve pattern and curve size. Spine 2003;28:74–78
38. D'Andrea LP, Betz RR, Lenke LG, et al. Do radiographic parameters correlate with clinical outcomes in adolescent idiopathic scoliosis? Spine 2000;25:1795–1802
39. Watanabe K, Hasegawa K, Hirano T, Uchiyama S, Endo N. Evaluation of postoperative residual spinal deformity and patient outcome in idiopathic scoliosis patients in Japan using the scoliosis research society outcomes instrument. Spine 2007;32: 550–554
40. Engsberg JR, Lenke LG, Reitenbach AK, Hollander KW, Bridwell KH, Blanke K. Prospective evaluation of trunk range of motion in adolescents with idiopathic scoliosis undergoing spinal fusion surgery. Spine 2002;27:1346–1354
41. Engsberg JR, Bridwell KH, Reitenbach AK, et al. Preoperative gait comparisons between adults undergoing long spinal deformity fusion surgery (thoracic to L4, L5, or sacrum) and controls. Spine 2001;26:2020–2028
42. Stokes IA, Ronchetti PJ, Aronsson DD. Changes in shape of the adolescent idiopathic scoliosis curve after surgical correction. Spine 1994;19:1032–1037, discussion 1037–1038
43. Palmer ML, Epler ME. Clinical assessment procedures in physical therapyed. Philadelphia: JB Lippincott; 1990
44. Marks MC, Newton PO, Betz RR, et al. Post-operative trunk motion in adolescent idiopathic scoliosis: Does the region of fusion affect motion? Presented at: IMAST annual meeting. Banff, Canada, 2005:E-poster #512
45. Marks MCN. PO, Petcharaporn M, Bastrom T, Shah, SA, Betz RR, Lonner BS, Miyanji F. A more distal fusion is associated with increased motion at L4/L5: A set up for degeneration? SRS/IMAST, 2009
46. Theologis TN, Jefferson RJ, Simpson AH, Turner-Smith AR, Fairbank JC. Quantifying the cosmetic defect of adolescent idiopathic scoliosis. Spine 1993;18:909–912
47. Buchanan R, Birch JG, Morton AA, Browne RH. Do you see what I see? Looking at scoliosis surgical outcomes through orthopedists' eyes. Spine 2003;28:2700–2704, discussion 2705
48. Goldberg CJ, Grove D, Moore DP, Fogarty EE, Dowling FE. Surface topography and vectors: A new measure for the three dimensional quantification of scoliotic deformity. Stud Health Technol Inform 2006;123:449–455
49. Smith PL, Donaldson S, Hedden D, et al. Parents' and patients' perceptions of postoperative appearance in adolescent idiopathic scoliosis. Spine 2006;31:2367–2374
50. Koch KDBR, Buchanan R, Birch JG, Morton AA, Gatchel RJ, Browne RH. Adolescents undergoing surgery for idiopathic scoliosis: How physical and psychological characteristics relate to patient satisfaction with the cosmetic result. Spine 2001;26: 2119–2124
51. Asher M, Lai SM, Burton D, Manna B. Spine deformity correlates better than trunk deformity with idiopathic scoliosis patients' quality of life questionnaire responses. Stud Health Technol Inform 2002;91:462–464
52. Clements DH, Marks M, Porter ST, et al. Trunk shape correction and patient satisfaction in adolescent idiopathic scoliosis. Paper presented at: 40th Annual Meeting of the Scoliosis Research Society, Miami, FL, Oct 27–30, 2005
53. Portney LG, Watkins MP. Foundations of Flinical Research: Applications to Practice ed. Norwalk, CT: Appleton & Lange; 1993
54. Hellman S, Hellman DS. Of mice but not men. Problems of the randomized clinical trial. N Engl J Med 1991;324(22):1585–1589
55. Gigerenzer G, Swijtink Z, Porter T, et al. The Empire of Chance ed. Cambridge, UK: Cambridge University Press; 1989
56. Marks MC, Stanford CF, Mahar AT, Newton PO. Standing lateral radiographic positioning does not represent customary standing balance. Spine 2003;28:1176–1182
57. Faro FD, Marks MC, Pawelek J, Newton PO. Evaluation of a functional position for lateral radiograph acquisition in adolescent idiopathic scoliosis. Spine 2004;29:2284–2289
58. Spinal Deformity Study Group. In: Lenke LG, ed. Radiographic Measurement Manual: Medtronic Sofamor Danek Memphis, TN, USA, Inc., 2004:110
59. The Harms Study Group Data Collection Standardization Manual, 2008
60. Newton PO, Parent S, Marks M, Pawelek J. Prospective evaluation of 50 consecutive scoliosis patients surgically treated with thoracoscopic anterior instrumentation. Spine 2005;30(17, suppl): S100–S109
61. Wiggin NJB, Bailor JC, McPeek B, et al. Writing for Publication, ed. 2. In Principles and Practices of Research, 2nd ed. New York: Springer-Verlag; 1991

# 22 Complications in Surgery for Spinal Deformity

*HoSun Hwang, Angel Macagno, Munish C. Gupta, and Michael F. O'Brien*

Many pitfalls are encountered in surgery for spinal deformity. The procedures are physiologically demanding for the patient and technically challenging for the surgeon. Not surprisingly, complications accompany this complex endeavor.

The variety of complications encountered in spine surgery and catalogued in the literature is extensive, and ranges from insignificant to severe.[1–3] Pulmonary complications predominate, accounting for more than 50% of the morbidity associated with anterior approaches to the thoracic and the thoracoabdominal spine.[4] Other reported complications include great-vessel injuries, retroperitoneal hematoma and fibrosis, ureteral injury, chylous-fluid leakage, and spinal-cord injury, to name but a few.[5] Added to this are isolated reports of unusual complications such as splenic injuries, empyema, bronchopleural fistula, chylothorax, and chyloperitoneum.[6–8] However, the incidence of major complications in surgery for spinal deformity is low, with death occurring in 0.3% of cases, paraplegia in 0.2%, and deep wound infection in 0.6%.[9]

Reported rates of morbidity for spine surgery in the adult population range from 18 to 86%.[3,10,11] Anderson and co-workers[12] have reported low rates of morbidity in their adult populations, citing nonidiopathic scoliosis, mental retardation, anterior spinal procedures, hypoxemia, and obstructive pulmonary disease as common denominators in the development of complications. In the pediatric population, morbidity from spinal procedures is reported to range from 10 to 74%.[13,14]

Idiopathic and acquired spinal deformity and congenital anomalies of the spine are the typical indications for spine surgery in the pediatric population. Degenerative disease of the discs, infections, trauma, degenerative deformities, and tumors are the typical indications for spinal surgery in adults.[10,15–21] The difference in pathology directly affects the surgical exposures for these two groups of patients. Pediatric patients typically require longer exposures to provide access to extensive deformities, whereas exposures in adults may be more focal. Naunheim et al[15] reported 4.5 vertebral segments exposed per patient and McElvein et al[10] reported ~5 vertebral segments exposed per patient in a mixed population of patients who were primarily adults with a mean age of 40 years. Janik and co-workers[22] reported 8.2 vertebrae exposed per patient in a primarily pediatric population. Patients with neuromuscular pathologies required slightly larger incisions, with an average exposure of 9.6 vertebral segments. In the adult population, from 21 to 26% of patients will require a thoracoabdominal approach with incision of the diaphragm.[4,10,12] In the pediatric population, from 58 to 82% of patients were found to require thoracoabdominal exposure.[22,23] Patients with syndromic conditions (e.g., neuromuscular disease, Ehlers–Danlos syndrome, etc.) often require longer incisions than are typical, even in the pediatric population. Series of both adult and pediatric patients typically record a higher incidence of complications for thoracic and thoracoabdominal approaches than for retroperitoneal or transperitoneal lumbar approaches.

Grossfeld and coworkers's review of 550 pediatric patients undergoing a total of 599 spinal procedures documents 45 major complications (**Table 22.1**) for a rate of major complications of 7.5%.[24] These complications included reintubation for pneumonia and respiratory distress, chylous effusion requiring chest tube drainage, paralysis, and death. Major complications were seen more often in patients older than 14 years of age (10.4%) than in those younger than 14 years (5.7%). Boys had a significantly higher complication rate of 11.7% than did girls, for whom the rate of complications was 4.7%. The combined effect of gender and age resulted in a greater complication rate of 15.5% among boys older than 14 years than among boys younger than 14 years, for whom the rate of complications was 8.1%. Girls had a complication rate of 5.3%. Major complications were more frequently seen in patients with kyphosis (16.3%) than in patients with scoliosis (4.2%). A major complication rate of 17.8% occurred in surgery for curves >100 degrees, as compared with complication rates of 6.8% and 5.2%, respectively, in surgery for moderate and small curves. Anterior-only procedures had a 9.7% major complication rate as compared with a 6.3% rate for combined anterior–posterior procedures and a rate of 7.3% for staged anterior–posterior procedures. Detachment of the diaphragm did not seem to increase the rate of major complications. However, as documented in other series, thoracotomy either alone or as part of a thoracoabdominal procedure is associated with a significantly higher rate of major complications of 8.2% versus 1.5% for anterior spinal surgery without thoracotomy. In both pediatric and adult populations, pre-existing

**Table 22.1 Major Complications Associated with Anterior Spinal Procedures**

| | % |
|---|---|
| Cardiac | 0.4 |
| Chylous effusion | 0.33 |
| Congestive heart failure | 0.17 |
| Cerebrovascular accident | 0.25 |
| Death | 0.33–8.2 |
| Deep wound infection | 1.17 |
| Gastroenterologic | 1.1 |
| Genitourinary | 0.4 |
| Hemothorax (requiring intubation) | 0.33 |
| Large intraoperative blood loss | 0.33 |
| Myocardial infarction | 0.17 |
| Paralysis | 0.33 |
| Perforated bowel | 0.50 |
| Pneumonia (requiring intubation) | 0.83 |
| Pneumothorax (requiring intubation) | 0.17 |
| Postoperative bleeding (requiring return to operating room) | 0.17 |
| Pulmonary | 4.9 |
| Pulmonary edema | 0.17 |
| Pulmonary embolism | 2.2 |
| Pulmonary hemorrhage | 0.17 |
| Respiratory distress (requiring intubation) | 2.00 |
| Respiratory distress syndrome (without intubation) | 0.33 |
| Sepsis | 0.17 |
| Ureteral laceration | 0.1 |

pulmonary disease increases the complication rate. Patients with pulmonary function of <40% of predicted values had a major complication rate of 14.8%, compared with 9% for patients with pulmonary function values of ≥40% of the predicted values.

Grossfeld and colleagues[24] also cited 193 minor complications in 145 surgical procedures for spinal deformity, or a rate of 32.6% (**Table 22.2**) Ileus, atelectasis, superior mesenteric artery syndrome, and pleural effusions were considered minor complications. Minor complications were more frequent in patients older than 14 years of age (41.7%) than in younger patients (26%). Gender did not significantly affect the rate of minor complications, with males (36%) and females (30.3%) having roughly equivalent rates. When age and gender were combined, boys older than 14 years typically had a higher rate of minor complications (49.1%) than

**Table 22.2 Minor Complications Associated with Anterior Spinal Procedures**

| Complications | % |
|---|---|
| Abdominal hernia | 1.18 |
| Arrhythmia | 0.33 |
| Atelectasis | 4.67 |
| Cardiac | 0.90 |
| Esophagitis | 0.33 |
| Genitourinary | 11.6 |
| Halo-pin infection | 0.33 |
| Hemothorax (without intubation or thoracotomy) | 0.17 |
| Horner syndrome | 0.17 |
| Ileus | 3.50 |
| Impotence | 0.8 |
| Intestinal ulcers/gastritis | 0.33 |
| Lumbar-plexus injury | 0.10 |
| Meralgia paresthetica | 1.67 |
| Neuropraxia | 0.54 |
| Parascapular pain | 1.00 |
| Pleural effusion | 2.67 |
| Pneumonia | 2.50 |
| Pneumothorax (without intubation or chest tube) | 2.17 |
| Postsympathectomy syndrome | 0.43 |
| Post-thoracotomy pain | 9.17 |
| Pressure sore or skin ulcer | 5.18 |
| Pulmonary | 2.2 |
| Retrograde ejaculation | 0.54 |
| Retroperitoneal lymphocele | 0.10 |
| SIADH | 1.50 |
| Superior mesentery artery syndrome | 0.83 |
| Thigh and knee pain | 0.33 |
| Thoracotomy | 2.7 |
| Thrombophlebitis | 0.9 |
| Transient ischemia of foot | 0.17 |
| Transient paresis | 0.50 |
| Urinary retention | 0.17 |
| Urinary tract infection | 0.67 |
| Vascular injury (requiring repair) | 15.6 |
| Wound infection (superficial) | 2.7 |

*Abbreviation:* SIADH, syndrome of inappropriate secretion of antidiuretic hormone did younger boys or girls in either group (23.6% and 36.8%, respectively). The rate of minor complications did not appear to be related to the type of spinal pathology, although patients with curves >100 degrees had higher minor-complication rates (45.2%) than did patients with curves of moderate size (34.7%) or small curves (27%). Minor complications were seen more often in patients with a marginal preoperative pulmonary vital capacity (59.2%) than in patients with a vital capacity >40% of the predicted value. Minor complications were seen more often in patients with staged anterior–posterior procedures (38%) than in combined anterior–posterior procedures (22%) or anterior procedures alone (33.9%). The minor-complication rate was not affected by thoracotomy or by detachment of the diaphragm.[24]

The theme that older patients experience more complications than younger ones is reinforced by Faciszewski and colleagues' study of 1152 adult patients[9] in which patients over the age of 60 years had a greater risk for complications, of 1.96 than for patients younger than 40 years. In Naunheim and coworkers' study,[15] patients under 39 years of age fared statistically better with fewer complications than did patients older than 60 years. Patients with more than two comorbidities have a higher risk of complications than do those with fewer than two comorbidities.[9] When cancer or osteomyelitis is the underlying pathology requiring surgery, there is a significantly greater risk of both operative morbidity (30%) and mortality (8.2%).[15,21] For patients undergoing a combined anterior–posterior procedure, the odds of complications occurring increase by a factor of 1.61 over that for patients undergoing a staged, anterior, or posterior procedure. Patients undergoing thoracotomy are at greater risk for having a complication by a factor of 1.6 over that for patients undergoing surgery via a retroperitoneal approach. Unlike Grossfeld et al's[24] review of a pediatric population undergoing spine surgery, Faciszewski et al's[9] review of an adult population suggests that the risk of a complication is greater for an adult female than for an adult male by a factor of 1.3.

McDonnell et al[25] reviewed 447 adolescent and adult patients undergoing anterior spinal surgery of the thoracic, thoracolumbar, and lumbar spine to determine the incidence of perioperative complications. Diagnostic groups included idiopathic, neuromuscular, and congenital scoliosis; kyphosis; fracture, trauma, or both; anterior revision surgery; tumor; vertebral osteomyelitis; and discitis. One hundred forty complications occurred in McDonnell and colleagues' 447 patients, for a complication rate of 31%. There were 60 major complications and 120 minor complications. The most common major complication was related to pulmonary function. The most common minor complication was genitourinary. Forty-seven patients (11%) had at least one major complication. At least one minor complication was identified in 109 patients (24%). Sixteen patients (4%) had both major and minor complications. Seven patients (2%) had more than one major complication and twelve patients (3%) had more than one minor complication. Two deaths occurred in this series of patients, resulting in a 0.4% mortality rate. Both deaths were the result of major postoperative pulmonary complications. There were no intraoperative deaths. Adolescents had the lowest complication rate (**Table 22.3**), And patients over 60 years of age had a higher risk of complications. Patients with neuromuscular scoliosis, tumor, and infection had the highest overall complication rates (**Table 22.4**).

In contrast to the findings in most other series, McDonnell and colleagues[25] report a higher complication rate for same-day combined anterior/posterior procedures than for staged procedures.[23,24,26] Also contrasting with the findings in other series was the lack of a statistical difference in the complication rate among patients undergoing thoracic, thoracolumbar, and lumbar anterior approaches. When patients were compared with respect to blood loss, no statistical difference in complication rate could be attributed to the loss of <500 mL, 500 to 1000 mL, 1000 to 1500 mL, or more than 1500 mL. However, if considered as a continuous variable, blood loss >520 mL was an important factor in predicting increasing complication rates. There was also a significant correlation between the amount of blood lost and the duration of surgery, but again there was no specific

**Table 22.3 Complications by Diagnosis**

| Diagnosis | Major (%) | Minor (%) |
|---|---|---|
| AIS | 3 | 14 |
| Congenital scoliosis | 8 | 31 |
| Adult scoliosis | 13 | 33 |
| Fracture | 13 | 21 |
| Revision procedure | 13 | 28 |
| Kyphosis | 18 | 16 |
| Neuromuscular scoliosis | 18 | 38 |
| Tumor | 21 | 16 |
| Osteomyelitis/ discitis | 38 | 50 |

**Table 22.4 Complications by Age Group**

| Age (Years) | Major (%) | Minor (%) |
|---|---|---|
| 3–20 | 9 | 20 |
| 21–40 | 6 | 21 |
| 41–60 | 14 | 27 |
| 61–85 | 32 | 44 |

*Abbreviation:* AIS, adolescent idiopathic scoliosis

correlation between the duration of surgery and increasing complication rate.[25]

The most comprehensive data for prospective complications of surgery for adolescent idiopathic scoliosis (AIS) comes from the Harms Study Group (HSG) database of 1800 patients. The "gold standard" data among these are prospective data, approved by institutional review boards, for consecutive patients. These data about complications are compiled cumulatively and inclusively in **Table 22.5**. The data are grouped according to complications associated with anterior and posterior spinal procedures in **Tables 22.6** and **22.7**, and are subdivided into major and minor complications in anterior

**Table 22.5 Total Complication Data in Surgery for Adolescent Idiopathic Scoliosis: Harms Study Group**

| Complication Type | Total Complications | Percent ($n = 1748$ Patients) | Anterior Complications | Percent ($n = 379$ Patients) | Posterior Complications | Percent ($n = 1369$ Patients) |
|---|---|---|---|---|---|---|
| **22.5A Total Complications** | | | | | | |
| Medical | 255 | 14.59% | 75 | 19.79% | 180 | 13.15% |
| Gastrointestinal | 69 | 3.95% | 23 | 6.07% | 46 | 3.36% |
| Pulmonary | 331 | 18.94% | 191 | 50.40% | 140 | 10.23% |
| Neurological | 120 | 6.86% | 47 | 12.40% | 73 | 5.33% |
| Instrumentation | 136 | 7.78% | 66 | 17.41% | 70 | 5.11% |
| Pseudarthrosis | 14 | 0.80% | 8 | 2.11% | 6 | 0.44% |
| Wound | 124 | 7.09% | 49 | 12.93% | 75 | 5.48% |
| Transfusion | 39 | 2.23% | 5 | 1.32% | 34 | 2.48% |
| **Total** | **1088** | **62.24%** | **464** | **122.43%** | **624** | **45.58%** |
| **22.5B Major Complications** | | | | | | |
| Medical | 5 | 0.29% | 1 | 0.26% | 4 | 0.29% |
| Gastrointestinal | 0 | 0.00% | 0 | 0.00% | 0 | 0.00% |
| Pulmonary | 12 | 0.69% | 1 | 0.26% | 11 | 0.80% |
| Neurological | 7 | 0.40% | 2 | 0.53% | 5 | 0.37% |
| Instrumentation | 34 | 1.95% | 12 | 3.17% | 22 | 1.61% |
| Pseudarthrosis | 14 | 0.80% | 8 | 2.11% | 6 | 0.44% |
| Wound | 20 | 1.14% | 3 | 0.79% | 17 | 1.24% |
| Transfusion | 0 | 0.00% | 0 | 0.00% | 0 | 0.00% |
| **Total** | **92** | **5.26%** | **27** | **7.12%** | **65** | **4.75%** |
| **22.5C Minor Complications** | | | | | | |
| Medical | 250 | 14.30% | 74 | 19.53% | 176 | 12.86% |
| Gastrointestinal | 69 | 3.95% | 23 | 6.07% | 46 | 3.36% |
| Pulmonary | 319 | 18.25% | 190 | 50.13% | 129 | 9.42% |
| Neurological | 113 | 6.46% | 45 | 11.87% | 68 | 4.97% |
| Instrumentation | 102 | 5.84% | 54 | 14.25% | 48 | 3.51% |
| Pseudarthrosis | 0 | 0.00% | 0 | 0.00% | 0 | 0.00% |
| Wound | 104 | 5.95% | 46 | 12.14% | 58 | 4.24% |
| Transfusion | 39 | 2.23% | 5 | 1.32% | 34 | 2.48% |
| **Total** | **996** | **56.98%** | **437** | **115.30%** | **559** | **40.83%** |

**Table 22.6 Total Complications Associated with Anterior Spinal Surgery in Patients with Adolescent Idiopathic Scoliosis***

| Medical complications | 75 | 19.79% |
|---|---|---|
| Back pain | 29 | 7.65% |
| Burn | 1 | 0.26% |
| Chest-wall pain | 9 | 2.37% |
| Costochondritis | 1 | 0.26% |
| Decreased blood pressure | | |
| DVT | 1 | 0.26% |
| Fever | 2 | 0.53% |
| Headaches | | |
| Low back pain | 9 | 2.37% |
| Muscle tenderness | | |
| Nausea | | |
| Nocturnal enuresis | 1 | 0.26% |
| Pain and stiffness | 3 | 0.79% |
| Pancreatis | | |
| Paraphimosis | | |
| Paraspinal pain | | |
| Residual levoscoliosis | | |
| Rib pain | 6 | 1.58% |
| Severe itching | | |
| Shoulder discomfort | 7 | 1.85% |
| Skin abrasions | | |
| Stress alopecia | | |
| Swelling | 1 | 0.26% |
| UTI | 2 | 0.53% |
| Visual changes | 1 | 0.26% |
| Vocal cord paresis | | |
| Yeast infection | | |
| Other | 2 | 0.53% |

| Gastrointestinal complications | 23 | 6.07% |
|---|---|---|
| Abdominal discomfort | 2 | 0.53% |
| Cholecystitis | | |
| Emesis | 3 | 0.79% |
| Gastroparesis | | |
| Gastrointestinal upset | 2 | 0.53% |
| Ileus | 5 | 1.32% |
| Pancreatitis | 1 | 0.26% |
| SMA syndrome | 4 | 1.06% |
| Vomiting | 6 | 1.58% |

| Instrumentation complications | 66 | 17.41% |
|---|---|---|
| Adding on | 10 | 2.64% |
| Broken rods | 13 | 3.43% |
| Broken screws | 4 | 1.06% |
| Crankshaft | | |
| Cross-link problem | | |
| Curve progression | 1 | 0.26% |
| Disengaged construct | 3 | 0.79% |
| Dislodged screw, hook, wire | 6 | 1.58% |
| Distal junctional kyphosis | | |
| Halo | 1 | 0.26% |
| Hook pullout | | |
| Increased lumbar lordosis | | |
| Low back pain | 1 | 0.26% |
| Lumbar curve progression | 1 | 0.26% |
| Misplaced screws | 1 | 0.26% |
| Perinstrument bursitis | | |
| Postoperative pain over prominent hardware | | |
| Progressive proximal kyphosis | 4 | 1.06% |
| Prominent hardware | 1 | 0.26% |
| Proximal junctional kyphosis | | |
| Screw impingement | | |
| Screw loosening | 5 | 1.32% |
| Screw pullout | 10 | 2.64% |
| Vertebral-body fracture | 3 | 0.79% |
| Other | 2 | 0.53% |

| Pseudarthosis | 8 | 2.11% |
|---|---|---|

| Wound problems | 49 | 12.93% |
|---|---|---|
| Abcess | 2 | 0.53% |
| Deep infection | | |
| Dehiscence | 9 | 2.37% |
| Dermatitis | 2 | 0.53% |
| Erythema, drainage | 6 | 1.58% |
| Hematoma | 1 | 0.26% |
| Hypertrophic scar | 11 | 2.90% |
| Keloid scar | 8 | 2.11% |
| Nevus excised | | |
| Pain | 3 | 0.79% |

**Table 22.6** *(Continued)* **Total Complications Associated with Anterior Spinal Surgery in Patients with Adolescent Idiopathic Scoliosis***

| **Wound problems** | **49** | **12.93%** |
|---|---|---|
| Other | | |
| **Pulmonary complications** | **191** | **50.40%** |
| Atelectasis | 81 | 21.37% |
| Chest-tube break | | |
| Insertion of test tube | | |
| Interstitial edema | | |
| Narcotic-related respiratory depression | | |
| PE | | |
| Pleural effusion | 66 | 17.41% |
| Pneumonia | 4 | 1.06% |
| Pneumothorax | 37 | 9.76% |
| Pulmonary edema | 3 | 0.79% |
| Respiratory failure | | |
| Other | | |
| **Neurological complications** | **47** | **12.40%** |
| Decreased tcMEP/SSEP | 1 | 0.26% |
| Dorsal/plantar foot paresthesia | | |
| Femoral cutaneous neuralgia | 4 | 1.06% |
| Foot drop | 1 | 0.26% |
| Hyperesthesia | | |
| Hypersensitivity | 4 | 1.06% |
| LLE weakness | | |
| Loss of sensation | 8 | 2.11% |
| Numbness | 18 | 4.75% |
| Pain | 2 | 0.53% |
| Paresthesia | 2 | 0.53% |
| Post-thoracotomy syndrome | 2 | 0.53% |
| Radiculopathy | 1 | 0.26% |
| SCI | | |
| Weakness | 4 | 1.06% |
| Other | | |
| Pleural tear | | |
| Seroma | | |
| Superficial infection | 2 | 0.53% |
| Swelling at incision | | |
| Unsightly scar | 1 | 0.26% |
| Wound infection | 1 | 0.26% |
| Other | 3 | 0.79% |
| **Transfusion** | **5** | **1.32%** |
| Reaction | | |
| Blood transfusion | 3 | 0.79% |
| Excessive blood loss | 2 | 0.53% |

*$n = 339$ patients

*Abbreviations:* DVT, deep-vein thrombosis; LLE, left lower extremity; PE, pulmonary embolism; SCI, spinal-cord ischemia; SMA, superior mesenteric artery; SSEP, somatosensory evoked potential; tcMEP, transcortical muscle evoked potential; UTI, urinary tract infection

(**Tables 22.8** and **22.9**) and posterior (**Tables 22.10** and **22.11**) spinal procedures for idiopathic scoliosis. Complications of instrumentation (3.17%) and pseudarthrosis (2.1%) were the most common major complications associated with anterior spinal surgery (**Table 22.8**). Pulmonary complications (50%) and complications associated with instrumentation (14.25%) were the most common minor complications (**Table 22.9**). For posterior procedures, instrumentation (1.61%) and wound complications (1.24%) were the most common major complications (**Table 22.11**). The most common minor complications associated with posterior procedures were medical (12.86%) and pulmonary (9.42%) (**Table 22.10**).

**Table 22.7 Total Complications Associated with Posterior Spinal Surgery in Patients with Adolescent Idiopathic Scoliosis***

| **Medical complications** | **180** | **13.15%** |
|---|---|---|
| Back pain | 59 | 4.31% |
| Burn | | |
| Chest-wall pain | 6 | 0.44% |
| Costochondritis | 1 | 0.07% |
| Decreased blood pressure | 4 | 0.29% |
| DVT | 1 | 0.07% |
| Fever | 1 | 0.07% |
| Headaches | 2 | 0.15% |
| Low back pain | 10 | 0.73% |
| Muscle tenderness | 1 | 0.07% |
| Nausea | 2 | 0.15% |
| Nocturnal enuresis | | |
| Pain and stiffness | 10 | 0.73% |
| Pancreatis | 1 | 0.07% |
| Paraphimosis | 1 | 0.07% |
| Paraspinal pain | 2 | 0.15% |
| Residual levoscoliosis | 1 | 0.07% |
| Rib pain | 10 | 0.73% |
| Severe itching | 1 | 0.07% |
| Shoulder discomfort | 19 | 1.39% |
| Skin abrasions | 1 | 0.07% |
| Stress alopecia | 1 | 0.07% |
| Swelling | 5 | 0.37% |
| UTI | 3 | 0.22% |
| Visual changes | 2 | 0.15% |
| Vocal cord paresis | 1 | 0.07% |
| Yeast infection | 1 | 0.07% |
| Other | 34 | 2.48% |
| **Gastrointestinal complications** | **46** | **3.36%** |
| Abdominal discomfort | 6 | 0.44% |
| Cholecystitis | 2 | 0.15% |
| Emesis | | |
| Gastroparesis | 1 | 0.07% |
| Gastrointestinal upset | 6 | 0.44% |
| Ileus | 18 | 1.31% |
| Pancreatitis | | |
| SMA syndrome | 7 | 0.51% |
| Vomiting | 6 | 0.44% |
| Other | | |

| **Instrumentation complications** | **70** | **5.11%** |
|---|---|---|
| Adding on | 7 | 0.51% |
| Broken rods | 3 | 0.22% |
| Broken screws | 1 | |
| Crankshaft | 1 | 0.07% |
| Cross-link problem | 1 | 0.07% |
| Curve progression | | |
| Disengaged construct | 6 | 0.44% |
| Dislodged screw, hook, wire | 4 | 0.29% |
| Distal junctional kyphosis | 5 | 0.37% |
| Halo | 3 | 0.22% |
| Hook pullout | 1 | 0.07% |
| Increased lumbar lordosis | 2 | 0.15% |
| Low back pain | 3 | 0.22% |
| Lumbar curve progression | 1 | 0.07% |
| Misplaced screws | 2 | 0.15% |
| Perinstrument bursitis | 1 | 0.07% |
| Postoperative pain over prominent hardware | 12 | 0.88% |
| Progressive proximal kyphosis | 1 | 0.07% |
| Prominent hardware | 3 | 0.22% |
| Proximal junctional kyphosis | 3 | 0.22% |
| Screw impingement | 3 | 0.22% |
| Screw loosening | 3 | 0.22% |
| Screw pullout | 2 | 0.15% |
| Vertebral-body fracture | | |
| Other | 2 | 0.15% |
| **Pseudarthosis** | **6** | **0.44%** |
| **Wound problems** | **75** | **5.48%** |
| Abcess | 2 | 0.15% |
| Deep infection | 6 | 0.44% |
| Dehiscence | 9 | 0.66% |
| Dermatitis | | |
| Erythema, drainage | 9 | 0.66% |
| Hematoma | 4 | 0.29% |
| Hypertrophic scar | 10 | 0.73% |
| Keloid scar | 3 | 0.22% |
| Nevus excised | 1 | 0.07% |
| Pain | 2 | 0.15% |
| Pleural tear | 1 | 0.07% |
| Seroma | 4 | 0.29% |

**Table 22.7** *(Continued)* **Total Complications Associated with Posterior Spinal Surgery in Patients with Adolescent Idiopathic Scoliosis***

| **Pulmonary complications** | **140** | **10.23%** |
|---|---|---|
| Atelectasis | 64 | 4.67% |
| Chest-tube break | 1 | 0.07% |
| Insertion of test tube | 1 | 0.07% |
| Interstitial edema | 1 | 0.07% |
| Narcotic-related respiratory depression | 1 | 0.07% |
| PE | 3 | 0.22% |
| Pleural effusion | 55 | 4.02% |
| Pneumonia | | |
| Pneumothorax | 1 | 0.07% |
| Pulmonary edema | 5 | 0.37% |
| Respiratory failure | 5 | 0.37% |
| Other | 3 | 0.22% |
| **Neurological complications** | **73** | **5.33%** |
| Decreased tcMEP/SSEP | 3 | 0.22% |
| Dorsal/plantar foot paresthesia | 1 | 0.07% |
| Femoral cutaneous neuralgia | 4 | 0.29% |
| Foot drop | | 0.00% |
| Hyperesthesia | 1 | 0.07% |
| Hypersensitivity | 3 | 0.22% |
| LLE weakness | 1 | 0.07% |
| Loss of sensation | 13 | 0.95% |
| Numbness | 28 | 2.05% |
| Pain | 5 | 0.37% |
| Paresthesia | 3 | 0.22% |
| Post-thoracotomy syndrome | | |
| Radiculopathy | 3 | 0.22% |
| SCI | 1 | 0.07% |
| Weakness | 1 | 0.07% |
| Other | 6 | 0.44% |
| Superficial infection | 11 | 0.80% |
| Swelling at incision | 3 | 0.22% |
| Unsightly scar | 5 | 0.37% |
| Wound infection | 3 | 0.22% |
| Other | 2 | 0.15% |
| **Transfusion-related complications** | **34** | **2.48%** |
| Reaction | 1 | 0.07% |
| Blood transfusion | 11 | 0.80% |
| Excessive blood loss | 22 | 1.61% |
| Other | | |

*$n = 1369$ patients

*Abbreviations:* DVT, deep-vein thrombosis; LLE, left lower extremity; PE, pulmonary embolism; SCI, spinal cord injury; SMA, superior mesenteric artery; SSEP; somatosensory evoked potential; tcMEP, transcortical muscle evoked potential; UTI, urinary tract infection

## Medical Complications

The incidence of perioperative medical complications following combined anterior and posterior procedures for the correction of spinal deformity has been as high as 70% in some series.[27] A lower incidence of complications is typically associated with purely posterior surgery for spinal deformity, owing to a diminished surgical insult. Medical complications may not be directly related to the operative technique used in spine surgery.

### Deep-vein Thrombosis and Pulmonary Embolism

Venous thrombosis and pulmonary embolism (PE) have been noted after spinal surgery. These are more typically identified in the adult population. Dearborn and co-workers[28] reported

**Table 22.8 Major Complications Associated with Anterior Spinal Surgery in Patients with Adolescent Idiopathic Scoliosis***

| | *n* | % | Reoperation | % |
|---|---|---|---|---|
| **Medical complications** | **1** | **0.26%** | | |
| Blindness | | | | |
| Death | | | | |
| MI | | | | |
| Pancreatis | | | | |
| Visual changes | 1 | 0.26% | | |
| Vocal-cord paresis | | | | |
| **Gastrointestinal complications** | **0** | **0.00%** | | |
| Toxic megacolon | | | | |
| **Pulmonary complications** | **1** | **0.26%** | | |
| ARDS | | | | |
| Chest-tube break | | | | |
| Insertion of test tube | | | | |
| PE | | | | |
| Pneumothorax | 1 | 0.26% | 1 | 0.26% |
| Respiratory failure | | | | |
| **Neurological complications** | **2** | **0.53%** | | |
| Brachial-plexus injury | | | | |
| Foot drop | 1 | 0.26% | | |
| Radiculopathy | 1 | 0.26% | 1 | 0.26% |
| SCI | | | | |
| Weakness | | | | |
| **Instrumentation complications** | **12** | **3.17%** | | |
| Adding on | 1 | 0.26% | 1 | 0.26% |
| Broken rods | 6 | 1.58% | 6 | 1.58% |
| Broken screws | 1 | 0.26% | 1 | 0.26% |
| Cross-link problem | | | | |
| Disengaged construct | 1 | 0.26% | 1 | 0.26% |
| Dislodged screw, hook, wire | 1 | 0.26% | 1 | 0.26% |
| Distal junctional kyphosis | | | | |
| Misplaced screws | | | | |
| Postoperative pain over prominent hardware | | | | |
| Prominent hardware | 1 | 0.26% | 1 | 0.26% |
| Proximal junctional kyphosis | | | | |
| Screw impingement | | | | |
| Screw loose | | | | |
| Screw pullout | 1 | | 1 | 0.26% |
| **Pseudarthosis** | **8** | **2.11%** | **5** | **1.32%** |

**Table 22.8** *(Continued)* **Major Complications Associated with Anterior Spinal Surgery in Patients with Adolescent Idiopathic Scoliosis***

| | *n* | % | Reoperation | % |
|---|---|---|---|---|
| **Wound problems** | **3** | **0.79%** | | |
| Deep infection | | | | |
| Dehiscence | 3 | 0.79% | 3 | 0.79% |
| Erythema, drainage | | | | |
| Hematoma | | | | |
| Seroma | | | | |
| Superficial infection | | | | |
| Wound infection | | | | |
| Total | 27 | 7.12% | 22 | 5.80% |

**n* = 379 patients

*Abbreviations:* ARDS, acute respiratory distress syndrome; MI, myocardial infarction; PE, pulmonary embolism; SCI, spinal-cord injury

**Table 22.9 Minor Complications Associated with Anterior Spinal Surgery in Patients with Adolescent Idiopathic Scoliosis***

| **Medical complications** | **74** | **19.53%** | **Instrumentation complications** | **54** | **14.25%** |
|---|---|---|---|---|---|
| Back pain | 29 | 7.65% | Adding on | 9 | 2.37% |
| Burn | 1 | 0.26% | Broken rods | 7 | 1.85% |
| Chest-wall pain | 9 | 2.37% | Broken screws | 3 | 0.79% |
| Coagulopathy | | | Crankshaft | | |
| Costochondritis | 1 | 0.26% | Cross-link problem | | |
| Decreased blood pressure | | | Curve progression | 1 | 0.26% |
| DVT | 1 | 0.26% | Disengaged construct | 2 | 0.53% |
| Fever | 2 | 0.53% | Dislodged screw, hook, wire | 5 | 1.32% |
| Headaches | | | Distal junctional kyphosis | | |
| Low back pain | 9 | 2.37% | Fretting/corrosion | | |
| Muscle tenderness | | | Halo | 1 | 0.26% |
| Nausea | | | Hook pullout | | |
| Nocturnal enuresis | 1 | 0.26% | Increased lumbar lordosis | | |
| Pain and stiffness | 3 | 0.79% | Loss of Correction | | |
| Paraphimosis | | | Low Back Pain | 1 | 0.26% |
| Paraspinal pain | | | Lumbar Curve Progression | 1 | 0.26% |
| Residual levoscoliosis | | | Misplaced screws | 1 | 0.26% |
| Rib pain | 6 | 1.58% | Perinstrument bursitis | | |
| Seizure | | | Postoperative pain over prominent hardware | | |
| Severe itching | | | Progressive proximal kyphosis | 4 | 1.06% |
| Shoulder discomfort | 7 | 1.85% | Prominent hardware | | |
| SIADH | | | Proximal junctional kyphosis | | |
| Skin abrasions | | | Screw impingement | | |
| Stress alopecia | | | Screw loosening | 5 | 1.32% |

*(Continued on page 294)*

**Table 22.9** (*Continued*) **Minor Complications Associated with Anterior Spinal Surgery in Patients with Adolescent Idiopathic Scoliosis***

| **Medical complications** | **74** | **19.53%** |
|---|---|---|
| Swelling | 1 | 0.26% |
| Ulcers | | |
| UTI | 2 | 0.53% |
| Yeast Infection | | |
| Other | 2 | 0.53% |
| **Gastrointestinal complications** | **23** | **6.07%** |
| Abdominal discomfort | 2 | 0.53% |
| Cholecystitis | | |
| Emesis | 3 | 0.79% |
| Gastroparesis | | |
| Gastrointestinal upset | 2 | 0.53% |
| Ileus | 5 | 1.32% |
| Pancreatitis | 1 | 0.26% |
| SMA syndrome | 4 | 1.06% |
| Vomiting | 6 | 1.58% |
| Other | | |
| **Pulmonary complications** | **190** | **50.13%** |
| Aspiration | | |
| Atelectasis | 81 | 21.37% |
| Hemothorax | | |
| Interstital edema | | |
| Narcotic-related respiratory depression | | |
| Pleural effusion | 66 | 17.41% |
| Pneumonia | 4 | 1.06% |
| Pneumothorax | 36 | 9.50% |
| Pulmonary edema | 3 | 0.79% |
| Other | | |
| **Neurological complications** | **45** | **11.87%** |
| Decreased tcMEP/SSEP | 1 | 0.26% |
| Dorsal/plantar foot paresthesia | | |
| Femoral cutaneous neuralgia | 4 | 1.06% |
| Hyperesthesia | | |
| Hypersensitivity | 4 | 1.06% |
| LLE weakness | | |
| Loss of sensation | 8 | 2.11% |
| Numbness | 18 | 4.75% |
| Pain | 2 | 0.53% |

| **Instrumentation complications** | **54** | **14.25%** |
|---|---|---|
| Screw pullout | 9 | 2.37% |
| Vertebral-body fracture | 3 | 0.79% |
| Other | 2 | 0.53% |
| **Wound problems** | **46** | **12.14%** |
| Abcess | 2 | 0.53% |
| Dehiscence | 6 | 1.58% |
| Dermatitis | 2 | 0.53% |
| Erythema, drainage | 6 | 1.58% |
| Hematoma | 1 | 0.26% |
| Hernia | | |
| Hypertrophic scar | 11 | 2.90% |
| Keloid scar | 8 | 2.11% |
| Nevus excised | | |
| Pain | 3 | 0.79% |
| Pleural tear | | |
| Seroma | | |
| Superficial infection | 2 | 0.53% |
| Swelling at incision | | |
| Unsightly scar | 1 | 0.26% |
| Wound infection | 1 | 0.26% |
| Other | 3 | 0.79% |
| **Transfusion-related complications** | **5** | **1.32%** |
| Aquired illness | | |
| Blood transfusion | 3 | 0.79% |
| Excessive blood loss | 2 | 0.53% |
| Reaction | | |
| Other | | |

**Table 22.9** *(Continued)* **Minor Complications Associated with Anterior Spinal Surgery in Patients with Adolescent Idiopathic Scoliosis***

| **Neurological complications** | **45** | **11.87%** |
|---|---|---|
| Paresthesia | 2 | 0.53% |
| Post-thoracotomy syndrome | 2 | 0.53% |
| Weakness | 4 | 1.06% |
| Other | | |

**n* = 379 patients

*Abbreviations:* DVT, deep-vein thrombosis; LLE, left lower extremity; PE, pulmonary embolism; SCI, spinal-cord injury; SIADH, syndrome of inappropriate secretion of antidiuretic hormone; SMA, superior mesenteric artery; tcMEP, transcortical muscle evoked potential; SSEP, somatosensory evoked potential; UTI, urinary tract infection

**Table 22.10 Minor Complications Associated with Posterior Spinal Surgery in Patients with Adolescent Idiopathic Scoliosis***

| **Medical complications** | **176** | **12.86%** |
|---|---|---|
| Back pain | 59 | 4.31% |
| Burn | | |
| Chest-wall pain | 6 | 0.44% |
| Coagulopathy | | |
| Costochondritis | 1 | 0.07% |
| Decreased blood pressure | 4 | 0.29% |
| DVT | 1 | 0.07% |
| Fever | 1 | 0.07% |
| Headaches | 2 | 0.15% |
| Low back pain | 10 | 0.73% |
| Muscle tenderness | 1 | 0.07% |
| Nausea | 2 | 0.15% |
| Nocturnal enuresis | | |
| Pain and stiffness | 10 | 0.73% |
| Paraphimosis | 1 | 0.07% |
| Paraspinal pain | 2 | 0.15% |
| Residual levoscoliosis | 1 | 0.07% |
| Rib pain | 10 | 0.73% |
| Seizure | | |
| Severe itching | 1 | 0.07% |
| Shoulder discomfort | 19 | 1.39% |
| SIADH | | |
| Skin abrasions | 1 | 0.07% |
| Stress alopecia | 1 | 0.07% |
| Swelling | 5 | 0.37% |
| Ulcers | | |
| UTI | 3 | 0.22% |
| Yeast infection | 1 | 0.07% |
| Other | 34 | 2.48% |

| **Instrumentation complications** | **48** | **3.51%** |
|---|---|---|
| Adding on | 7 | 0.51% |
| Broken rods | 1 | |
| Broken screws | | |
| Crankshaft | 1 | 0.07% |
| Cross-link problem | | |
| Curve progression | | |
| Disengaged construct | 3 | 0.22% |
| Dislodged screw, hook, wire | 2 | 0.15% |
| Distal junctional kyphosis | 3 | 0.22% |
| Fretting/corrosion | | |
| Halo | 3 | 0.22% |
| Hook pullout | 1 | 0.07% |
| Increased lumbar lordosis | 2 | 0.15% |
| Loss of correction | | |
| Low Back Pain | 3 | 0.22% |
| Lumbar curve progression | 1 | 0.07% |
| Misplaced screws | 1 | 0.07% |
| Perinstrument bursitis | 1 | 0.07% |
| Postoperative pain over prominent hardware | 8 | 0.58% |
| Progressive proximal kyphosis | 1 | 0.07% |
| Prominent hardware | | |
| Proximal junctional kyphosis | 2 | 0.15% |
| Screw impingement | 2 | 0.15% |
| Screw loosening | 2 | 0.15% |
| Screw pullout | 2 | 0.15% |
| Vertebral-body fracture | | |
| Other | 2 | 0.15% |

| **Wound problems** | **58** | **4.24%** |
|---|---|---|
| Abcess | 2 | 0.15% |

*(Continued on page 296)*

**Table 22.10** (*Continued*) **Minor Complications Associated with Posterior Spinal Surgery in Patients with Adolescent Idiopathic Scoliosis***

| | | |
|---|---|---|
| **Gastrointestinal complications** | **46** | **3.36%** |
| Abdominal discomfort | 6 | 0.44% |
| Cholecystitis | 2 | 0.15% |
| Emesis | | |
| Gastroparesis | 1 | 0.07% |
| Gastrointestinal upset | 6 | 0.44% |
| Ileus | 18 | 1.31% |
| Pancreatitis | | |
| SMA syndrome | 7 | 0.51% |
| Vomiting | 6 | 0.44% |
| Other | | |
| **Pulmonarycomplications** | **129** | **9.42%** |
| Aspiration | | |
| Atelectasis | 64 | 4.67% |
| Hemothorax | | |
| Interstital edema | 1 | 0.07% |
| Narcotic-related respiratory depression | 1 | 0.07% |
| Pleural effusion | 55 | 4.02% |
| Pneumonia | | |
| Pneumothorax | | |
| Pulmonary edema | 5 | 0.37% |
| Other | 3 | 0.22% |
| **Neurological complications** | **68** | **4.97%** |
| Decreased tcMEP/SSEP | 3 | 0.22% |
| Dorsal/plantar foot paresthesia | 1 | 0.07% |
| Femoral cutaneous neuralgia | 4 | 0.29% |
| Hyperesthesia | 1 | 0.07% |
| Hypersensitivity | 3 | 0.22% |
| LLE weakness | 1 | 0.07% |
| Loss of sensation | 13 | 0.95% |
| Numbness | 28 | 2.05% |
| Pain | 5 | 0.37% |
| Paresthesia | 3 | 0.22% |
| Post-thoracotomy syndrome | | |
| Weakness | | |
| Other | 6 | 0.44% |
| Dehiscence | 6 | 0.44% |
| Dermatitis | | |
| Erythema, drainage | 7 | 0.51% |
| Hematoma | 2 | 0.15% |
| Hernia | | |
| Hypertrophic scar | 10 | 0.73% |
| Keloid scar | 3 | 0.22% |
| Nevus excised | 1 | 0.07% |
| Pain | 2 | 0.15% |
| Pleural tear | 1 | 0.07% |
| Seroma | 3 | 0.22% |
| Superficial infection | 10 | 0.73% |
| Swelling at incision | 3 | 0.22% |
| Unsightly scar | 5 | 0.37% |
| Wound infection | 1 | 0.07% |
| Other | 2 | 0.15% |
| **Transfusion-related complications** | **34** | **2.48%** |
| Acquired illness | | |
| Blood transfusion | 11 | 0.80% |
| Excessive blood loss | 22 | 1.61% |
| Reaction | 1 | 0.07% |
| Other | | |

*$n$ = 1369 patients

*Abbreviations:* DVT, deep-vein thrombosis; LLE, left lower extremity; PE, pulmonary embolism; SCI, spinal-cord injury; SIADH, syndrome of inappropriate secretion of antidiuretic hormone; SMA, superior mesenteric artery; tcMEP, transcortical muscle evoked potential; SSEP, somatosensory evoked potential; UTI, urinary tract infection

**Table 22.11 Major Complications Associated with Posterior Spinal Surgery in Patients with Adolescent Idiopathic Scoliosis***

| | *n* | % | Re-Op | % |
|---|---|---|---|---|
| **Medical complications** | **4** | **0.29%** | | |
| Blindness | | | | |
| Death | | | | |
| MI | | | | |
| Pancreatis | 1 | 0.07% | | |
| Visual changes | 2 | 0.15% | | |
| Vocal-cord paresis | 1 | 0.07% | | |
| Gastrointestinal complications | 0 | 0.00% | | |
| Toxic megacolon | | | | |
| **Pulmonary complications** | **11** | **0.80%** | | |
| ARDS | | | | |
| Chest-tube break | 1 | 0.07% | 1 | 0.07% |
| Insertion of test tube | 1 | 0.07% | 1 | 0.07% |
| PE | 3 | 0.22% | 1 | 0.07% |
| Pneumothorax | 1 | 0.07% | 1 | 0.07% |
| Respiratory Failure | 5 | 0.37% | | |
| **Neurologic complications** | **5** | **0.37%** | | |
| Brachial-plexus injury | | | | |
| Foot drop | | | | |
| Radiculopathy | 3 | 0.22% | 1 | 0.07% |
| SCI | 1 | 0.07% | | |
| Weakness | 1 | 0.07% | 1 | 0.07% |
| **Instrumentation complications** | **22** | **1.61%** | | |
| Adding on | | | | |
| Broken rods | 2 | 0.15% | 2 | 0.15% |
| Broken screws | 1 | | 1 | 0.07% |
| Cross-link problem | 1 | 0.07% | 1 | 0.07% |
| Disengaged construct | 3 | 0.22% | 3 | 0.22% |
| Dislodged screw, hook, wire | 2 | 0.15% | 2 | 0.15% |
| Distal junctional kyphosis | 2 | 0.15% | 2 | 0.15% |
| Misplaced screws | 1 | 0.07% | 1 | 0.07% |
| Postoperative pain over prominent hardware | 4 | 0.29% | 4 | 0.29% |
| Prominent hardware | 3 | 0.22% | 3 | 0.22% |
| Proximal junctional kyphosis | 1 | 0.07% | 1 | 0.07% |
| Screw impingement | 1 | 0.07% | 1 | 0.07% |
| Screw loosening | 1 | 0.07% | 1 | 0.07% |
| Screw pullout | | | | |
| Pseudarthosis | 6 | 0.44% | 5 | 0.37% |

(*Continued on page 298*)

**Table 22.11** *(Continued)* **Major Complications Associated with Posterior Spinal Surgery in Patients with Adolescent Idiopathic Scoliosis***

| | *n* | % | Re-Op | % |
|---|---|---|---|---|
| **Instrumentation complications** | **22** | **1.61%** | | |
| Wound problems | 17 | 1.24% | | |
| Deep Infection | 6 | 0.44% | 6 | 0.44% |
| Dehiscence | 3 | 0.22% | 3 | 0.22% |
| Erythema, drainage | 2 | 0.15% | 2 | 0.15% |
| Hematoma | 2 | 0.15% | 2 | 0.15% |
| Seroma | 1 | 0.07% | 1 | 0.07% |
| Superficial infection | 1 | 0.07% | 1 | 0.07% |
| Wound infection | 2 | 0.15% | 2 | 0.15% |
| Total | 65 | 4.75% | 50 | 3.65% |

*$n = 1369$ patients

*Abbreviations:* DVT, deep-vein thrombosis; LLE, left lower extremity; PE, pulmonary embolism; SCI, spinal-cord injury; SIADH, syndrome of inappropriate secretion of antidiuretic hormone; SMA, superior mesenteric artery; tcMEP, transcortical muscle evoked potential; SSEP, somatosensory evoked potential; UTI, urinary tract infection

on thromboembolic complications in 116 adult patients undergoing major reconstructive spine surgery who were investigated with duplex ultrasound and lung perfusion scans. One patient was identified with an asymptomatic iliac thrombosis and seven patients had symptomatic PEs. Six of these embolisms occurred after combined anterior–posterior surgeries. Smith et al[29] reported a prospective study involving 317 patients undergoing anterior thoracoabdominal surgery in which 126 patients were investigated with Doppler ultrasound so as not to miss clinically asymptomatic thromboembolism. All of the ultrasound tests for embolism were negative, yet despite this, one patient in the tested group developed a deep-vein thrombosis (DVT), which was successfully treated. A fatal PE occurred in one of the untested patients. The incidence of thromboembolism was 0.9%. Smith and colleagues concluded that because of the low incidence of clinically significant thromboembolism, intensive prophylactic screening was unwarranted in anterior thoracoabdominal surgery. Faciszewski and co-workers[9] identified 10 patients (0.8%) with PE, of whom 2 patients ultimately died. The remaining eight patients were treated with anticoagulation, with one patient experiencing a cerebrovascular accident (CVA) secondary to the treatment. Seven patients had no long-term sequelae. The authors reported one fatal PE in a patient who was completely asymptomatic for 18 days after surgery. On the morning of her discharge from rehabilitation therapy, the patient succumbed to a massive PE without warning.

Although there is considerable emphasis on the prevention of perioperative DVT, limiting the occurence of PE should be the objective of any preventive intervention in spine surgery. In a study that followed 116 patients prospectively for subclinical DVTs and 318 patients retrospectively for symptomatic thromboembolism after major thoracolumbar spine surgery, patients who had purely posterior surgery had a 0.5% incidence of PE, as compared with an incidence of 6% among patients who had anterior and posterior fusion.[28] Another study, of 317 patients undergoing major reconstructive surgery of the spine, included 77 patients undergoing corrections of scoliosis.[29] None of the scoliosis patients experienced thromboembolic events, and the overall incidence of PE was 0.3%. Another study did report a 14% incidence of DVT, but this study included a large proportion of patients with spinal cord injuries.[30] Pneumatic compression devices and thrombosis-deterrent stockings should be used routinely for patients undergoing spine surgery.[31] We do not recommend routine chemical prophylaxis for patients undergoing purely posterior surgery.

## Renal Complications

Urinary tract infections (UTIs) are the most common postoperative medical complications after surgery for scoliosis in adults.[27] Although such UTIs are typically benign, mortality from these infections is three times greater among patients with bacteriuria.[32] The Foley catheter is the common culprit, and efforts should be made to remove this as soon as possible.

Acute renal failure is relatively uncommon in patients having spine surgery. The typical etiology is hypovolemia or hypotension resulting in prerenal failure. If untreated, prerenal failure may progress to acute tubular necrosis, an intrarenal disorder. One medical cause of perioperative hypotension is the continuation of angiotensin converting enzyme inhibitors, which may blunt the renin–angiotensin system.[33]

### Ureteral Complications

The ureters are located to the left of the aorta and to the right of the vena cava, respectively, and are adherent to the posterior peritoneum. They are typically mobilized with the peritoneal sac during an anterior retroperitoneal approach unless the approach is complicated by inflammatory disease, tumor, morbid obesity, or previous retroperitoneal surgery.[34,35] During revision surgery for spinal deformities the ureters may be found embedded in scar tissue between the psoas and the great vessels. Ureteral injury may occur during urgent repair of an injured major vessel.

In Faciszewski and colleagues' study, one patient in 1223 procedures sustained a ureteral laceration. This patient was undergoing anterior revision surgery for repair of a pseudarthrosis. Intraoperative repair of the ureter did not result in any long-term sequel for the patient.[9]

### Cardiac Complications

Cardiac complications among patients undergoing deformity surgery are not well characterized in the literature. A study of 46 patients over the age of 60 years who were undergoing spinal-deformity surgery, of whom half had solely posterior procedures, reported myocardial infarction in one patient.[36] In this study, patients over the age of 69 years had nine times as many major complications as did those under the age of 69. However, patients undergoing pedicle subtraction osteotomy had a 7-fold greater frequency of at least one major complication than did those not undergoing this procedure. In contrast to other studies, this study also reported that postoperative complications were unrelated to preoperative comorbidities. Another study, of 149 patients over 60 years of age who were undergoing various surgical procedures on the thoracolumbar spine, including 48 procedures for deformity, reported 3 cases of myocardial infarction.[37] Faciszewski and co-workers[9] reported cardiac arrests in 4 of 1152 patients (0.3%), with only 1 patient successfully resuscitated. Three of the 1152 patients (0.3%) suffered CVAs. The authors did not encounter either of these complications in conjunction with anterior spinal surgery.

Perioperative arrhythmias occur in 0.6 to 0.9% of patients having surgery for a spinal deformity, although the higher rate of 0.9% was reported for anterior procedures.[25,37] Patients with cardiac complications must be closely monitored in the intensive care unit. Those with infarction from coronary artery disease must be treated appropriately with antiplatelet therapy, anticoagulation, or even thrombolytic therapy regardless of the potential for complications of such treatment.

### Vision Loss

Postoperative loss of vision, although not affecting global cerebral function, is another central nervous system complication with a predilection for spine surgery. Its incidence ranges from 0.02 to 0.2%.[38] Prone positioning, particularly in the Trendelenburg position, has been noted to increase intraocular pressure, which is hypothesized to be a risk factor for postoperative loss of vision as the result of decreased perfusion of the optic nerve.[39] A retrospective review of 37 cases of postoperative vision loss identified surgery on patients in the prone position, long operative times, and large intraoperative blood loss as potential risk factors for this complication. Most of the patients who experienced loss of vision manifested their deficit within 2 days after surgery. Most of the deficits were permanent.

## ■ Gastrointestinal Complications

Perioperative gastrointestinal complications include ileus, superior mesenteric artery (SMA) syndrome, pancreatitis, and cholecystitis. Ileus is a common finding after spine surgery, occurring in 5 to 12% of all patients.[40] One etiology for such ileus may be stretching of the posterior peritoneal innervation during deformity correction, causing a reactive ileus.[41] Patients who experience gastrointestinal complications of spine surgery are often elderly, immobile, and taking large quantities of narcotics for postoperative pain. Grossfeld et al[24] reported a 3.5% incidence of ileus, and Rajaraman and colleagues[42] reported three patients (5%) who developed persistent ileus, which prolonged their postoperative hospitalization by an additional 7 days. Prokinetic agents have recently been introduced to help with this group of patients, but we believe that these agents are of unproven benefit and may be harmful.[43] Ileus is treated with bowel rest, intravenous hydration, and correction of any electrolyte deficiencies.

SMA syndrome occurs when the third part of the duodenum becomes compressed between the SMA and the aorta, and is often associated with scoliosis surgery.[44] It may occur after reduction of a spinal deformity or manipulation of the peritoneal contents. An incidence of SMA syndrome of 1.5% reported in Janik and colleagues' study is consistent with that in other series. The clinical symptoms of SMA syndrome following spine surgery include prolonged ileus or the development of bilious vomiting. Patients should be treated with nasogastric decompression, alimentation via feeding tubes or intravenous hyperalimentation. In Janik and colleagues' series, all patients recovered from SMA syndrome and none required surgical intervention.[22] In the elderly, Ogilvie syndrome may be more difficult to treat, but nonoperative regimens for its treatment are typically successful.

A retrospective review of 2939 charts yielded a 0.5% incidence of SMA syndrome with an average onset of 7.2 days postoperatively.[45] Another study reported a 1.1% incidence following scoliosis surgery with an average onset of 5 days postoperatively.[46] A case–control study of 364 patients with a 4.7% incidence of SMA syndrome identified risk factors for the syndrome as short stature, low body mass index, more lumbar lateralization, and a lower percent correction of the thoracic curve on bending.[47] SMA syndrome can be distinguished from ileus through the presence of bowel sounds[48] and the characteristic appearance of the syndrome in an upper gastrointestinal barium series. The syndrome is typically treated with suction through a nasogastric tube and either parenteral or nasojejunal nutrition. Pancreatitis and cholecystitis have also been noted after surgery for spinal deformity.[41,49]

### Bowel Complications

Intraoperative bowel perforation has been reported in a few patients undergoing surgical correction of spinal deformities.[24,42] If perforation of the bowel is identified intraoperatively, immediate repair is required. If significant contamination occurs, fusion and instrumentation should be abandoned. Missed bowel perforations can be fatal.[24]

During surgery via a retroperitoneal approach, it is not uncommon to create a rent in the peritoneum. Immediate repair with resorbable suture is ideal but often impractical. After such a tear, intraperitoneal air may appear on postoperative radiographs and cause undue concern. Complications from unrepaired peritoneal defects have not been reported.

## Pulmonary Complications

Overall, pulmonary problems represent the most common potentially life-threatening perioperative medical complications of spine surgery.[27] Pulmonary complications of such surgery span a range from well-tolerated events detectable only on radiographs, such as small pleural effusions, to potentially life-threatening conditions such as acute respiratory distress syndrome (ARDS). Pulmonary pathology is the most commonly reported postoperative complication of anterior spine surgery (**Table 22.5**). Atelectasis (4.8%) and respiratory distress (2%) are also commonly reported.[24] Janik et al[22] reported complications occurring in 51 patients (9.8%) undergoing anterior spine surgery. More than 50% of the morbidity from these complications was related to respiratory complications including effusion, pneumothorax, atelectasis, and excessive chest-tube drainage. Karol and co-workers[50] reported sudden intraoperative hemodynamic collapse in six patients with myelomeningocele who were undergoing spine surgery in the lateral decubitus position. Severe acute respiratory impairment of the dependent lung has been postulated as one of the possible etiologies of pulmonary complications following spine surgery. Almond et al[23] reported 65 complications in 29 of 39 adolescent patients. Forty-five of the complications were pulmonary or respiratory. They included atelectasis ($n = 15$), pneumothorax ($n = 10$), effusion ($n = 8$), pneumonia ($n = 5$), bronchopleural fistula ($n = 3$), respiratory failure ($n = 2$), asthma ($n = 1$), and laryngospasm ($n = 1$).

### Pneumothorax

Tension pneumothorax in the contralateral lung is an infrequently reported intraoperative complication. We are aware of two such cases, of which the exact etiology is unclear. It is possible that the pneumothorax in these cases came from high airway pressures that caused the rupture of a bleb in the contralateral lung. The clinical symptoms were decreasing blood pressure and oxygen saturation. Both patients were successfully treated by placement of a chest tube.

In Faciszewski and colleagues' study, 12 patients (1.8%) required reinsertion of a chest tube to evacuate a pneumothorax that formed during removal of an original chest tube.[9] An additional 20 patients (3%) required reinsertion of a chest tube or thoracentesis to drain a persistent pleural effusion. Chest tubes themselves may induce a sympathetic effusion. Clinical symptoms suggestive of both pneumothorax and pleural effusion are dyspnea and tachypnea. Retained hemothorax is typically not a problem with the use of a chest tube. Hsieh et al[51] report an unusual case of a symptomatic hemothorax on the contralateral side from laceration of the diaphragm by an excessively long T11 vertebral body screw. The patient required a right-sided thoracotomy for drainage of the resulting hematoma, repair of the diaphragmatic laceration, and trimming of the screw.

### Pneumonia

Pneumonia acquired in the postoperative period is typically a nosocomial infection. The clinical symptoms are fever and sputum production. Chest auscultation is abnormal, and there is evidence of leukocytosis, and of infiltrates on chest radiographs. The incidence of pneumonia following surgery for spinal deformity ranges from 1.0 to 2.2%.[36,52] This can be minimized with smoking cessation for 8 to 10 weeks preoperatively. Aggressive postoperative pulmonary toilet, incentive spirometry, early sitting, and early ambulation are also effective at decreasing pneumonia after spine surgery. Keeping patients in the supine position for prolonged periods significantly reduces functional residual capacity and may contribute to pneumonia.[53]

### Respiratory Failure

Acute pulmonary injury leading to postoperative respiratory failure is hypothesized to result from various events including blood-transfusion reactions and microembolism of fat and surgical debris. Noncardiogenic pulmonary edema caused by blood transfusion, with resultant acute hypoxemia is known as transfusion-related acute lung injury (TRALI),[54] and is the most frequent cause of death following blood transfusion.[55] Diagnosis of TRALI requires that its signs and symptoms begin within 6 hours after a blood transfusion. Treatment is supportive. ARDS is an infrequent complication following deformity surgery, but can result in mortality in >30% of cases.[56]

### Predicting Pulmonary Complications

Zhang and coworkers evaluated the role of preoperative pulmonary function tests (PFTs) in predicting postoperative pulmonary complications in 298 patients undergoing correction of spinal deformities.[52] Preoperative respiratory symptoms were predictive of abnormal PFT values but not of postoperative pulmonary complications. Abnormal PFT values did not correlate significantly with pulmonary complications. Zhang and colleagues found that transthoracic procedures produce 18 times as many pulmonary complications as purely posterior spine surgery.

## Neurological Complications

Short of perioperative mortality, spinal-cord injury during surgery for spinal deformity is one of the most feared of its complications by both patients and surgeons.[57,58] Significant progress in the technology of intraoperative neurophysiological monitoring has given the surgeon real-time feedback about the neurological effects of their intraoperative actions. This allows the surgeon to take corrective action more quickly and thus minimize the potential for permanent neurological injury. Neurological injury may occur at any level of the neuraxis including the spinal cord, conus medullaris, cauda equina, and nerve roots. A severe cord-level injury may cause either tetraplegia or paraplegia, depending on the location of the injury, and may portend a poor prognosis similar to that in traumatic spinal-cord injury.[59] Injury to the cauda equina may cause saddle anesthesia, bowel and bladder dysfunction, and weakness of the lower extremities. Nerve-root injuries are less morbid and have a better prognosis for recovery. Correction of deformity in the thoracic spine, such as kyphosis, carries a potential for greater morbidity with respect to neurological injury than does surgery on other regions of the spine.

### Delirium and Stroke

Central nervous system embarrassments following spinal surgery are more common among elderly patients. Delirium is a depressed state of mental function with a fluctuating course. One study of 341 patients undergoing a variety of procedures on the spine including decompression alone included 104 patients over 70 years old. Delirium occurred in this population with an incidence of 12.5%.[60] Another risk factor for delirium in this study were low values of hemoglobin and hematocrit on postoperative day 1. In this study delirium resolved in all but one patient, who had persistent cognitive dysfunction. The incidence of perioperative CVAs in surgery for spinal deformity is not well quantified. In a study of 1223 anterior procedures for spinal deformity, the incidence of stroke was 0.25%.[9]

### Spinal Cord

The incidence of perioperative neurological injury in surgery for spinal deformity is related to the nature of the deformity. Among patients undergoing spinal fusion for AIS, the incidence of neurological injury was found to be relatively low, at 0.32 to 0.69%.[61,62] This is comparable to the incidence of such injury reported more than 30 years ago.[63] The incidence of neurological injury increases in surgery for other deformities. The incidence of spinal-cord injury in spinal fusion for Scheuermann's kyphosis is 1.8%.[64] Neurological deficit following corrective fusion for congenital scoliosis with a Cobb angle >90 degrees was reported in one study to occur in 7.23% of patients.[65] This same study identified congenital scoliosis, scoliosis with hyperkyphosis, scoliosis with a Cobb angle >90 degrees, revision surgery, and combined anterior and posterior procedures as risk factors for postoperative neurological deficit.[65] In contrast, a retrospective review of 40 pediatric patients under the age of 8 years who had either congenital kyphosis or scoliosis and underwent a variety of corrective instrumented fusions revealed no instances of postoperative neurological injury.[66]

Surgical treatment of spinal dysraphism, such as diastematomyelia and syringomyelia, is accompanied by an increased risk of neurological injury during deformity correction.[67,68]

In a retrospective review of nine patients with diastematomyelia and two patients with syringomyelia with a tethered spinal cord who underwent posterior surgery for spinal deformity, two patients (18%) had neurological injury.[69] One of these patients had a transient worsening of monoplegia following the simultaneous excision of a bone spur from diastematomyelia and correction of a spinal deformity. The other patient, who had undergone previous excision of an osseous T11 diastematomyelia, sustained transient paraplegia when pedicle screws in T2 of his spine migrated into the spinal canal during correction of a deformity. Despite the high incidence of neurological injury in this study, other studies reported no neurological injuries after instrumented fusion among patients with syringomyelia.[66]

Aside from being influenced by the nature of an underlying spinal deformity, the incidence of neurological injury in the surgical correction of deformities also depends on the specific type of corrective procedure being used. A retrospective review of 108 consecutive lumbar pedicle subtraction osteotomies revealed an 11.1% incidence of postoperative neurological deficit manifested as either motor or bowel/bladder dysfunction; the incidence of permanent deficit was 2.8%.[70] A retrospective review of 25 consecutive posterior-vertebral column resections in the lower lumbar spine revealed 2 patients (8%) with transient motor weakness of toe and ankle dorsiflexion that resolved by 6 months postoperatively.[71] Another retrospective review, of 407 surgical procedures for spinal deformities in adults, revealed an overall incidence of lumbar nerve-root palsy of 2.9%, which increased to 7.4% among patients who underwent fusion of more than 10 vertebral levels.[72] The incidence of such palsy was lower, at 1.3%, in the subset of patients who underwent purely posterior surgery. Overall, single anterior or posterior approaches to fusion result in similar rates of neurological injury; combined anterior and posterior fusion results in an increased rate of neurological injury.[73]

The underlying mechanism of neurological injury in the surgical correction of spinal deformity can include mechanical trauma, stretching or compression of neurological structures, or vascular ischemia.[74] Iatrogenic injury from inadvertent misplacement of hardware is discussed in the section on spinal instrumentation. Stretching of the spinal cord may result from distraction following instrumentation. Mechanical compression of the spinal cord or cauda equina may follow the correction of a deformity as the result of protrusion of an intervertebral disc, formation of an epidural hematoma, or infolding of the ligamentum flavum, dura mater, or posterior longitudinal ligament. Vascular insult resulting from ischemic injury to the spinal cord is more commonly reported during anterior spinal exposures with ligation of the segmental arteries and in vascular surgical procedures than in other types of procedures.[75–77]

Intraoperative hypotension induces spinal-cord ischemia in animal studies.[74] However, there is no definitive clinical series in which controlled hypotension has induced spinal-cord injury. The literature does carry case reports of high-cervical-cord infarction resulting in tetraplegia following posterior spine surgery.[78,79]

Even when the spinal cord is not exposed, it is at risk for injury during the reduction of deformities and during the ligation of segmental vessels, which can precipitate an ischemic event in the spinal cord. Decreased blood flow in the anterior spinal artery can result in infarction of a significant portion of the spinal cord. Cadaveric investigations suggest that the anterior spinal artery typically appears to be a continuous structure. However, because of the wide range of its luminal size, functional discontinuities may occur in blood flow through this vessel.[80] Because of the variations in its diameter (0.23 to 0.94 mm), variability in resistance to blood flow through the anterior spiunal artery is likely. Variations in luminal diameter may result in a resistance to flow of as great as 278 times normal in vessels with narrow lumens. This in turn may result in regions of functionally decreased blood flow to the spinal-cord blood.[80] Patients experiencing ischemic events in the spinal cord after aortic surgery typically have predisposing risk factors for this, such as hypertension, diabetes mellitus, atherosclerosis, chronic obstructive pulmonary disease, or a history of CVAs.[81] These underlying risk factors may also predispose patients undergoing spine surgery to ischemic events in the spinal cord. Disruption of blood flow in the artery of Adamkiewicz has often been implicated in such events.

Three major neurological patterns can emerge during an ischemic event originating in the anterior spinal-cord artery: (1) Transient ischemic attacks in the spinal cord, manifested by transient motor deficits and sphincter dysfunction, which resolve without neurological deficit; (2) reversible spinal-cord ischemia with significant neurological symptoms that resolve slowly, leaving minor residual neurological deficits; and (3) complete spinal-cord injury with flaccid paralysis and complete sphincter dysfunction.[81]

The distribution of abnormalities in magnetic resonance imaging (MRI) signals seems to correlate with the severity of spinal-cord injury. Increased signal intensity limited to the anterior horn of the gray matter is often seen in injuries of type 1 and type 2 in which there is some preservation of motor function and a better clinical outcome. Patients with type 3 injury have more diffuse involvement including the anterior horns, central gray, and posterior gray matter of the cord, and typically have complete and irreversible neurological deficits.[81]

Spinal-cord injury resulting from either a vascular or an embolic event in the cervical spine above the level of surgical intervention has been reported in two cases of surgery for thoracic deformity (AIS, $n = 1$; neuromuscular scoliosis, $n = 1$).[82] In the patient with AIS the cord insult was focal and resulted in a Brown–Sequard-like syndrome that resolved over several weeks. In the patient with neuromuscular scoliosis the insult was massive. Changes in the patient's MRI scan were noted within the entire cervical cord and were associated with complete loss of motor and sensory function in all four extremities. Minimal return of sensory function occurred in the upper extremities. Useful motor function did not return in either the upper or lower extremities. A case report of transient hemiplegia following posterior instrumentation for idiopathic scoliosis has also been reported. In this patient it was felt that engorgement of an arteriovenous fistula was the cause of the hemiplegia.[83]

Most neurological injuries in the surgical correction of spinal deformity manifest in the immediate perioperative period. Insults from mechanical events related to the correction of a deformity usually have immediate effects, although deficits presenting up to 2 days postoperatively have been reported, particularly with the correction of kyphosis or severe scoliosis.[84,85] Vascular etiologies also may have a varied course of presentation. Acute, spinal-cord ischemia following anterior ligation of segmental arteries may be detected immediately through neurophysiological monitoring,[75,86] although this is a subject of debate.[87] Less commonly, formation of an epidural hematoma several days or up to 9 days postoperatively may create sufficient compression of the cord to cause a neural deficit.[88] Neurological deficit of late onset after instrumentation is even rarer and has only occasionally been reported such as in the case of an L2 laminar hook causing cauda equina syndrome 10 years after surgery.[89] In fact, this may represent a case of stenosis from junctional degeneration.

Historically, the Stagnara wake-up test has been the gold standard for the intraoperative detection of neural injury.[90] Although effective, it is cumbersome, causing a significant delay between the inciting event and performance of the test. This may delay corrective action. Moreover, the sensitivity of the test to weakness is questionable, because the level of sedation often limits the examination to the observation only of gross motion. Also, sensory-tract dysfunction is difficult to evaluate with the test, and young children may not appropriately follow the test commands. The ankle clonus test also has been described as a means of evaluating neurological function during spine surgery for scoliosis.[91] In current practice, neurophysiological monitoring is used during spine surgery because it is highly sensitive and has the ability to detect injury concurrent with the inducing event.[92] Neurophysiological monitoring in surgery for spinal deformity may include monitoring of somatosensory evoked potentials (SSEPs), neurogenic mixed evoked-potentials (NMEPs), transcranial electrical motor-evoked potentials (tcMEPs), and electromyography.[92] Successful intraoperative neurophysiological monitoring in spinal-deformity surgery requires total intravenous anesthesia because electrophysiological monitoring is sensitive to inhalational anesthesia.

In a retrospective study of 500 patients who underwent combined intraoperative monitoring of tcMEPs and SSEPs, the sensitivity of the monitoring was 98.6% and the specificity was 100%.[93] In this study the false-positive rate of significant signal change without postoperative neurological deficit was 0.014%, and there were no false-negative results.

The tcMEP is an important component of neurophysiological monitoring because it is a measure of anterior motor-tract function, whereas the SSEP is a measure of afferent function in the posterior column.[94] In a review of 1121 patients with AIS who underwent corrective surgery with SSEP and MEP monitoring, 38 patients had significant intraoperative signal changes.[94] Of these 38 patients, 45% (17) had a significant decrease only in tcMEP amplitude, with normal SSEP signals. Moreover, when the amplitudes of both tcMEPs and SSEPs were abnormal, the onset of the decrease in SSEP amplitude lagged behind that of the tcMEP amplitude by an average of 5 minutes.

It is important for the surgeon to assess changes in the data provided by neurophysiological monitoring. The disappearance of an initially present tcMEP, for example, represents a highly significant finding that requires corrective action. On the other hand, if the tcMEP was either absent or misinterpreted as being present before a surgical procedure was begun, its absence later on may not be significant.

When a neurological deficit is identified, corrective action must be undertaken immediately to minimize the potential for permanent injury. Corrective action begins with medical management and may subsequently include surgical intervention.

The stability of the spine at the time of detection of a neurological deficit will influence the appropriate surgical treatment. In a relatively stable spine, such as one treated with posterior instrumention and fusion for idiopathic scoliosis without destabilizing osteotomies, complete removal of the instrumentation is a viable option. The surgeon may then return at a later time to reapply the instrumentation for internal fixation. On the other hand, an unstable spine, such as one that has had a vertebral-column resection, will not tolerate the complete removal of instrumentation. In this circumstance, removal of the instrumentation may exacerbate a neurological injury by allowing hypermobility of the spine.

Medical management of a neurological deficit identified intraoperatively begins with a series of corrective actions.[92] First, the patients mean arterial blood pressure (MABP) should be elevated to ≥90 mmHg together with the administration of an increased concentration of inspired oxygen. Concurrently, the patient's surgical wound may be irrigated with warm saline in an effort to increase perfusion. Second, the patient's arterial blood gases should be assayed to detect an unrecognized low hemoglobin concentration or other metabolic abnormality. If a deficit remains despite these corrective actions, initiation of high-dose methylprednisolone in accord with the protocol for its use in acute spinal-cord injury (30 mg/kg given over a period of 45 minutes, followed by a continuous infusion of 5.4 mg/kg/hour for 24 hours) may be warranted. This has not been studied in the setting of corrective surgery for spinal deformity.

Failing appropriate medical action for an intraoperative neurological deficit, the spinal deformity should be recreated either completely or in part by releasing the instrumentation for correcting it. If this does not reverse the deficit, the surgeon must assess the relative stability of the spine. In a relatively stable situation, all hardware should be removed, including screws, hooks, and wires. In an unstable situation, the hardware should not be completely removed.

Appropriate intraoperative action may prevent permanent neurological injury. In a retrospective review, all of 9 pediatric patients who experienced complete loss of NMEPs during the correction of kyphosis had a return of NMEPs with normal results of postoperative neurological examination.[95] In this study, one patient improved through blood-pressure elevation alone, one patient required further decompression alone, six patients required some sort of adjustment or release of the instrumentation for correction of their deformities, and one patient required placement of an anterior interbody strut to restore the height of the anterior column.

Neurological dysfunction presenting in the postoperative period requires emergent identification of the causative factor. This includes appropriate diagnostic imaging and medical management.

The medical management of neurological dysfunction presenting postoperatively is similar in concept to the intraoperative management described above. As noted, hypoperfusion from hypotension or a low hemoglobin concentration must be identified and corrected. High-dose methylprednisolone infusion may also be indicated as well, but steroid-treatment protocols for spinal-cord injury have not been studied in this setting. In a case report of monoplegia that developed 2 days after the correction of kyphosis, there was complete recovery with medical management alone, including the intravenous administration of fluids, vasopressors, and methylprednisolone.[84]

In the postoperative setting, diagnostic imaging of the spine is imperative for identifying a surgically correctable etiology for a neurological deficit. Although MRI is a useful noninvasive preoperative modality, the presence of significant metallic instrumentation along much of the area of interest limits the utility of this procedure in the immediate postoperative period. Instead, emergent myelography with computed tomography (CT) is the preferred method for evaluating compression of the neural axis. The presence of a significant stenosis may require emergent osseous decompression or modification of the instrumentation for deformity correction according to the principles of stability discussed above. In a case report of paraparesis that presented 30 hours after correction of a scoliosis, the patient had complete neurological recovery with decompression and removal of the corrective instrumentation.[85]

Dural buckling resulting in neurological deficit after acute correction of a spinal deformity is another known complication that may manifest in the postoperative period.[96] In our experience and as reflected in the literature, duraplasty with untethering of any associated arachnoid adhesions is an effective treatment for such buckling, resulting in improvement of neural function.[96]

## Superior and Inferior Hypogastric Plexus

A clear distinction must be made between sterility and impotence. Sterility implies the inability of a male to deliver an adequate number of spermatozoa to impregnate a female. This may be the consequence of retrograde ejaculation,[97] and this does not imply impotence. The autonomic nerve supply (superior hypogastric plexus) to the internal vesicular sphincters lies in the retroperitoneal space anterior to the vertebral bodies of L4, L5, S1. These nerves may be injured during a retroperitoneal dissection.[98] Retrograde ejaculation has also been reported in patients undergoing retroperitoneal dissection for the placement of aortic grafts.[99] Dissection in the retroperitoneal space over the sacral promontory is the common factor in these surgeries. Rough handling of soft tissue and electrocautery have been implicated in the problem of retrograde ejaculation. Gentle, blunt dissection, using only bipolar cautery for hemostasis, seems to prevent this problem. Retrograde ejaculation may be more common after bilateral sympathectomies.

A review of 4500 anterior lumbosacral spinal surgeries, the experience of 20 surgeons worldwide,[100] suggests that sterility (retrograde ejaculation) is seen in 0.42% of all cases (19/4500) and impotence is seen in 0.44% (20/4500). Retrograde ejaculation resolved in 25% of the patients and normal function ultimately returned without any intervention. Impotence was felt to be nonorganic. Corroborating Flynn's findings in the 1990s, Faciszewski et al[9] reported retrograde ejaculation in only 2 of 371 males undergoing retroperitoneal dissection for an anterior approach to the lumbar spine (0.5%). In the same population, three patients (0.8%) reported impotence.[9] Humphries et al[99] reported a 10% incidence of retrograde ejaculation in patients undergoing retroperitoneal dissections for the placement of aortic grafts. In one-third of these patients normal ejaculation returned over a period of 2 to 3 years without any specific intervention. This suggests that alternate paths are either available or develop to re-establish ejaculatory function. In a transperitoneal approach, entering the retroperitoneal space on the right side may be of some benefit because the superior hypogastric plexus tends to be more left-sided. Because the superior hypogastric plexus is typically elevated with the peritoneum and great vessels during a retroperitoneal dissection, the side on which an approach is made may be less important in this instance.

True impotence is not caused by anterior spinal surgery. The inferior hypogastric plexus is responsible for the parasympathetic input that regulates blood flow into the penis, which controls erection (i.e., potency). This plexus is located deep within the pelvis. The fibers emanating from the anterior sacral foramen below S1 are outside of the surgical field of dissection. For this reason, it is highly unlikely that impotence could be caused either by a retroperitoneal or a transperitoneal approach to L5/S1 or higher.[100] Impotence following the surgical correction of a spinal deformity is typically transitory, and most authors feel that it is not physiologically related to the reproductive system. It is more likely psychological in origin. Time and psychotherapy or both generally resolve the problem.[101]

### Injury to the Brachial Plexus

Injury to the brachial plexus is uncommon in anterior approaches to the spine. However, compressive injury may result from positioning of the patient if an axillary roll is not used. Faciszewski et al.[9] reported that 2 of 1152 patients undergoing anterior spinal fusion had partial brachial plexus neurapraxias. These resolved within several days. A further two patients had partial ulnar-nerve or brachial-plexus neurapraxias that resolved within several months. All of these cases of injury to the brachial plexus were felt to have resulted from patient positioning.[9] We have reported transient ulnar-nerve and brachial-plexus neurapraxias in adolescent idiopathic scoliosis resulting from the positioning of patients with AIS.[102] Occasionally such neurapraxias will be detected with electrophysiological monitoring. If they are detected intraoperatively, repositioning of the patient's upper extremities often reverses the electrical abnormality. However, even when such neurapraxias were undetected intraoperatively, all of the postoperative deficits resolved within several months.[102]

### Injury to the Sympathetic Chain

A standard retroperitoneal approach to the spine exposes the ipsilateral sympathetic chain. It is worth trying to avoid injury to this structure. However, it is often difficult to move this part of the spinal cord out of the field of dissection. This is especially true in patients who have had previous retroperitoneal dissections and in those with significant scoliotic deformities and lumbar spondylosis with large anterior osteophytes. Even if spared early in the dissection, the sympathetic chain ipsilateral to the side of surgery is often damaged by continued manipulation during the course of discectomy and fusion, especially when lateral annular releases are required to achieve reduction of the deformity. The practical consequences of disruption of this neurologic structure are usually limited to increased blood flow in the ipsilateral lower extremity. This is typically experienced by patients and caregivers as increased warmth in the ipsilateral lower extremity, or is mistakenly interpreted as coolness, possibly from an arterial thrombotic event, in the contralateral lower extremity. Rajaraman and co-workers[42] report 6 of 60 patients as having had sympathetic dysfunction including temperature variation, dysesthesia, skin discoloration, and swelling of the ipsilateral foot without DVT after retroperitoneal approaches to surgery for scoliosis. Most of these symptoms dissipated within 3 to 4 months. However, one patient continued to have persistent swelling and discoloration of the foot at 6 months. One patient had a persistent burning dysesthesia that was not disabling, and another had similar symptoms in the thigh. Prolonged sympathetic symptoms are unusual in surgery for spinal deformity, but may be a significant management problem if persistent.[103]

An unusual complication of high thoracotomies (fourth rib) for approach to T1 and T2 is injury to the stellate ganglion of the sympathetic chain resulting in Horner syndrome. Faciszewski et al reported 3 such cases in a group of 42 high thoracotomies (7%). The resulting unilateral ptosis, anhidrosis, and myosis did not resolve.[9]

## Injury from Instrumentation

Despite the continuous evolution of the design of posterior spinal instrumentation, hardware failure persists in surgery for spinal deformity. Spinal instrumentation may fail acutely following implantation, or in a delayed fashion. Although one typically envisions broken rods and screws in the discussion of instrumentation failure, the iatrogenic malpositioning of hardware is also considered a mode of failure in surgery to correct spinal deformity.

### Implant Material

Posterior spinal instrumentation is typically manufactured from titanium (Ti) alloy or stainless steel (SS). In an in vitro cyclic loading test of posterior spinal instrumentation made of Ti and SS, the fatigue life of the instrumentation was not related to the implant material.[104] As expected, implants made of SS were stiffer than their Ti counterparts. Another cyclic loading test revealed that although SS and Ti implants had similar ultimate static strengths, Ti was sensitive to load frequency.[105] In this study, Ti implants had endurance limits similar to those of SS implants when loaded at 16 Hz. However, Ti implants performed better when loaded at 4 Hz. Implants made of Ti are also less ferromagnetic than their SS counterparts, and show less distortion on MRI scanning.[106] Implant material is thought to influence the risk of surgical site infection. Plates made of Ti were shown to be associated with a significantly lower incidence of surgical-site infection than plates made of SS in a rabbit model of bacterial inoculation.[107] Limited data in human in vivo studies have not shown a statistically significant difference in infection rates with the use of Ti versus SS.[108] Moreover, no clinical studies of this topic have been done in relation to spine implants.

In general, systemic complications from increased metal ion concentrations are a concern following the implantation of metal hardware in the body. A retrospective study of 30 patients at a mean of 26 months after the implantation of spinal instrumentation made of Ti showed significantly increased serum Ti levels as compared with those in control patients who had no metal implants.[109] Although there was wide variability in the serum Ti concentration among the study subjects, patients with a greater number of pedicle screws tended to have higher serum Ti concentrations, although not significantly so. The consequences of these findings remain unclear.

## Early Failure

Acute failures of instrumentation in surgery for the correction of spinal deformity may result from breakage or malpositioning of the hardware itself or from underlying patient comorbidity. Osteoporosis is one such comorbidity, and may result in loss of implant fixation.[110] In a biomechanical comparison of pedicle screw, laminar hook, and spinous-process wiring in osteoporotic cadaveric spines, the laminar hook had the greatest pullout strength.[61] In contrast to the other fixation methods, the strength of laminar-hook fixation also did not depend on the bone mineral density. Many biomechanical studies have evaluated the efficacy of polymethylmethacrylate (PMMA) cement for augmenting the anchoring of pedicle screws; one such study reported a doubling of the pullout strength of such screws in osteoporotic bone with cement augmentation.[111] A clinical evaluation of 291 pedicle screws augmented with PMMA cement in 41 patients with osteoporosis revealed satisfactory outcomes and no instances of symptomatic extravasations of cement.[112]

Patients with poor bone stock may also experience acute junctional failures. In a retrospective study of 47 multilevel fusions for adult spinal deformities among patients over the age of 65 years, there were three compression fractures of the last instrumented cephalad vertebrae and two compression fractures of the vertebra adjacent to the last instrumented vertebra.[113] This mode of failure is uncommon in pediatric and young adult patients. The fractures occurred in the early postoperative period with three additional compression fractures presenting more than 3 months after surgery.

There is a paucity of published information on implant breakage and disengagement in the period immediately following posterior surgical procedures for spinal deformity. In our personal experience we have encountered disengagement at the rod–screw interface. The usual location of such failure is at the ends of long constructs, such as the most cephalad or caudal fixation points.

Implant malpositioning may also be considered a complication. Pedicle-screw placement in the lumbar spine is generally recognized as a safe method of internal fixation. One report of 20 patients undergoing lumbar pedicle-screw placement noted no acute complications attributable to the pedicle screws.[114] In contrast, an earlier study based on responses to questionnaires revealed a 5.2% rate of screw misplacement and 2.3% rate of permanent nerve root injury.[115]

Medial breach of the pedicle wall by a screw does not necessarily cause neurological injury. In the thoracic spine, a computer-aided modeling study revealed that up to 4 mm of intrusion into the medial canal by a pedicle screw may have no neurological sequelae.[116]

The use of pedicle-screw fixation in the thoracic spine has become increasingly popular. A retrospective study of 112 thoracic pedicle screws identified placement in the concavity of the deformity and in levels at or above T8 as risk factors for misplacement.[117] A retrospective review of 1035 thoracic pedicle screws, evaluated by postoperative CT scans only if plain radiographs revealed questionable pedicle screw placement, revealed 18 (1.7%) misplaced screws in 13 patients. Only one screw caused a symptomatic problem, from pleural effusion.[118] In this study, intraoperative pedicle fracture occurred in 15 patients, in 3 of whom it occurred at the time of rod rotation. The remaining pedicle fractures resulted from repeated attempts at screw placement. An earlier study of thoracic pedicle-screw placement revealed a 3% incidence of asymptomatically malpositioned screws.[119] In contrast to these studies, a prospective CT scan evaluation of 120 thoracic pedicle screws placed for idiopathic scoliosis revealed an overall penetration rate into the pedicle cortex, anterior vertebral body, or both of 25%.[120] The rate of penetration into the medial pedicle wall was 8.3%. As in the other studies, however, there were no neurological complications from these malpositioned screws.

In 60 pediatric patients with spinal deformities, a postoperative CT scan study of 1023 pedicle screws placed by freehand technique revealed significant mediolateral pedicle-wall violations in 10.5% of the screws.[121] There was a statistically higher rate of pedicle-wall violations in patients with kyphosis other than those with scoliosis. Importantly, none of the patients with malpositioned screws exhibited neurological, vascular, or visceral complications. An earlier study of 759 pedicle screws placed in pediatric thoracic and lumbar spines revealed a 0.8% clinical complication rate attributable to screw placement.[122] Subjects in this study did not undergo routine postoperative CT scans.

Pedicle-screw placement may be more difficult in revision surgery for spinal deformities than in initial surgery, because of obliteration of the usual anatomical landmarks. A retrospective study of 308 pedicle screws placed by freehand technique into areas of prior posterior fusion surgery revealed 9 malpositioned screws upon radiographic evaluation and 4 malpositioned screws upon triggered electromyographic evaluation.[123] No patient experienced neurological deficit from pedicle-screw placement.

Intraoperative neurophysiological monitoring is a useful aid in determining safe pedicle-screw positioning. A prospective study of 512 lumbar pedicle screws that were subjected to intraoperative electrodiagnostic screw stimulation through triggered electromyographic (EMG) monitoring along with postoperative CT scanning revealed safe screw positioning with 98% confidence when the screw-stimulation threshold was >15 mA.[124] In this study, pedicle exploration was recommended if the threshold for screw stimulation was between 10 and 15 mA. A more recent study of 4857 lumbar pedicle screws tested with triggered EMG found a specificity of 94% and sensitivity of 86% in detecting medial pedicle-wall breaching at 8.0 mA.[125] The study investigators therefore recommended a stimulation threshold of >8.0 mA for determining the presence of an intact pedicle. In our practice, we use 8.0 mA as the threshold for pedicle exploration. In cases in which the probed path of a pedicle screw stimulates the nerve root at a low threshold, but in which the probed path feels intact, direct stimulation of the superior facet joint of the inferior vertebra can serve as a "control baseline" for nerve-root stimulation. If in this case the direct facet EMG is similar to the pedicle EMG, the threhold for pedicle-screw stimulation probably represents a safe value.

Intraoperative fluoroscopy is often used to aid in accurate pedicle-screw placement.[126,127] Nonetheless, a low rate of pedicle-screw malpositioning in the cervical, thoracic, and lumbar spine has been reported without the use of intraoperative fluoroscopy.[128]

The use of computer-aided navigation in pedicle-screw placement is gaining popularity. A meta-analysis of pedicle-screw placement found a 95.2% overall median accuracy of placement with the use of navigation, as compared with a 90.3% accuracy without its use.[129] However, in the thoracic spine, the accuracy of pedicle-screw placement was equivalent for screws placed with and without navigation.

Sublaminar wires are another form of segmental fixation of instrumentation for correcting spinal deformities. Despite their deliberate penetration into the spinal canal, such wires have been shown to be safe. A study of 1366 sublaminar wires placed throughout the thoracic and lumbar spine did not find any permanent neurological deficits.[130] In this study, two patients undergoing revision surgery experienced leg dysesthesia that resolved within 2 weeks postoperatively. Luque reported that 7 of 78 patients undergoing segmental instrumentation for the correction of scoliosis experienced paresthesias, which also resolved within 2 weeks postoperatively.[131] Nonetheless, there are reports in the literature of spinal-cord injury rates of 0.8% to 3.5% with the use of sublaminar wires.[130] Therefore, others have explored the option of using transverse-process wiring.[132]

## Late Failure

Late failures of instrumentation for correcting spinal deformities may also occur. In a retrospective study of long fusions, the most common clinical presentation of nonunion was broken hardware. In a series of 16 patients with scoliosis from poliomyelitis who underwent posterior segmental instrumentation *without* fusion,[133] all but 1 of the patients had failure of the hardware within 3 years. Six of the patients had rod breakage, 4 patients had the L-rod cut out of the pelvis, and 5 patients had longitudinal rod migration.

Mechanically, the moment of inertia for a cylindrical rod is proportional to the fourth power of its radius. Therefore, the use of a slightly larger diameter rod, such as a rod of 6.35-mm versus 5.5-mm diameter, results in an exponentially stiffer construct that may better resist hardware breakage.

Aside from hardware breakage, the metal hardware used in a construct for correcting spinal deformity may undergo fretting and corrosion, resulting in areas of sterile inflammation. An ultrastructural analysis of tissue surrounding spinal instrumentation removed for late pain at the site of its surgical placement revealed abundant particular debris, especially around the connections between rods and transverse rod connectors.[134] A light- and electron-microscope analysis revealed wear in 75% and corrosion in 39% of the retrieved posterior instrumentation.[135] No implants made of Ti exhibited corrosion. Rods from long SS constructs had more wear and corrosion than did those from short SS constructs. A cell-culture study showed decreased osteoblast proliferation with exposure to electromagnetic fields such as those generated by corroding spinal hardware.[136] The investigators in the latter study concluded that osteoblast inhibition from corroding hardware may contribute to periprosthetic osteolysis.

There are case reports of delayed vascular injury from malpositioned pedicle screws. A case report and literature review identified a total of 10 patients with delayed aortic perforation caused by pedicle screws.[137] The report noted that even without perforation at the time of initial surgery, a prominent pedicle screw tip may eventually erode through a vessel wall.

Long instrumented fusions present problems with junctional segment failure and nonunion at the lumbosacral junction. A retrospective study of 47 patients undergoing posterior fusion for degenerative lumbar scoliosis, with an average of 3.8 years of follow-up, revealed 15 instances of degeneration of adjacent segments, with 10 occurring proximally and 5 distally.[138] This study included only symptomatic junctional failures. Proximal-segment failures included four spinal stenoses, three compression fractures, two junctional kyphoses, and one lateral translation. Distal-segment failures included two spinal stenoses, two junctional kyphoses, and one herniated intervertebral disc. Of the 24 patients who underwent fixation to the sacrum, 2 experienced nonunion at the lumbosacral junction. Neither of these two patients received inter-vertebral-body support at the lumbosacral junction.

A retrospective study of 54 patients undergoing long fusions to the sacrum (from at least T11 to the sacrum) reported results with three different sacral-fixation techniques including the Luque–Galveston technique, sacral screw fixation, and combined sacral and iliac screw fixation.[139] All 54 patients underwent anterior interbody fusion at the L5-to-S1 level. The incidence of nonunion at the lumbosacral junction was 36% in patients who underwent Luque–Galveston fixation and 11% in patients who underwent sacral and iliac screw fixation. Surprisingly, no patients with sacral screw fixation alone had nonunion. The investigators who conducted the study did note that sacral screw fixation alone is successful only with restoration of satisfactory sagittal alignment. A biomechanical comparison of multiple fixation techniques across the lumbosacral junction revealed that iliac fixation decreases the strain on the S1 screw by 70%.[140]

### Symptomatic Effects of Spinal Hardware

Posterior spinal instrumentation may become symptomatic for several reasons. Some authors have called this "late operative site pain."[141] One etiology of such pain is prominence of a construct component over an area with little muscle or fat coverage, as in the case of iliac screws placed in the posterior superior iliac spine. In one study, 15.2% of patients with posterior lumbosacral instrumentation underwent removal of painful hardware.[139] Eighty-nine percent of these patients had iliac screw fixation. Another etiology may be inflammation caused by metal-implant corrosion, although this may be difficult to differentiate from subacute infection.[134,141]

The removal of painful hardware leads to concern that correction of a deformity may be lost even without nonunion. This may affect sagittal and coronal correction.[142,143]

In a prospective analysis of 43 pediatric patients who underwent removal of posterior spinal instrumentation either because of painful hardware or infection, 56% of the patients had an increase in thoracic kyphosis of >10 degrees at an average of 9.5 years after implant removal.[142] Coronal-plane alignment was better maintained. Only 7% of the patients experienced an increase in scoliosis of >10 degrees. In this study, greater thoracic kyphosis before the initial fusion procedure and greater lumbar scoliosis before implant removal were risk factors for an increase of >20 degrees in thoracic kyphosis after implant removal. A retrospective study of adult patients undergoing symptomatic hardware removal also showed loss of sagittal alignment.[143] In contrast, another retrospective study found no significant change in sagittal curvature after hardware removal in patients with AIS.[144] This study did find a small loss of coronal correction, termed a *settling effect*, especially in patients who underwent hardware removal within 2 years after fusion surgery.

Although not a reasonable option in patients undergoing removal of painful hardware, re-instrumentation following hardware removal minimizes the loss of correction of a deformity. A retrospective review of patients undergoing removal of infected posterior spinal instrumentation found a significantly smaller loss of correction when re-instrumentation was done immediately or within 1.5 years.[145] Immediate re-instrumentation with Ti implants during irrigation and debridement for instrumentation-related spinal infections is becoming more common. The successful eradication of infection with this technique, and protection from a recurrence of deformity, makes it a promising technique.

## Pseudarthrosis

The failure of healing of spinal fusions has been described for nearly as long as techniques for fusion have existed.[146] Although the terms *nonunion* and *pseudarthrosis* are colloquially used interchangeably for such failure, they have distinct definitions. Nonunion of a spinal fusion is defined as failure of the fusion to heal by 1 year after surgery.[147] It may also be defined as failure of the fusion to heal without further intervention. Pseudarthrosis refers to significant motion and the development of a synovial membrane lining at a site of nonunion.

### Incidence

The true incidence of nonunion may be difficult to determine because some cases of nonunion are asymptomatic, which leads to underdiagnosis of this problem.[147] Moreover, many studies use different criteria in diagnosing nonunion. The incidence of nonunion also depends on the type of bone graft used and whether bone morphogenetic protein (BMP) is used.[148] Nonetheless, the reported incidence of nonunion in posterior spinal deformity surgery ranges from 1 to 15% following lumbar fusion in posterior surgery for spinal deformities,[148] and to as high as 83% in long thoracolumbar fusions to the sacrum.[149]

A lower incidence of nonunion following posterior spinal fusion occurs in children than in their adult counterparts. In the population with AIS, rates of nonunion range from nil to 7.3% with the use of allograft bone.[150–152]

Among pediatric patients with congenital abnormalities of the spine, such as hemivertebrae, bars, and kyphosis, the incidence of nonunion remains low. In a retrospective review of 107 pediatric spinal fusions for congenital spinal deformity, 2 of 49 patients (4%) undergoing purely posterior surgery experienced nonunion.[153] This occurred despite the use of freeze-dried corticocancellous allograft chips. One shortcoming of these studies is their limited follow-up period.[150–153]

Adults tend to have a higher overall incidence of nonunion following spine fusion. A retrospective review of 144 fusions to the sacrum (average patient age: 52 years) included 16 purely posterior fusions.[149] There were 5 nonunions within this posterior-only group, or a rate of nonunion of 31%. In contrast, the rate of nonunion in the 128 anterior and posterior fusions to the sacrum was 23%. In this study, patients with nonunion had significantly lower functional outcome scores on the Scoliosis Research Society (SRS)-24 instrument. In another study, of 46 patients over the age of 60 years and undergoing correction of spinal deformities, nonunion led to a reoperation rate of 19.5%. In this study, one-half of the patients had undergone purely posterior surgery.

Smaller case series of posterior spinal surgery for specific deformities report lower incidences of nonunion. A series of 17 patients who underwent Ponte osteotomies for Scheuermann's kyphosis had no instances of nonunion.[154] A series of 16 patients treated with transpedicular decancellation osteotomies for post-tuberculous kyphosis also had no instances of nonunion.[155]

## Diagnostic Criteria

Various criteria exist for the diagnosis of nonunion. They typically include loss of correction of a deformity, failure of instrumentation, or radiographic evidence of nonunion.[152] One such criterion suggests that a 10-degree loss of correction of a deformity implies the presence of a nonunion.[152,156]

Ten degrees is considered to be a meaningful change in the Cobb-angle measurement when taking into account the inter- and intraobserver reliability of the Cobb-angle method.[152] Another criterion is loss of fixation, including implant breakage, dislodgement, or haloes around pedicle screws.[149] The current procedural gold standard for ascertaining fusion is surgical exploration of the fusion mass to determine satisfactory union and stability.

Heggeness and Esses described a classification system for lumbar nonunion.[157] This system categorizes such nonunion into the four categories of atrophic, transverse, shingle, and complex. Atrophic nonunions exhibit bone-graft resorption and are associated with stress shielding from spinal instrumentation. Transverse nonunions typically occur in uninstrumented fusions and are seen as transverse discontinuities within the fusion mass. A shingle nonunion is an oblique discontinuity within the fusion mass. Complex nonunions occur in the presence of more than one adjacent nonunion site in the fusion mass.

## Diagnostic Imaging

Many imaging modalities exist for diagnosing nonunion of spinal fusion. Simple, plain radiographs provide useful information. Static plain radiographs may reveal lack of bone-graft consolidation, instrumentation failure, and loss of deformity correction. Dynamic plain radiographs may reveal areas of excessive motion. Various thresholds of angular motion exist for diagnosing nonunion. The U. S. Food and Drug Administration uses 4 degrees of motion in the lumbar spine to define failed fusion.[158] Others have used 10 degrees of angular motion as the threshold.[159]

Nuclear imaging studies, such as three-phase technetium-99m bone scans, show the vascularity and osteoblastic activity of fusion sites. Persistent activity beyond the expected period of healing may indicate nonunion. However, nuclear imaging studies lack sufficient specificity for the routine detection of nonunion.[160]

Conventional tomography is now an infrequently performed study. Historically, radiolucency at a fusion site, seen with anteroposterior (AP) tomographic imaging, has correlated well with the presence of nonunion upon surgical exploration.[161]

CT scanning is more readily available to the clinician for evaluating spinal fusion. The coronal view in CT imaging, like the AP plane in conventional tomography, is useful in identifying sites of nonunion. Metallic instrumentation can generate artifacts that may interfere with accurate imaging of the surrounding fusion mass. The use of 3D surface reconstruction has been reported to improve the detection of spinal nonunion.[162,163]

## Time to Clinical Presentation

With improvements in metallurgy and implant design resulting in stronger instrumentation, the time to clinical presentation of nonunions has increased. In a review of 40 cases of nonunion among 232 long fusions done with modern segmental instrumentation, the average time to presentation of nonunion was 3.5 years.[164] In 23% of the cases of nonunion, implant failure was detected 5 to 10 years postoperatively. The most common site of nonunion in this study was the thoracolumbar junction, followed by the lumbosacral junction. Higher rates of nonunion did not occur in fusions done in conjunction with osteotomies than in those done without osteotomies. The most common radiographic finding in cases of nonunion was rod breakage, followed by the progression of deformity. Risk factors for nonunion were age over 55 years, fusion of more than 12 vertebral levels, and preoperative thoracolumbar kyphosis. In an earlier study in which 41% of the subjects had Harrington rod instrumentation, nonunion was diagnosed at an average of 2.8 years after initial surgery.[165]

## Treatment

The treatment of nonunion following posterior fusion for spinal deformity requires identification of the etiology underlying the nonunion. Correction of metabolic abnormalities and appropriate treatment of chronic infection can assist in the ultimate healing of nonunions at sites of fusion.[147] Interestingly, and contrary to evidence about its other adverse effects, smoking was not significantly associated with nonunion in two recent studies of patients who had undergone multiple operatations.[164,166]

In cases of complicated nonunion following posterior spinal fusion, the traditional approach has been to perform an anterior fusion along with revision of the posterior fusion and instrumentation. A recent study retrospectively evaluated the outcomes of revision surgery in 132 adult patients with painful nonunions following fusions for scoliosis in adults.[166] This study used three different revision strategies depending upon the nature of the nonunion. Single-level nonunions without gross intraoperative instability were treated with posterior only revision surgery with a minimum of 6 points of fixation. Multiplanar nonunions at multiple vertebral levels were treated with anterior surgery. All nonunions in the L5 area were treated with both anterior and posterior revision surgery. With this strategy, the investigators who conducted the study achieved a 90% rate of fusion with a minimum follow-up of 40 months. Risk factors for persistent nonunion following revision surgery included thoracolumbar kyphosis >18 degrees (immediately following revision surgery), positive sagittal imbalance (a mean of 7.9 cm of positive sagittal alignment in failed revision fusions as compared with a mean of 3.8 cm in successful revision fusions), and three or more sites of nonunion. Coronal imbalance was not associated with failure of revision surgery. There was no comment about whether or not BMP was used in this study. Another study reported an 18% rate of persistent nonunion following revision surgery in 82 adult patients undergoing fusions for spinal deformities.[164]

The introduction of BMP into routine clinical practice provided the option of using purely posterior revision surgery with the use of BMP in cases of complex nonunion. Substantial data on clinical outcomes with this treatment option are not yet available.

## Surgical-site Infection

Despite modern antiseptic techniques and prophylactic antibiotics, postoperative surgical-site infection remains a source of morbidity and increased cost in spinal-deformity surgery. The U.S. Centers for Disease Control and Prevention has established the following criteria for a surgical-site infection in an instrumented spine: (1) an infection of the surgical site occurring within 1 year after the index operation and which appears to be related to it; and (2) the presence of one of the following: purulent drainage, identification of an organism from an aseptically obtained culture, presence of an abscess or other evidence of infection obtained on evaluation, or diagnosis of an infection by the surgeon.[167]

Surgical-site infections presenting acutely are theorized to result from bacterial seeding with a virulent organism at the time of the index surgery. Generally, acute infections present within several weeks after the index surgery. The reported incidence of infection following instrumented posterior spinal fusion ranges from 2.6 to 9.7%, with some reports of an incidence as high as 24% among patients with myelodysplasia.[168,169]

In contrast, infection rates following anterior spinal surgery are quite low approaching nil in some reports.[169] Diabetes, suboptimal timing of the use of prophylactic antibiotics, obesity, and two or more surgical residents participating in an operative procedure were found to be risk factors for surgical-site infection in a case–control study of orthopedic spinal surgery in which 72% of the cases included fusion with instrumentation.[170]

Infections presenting late after spine surgery with instrumentation are thought to result from the hematogenous seeding of pathogens; activation of previously seeded organisms by local inflammation, such as that caused by fretting of metallic instrumentation; or persistence of an acute infection.[171] Late infections typically present well beyond 1 year postoperatively. The incidence of late posterior spinal surgical-site infection is reported to range from 0.2 to 6.7%.[168] Some controversy exists about whether certain instances of delayed infection reported in the literature are actually cases of aseptic inflammation from metal corrosion.[172]

The prevention of surgical-site infection requires strict attention to surgical preparation. The appropriate selection and timing of administration of prophylactic antibiotics have been shown to be important factors in mitigating surgical-site infection.[173,174] It has been suggested that verification of the administration of appropriate prophylactic antibiotics be included in the "wrong-site-surgery time out" protocol. The use of hair clippers in skin preparation for surgery has become standard because the use of shavers has been shown to increase the incidence of postoperative surgical-site infections.[175]

Anterior deep-wound infections are uncommon in the surgical correction of spinal deformities. Janik et al[22] reported no deep wound infections in 20 years of experience. Faciszewski and colleagues[9] identified 7 of 1152 patients (0.57%) as having deep-wound infections. *Staphylococcus aureus* was the most common infecting organism in these cases. None of the infections resulted in osteomyelitis. Superficial infections were identified in an additional 12 procedures (0.98%).[9,24] Grossfeld et al[24] reported a similar deep-wound infection rate of 1.2%. We have not experienced any anterior deepwound infections in our spine surgery.

### Clinical Presentation

An acute postoperative surgical-site infection is often heralded by superficial wound erythema, drainage or fluctuance, and tenderness.[176] Wound dehiscence may follow.

The patient may also exhibit systemic findings such as fever, chills, malaise, and anorexia.

Delayed infection typically presents with spontaneous drainage of the surgical site after a prolonged period. A study of 489 patients who underwent posterior spinal instrumentation for idiopathic scoliosis revealed 23 cases (4.7%) of delayed infection presenting an average of 27 months after initial surgery.[172] The most common presenting sign in this study was spontaneous drainage, with fluctuance next in frequency. The least common presenting complaints were pain and fever.

## Laboratory Evaluation

The standard laboratory evaluation for surgical-site infection includes a peripheral white blood cell (WBC) count, erythrocyte sedimentation rate (ESR), and C-reactive protein (CRP). However, the ESR and CRP are also known to become elevated in the immediate postoperative period among patients without infection. Following uncomplicated spine surgery, the ESR peaks at day 5 and may remain elevated for 3 to 6 weeks.[177] CRP peaks earlier, on day 3, and typically normalizes in 1 to 2 weeks.[177] Therefore, CRP is a more suitable indicator of acute surgical-site infection.

In late infection, laboratory markers are often normal or in the upper range of normal. In a review of 7 instances of delayed infection among 101 cases of instrumented posterior fusion for idiopathic scoliosis, the ESR and CRP were normal in 2 patients.[178] Therefore, one cannot exclude late infection solely on the basis of normal laboratory values.

Wound cultures obtained from acute surgical-site infections most commonly reveal *Staphylococcus* species as pathogens.[168,179,180] Other isolated organisms include *Escherichia coli*. In late infections, propionibacteria becomes the predominant infecting organism.[168,172,178]

## Imaging Studies

The presence of spinal instrumentation often interferes with the detection of surgical-site infection in diagnostic imaging studies. Plain radiographs may show loss of deformity correction or instrumentation failure from nonunion caused by a postoperative infection. CT scanning with contrast medium provides better imaging of paraspinal soft tissues as well as of osseous structures than does plain radiography. MRI is the best modality for evaluating infections of the spine, although it is subject to interference by metallic implants[181] Although radionuclide studies including three-phase technetium-99m bone scans and gallium-67 citrate scans are sensitive in detecting de novo infection of the spine, their role in surgical-site infection in the literature remains unclear.[181]

## Treatment

Upon diagnosis of a surgical-site infection, several treatment options exist. For superficial wound infections such as cellulitis, nonoperative treatment with antibiotics and local wound care may be considered. Deep surgical-site infections must undergo incision and debridement along with antibiotic therapy based on the results of wound culture.

The issue of retention of spinal instrumentation in cases of surgical-site infection is a source of controversy, especially between surgeons and infectious disease specialists.[180] The retention of corrective instrumentation prevents the loss of correction of a deformity during the treatment of early and late surgical-site infections. The removal of instrumentation eliminates a source of continued wound inoculation from bacterial biofilm.[181] Lymphocytes have difficulty eliminating pathogens that are adherent to corrective spinal hardware, especially hardware made of SS.

Some authors report poor results when spinal instrumentation is retained in the face of acute surgical-site infection. Collins et al[168] reported a retrospective study of 74 posterior surgical-site infections diagnosed at a median of 14 months postoperatively among 1980 instrumented spinal fusions. After initial incision and debridement, their treatment protocol hinged on the presence of fusion. In infections in which there was nonunion at fusion sites, patients received 6 weeks of intravenous antibiotics followed by oral antibiotics until fusion took place. The patients' spinal instrumentation was removed upon fusion. Infections in cases in which there was union of fusions were further subdivided according to the infecting organisms. Infections caused by *Staphylococcus aureus* and gram-negative bacteria were treated with the removal of instrumentation and 6 weeks of intravenous antibiotics followed by 6 weeks of oral antibiotic therapy. Infections caused by propionibacteria and coagulase-negative *Staphylococcus* species were treated with the removal of instrumentation and 4 weeks of oral antibiotics. This protocol of retaining instrumentation until fusion occurred resulted in a 60% rate of persistent active infection at the time of the eventual removal of instrumentation. However, even with the eradication of infection, only 46% of patients were pain free. One patient underwent revision surgery for loss of correction of a deformity.

Among children, a retrospective review of 53 infections following instrumented spinal fusion for pediatric scoliosis revealed a nearly 50% rate of persistent infection, despite multiple incisions and debridements, if the hardware was retained.[179]

Contrastingly, other studies report good outcomes with retained instrumentation in the presence of acute surgical-site infection. In a single-surgeon experience of retained instrumentation in 19 of 22 infected spinal fusions in adults (average patient age: 57.2 years), no patient had recurrent or chronic infection when followed for more than 1 year.[176]

Deep surgical-site infections without union of fusions were treated with incision and debridement, with secondary wound closure 48 hours later. Six weeks of intravenous antibiotic therapy completed the patients' treatment regimen. In another report, of 26 deep-wound infections, 24 patients retained their corrective spinal instrumentation, with the successful resolution of infection accomplished through a protocol of multiple debridements and antibiotic therapy.[180]

With respect to final outcomes, a single-surgeon experience with 7 infections following posterior fusion in 236 cases of AIS found no difference in pain, function, self-image, satisfaction, or total score on the SRS-24 outcomes instrument among infected and noninfected patients at final follow-up.[182] In this study there was only one incidence of acute infection; the remaining 6 infections presented with back pain and local swelling at an average of 34.2 months after surgery.

With regard to delayed infections, a retrospective review evaluated 23 such infections presenting at an average of 27 months after initial surgery for idiopathic scoliosis.[172] These patients underwent removal of their instrumentation, intravenous antibiotic therapy for up to two weeks, and oral antibiotic therapy for an additional month. The most common infecting organism was *Propionibacterium acnes* followed by *Staphylococcus epidermidis*. All wounds healed uneventfully except in the case of one patient who required re-instrumentation for nonunion of a fusion. Another retrospective review, of 45 delayed infections, evaluated 35 patients who had only the removal of hardware and 10 patients who underwent single-stage removal of their hardware followed by re-instrumentation.[145] The patients who had re-instrumentation had significantly better maintenance of their deformity corrections. Immediate exchange of instrumentation made of SS for instrumentation made of Ti is gaining favor in this situation.

Every infection will have host-, organism-, and surgical-site-related factors that may dictate its treatment. A reasonable algorithim for treating deep surgical-site infection without a mature fusion involves irrigation and debridement with the retention of corrective spinal instrumentation. With the guidance of an infectious disease specialist, intravenous antibiotics are administered for 6 to 12 weeks with a prolonged ensuing course of oral antibiotics. Patients presenting with delayed infections and healed fusions may undergo incision and debridement with the removal of instrumentation. These patients should be monitored closely for loss of deformity correction.

## Complications of Surgical Approaches

### Vascular Complications

It is difficult to estimate the incidence of vascular injuries encountered during anterior lumbar and thoracic surgery. Mobilization of the great vessels and subsequent injury during anterior spinal procedures is uncommon. Incidental lacerations of major and minor vessels resulting from the approach are often not detailed clearly in the literature. Most surgeons consider hemorrhage from these vessels annoying, but view it as an expected occasional difficulty associated with a complex surgical procedure. In a retrospective review of anterior retroperitoneal lumbar dissections for corrective spinal surgery, Baker and colleagues[183] reported a 15.6% incidence of major vascular injuries. Westfall et al[184] reported a varying incidence of great-vessel injury depending on the surgical approach. On the other hand, Faciszewski and coworkers[9] reported a low incidence (0.08%) of great-vessel injury in retroperitoneal exposures of the lumbar spine.

The choice of a right- or a left-sided retroperitoneal approach is often dictated by the patient's spinal pathology, and may influence whether arterial or venous injuries predominate. Because it may be easier to repair arterial injuries (aorta vs. vena cava), it is probably reasonable to approach from the left side at levels below the midthoracic level. Right-sided approaches to the upper thoracic spine may be reasonable for avoiding retraction on the heart. Avoiding previously dissected areas if possible is always an advantage, especially on the right side, where the vena cava may be injured.[12] Ultimately, the number of vessel injuries will depend on the experience of the surgical team and the difficulty of the cases typically encountered.

#### Aorta

Aortic injury is a rarely reported complication of corrective surgery for spinal deformity. Janik et al[22] reported a single aortic laceration in their series. A single aortic laceration, which occurred in an attempt to remove a large neurofibroma from the spinal column, was also reported by Almond et al.[23] Vogel et al[217] reported several cases of segmental artery avulsions from the aorta in patients with Ehlers–Danlos syndrome. These aortic injuries are typically relatively easily repaired, without long-term sequelae.

#### Iliac Artery

Thrombosis is a rare event in anterior spinal surgery. Only a few cases are reported in the literature.[185,186] A high degree of suspicion is necessary to arrive at this diagnosis. Vascular insufficiency can easily be confused with neurological compromise. Thorough knowledge of the patient's pre- and postoperative vascular status is necessary to make the correct diagnosis in a timely manner. Early re-establishment of arterial blood flow will more likely facilitate full recovery in cases of thrombosis. Routine palpation of pulses in the lower extremities after anterior spinal surgery, particularly when the surgery involves mobilization of the iliac arteries, is probably prudent.[185]

In the evaluation of a patient for possible postoperative arterial injuries, attention should be paid to the hallmark features of vascular insufficiency, such as pulselessness, mottled skin, and temperature differences between the involved and uninvolved limbs. Patients with pre-existing vascular disease may have developed collateral circulation that modifies the expression of severe vascular compromise.

Marsicano et al[187] have reported a left common iliac artery occlusion after an anterior retroperitoneal approach to the lumbar spine. This was presumably the result of retraction of the vessels during the approach. An iliac-to-iliac arterial bypass was done 24 hours after the patient's spinal surgery, restoring the arterial blood flow. The patient regained excellent motor function, but continued to have left-leg pain, presumably from nerve ischemia, at several months after the index surgery.

## Segmental Artery

The artery of Adamkiewicz has been postulated to be the primary blood supply to the thoracic spinal cord. It is clear from numerous anatomical studies that the spine is supplied by three arterial watersheds distinguished by the number of afferent radicular spinal arteries. The cervicothoracic and the thoracolumbar areas are typified by numerous segmentally perforating afferent arteries, whereas the central thoracic region is more sparsely penetrated by afferent radicular arteries. This vascular anatomy may make some investigators' proposition that the anterior spinal artery is not a continuous structure into more than an academic point.[80,188,189] This critical zone for spinal-cord perfusion is an area of concern in anterior spinal surgery.

Standard anterior retroperitoneal and thoracotomy-based approaches to the spine sacrifice segmental vessels. The vast clinical experience in spine surgery over the past 30 years has not been marred by a significant rate of spinal-cord injury as a result of the surgical approach used.[87] However, the cardiothoracic literature suggests that during thoracolumbar aortic surgery, reconstruction of the intercostal arteries (ICAs) and lumbar arteries (LAs) is necessary to maintain flow through the artery of Adamkiewicz. Yet Lowell and co-workers[190] were unable to show any protective effect on the spinal cord of shunting to the ICAs upon aortic cross-clamping in a canine model. Seven of eight animals in both the control and the experimental groups developed irreversible spinal-cord injuries with such cross-clamping. Criteria for which of the ICAs or LAs or both must be reconstructed, and how many, are unclear. The rule of thumb has been to repair or reconstruct larger diameter ICAs and LAs.

Koshino and colleagues[191] have shown in anatomical dissections that the artery of Adamkiewicz does not necessarily arise from the larger ICAs and LAs. In addition, the artery of Adamkiewicz has a variable location. In 90 cadavers, a single artery of Adamkiewicz was found in 67 patients (74%), whereas more than two arteries of Adamkiewicz were found in 23 cadavers (26%). Of the identified arteries of Adamkiewicz, 72% originated from the ICAs or LAs or both on the left side, and 34 (28%) originated from these vessels on the right side. When two arteries of Adamkiewicz were identified, 57% were found unilaterally and 43% were found bilaterally. The artery was identified at T5 in 2% of patients, T6 in 2%, T7 in 3%, T8 in 5%, T9 in 19%, T10 in 23%, T11 in 25%, T12 in 12%, L1 in 8%, and L2 in 3%. Therefore, the artery of Adamkiewicz originates in more than 90% of patients between T8 and L1. The artery ranged in size from 0.5 to 1.5 mm in diameter, with a mean diameter of $0.77 \pm 0.24$ mm. Because there was no obvious correlation between the artery of Adamkiewicz and the size of the feeding vessels (ICAs/LAs), some credence must be given to the recent trend toward vessel preservation, although surgical preservation of these vessels is often difficult.

Proposed modifications in surgical technique have suggested the temporary ligation of prominent segmental vessels as a way to safeguard against accidental ligation of a prominent segmental afferent vessel to the anterior spinal artery. Temporary occulusion of segmental arteries may elicit changes in SSEPs and MEPs that could alert the surgeon to an important segmental contribution to spinal-cord blood flow. This technique may be particularly useful in severely angulated kyphoses or kyphoscolioses, which may mechanically deform the spinal cord and apply tension to extramedullary and intramedullary blood vessels, diminishing their functional diameters.

Unfortunately, reports document the delayed postoperative decline of neurological function despite normal intraoperative monitoring.[192–194] Pelosi et al[195] report the case of a patient with normal intraoperative SSEPs who developed asymmetrical weakness of the legs, worse on the right, with decreased sensation below T5, and which did not become evident until some 40 minutes after an anterior spinal procedure in which segmental vessels were ligated from T6 to 11. The paresis was worse proximally, with absent abdominal reflexes and suspended sensation between T5 and T12 on the left and hyperalgesia at the same levels on the right. Fortunately, the deficit showed gradual improvement, and the patient had essentially full recovery of neurological function at 3 months postoperatively. Others have reported similar episodes of delayed spinal cord injury presumably related to ischemia and occurring several hours after the conclusion of surgery.[192–194] These episodes are sometimes associated with postoperative hypovolemia or hypotension.[192,195]

Bassett and co-workers[196] used preoperative spinal angiography in an attempt to identify significant radicular afferent arteries supplying the spinal cord in 16 patients. None of the eight patients requiring intraoperative occlusion and subsequent ligation of these segmental afferents showed changes during SSEP monitoring, nor did any of these patients sustain a neurological injury as a result of the occlusion and ligation procedure. This echoes the vast clinical experience of spine surgeons around the world regarding the safety of segmental artery ligation during anterior spinal surgery.[87]

The importance of segmental vessels in any individual patient's spinal-cord perfusion will be difficult to ascertain. Scattered reports of neurological deficit after anterior spinal surgery without any obvious spinal-cord trauma suggests that caution be taken when ligating intercostal and segmental vessels. The technique of temporarily ligating larger penetrating segmental vessels and watching the electrophysiological consequences seems prudent. However, in the light of Koshino and colleagues'[191] study, larger vessels do not necessarily imply more prominent contribution to spinal-cord blood flow. Therefore, care should be taken in ligating any segmental vessels when performing anterior thoracic and lumbar surgery, particularly between T8 and L1 on the left side. When operating at the thoracolumbar junction, we routinely attempt to isolate and preserve segmental vessels if possible. When vessels must be sacrificed, ligation or electrocautery should be accomplished well away from the neuroforamen, to prevent injury or thrombosis of the anterior spinal artery. Ligation close to the aorta at the middle aspect of the vertebral-body is ideal.

## Venous Complications

The chief hazard during anterior approaches to the lumbar spine lies in the large and small venous structures.[20,197] Although injury to these vessels is documented in the literature from time to time, Baker and co-workers[183] suggest that its incidence is vastly underreported. In their series, they report an overall vascular injury rate of 15.6% during surgery on the lumbar spine. The injuries included both small- and large-vessel lacerations, all requiring at least a single suture for repair. In 26 patients undergoing surgery via an anterolateral approach there were 2 venous injuries, for an incidence of 7.7%. Seventy-six patients underwent surgery via a paramedian approach through a smaller incision, which resulted in 14 vascular complications for an incidence of 18.4%. Baker and coworkers felt that the learning curve for the retroperitoneal approach was not an issue because all of the surgeons involved were fellowship-trained vascular surgeons familiar with this technique. Interestingly, few of the venous injuries reported by Baker et al resulted from the "orthopedic" part of the procedure. They surmised that the approach to the retroperitoneal spine is the most hazardous part of an anterior lumbar procedure, and noted that the smaller skin incisions seemed predisposed to an increasing number of vascular injuries, perhaps because of the smaller surgical fields created.[183] Janik et al[22] reported 57% of all vessel injuries in anteruior approaches to the spine as occurring in patients with neuromuscular disease. This was three times the rate for other patients. Jarvik and colleagues felt that this was probably partly the result of the typically larger deformities in patients with neuromuscular disease and the more frequent need to dissect the low lumbar and hypogastric vessels in such cases. The clinical significance and consequences of these venous injuries are difficult to determine because they are not typically detailed in the literature. Thrombosis following repair of a spinal deformity is common. Despite this, symptomatic pulmonary embolism is rarely reported in the literature. However, postphlebitic syndrome has been noted to be a problem.[198]

## Cisterna Chyli and Thoracic Duct

Lymph vessels below the diaphragm drain the lower extremities, pelvis, retroperitoneum, and intestines, and join to form a saccular dilatation known as a cisterna chyli. Excess tissue fluid, extravasated proteins, and macromolecules from the intestinal space are channeled via the lymph vessels into the cisterna chyli. From there, powered by the negative pressure generated within the thoracic cavity during respiration, lymph is funneled into the thoracic duct. The cisterna chyli is typically located at the level of the first and second lumbar vertebrae, between the abdominal aorta and the vena cava. It is present in ~50% of the population. However, Propst-Proctor et al[199] reported positive identification of the cisterna chyli or thoracic duct in only 15 of 1000 orthopedic operations (1.5%). The reported incidence of significant chylous leakage is low. However, the identification of chylous leakage during a retroperitoneal or transthoracic dissection is common. Because of the fragility of the chylous vessels and their meandering course, it is often difficult to ligate or cauterize them.

Subclinical retroperitoneal chylous leakage and chylothorax probably often go unrecognized. However, chylothorax, chylous ascites, chylous pericardium, chylous urea, and chylous retroperitoneum can be major postoperative complications.[200,201] Because of the loss of significant nutritional elements and subsequent electrolyte depletion and lymphocytopenia, chronic chylous leakage may have a mortality rate as high as 50% without proper support. The amount of chyle produced and transported through the lymph system depends on the fat content of the diet, on activity, and on bowel function. Typically, between 1.5 and 2.5 L of fluid pass through the lymphatic system per day. Fluid and electrolyte loss via a chylous leak has the same metabolic impact as a corresponding volumetric loss of blood plasma. Because chyle contains a high number of lymphocytes (400 to 600 cells/mL), patients with chylous leakage may become lymphopenic. The loss of fat, protein, and fat-soluble vitamins can eventually cause severe metabolic complications.

Once identified, chylous leakage is typically treated conservatively. Principles of conservative management include changes in diet and nutritional support. The appropriate diet is a low-fat diet of medium-chain-length triglycerides that can be immediately absorbed into the circulation without being shunted into the lymphatic system.

DeHart et al, in their series of three intraoperatively recognized lymphatic leaks, reported good success with routine wound closure without the placement of a retroperitoneal drain.[7] This has also been our experience on numerous occasions. It seems reasonable then, even in the presence of an obvious chylous leak, to proceed with standard wound closure. If a collection of lymph persists or becomes apparent on postoperative radiography, or if drainage from a wound suggests a chylous leak, dietary alteration as noted above, and nutritional support, will probably result in spontaneous closure of the source of the leakage without long-term complications.[7] Faciszewski et al[9] reported one patient who sustained a significant retroperitoneal lymphocele requiring treatment. The index surgery was uneventful, but 4 months after surgery the patient developed clear drainage from the anterior surgical wound. Investigation identified a lymphocele, which was drained percutaneously and treated with sclerosing agents and an indwelling catheter without long-term sequelae. Surgical intervention in such cases is typically unnecessary and is controversial.[9]

Chylous ascites may result from an injury to the cisterna chyli with concomitant violation of the integrity of the peritoneum. Chylous ascites typically responds to a low-fat diet or hyperalimentation. Drainage of chylous ascites is rarely necessary.

Postoperative chylothorax is a well-documented but rare complication discussed in the cardiothoracic surgical literature. Its incidence after anterior spinal surgery is reported to range from 0.2 to 0.6%.[202] Propst-Proctor et al[199] identified only 3 chylothoraces in 1000 patients (0.3%). The thoracic duct originates from the cisterna chyli, penetrates the diaphragm to the right of the aorta, and comes to lie along the right side of the esophagus. It extends extrapleurally along the right anterior surface of the vertebral bodies rostrally to approximately T7. It then crosses to the left side and ascends rostrally from T5 to eventually enter the left internal jugular and subclavian veins. Chylothorax may be either right- or left-sided depending on the level and location of the injury causing it. Injury to the thoracic duct below T5 typically produces a right-sided chylothorax. Injury to the thoracic duct above T5 typically results in a left-sided chylothorax.[203,204] The clinical symptoms of chylothorax are slowly developing effusion, fatigue, depression, and a sense of heaviness. Symptoms of rapid onset may include respiratory distress, shock, tachycardia, and hypotension. Initially, mortality rates as high as 50% were reported in chylothorax. With newer treatment protocols, the current mortality rate is probably less than 10%.[205] Chylothorax may result in mediastinal shift, and the effusion may reduce vital capacity. Patients with preoperatively decreased vital capacity may be at risk for significant respiratory distress.[206] Interestingly, infection is rare in the presence of chylothorax because of the bacteriostatic properties of chyle, which has a high lymphocyte count.[207] The major complications with chylothorax are pulmonary compromise and metabolic depletion as results of the loss of up to 2500 mL of fluid containing important electrolytes and proteins.[208] Conservative management of chylothorax is usually successful. Thoracentesis or chest-tube drainage may be necessary. However, a low-fat diet of medium-chain triglycerides or total parenteral alimentation to avoid activation of the gut may be the only necessary treatment. Surgical intervention should be considered if there is excessive chylous leakage (1500 mL daily in adults and 100 mL per year of age daily in children).

Other reasons for considering surgical intervention for chylous leakage include persistent leakage or the development of complications.[209] Some have suggested that surgical intervention be instituted after 14 days of leakage if conservative measures to stop it have failed.[206] Ligation of the thoracic duct below the level of leakage has been suggested as one type of surgical intervention. However, this is often unsuccessful because of the great variation in anatomy of the thoracic duct and the number of possible collateral channels. More extreme solutions have included sewing an intercostal-muscle pedicle flap over the site of leakage, pleural peritoneal shunting, and chemical pleurodesis.[210] Some of these later techniques have been facilitated by video-assisted thoracoscopic surgery for minimally invasive placement of fibrin glues and endoscopic clips. Conservative management of chylous leakage is successful in 50% of cases. If conservative management is unsuccessful, surgical treatment should not be delayed.[206]

### Incisional and Diaphragmatic Hernia

Hernias thnrough the abdominal wall after anterior lumbar and thoracolumbar surgery are infrequent. Faciszewski et al[9] report 11 abdominal hernias as a consequence of 1223 such procedures (1%). Seven of these required operative repair. More commonly seen are pseudohernias secondary to abdominal-wall paralysis. Muscle denervation results in a patulous abdominal wall on the ipsilateral side. This complication is more often encountered with standard anterolateral oblique incisions, which involve transverse incision of the internal oblique and transversus abdominus muscles. This may be potentiated by injury to the ipsilateral iliohypogastric nerve, which supplies the internal, external, and transversus abdominus muscles. Diaphragmatic hernias are rare after thoracolumbar approaches to spine surgery. After 505 surgeries, Janik et al[22] reported no diaphragmatic hernias from surgical exposures crossing the diaphragm.

## Conclusion

Numerous authors have reported acceptable rates of complications of surgery for spinal deformity when it is done by well-trained spinal teams in both the adult and pediatric populations.[24,211–214] The reported complication rates compare favorably with those reported in other elective procedures. Gerhart et al[215] reported a 2% mortality rate (42 of 2091 patients) in the elective treatment of hip fractures. Lytle et al[216] reported a 1.4% mortality rate (14 of 1000 patients) in coronary bypass surgery. The mortality rate in both the adult and pediatric populations undergoing spinal surgeries is documented in the literature at ~0.3%.[9,24] The mortality rate for a heterogenous population of adolescents and adults with a wide variety of spinal pathologies has been documented at 0.4%.[25] The very detailed prospective accounting by the HSG of complications in a group of adolescent and pediatric patients showed a rate of major complications of 5.26% and of minor complications of 56% (**Table 22.5**). Although these figures appear somewhat higher than those in previous reports, it is likely that they are a more accurate representation of the real complication rates because they are based on data collected prospectively rather than retrospectively. Review of these data are meant to help identify patients undergoing spinal surgery who have an above-average risk for experiencing complications. An increased risk of perioperative morbidity can be expected for patients over 60 years of age and for those patients with neuromuscular scoliosis and medical comorbidities. The overall incidence of complication is related to the surgical approach used in spine surgery.[23] Thoracic and thoracoabdominal approaches generally have a higher complication rate. In Janik's[22] review, complications occurred in 12% of thoracic approaches, in 9.3% of thoracoabdominal approaches, in 7% of retroperitoneal approaches, and in 0% of transperitoneal approaches.

The number of vertebral levels fused in corrective surgery on the spine is not a significant predictor of perioperative mortality or morbidity. However, blood loss (>520 mL) seems to be associated with an increased risk of complications. Adult male patients tend to have a lower incidence (1.6%) of perioperative morbidity or mortality or both than do adult female patients (4.6%). Besides patients with obvious comorbidities such as cardiac and pulmonary disease, physiologically fragile patients, such as those with neuromuscular diseases and Ehlers–Danlos syndrome, may be at greater risk for complications.[15,217] The high incidence of pulmonary and genitourinary complications in spine surgery must be recognized.

The authors of this chapter, after reviewing the available literature and their own clinical experience, feel that although complex spine surgery is demanding, it can be performed in 95% of cases without major complications in the hands of a well-trained team of surgeons, with appropriate medical and intensive care support.

## References


1. Betz RR, Iorio R, Lombardi AV, Clancy M, Steel HH. Scoliosis surgery in neurofibromatosis. Clin Orthop Relat Res 1989;245:53–56
2. Weis JC, Betz RR, Clements DH III, Balsara RK. Prevalence of perioperative complications after anterior spinal fusion for patients with idiopathic scoliosis. J Spinal Disord 1997;10:371–375
3. Riseborough EJ. The anterior approach to the spine for the correction of deformities of the axial skeleton. Clin Orthop Relat Res 1973;93:207–214
4. Anderson PR, Puno MR, Lovell SL, Swayze CR. Postoperative respiratory complications in non-idiopathic scoliosis. Acta Anaesthesiol Scand 1985;29:186–192
5. Chan FL, Chow SP. Retroperitoneal fibrosis after anterior spinal fusion. Clin Radiol 1983;34:331–335
6. Hodge WA, DeWald RL. Splenic injury complicating the anterior thoracoabdominal surgical approach for scoliosis. A report of two cases. J Bone Joint Surg Am 1983;65:396–397
7. DeHart MM, Lauerman WC, Conely AH, Roettger RH, West JL, Cain JE. Management of retroperitoneal chylous leakage. Spine 1994;19:716–718
8. Nakai S, Zielke K. Chylothorax: A rare complication after anterior and posterior spinal correction. Report on six cases. Spine 1986;11:830–833
9. Faciszewski T, Winter RB, Lonstein JE, Denis F, Johnson L. The surgical and medical perioperative complications of anterior spinal fusion surgery in the thoracic and lumbar spine in adults. A review of 1223 procedures. Spine 1995;20:1592–1599
10. McElvein RB, Nasca RJ, Dunham WK, Zorn GL Jr. Transthoracic exposure for anterior spinal surgery. Ann Thorac Surg 1988;45:278–283
11. Tiusanen H, Seitsalo S, Osterman K, Soini J. Anterior interbody lumbar fusion in severe low back pain. Clin Orthop Relat Res 1996;324:153–163
12. Anderson TM, Mansour KA, Miller JI Jr. Thoracic approaches to anterior spinal operations: Anterior thoracic approaches. Ann Thorac Surg 1993;55:1447–1451, discussion 1451–1452
13. Burrington JD, Brown C, Wayne ER, Odom J. Anterior approach to the thoracolumbar spine: Technical considerations. Arch Surg 1976;111:456–463
14. Perry J. The total care of spinal cord injuries. In: Pierce N, V Neds. Surgical Approaches to the Spine. Boston: Little Brown; 1977:53–79
15. Naunheim KS, Barnett MG, Crandall DG, Vaca KJ, Burkus JK. Anterior exposure of the thoracic spine. Ann Thorac Surg 1994;57:1436–1439
16. Dwyer AF, Newton NC, Sherwood AA. An anterior approach to scoliosis. A preliminary report. Clin Orthop Relat Res 1969;62:192–202
17. Dwyer AF, Schafer MF. Anterior approach to scoliosis. Results of treatment in fifty-one cases. J Bone Joint Surg Br 1974;56:218–224
18. Smith TK, Stallone RJ, Yee JM. The thoracic surgeon and anterior spinal surgery. J Thorac Cardiovasc Surg 1979;77:925–928
19. Harmon PH. Anterior extraperitoneal lumbar disc excision and vertebral body fusion. Clin Orthop Relat Res 1960;18:169–182

20. Harmon PH. A simplified surgical technic for anterior lumbar diskectomy and fusion; avoidance of complications; anatomy of the retroperitoneal veins. Clin Orthop Relat Res 1964;37:130–144
21. Walsh GL, Gokaslan ZL, McCutcheon IE, et al. Anterior approaches to the thoracic spine in patients with cancer: Indications and results. Ann Thorac Surg 1997;64:1611–1618
22. Janik JS, Burrington JD, Janik JE, Wayne ER, Chang JHT, Rothenberg SS. Anterior exposure of spinal deformities and tumors: A 20-year experience. J Pediatr Surg 1997;32:852–859
23. Almond PS, Pesson C, MacEwen D, et al. Analysis of the two-team approach to anterior spinal fusion. South Med J 1990;83:1273–1276
24. Grossfeld S, Winter RB, Lonstein JE, Denis F, Leonard A, Johnson L. Complications of anterior spinal surgery in children. J Pediatr Orthop 1997;17:89–95
25. McDonnell MF, Glassman SD, Dimar JR II, Puno RM, Johnson JR. Perioperative complications of anterior procedures on the spine. J Bone Joint Surg Am 1996;78:839–847
26. O'Brien T, Akmakjian J, Ogin G, Eilert R. Comparison of one-stage versus two-stage anterior/posterior spinal fusion for neuromuscular scoliosis. J Pediatr Orthop 1992;12:610–615
27. Baron EM, Albert TJ. Medical complications of surgical treatment of adult spinal deformity and how to avoid them. Spine 2006; 31(19, suppl):S106–S118
28. Dearborn JTHS, Hu SS, Tribus CB, Bradford DS. Thromboembolic complications after major thoracolumbar spine surgery. Spine 1999;24:1471–1476
29. Smith MD, Bressler EL, Lonstein JE, Winter R, Pinto MR, Denis F. Deep venous thrombosis and pulmonary embolism after major reconstructive operations on the spine. A prospective analysis of three hundred and seventeen patients. J Bone Joint Surg Am 1994; 76:980–985
30. West JL III, Anderson LD. Incidence of deep vein thrombosis in major adult spinal surgery. Spine 1992;17(8, suppl):S254–S257, S27
31. Rokito SE, Schwartz MC, Neuwirth MG. Deep vein thrombosis after major reconstructive spinal surgery. Spine 1996;21:853–858, discussion: 859
32. Hashmi S, Kelly E, Rogers SO, Gates J. Urinary tract infection in surgical patients. Am J Surg 2003;186:53–56
33. Coriat P, Richer C, Douraki T, et al. Influence of chronic angiotensin-converting enzyme inhibition on anesthetic induction. Anesthesiology 1994;81:299–307
34. Johnson RM, McGuire EJ. Urogenital complications of anterior approaches to the lumbar spine. Clin Orthop Relat Res 1981;154: 114–118
35. Kern HB, Barnes W, Malament M. Lumbar laminectomy and associated ureteral injury. J Urol 1969;102:675–677
36. Daubs MD, Lenke LG, Cheh G, Stobbs G, Bridwell KH. Adult spinal deformity surgery: Complications and outcomes in patients over age 60. Spine 2007;32:2238–2244
37. Fujita T, Kostuik JP, Huckell CB, Sieber AN. Complications of spinal fusion in adult patients more than 60 years of age. Orthop Clin North Am 1998;29:669–678
38. Baig MN, Lubow M, Immesoete P, Bergese SD, Hamdy EA, Mendel E. Vision loss after spine surgery: Review of the literature and recommendations. Neurosurg Focus 2007;23:E15
39. Walick KS, Kragh JE Jr, Ward JA, Crawford JJ. Changes in intraocular pressure due to surgical positioning: Studying potential risk for postoperative vision loss. Spine 2007;32:2591–2595
40. Althausen PL, Gupta MC, Benson DR, Jones DA. The use of neostigmine to treat postoperative ileus in orthopedic spinal patients. J Spinal Disord 2001;14:541–545
41. Shapiro G, Green DW, Fatica NS, Boachie-Adjei O. Medical complications in scoliosis surgery. Curr Opin Pediatr 2001;13: 36–41
42. Rajaraman V, Vingan R, Roth P, Heary RF, Conklin L, Jacobs GB. Visceral and vascular complications resulting from anterior lumbar interbody fusion. J Neurosurg 1999; 91(1, suppl):60–64
43. Bungard TJ, Kale-Pradhan PB. Prokinetic agents for the treatment of postoperative ileus in adults: A review of the literature. Pharmacotherapy 1999;19:416–423
44. Akin JT Jr, Skandalakis JE, Gray SW. The anatomic basis of vascular compression of the duodenum. Surg Clin North Am 1974;54: 1361–1370
45. Altiok H, Lubicky JP, DeWald CJ, Herman JE. The superior mesenteric artery syndrome in patients with spinal deformity. Spine 2005;30:2164–2170
46. Zhu ZZ, Qiu Y. Superior mesenteric artery syndrome following scoliosis surgery: Its risk indicators and treatment strategy. World J Gastroenterol 2005;11:3307–3310
47. Braun SV, Hedden DM, Howard AW. Superior mesenteric artery syndrome following spinal deformity correction. J Bone Joint Surg Am 2006;88:2252–2257
48. Crowther MA, Webb PJ, Eyre-Brook IA. Superior mesenteric artery syndrome following surgery for scoliosis. Spine 2002;27: E528–E533
49. Floman Y, Micheli LJ, Barker WD, Hall JE. Acute cholecystitis following the surgical treatment of spinal deformities in the adult: A report of three cases. Clin Orthop Relat Res 1980;151: 205–209
50. Karol LA, Richards BS, Prejean E, Safavi F. Hemodynamic instability of myelomeningocele patients during anterior spinal surgery. Dev Med Child Neurol 1993;35:261–267
51. Hsieh PH, Chen WJ, Chen LH, Niu CC. An unusual complication of anterior spinal instrumentation: Hemothorax contralateral to the side of the incision. A case report. J Bone Joint Surg Am 1999; 81:998–1001
52. Zhang JG, Wang W, Qiu GX, Wang YP, Weng XS, Xu HG. The role of preoperative pulmonary function tests in the surgical treatment of scoliosis. Spine 2005;30:218–221
53. Brooks JA. Postoperative nosocomial pneumonia: Nurse-sensitive interventions. AACN Clin Issues 2001;12:305–323
54. Cherry T, Steciuk M, Reddy VV, Marques MB. Transfusion-related acute lung injury: past, present, and future. Am J Clin Pathol 2008;129:287–297
55. Toy P, Popovsky MA, Abraham E, et al; National Heart, Lung and Blood Institute Working Group on TRALI. Transfusion-related acute lung injury: Definition and review. Crit Care Med 2005; 33:721–726
56. Santacruz JF, Diaz Guzman Zavala E, Arroliga AC. Update in ARDS management: recent randomized controlled trials that changed our practice. Cleve Clin J Med 2006;73:217–219, 223–225, 229 passim
57. Lonstein JE, Winter RB, Moe JH, Bradford DS, Chou SN, Pinto WC. Neurologic deficits secondary to spinal deformity. A review of the literature and report of 43 cases. Spine 1980;5:331–355
58. Winter RB. Congenital kyphoscoliosis with paralysis following hemivertebra excision. Clin Orthop Relat Res 1976;119:116–125

59. Turgut M, Akpinar G, Akalan N, Ozcan OE. Spinal injuries in the pediatric age group: A review of 82 cases of spinal cord and vertebral column injuries. Eur Spine J 1996;5:148–152
60. Kawaguchi Y, Kanamori M, Ishihara H, et al. Postoperative delirium in spine surgery. Spine J 2006;6:164–169
61. Coe JD, Warden KE, Herzig MA, McAfee PC. Influence of bone mineral density on the fixation of thoracolumbar implants. A comparative study of transpedicular screws, laminar hooks, and spinous process wires. Spine 1990;15:902–907
62. Diab M, Smith AR, Kuklo TR ; Spinal Deformity Study Group. Neural complications in the surgical treatment of adolescent idiopathic scoliosis. Spine 2007;32:2759–2763
63. MacEwen GD, Bunnell WP, Sriram K. Acute neurological complications in the treatment of scoliosis. A report of the Scoliosis Research Society. J Bone Joint Surg Am 1975;57:404–408
64. Tribus CB. Transient paraparesis: A complication of the surgical management of Scheuermann's kyphosis secondary to thoracic stenosis. Spine 2001;26:1086–1089
65. Qiu Y, Wang S, Wang B, Yu Y, Zhu F, Zhu Z. Incidence and risk factors of neurological deficits of surgical correction for scoliosis: Analysis of 1373 cases at one Chinese institution. Spine 2008;33: 519–526
66. Hedequist DJ, Hall JE, Emans JB. The safety and efficacy of spinal instrumentation in children with congenital spine deformities. Spine 2004;29:2081–2086, discussion 2087
67. Lewandrowski KU, Rachlin JR, Glazer PA. Diastematomyelia presenting as progressive weakness in an adult after spinal fusion for adolescent idiopathic scoliosis. Spine J 2004;4: 116–119
68. Noordeen MH, Taylor BA, Edgar MA. Syringomyelia. A potential risk factor in scoliosis surgery. Spine 1994;19:1406–1409
69. Ayvaz M, Alanay A, Yazici M, Acaroglu E, Akalan N, Aksoy C. Safety and efficacy of posterior instrumentation for patients with congenital scoliosis and spinal dysraphism. J Pediatr Orthop 2007; 27:380–386
70. Buchowski JM, Bridwell KH, Lenke LG, et al. Neurologic complications of lumbar pedicle subtraction osteotomy: A 10-year assessment. Spine 2007;32:2245–2252
71. Suk SI, Chung ER, Lee SM, Lee JH, Kim SS, Kim JH. Posterior vertebral column resection in fixed lumbosacral deformity. Spine 2005;30:E703–E710
72. Pateder DB, Kostuik JP. Lumbar nerve root palsy after adult spinal deformity surgery. Spine 2005;30:1632–1636
73. Coe JD, Arlet V, Donaldson W, et al. Complications in spinal fusion for adolescent idiopathic scoliosis in the new millennium. A report of the Scoliosis Research Society Morbidity and Mortality Committee. Spine 2006;31:345–349
74. Bridwell KH, Lenke LG, Baldus C, Blanke K. Major intraoperative neurologic deficits in pediatric and adult spinal deformity patients. Incidence and etiology at one institution. Spine 1998;23:324–331
75. Apel DM, Marrero G, King J, Tolo VT, Bassett GS. Avoiding paraplegia during anterior spinal surgery. The role of somatosensory evoked potential monitoring with temporary occlusion of segmental spinal arteries. Spine 1991;16(8, suppl):S365–S370
76. Rosenthal D. Spinal cord ischemia after abdominal aortic operation: Is it preventable? J Vasc Surg 1999;30:391–397
77. Orchowski J, Bridwell KH, Lenke LG. Neurological deficit from a purely vascular etiology after unilateral vessel ligation during anterior thoracolumbar fusion of the spine. Spine 2005;30: 406–410
78. Langmayr JJ, Ortler M, Obwegeser A, Felber S. Quadriplegia after lumbar disc surgery. A case report. Spine 1996;21:1932–1935
79. Deen HG Jr. Healthy young man who developed high cervical cord infarction with quadriplegia and occipital lobe infarction with visual disturbance after lumbar disc surgery. Spine 1997; 22:464
80. Parke WW, Whalen JL, Bunger PC, Settles HE. Intimal musculature of the lower anterior spinal artery. Spine 1995;20:2073–2079
81. Mawad ME, Rivera V, Crawford S, Ramirez A, Breitbach W. Spinal cord ischemia after resection of thoracoabdominal aortic aneurysms: MR findings in 24 patients. AJR Am J Roentgenol 1990;155:1303–1307
82. O'Brien MF. Personal communication.
83. Schulte TL, Lerner T, Berendes E, et al. Transient hemiplegia in posterior instrumentation of scoliosis. Spine 2004;29:E394–E398
84. Keyoung HM, Kanter AS, Mummaneni PV. Delayed-onset neurological deficit following correction of severe thoracic kyphotic deformity. J Neurosurg Spine 2008;8:74–79
85. Mineiro J, Weinstein SL. Delayed postoperative paraparesis in scoliosis surgery. A case report. Spine 1997;22:1668–1672
86. Leung YL, Grevitt M, Henderson L, Smith J. Cord monitoring changes and segmental vessel ligation in the "at risk" cord during anterior spinal deformity surgery. Spine 2005;30:1870–1874
87. Winter RB, Lonstein JE, Denis F, Leonard AS, Garamella JJ. Paraplegia resulting from vessel ligation. Spine 1996;21(10):1232–1233, discussion 1233–1234
88. Neo M, Sakamoto T, Fujibayashi S, Nakamura T. Delayed postoperative spinal epidural hematoma causing tetraplegia. Case report. J Neurosurg Spine 2006;5:251–253
89. Rittmeister M, Leyendecker K, Kurth A, Schmitt E. Cauda equina compression due to a laminar hook: A late complication of posterior instrumentation in scoliosis surgery. Eur Spine J 1999;8: 417–420
90. Vauzelle C, Stagnara P, Jouvinroux P. Functional monitoring of spinal cord activity during spinal surgery. Clin Orthop Relat Res 1973;93:173–178
91. Hoppenfeld S, Gross A, Andrews C, Lonner B. The ankle clonus test for assessment of the integrity of the spinal cord during operations for scoliosis. J Bone Joint Surg Am 1997;79:208–212
92. Devlin VJ, Schwartz DM. Intraoperative neurophysiologic monitoring during spinal surgery. J Am Acad Orthop Surg 2007;15: 549–560
93. Padberg AM, Wilson-Holden TJ, Lenke LG, Bridwell KH. Somatosensory- and motor-evoked potential monitoring without a wake-up test during idiopathic scoliosis surgery. An accepted standard of care. Spine 1998;23:1392–1400
94. Schwartz DM, Auerbach JD, Dormans JP, et al. Neurophysiological detection of impending spinal cord injury during scoliosis surgery. J Bone Joint Surg Am 2007;89:2440–2449
95. Cheh G, Lenke LG, Padberg AM, et al. Loss of spinal cord monitoring signals in children during thoracic kyphosis correction with spinal osteotomy: Why does it occur and what should you do? Spine 2008;33:1093–1099
96. O'Shaughnessy BA, Koski TR, Ondra SL. Reversal of neurologic deterioration after vertebral column resection by spinal cord untethering and duraplasty. Spine 2008;33:E50–E54

97. Lipshultz LI, McConnell J, Benson GS. Current concepts of the mechanisms of ejaculation. Normal and abnormal states. J Reprod Med 1981;26:499–507
98. Duncan HJM, Jonch IM. The presacral plexus in anterior fusion of the lumbar spine. S Afr J Surg 1965;9:93
99. Humphries AW, Hawk WA, Berndt AL. Anterior fusion of lumbar vertebrae. A surgical technique. Surg Clin North Am 1961;41: 1685–1700
100. Flynn JC, Price CT. Sexual complications of anterior fusion of the lumbar spine. Spine 1984;9:489–492
101. Flynn JC, Hoque MA. Anterior fusion of the lumbar spine. End-result study with long-term follow-up. J Bone Joint Surg Am 1979;61:1143–1150
102. O'Brien MF, Lenke LG, Bridwell KH, Padberg A, Stokes M. Evoked potential monitoring of the upper extremities during thoracic and lumbar spinal deformity surgery: a prospective study. J Spinal Disord 1994;7:277–284
103. McMahon SB. Mechanisms of sympathetic pain. Br Med Bull 1991;47:584–600
104. Pienkowski D, Stephens GC, Doers TM, Hamilton DM. Multicycle mechanical performance of titanium and stainless steel transpedicular spine implants. Spine 1998;23:782–788
105. Stambough JL, Genaidy AM, Huston RL, Serhan H, El-khatib F, Sabri EH. Biomechanical assessment of titanium and stainless steel posterior spinal constructs: effects of absolute/relative loading and frequency on fatigue life and determination of failure modes. J Spinal Disord 1997;10:473–481
106. Rupp R, Ebraheim NA, Savolaine ER, Jackson WT. Magnetic resonance imaging evaluation of the spine with metal implants. General safety and superior imaging with titanium. Spine 1993; 18:379–385
107. Arens S, Schlegel U, Printzen G, Ziegler WJ, Perren SM, Hansis M. Influence of materials for fixation implants on local infection. An experimental study of steel versus titanium DCP in rabbits. J Bone Joint Surg Br 1996;78:647–651
108. Pieske O, Geleng P, Zaspel J, Piltz S. Titanium alloy pins versus stainless steel pins in external fixation at the wrist: A randomized prospective study. J Trauma 2008;64:1275–1280
109. Richardson TD, Pineda SJ, Strenge KB, et al. Serum titanium levels after instrumented spinal arthrodesis. Spine 2008;33: 792–796
110. Okuyama K, Abe E, Suzuki T, Tamura Y, Chiba M, Sato K. Influence of bone mineral density on pedicle screw fixation: A study of pedicle screw fixation augmenting posterior lumbar interbody fusion in elderly patients. Spine J 2001;1:402–407
111. Soshi S, Shiba R, Kondo H, Murota K. An experimental study on transpedicular screw fixation in relation to osteoporosis of the lumbar spine. Spine 1991;16:1335–1341
112. Chang MC, Liu CL, Chen TH. Polymethylmethacrylate augmentation of pedicle screw for osteoporotic spinal surgery: A novel technique. Spine 2008;33:E317–E324
113. DeWald CJ, Stanley T. Instrumentation-related complications of multilevel fusions for adult spinal deformity patients over age 65: Surgical considerations and treatment options in patients with poor bone quality. Spine 2006;31(19, suppl):S144–S151
114. Barr SJ, Schuette AM, Emans JB. Lumbar pedicle screws versus hooks. Results in double major curves in adolescent idiopathic scoliosis. Spine 1997;22:1369–1379
115. Esses SI, Sachs BL, Dreyzin V. Complications associated with the technique of pedicle screw fixation. A selected survey of ABS members. Spine 1993;18:2231–2238, discussion 2238–2239
116. Polly DW Jr, Potter BK, Kuklo T, Young S, Johnson C, Klemme WR. Volumetric spinal canal intrusion: A comparison between thoracic pedicle screws and thoracic hooks. Spine 2004; 29:63–69
117. Smorgick Y, Millgram MA, Anekstein Y, Floman Y, Mirovsky Y. Accuracy and safety of thoracic pedicle screw placement in spinal deformities. J Spinal Disord Tech 2005;18:522–526
118. Di Silvestre M, Parisini P, Lolli F, Bakaloudis G. Complications of thoracic pedicle screws in scoliosis treatment. Spine 2007;32: 1655–1661
119. Suk SI, Lee CK, Kim WJ, Chung YJ, Park YB. Segmental pedicle screw fixation in the treatment of thoracic idiopathic scoliosis. Spine 1995;20:1399–1405
120. Liljenqvist UR, Halm HF, Link TM. Pedicle screw instrumentation of the thoracic spine in idiopathic scoliosis. Spine 1997;22: 2239–2245
121. Lehman RA Jr, Lenke LG, Keeler KA, Kim YJ, Cheh G. Computed tomography evaluation of pedicle screws placed in the pediatric deformed spine over an 8-year period. Spine 2007;32:2679–2684
122. Brown CA, Lenke LG, Bridwell KH, Geideman WM, Hasan SA, Blanke K. Complications of pediatric thoracolumbar and lumbar pedicle screws. Spine 1998;23:1566–1571
123. Kim YW, Lenke LG, Kim YJ, et al. Free-hand pedicle screw placement during revision spinal surgery: Analysis of 552 screws. Spine 2008;33:1141–1148
124. Glassman SD, Dimar JR, Puno RM, Johnson JR, Shields CB, Linden RD. A prospective analysis of intraoperative electromyographic monitoring of pedicle screw placement with computed tomographic scan confirmation. Spine 1995;20:1375–1379
125. Raynor BL, Lenke LG, Bridwell KH, Taylor BA, Padberg AM. Correlation between low triggered electromyographic thresholds and lumbar pedicle screw malposition: Analysis of 4857 screws. Spine 2007;32:2673–2678
126. Kuntz C IV, Maher PC, Levine NB, Kurokawa R. Prospective evaluation of thoracic pedicle screw placement using fluoroscopic imaging. J Spinal Disord Tech 2004;17:206–214
127. Chen J, Shufflebarger HL, O'Brien MF, Quevedo F. Surgical Technique: Pedicle Screw Insertion Technique. Raynam, MA: DePuy Spine; 2006
128. Kotil K, Bilge T. Accuracy of pedicle and mass screw placement in the spine without using fluoroscopy: A prospective clinical study. Spine J 2008;8:591–596
129. Kosmopoulos V, Schizas C. Pedicle screw placement accuracy: A meta-analysis. Spine 2007;32:E111–E120
130. Girardi FP, Boachie-Adjei O, Rawlins BA. Safety of sublaminar wires with Isola instrumentation for the treatment of idiopathic scoliosis. Spine 2000;25:691–695
131. Luque ER. Segmental spinal instrumentation for correction of scoliosis. Clin Orthop Relat Res 1982;163:192–198
132. Erel N, Sebik A, Karapinar L, Gürbulak E. Transverse process wiring for thoracic scoliosis: A new technique. Acta Orthop Scand 2003;74:312–321
133. Eberle CF. Failure of fixation after segmental spinal instrumentation without arthrodesis in the management of paralytic scoliosis. J Bone Joint Surg Am 1988;70:696–703

134. Senaran H, Atilla P, Kaymaz F, Acaroglu E, Surat A. Ultrastructural analysis of metallic debris and tissue reaction around spinal implants in patients with late operative site pain. Spine 2004; 29:1618–1623, discussion 1623
135. Villarraga ML, Cripton PA, Teti SD, et al. Wear and corrosion in retrieved thoracolumbar posterior internal fixation. Spine 2006;31: 2454–2462
136. Denaro V, Papapietro N, Sgambato A, et al. Periprosthetic electrochemical corrosion of titanium and titanium-based alloys as a cause of spinal fusion failure. Spine 2008;33:8–13
137. Kakkos SK, Shepard AD. Delayed presentation of aortic injury by pedicle screws: Report of two cases and review of the literature. J Vasc Surg 2008;47:1074–1082
138. Cho KJ, Suk SI, Park SR, et al. Complications in posterior fusion and instrumentation for degenerative lumbar scoliosis. Spine 2007; 32:2232–2237
139. Emami A, Deviren V, Berven S, Smith JA, Hu SS, Bradford DS. Outcome and complications of long fusions to the sacrum in adult spine deformity: Luque-Galveston, combined iliac and sacral screws, and sacral fixation. Spine 2002;27:776–786
140. Alegre GM, Gupta MC, Bay BK, Smith TS, Laubach JE. S1 screw bending moment with posterior spinal instrumentation across the lumbosacral junction after unilateral iliac crest harvest. Spine 2001;26:1950–1955
141. Gaine WJ, Andrew SM, Chadwick P, Cooke E, Williamson JB. Late operative site pain with isola posterior instrumentation requiring implant removal: Infection or metal reaction? Spine 2001;26:583–587
142. Rathjen KWM, Wood M, McClung A, Vest Z. Clinical and radiographic results after implant removal in idiopathic scoliosis. Spine 2007;32:2184–2188
143. Deckey JECC, Court C, Bradford DS. Loss of sagittal plane correction after removal of spinal implants. Spine 2000;25:2453–2460
144. Potter BK, Kirk KL, Shah SA, Kuklo TR. Loss of coronal correction following instrumentation removal in adolescent idiopathic scoliosis. Spine 2006;31:67–72
145. Muschik M, Lück W, Schlenzka D. Implant removal for late-developing infection after instrumented posterior spinal fusion for scoliosis: Reinstrumentation reduces loss of correction. A retrospective analysis of 45 cases. Eur Spine J 2004;13:645–651
146. Thompson WA, Ralston EL. Pseudarthrosis following spine fusion. J Bone Joint Surg Am 1949;31A:400–405
147. Lee C, Dorcil J, Radomisli TE. Nonunion of the spine: A review. Clin Orthop Relat Res 2004;419:71–75
148. Hsu WK, Wang JC. The use of bone morphogenetic protein in spine fusion. Spine J 2008;8:419–425
149. Kim YJ, Bridwell KH, Lenke LG, Rhim S, Cheh G. Pseudarthrosis in long adult spinal deformity instrumentation and fusion to the sacrum: prevalence and risk factor analysis of 144 cases. Spine 2006;31(20):2329–2336
150. Blanco JS, Sears CJ. Allograft bone use during instrumentation and fusion in the treatment of adolescent idiopathic scoliosis. Spine 1997;22:1338–1342
151. Jones KC, Andrish J, Kuivila T, Gurd A. Radiographic outcomes using freeze-dried cancellous allograft bone for posterior spinal fusion in pediatric idiopathic scoliosis. J Pediatr Orthop 2002;22:285–289
152. Price CT, Connolly JF, Carantzas AC, Ilyas I. Comparison of bone grafts for posterior spinal fusion in adolescent idiopathic scoliosis. Spine 2003;28:793–798
153. Hedequist D, Yeon H, Emans J. The use of allograft as a bone graft substitute in patients with congenital spine deformities. J Pediatr Orthop 2007;27:686–689
154. Geck MJ, Macagno A, Ponte A, Shufflebarger HL. The Ponte procedure: posterior only treatment of Scheuermann's kyphosis using segmental posterior shortening and pedicle screw instrumentation. J Spinal Disord Tech 2007;20:586–593
155. Bezer M, Kucukdurmaz F, Guven O. Transpedicular decancellation osteotomy in the treatment of posttuberculous kyphosis. J Spinal Disord Tech 2007;20:209–215
156. Roberto RF, Lonstein JE, Winter RB, Denis F. Curve progression in Risser stage 0 or 1 patients after posterior spinal fusion for idiopathic scoliosis. J Pediatr Orthop 1997;17:718–725
157. Heggeness MH, Esses SI. Classification of pseudarthroses of the lumbar spine. Spine 1991; 16 (8,suppl):S449–S454
158. Hipp JA, Reitman CA, Wharton N. Defining pseudoarthrosis in the cervical spine with differing motion thresholds. Spine 2005;30: 209–210
159. Steinmann JC, Herkowitz HN. Pseudarthrosis of the spine. Clin Orthop Relat Res 1992;284:80–90
160. Hilibrand AS, Dina TS. The use of diagnostic imaging to assess spinal arthrodesis. Orthop Clin North Am 1998;29:591–601
161. Dawson EG, Clader TJ, Bassett LW. A comparison of different methods used to diagnose pseudarthrosis following posterior spinal fusion for scoliosis. J Bone Joint Surg Am 1985;67: 1153–1159
162. Zinreich SJ, Long DM, Davis R, Quinn CB, McAfee PC, Wang H. Three-dimensional CT imaging in postsurgical "failed back" syndrome. J Comput Assist Tomogr 1990;14:574–580
163. Lang P, Genant HK, Chafetz N, Steiger P, Morris JM. Three-dimensional computed tomography and multiplanar reformations in the assessment of pseudarthrosis in posterior lumbar fusion patients. Spine 1988;13:69–75
164. Kim YJ, Bridwell KH, Lenke LG, Cho KJ, Edwards CC II, Rinella AS. Pseudarthrosis in adult spinal deformity following multisegmental instrumentation and arthrodesis. J Bone Joint Surg Am 2006; 88:721–728
165. Lauerman WC, Bradford DS, Transfeldt EE, Ogilvie JW. Management of pseudarthrosis after arthrodesis of the spine for idiopathic scoliosis. J Bone Joint Surg Am 1991;73:222–236
166. Pateder DB, Park YS, Kebaish KM, et al. Spinal fusion after revision surgery for pseudarthrosis in adult scoliosis. Spine 2006;31: E314–E319
167. Mangram AJ, Horan TC, Pearson ML, Silver LC, Jarvis WR ; Centers for Disease Control and Prevention (CDC) Hospital Infection Control Practices Advisory Committee. Guideline for Prevention of Surgical Site Infection, 1999. Am J Infect Control 1999;27:97–132; quiz: 133–134, discussion: 96
168. Collins I, Wilson-MacDonald J, Chami G, et al. The diagnosis and management of infection following instrumented spinal fusion. Eur Spine J 2008;17:445–450
169. Labbé AC, Demers AM, Rodrigues R, Arlet V, Tanguay K, Moore DL. Surgical-site infection following spinal fusion: A case-control study in a children's hospital. Infect Control Hosp Epidemiol 2003;24:591–595
170. Olsen MA, Nepple JJ, Riew KD, et al. Risk factors for surgical site infection following orthopaedic spinal operations. J Bone Joint Surg Am 2008;90:62–69

171. Bose B. Delayed infection after instrumented spine surgery: Case reports and review of the literature. Spine J 2003;3:394–399
172. Richards BR, Emara KM. Delayed infections after posterior TSRH spinal instrumentation for idiopathic scoliosis: Revisited. Spine 2001;26:1990–1996
173. Kanayama M, Hashimoto T, Shigenobu K, Oha F, Togawa D. Effective prevention of surgical site infection using a Centers for Disease Control and Prevention guideline-based antimicrobial prophylaxis in lumbar spine surgery. J Neurosurg Spine 2007;6:327–329
174. Rosenberg AD, Wambold D, Kraemer L, et al. Ensuring appropriate timing of antimicrobial prophylaxis. J Bone Joint Surg Am 2008;90:226–232
175. Celik SE, Kara A. Does shaving the incision site increase the infection rate after spinal surgery? Spine 2007;32:1575–1577
176. Weinstein MA, McCabe JP, Cammisa FP Jr. Postoperative spinal wound infection: A review of 2,391 consecutive index procedures. J Spinal Disord 2000;13:422–426
177. Thelander U, Larsson S. Quantitation of C-reactive protein levels and erythrocyte sedimentation rate after spinal surgery. Spine 1992;17:400–404
178. Hahn F, Zbinden R, Min K. Late implant infections caused by *Propionibacterium acnes* in scoliosis surgery. Eur Spine J 2005;14: 783–788
179. Ho C, Skaggs DL, Weiss JM, Tolo VT. Management of infection after instrumented posterior spine fusion in pediatric scoliosis. Spine 2007;32:2739–2744
180. Picada R, Winter RB, Lonstein JE, et al. Postoperative deep wound infection in adults after posterior lumbosacral spine fusion with instrumentation: Incidence and management. J Spinal Disord 2000;13:42–45
181. An HS, Seldomridge JA. Spinal infections: Diagnostic tests and imaging studies. Clin Orthop Relat Res 2006;444:27–33
182. Rihn JA, Lee JY, Ward WT. Infection after the surgical treatment of adolescent idiopathic scoliosis: Evaluation of the diagnosis, treatment, and impact on clinical outcomes. Spine 2008;33:289–294
183. Baker JK, Reardon PR, Reardon MJ, Heggeness MH. Vascular injury in anterior lumbar surgery. Spine 1993;18:2227–2230
184. Westfall SH, Akbarnia BA, Merenda JT, et al. Exposure of the anterior spine. Technique, complications, and results in 85 patients. Am J Surg 1987;154:700–704
185. Raskas DS, Delamarter RB. Occlusion of the left iliac artery after retroperitoneal exposure of the spine. Clin Orthop Relat Res 1997;(338):86–89
186. Stambough JL, Simeone FA. Vascular complications in spine surgery. In: Rothman RH, Simeone FA, eds. The Spine. Philadelphia: WB Saunders; 1992:1877–1885.
187. Marsicano J, Mirovsky Y, Remer S, Bloom N, Neuwirth M. Thrombotic occlusion of the left common iliac artery after an anterior retroperitoneal approach to the lumbar spine. Spine 1994;19:357–359
188. Lazorthes G, Gouaze A, Zadeh JO, Santini JJ, Lazorthes Y, Burdin P. Arterial vascularization of the spinal cord. J Neurosurg 1971; 35:253–262
189. Dommisse GF. The blood supply of the spinal cord. A critical vascular zone in spinal surgery. J Bone Joint Surg Br 1974;56:225–235
190. Lowell RC, Gloviczki P, Bergman RT, et al. Failure of selective shunting to intercostal arteries to prevent spinal cord ischemia during experimental thoracoabdominal aortic occlusion. Int Angiol 1992;11:281–288
191. Koshino T, Murakami G, Morishita K, Mawatari T, Abe T. Does the Adamkiewicz artery originate from the larger segmental arteries? J Thorac Cardiovasc Surg 1999;117:898–905
192. Taylor BA, Webb PJ, Hetreed M, Mulukutla RD, Farrell J. Delayed postoperative paraplegia with hypotension in adult revision scoliosis surgery. Spine 1994;19:470–474
193. Lesser RP, Raudzens P, Lüders H, et al. Postoperative neurological deficits may occur despite unchanged intraoperative somatosensory evoked potentials. Ann Neurol 1986;19:22–25
194. Ginsburg HH, Shetter AG, Raudzens PA. Postoperative paraplegia with preserved intraoperative somatosensory evoked potentials. Case report. J Neurosurg 1985;63:296–300
195. Pelosi L, Jardine A, Webb JK. Neurological complications of anterior spinal surgery for kyphosis with normal somatosensory evoked potentials (SEPs). J Neurol Neurosurg Psychiatry 1999;66:662–664
196. Bassett G, Johnson C, Stanley P. Comparison of preoperative selective spinal angiography and somatosensory-evoked potential monitoring with temporary occlusion of segmental vessels during anterior spinal surgery. Spine 1996;21:1996–1999, discussion 2000
197. Hobson RW II, Yeager RA, Lynch TG, et al. Femoral venous trauma: Techniques for surgical management and early results. Am J Surg 1983;146:220–224
198. Immelman EJ, Jeffery PC. The postphlebitic syndrome. Pathophysiology, prevention and management. Clin Chest Med 1984;5: 537–550
199. Propst-Proctor SL, Rinsky LA, Bleck EE. The cisterna chyli in orthopaedic surgery. Spine 1983;8:787–792
200. Shen YS, Cheung CY, Nilsen PT. Chylous leakage after arthrodesis using the anterior approach to the spine. Report of two cases. J Bone Joint Surg Am 1989;71:1250–1251
201. Cevese PG, Vecchioni R, D'Amico DF, et al. Postoperative chylothorax. Six cases in 2,500 operations, with a survey of the world literature. J Thorac Cardiovasc Surg 1975;69:966–971
202. Marts BC, Naunheim KS, Fiore AC, Pennington DG. Conservative versus surgical management of chylothorax. Am J Surg 1992;164:532–534; discussion: 534–535
203. Bessone LN, Ferguson TB, Burford TH. Chylothorax. Ann Thorac Surg 1971;12:527–550
204. Watkins RD. Surgical Approaches to the Spine ed. New York: Springer-Verlag, 1983.
205. Dulchavsky SA, Ledgerwood AM, Lucas CE. Management of chylothorax after blunt chest trauma. J Trauma 1988;28:1400–1401
206. Verhoeven W, Low CO, See HF, Chacha PB, Tan NC. Massive chylothorax after anterior fusion of the thoracic spine. Ann Acad Med Singapore 1996;25:286–288
207. Selle JG, Snyder WH III, Schreiber JT. Chylothorax: Indications for surgery. Ann Surg 1973;177:245–249
208. Colletta AJ, Mayer PJ. Chylothorax: An unusual complication of anterior thoracic interbody spinal fusion. Spine 1982;7:46–49
209. Milsom JW, Kron IL, Rheuban KS, Rodgers BM. Chylothorax: an assessment of current surgical management. J Thorac Cardiovasc Surg 1985;89:221–227
210. Aoki M, Kato F, Saito H, Mimatsu K, Iwata H. Successful treatment of chylothorax by bleomycin for Gorham's disease. Clin Orthop Relat Res 1996;330:193–197
211. Byrd JA III, Scoles PV, Winter RB, Bradford DS, Lonstein JE, Moe JH. Adult idiopathic scoliosis treated by anterior and posterior spinal fusion. J Bone Joint Surg Am 1987;69:843–850

212. Floman Y, Micheli LJ, Penny JN, Riseborough EJ, Hall JE. Combined anterior and posterior fusion in seventy-three spinally deformed patients: Indications, results and complications. Clin Orthop Relat Res 1982;164:110–122
213. Shufflebarger HL, Grimm JO, Bui V, Thomson JD. Anterior and posterior spinal fusion. Staged versus same-day surgery. Spine 1991; 16:930–933
214. Spivak JM, Neuwirth MG, Giordano CP, Bloom N. The perioperative course of combined anterior and posterior spinal fusion. Spine 1994;19:520–525
215. Gerhart TN, Yett HS, Robertson LK, Lee MA, Smith M, Salzman EW. Low-molecular-weight heparinoid compared with warfarin for prophylaxis of deep-vein thrombosis in patients who are operated on for fracture of the hip. A prospective, randomized trial. J Bone Joint Surg Am 1991;73:494–502
216. Lytle BW, Cosgrove DM III. Coronary artery bypass surgery. Curr Probl Surg 1992;29:735–807
217. Vogel LC, Lubicky JP. Neurologic and vascular complications of scoliosis surgery in patients with Ehlers-Danlos syndrome. A case report. Spine 1996;21:2508–2514

# 23 Spinopelvic Fixation in Idiopathic Scoliosis

*Mark F. Abel, Michael F. O'Brien, and Burt Yaszay*

Spinopelvic fixation (SPF) and fusion are done for a variety of clinical conditions including neuromuscular scoliosis, spondylolisthesis, traumatic injury, and neoplasm.[1] In this chapter, SPF will be considered as a procedure for the salvage of decompensating spinal deformity in adults who had adolescent idiopathic scoliosis (AIS). These older former AIS patients develop lumbosacral deformities with time, as a consequence of pre-existing coronal and sagittal truncal imbalance, and often present with concurrent disc degeneration, spinal arthrosis, stenosis, back pain, or leg pain. The surgical procedures needed to address these problems may require linking into older spinal fixations, revision instrumentation, spinal decompression for degenerative changes, and osteotomies for truncal imbalance. However, this chapter will focus on the frequently required surgical technique of SPF in this setting. The large bone area of the pelvis and sacrum is used as a foundation for instrumentation and the correction of deformity to restore truncal balance. The chapter will review the anatomy and biomechanics of the lumbosacral spine as they relate to fixation techniques, and will present a summary of outcome studies of SPF.

## Historical Overview

Fusions from the spine to the pelvis have historically been difficult to achieve because of the high stresses produced at this pivot point between the trunk and lower body.[2] The evolution of surgical techniques for SPF largely reflect attempts to prevent implant failures, pseudarthrosis, and truncal imbalance. Before the era of Harrington instrumentation, SPFs were done with autologous bone grafting and body casting, with resultant pseudarthrosis in up to 83% of cases.[2–4] In the 1970s and 1980s, Harrington distraction instrumentation was used with sacral hooks or a transiliac bar in an attempt to obtain SPF. The distraction technique frequently led to a loss of lumbar lordosis (flat back) in up to 49% of cases and pseudarthrosis in 20 to 40% of cases (**Fig. 23.1**).[5] The modified Luque technique for SPF with sublaminar wires and a contoured L-rod driven into the ilium for SPF[6,7] overcame the problem of inducing flat back by distraction, and introduced segmental fixation; however, the wire and pelvic anchors used in this technique lacked sufficient bending and torsional rigidity to consistently overcome scoliosis and pelvic obliquity.[8] Therefore, early techniques of fixation to the pelvis had low rates of successful fusion and the restoration of global balance.

The SPF techniques developed by Dubousset and Cotrel, Jackson, and Allen and Fergusen are the foundations of modern iliac fixation (**Fig. 23.2**).[9–12] Dubousset and Cotrel utilized iliosacral screws directed across the posterior part of the sacroiliac (SI) joint and into the S1 centrum for distal fixation, and coupled these screws to rods on either side of the midline of the spine with subsequent cross-linking to provide further rigidity.[12] Jackson's technique placed rods within the sacral ala and used the posterior sacral cortex and overhanging posterior iliac wings as a buttress to neutralize bending stress.[9] The insertion point of the rod was caudal to S1 so that the rod could be coupled to S1 pedicle screws. The Jackson technique is technically demanding and more susceptible to bending failure than coupling of the rod to iliac screws or to parts of sacral screw.[13] The Galveston technique, introduced by Allen and Ferguson, uses bilateral L-shaped rods with the horizontal part of the "L" driven into the iliac wings for pelvic fixation, whereas the vertical component provides the spinal fixation.[11] Variations of this technique, using rods or screws passed between the iliac tables, have been used extensively for SPF with long fusions in neuromuscular and adult deformities.[1] McCarthy and colleagues developed an S-shaped rod positioned with the short arm of the "S"-rod placed over the sacral ala from posterior to anterior and coming to rest on the anterior ala, whereas the long arm of the "S" ran along the spinal axis. This S-rod was specifically designed to resist flexion in patients with neuromuscular conditions, particularly meningomyelocele associated with lumbar or thoracolumbar kyphosis.[10]

The specific aspects of these older SPF techniques that persist today include multiple points of fixation (segmental fixation), chiefly with iliac and sacral screw-anchored rods, augmented anterior column support, and cross-linking of rods to increase rigidity of the construct. Compression forces and restoration of coronal and sagittal truncal balance are recognized as crucial for minimizing complications with such techniques. Nevertheless, despite the use of modern

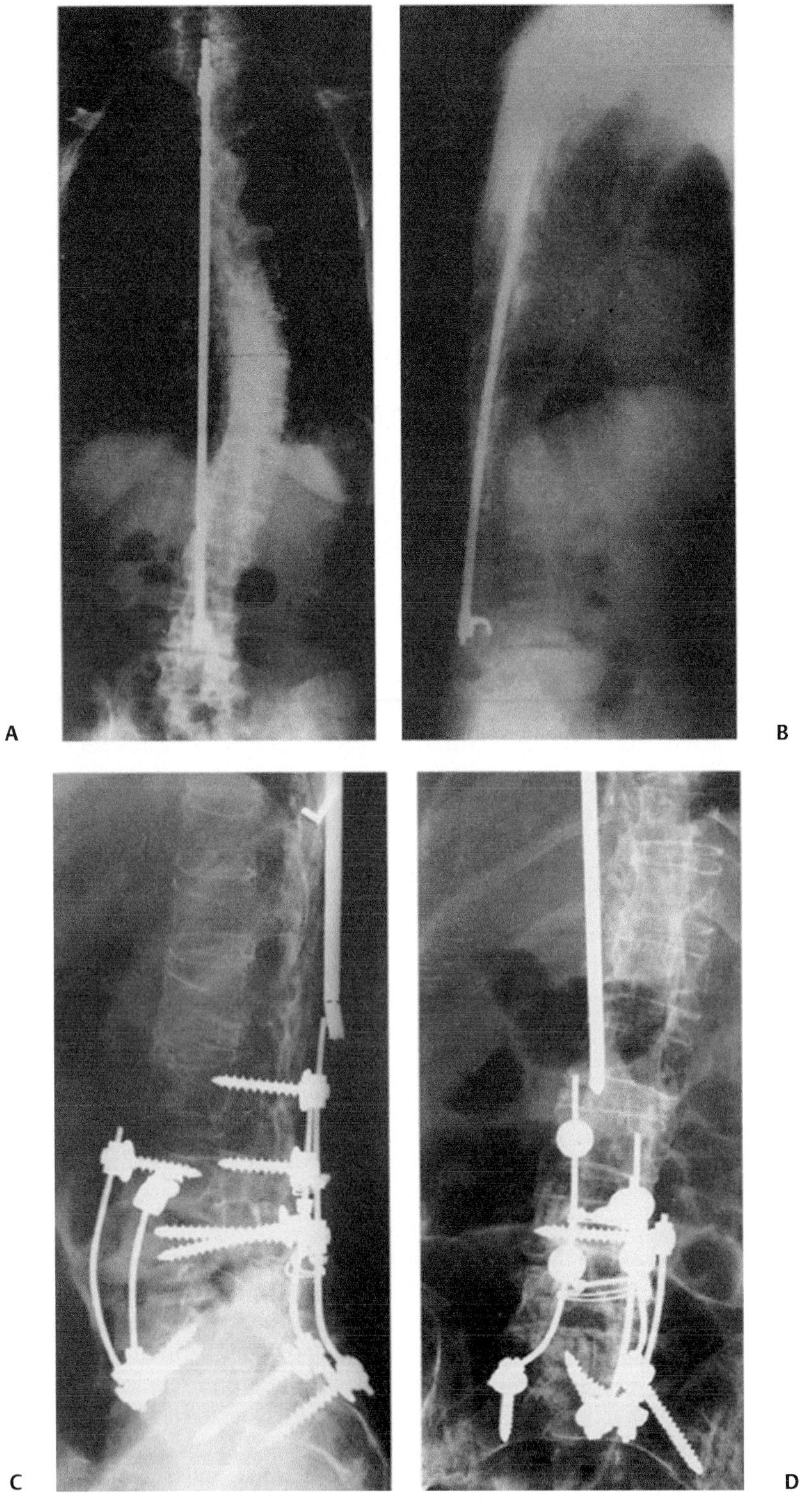


**Fig. 23.1** Radiographs of a 30-year-old woman. **(A)** The anteroposterior view shows previous fusion to L3, done 12 years previously. **(B)** The lateral view shows marked disc narrowing with loss of lordosis within the area of previous fusion and distally. **(C)** Radiograph showing that fusion has been extended to the sacrum with Zielke instrumentation and anterior inter-vertebral-body grafts of iliac crest bone (blocks). **(D)** Radiograph showing that an osteotomy through the pars interarticularis at L4 was done to increase lordosis. (From Kostuik JP, Musha Y. Extension to the sacrum of previous adolescent scoliosis fusions in adult life. Clinical Orthopaedics & Related Research (364):53-60, 1999. Reprinted with permission.)

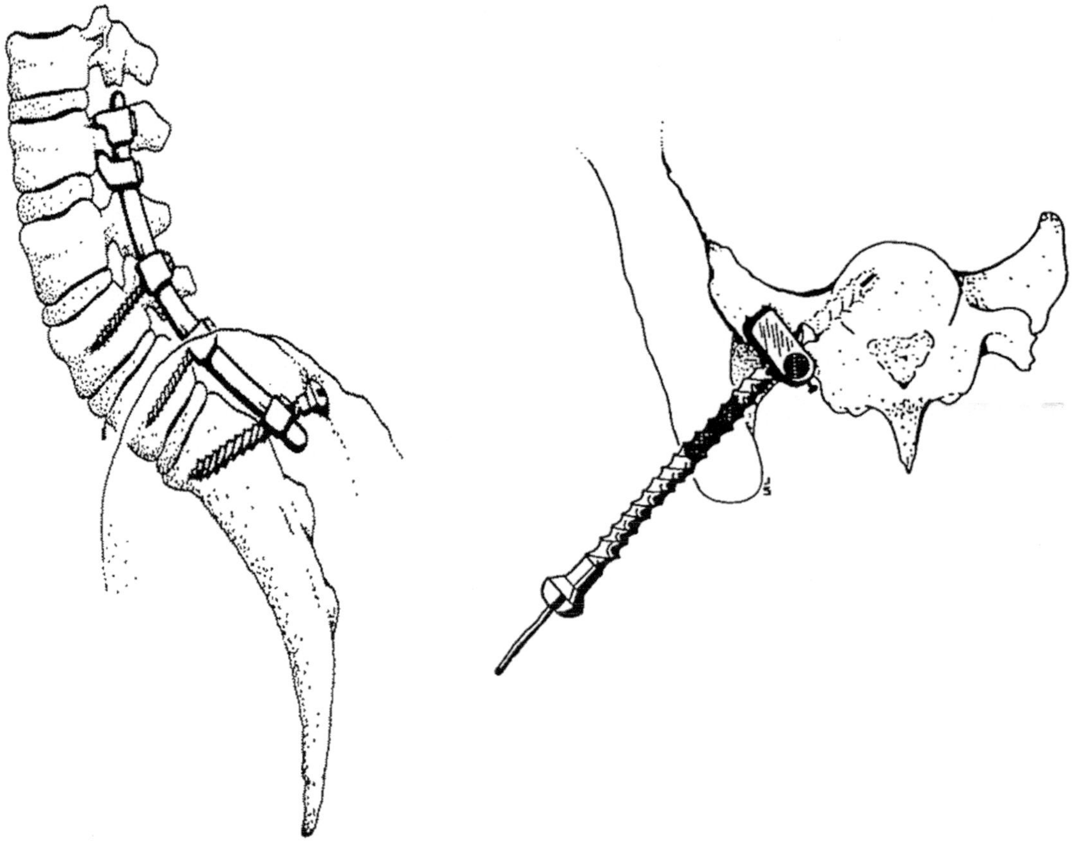

A

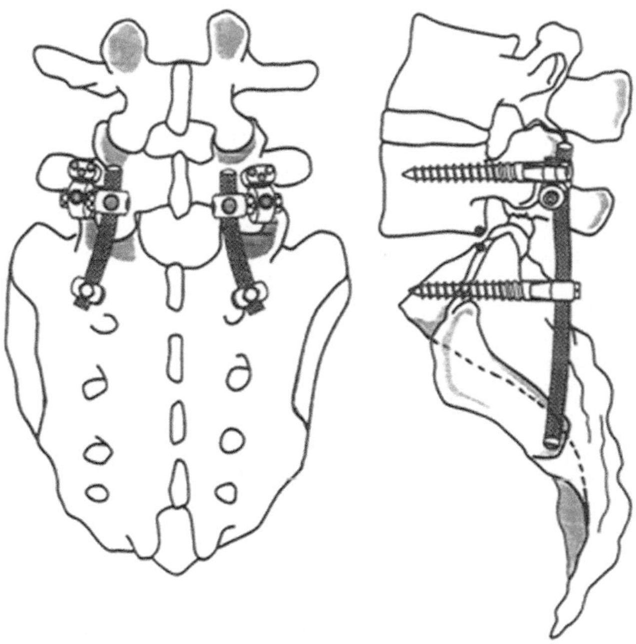

B

**Fig. 23.2** Lumbosacral fixation techniques. **(A)** Iliosacral screw and rods. **(B)** Jackson intrasacral rods.

(*Continued on page 326*)

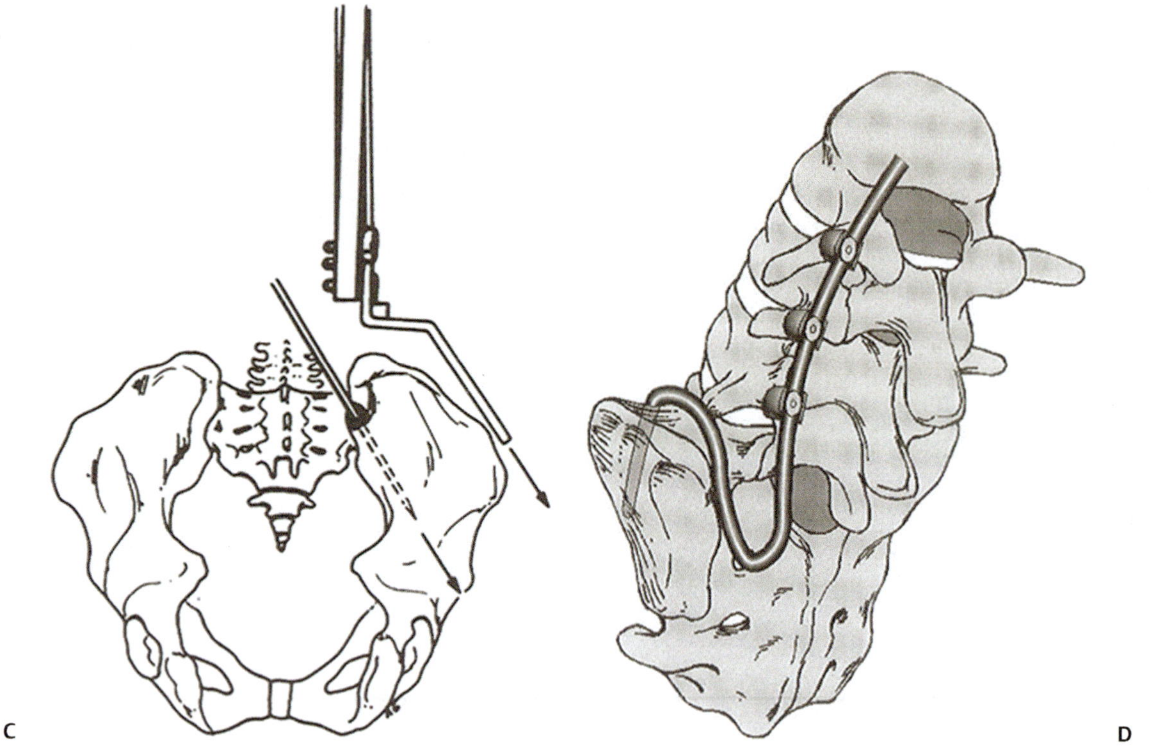


**Fig. 23.2** (*Continued*) Lumbosacral fixation techniques. **(C)** Modified Galveston technique. **(D)** McCarthy–Dunn technique. (**[B–D]** from O'Brien MF. Sacropelvic fixation in spinal deformity. In: DeWald RL, ed. Spinal Deformities: The Comprehensive Text. New York: Thieme Medical Publishers; 2003: 602,605. Reprinted with permission.)

techniques, fixation to the pelvis remains a challenge. As will be discussed, even in the most recent series, rates of pseudarthrosis and complication remain above 20%.[14–18] As a starting point, the anatomy and biomechanics of lumbosacral fixation will be considered.

## Anatomy

The keystone configuration of the sacrum between the iliac wings provides stability in the face of extremely high stresses as weight is transferred from the spine to the pelvis and lower limbs (**Fig. 23.3**). In the sagittal plane, the C7 plumbline falls near the posterior aspect of the L5–S1 disc, defining it as the instantaneous axis of rotation (IAR) for flexion and extension in the lumbosacral spine. The L5–S1 disc is the most vertical intervertebral segment, with the superior endplate of S1 tilted an average of 40 degrees to the horizontal. Consequently, the lumbosacral junction is subject to an enormous amount of stress including bending, shear, and rotational stresses. Consequently, it is logical that the L5–S1 intervertebral segment and lumbosacral junction are not only the areas of the spine most commonly developing degenerative changes, but also the hardest areas to fuse.

The SI joint allows relief of stress from forces coming across the upper three sacral segments and the ilium. Strong ligamentous connections between the spine, sacrum, and ilium include the iliolumbar ligaments, sacroiliac ligaments (posterior and anterior sacroiliac ligaments), and sacrospinous and sacrotuberous ligaments. The SI joint is stabilized anteriorly by the ventral SI ligaments and the sacrospinous ligament and posteriorly by the sacrotuberous and dorsal SI ligaments. The dorsal portion of the SI joint is fibrocartilaginous and is the preferred site into which to pass iliosacral screws (**Fig. 23.4** and **Fig. 23.2A**).[19] An iliosacral screw typically enters the outer table of the ilium at 1 cm below the iliac crest and in line with the S1 superior articular facet, and is directed at a 45-degree angle to the sagittal plane, exiting in the iliosacral space posterior to the SI joint (**Fig. 23.2A**). The screw then proceeds into the S1 pedicle, parallel to the S1 endplate and toward the promontory.[1]

The sacrum is initially composed of five vertebrae, which fuse together as a solid bone in adults (**Fig. 23.5**). Caudally, the sacrum articulates with the coccyx, which has from three to five segments. The sacrum is thickest in the midsagittal plane at S1, where it averages 50 mm thick, but tapers to a thickness of 20 to 30 mm at S3. The sacral canal

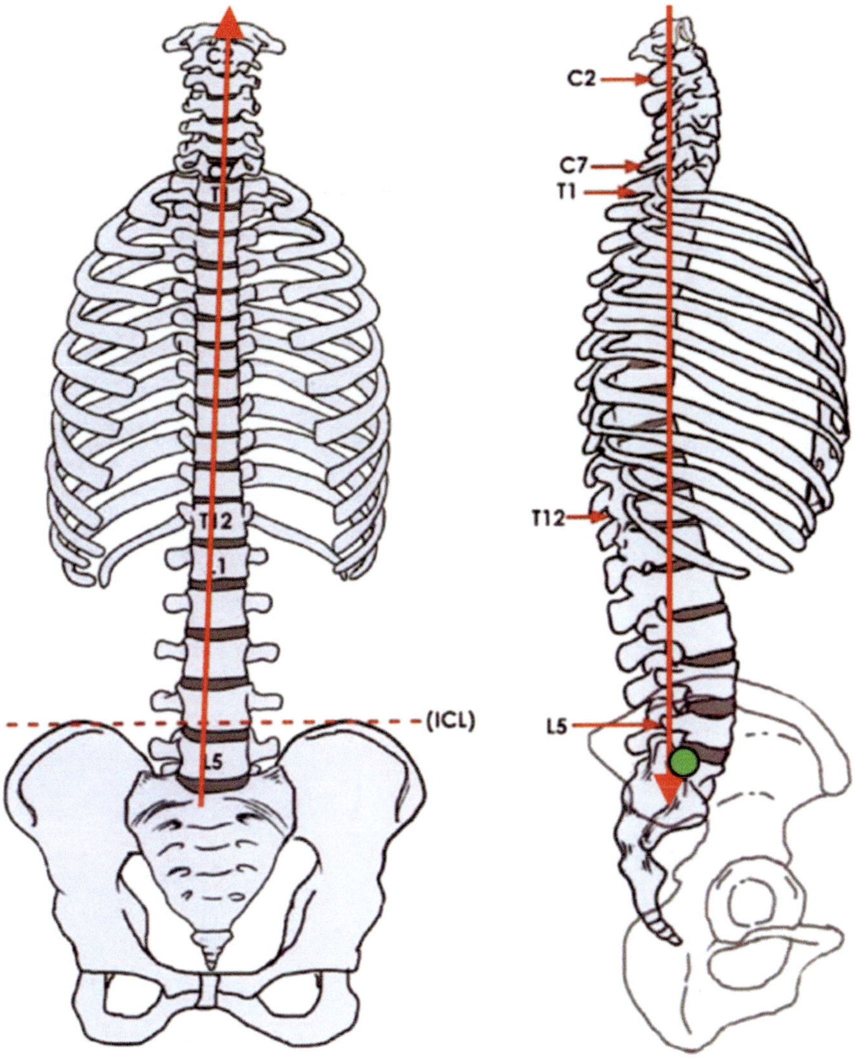


**Fig. 23.3** Frontal and sagittal projections of the spine and pelvis showing the central sacral vertical line (CSVL) and the sagittal plumbline. Normal coronal balance is achieved when C2 is balanced over the midsacrum and all vertebrae are bisected by the CSVL. In the sagittal plane the C2 plumbline falls near the junction of the L5–S1 posterior disc, which is the IAR (shown as a *green circle*) between the spine and pelvis.

is continuous with the lumbar canal and is covered by the lamina. The laminae typically join in the midline to form the spinous processes; however, ~10% of patients have a bifid S1 or S2.

The sacrum has five posterior crests (**Fig. 23.5**). The median sacral crest is the midline ridge of the spinous processes, which extends down to the sacral hiatus and the termination of the dural sac at S3. The rudimentary facets form the two intermediate crests or ridges with four neuroforamina located just lateral to them. Dorsal sensory rami with vessels penetrate the dorsal neuroforamina of the sacrum. There are also two lateral sacral crests, located lateral to the neuroforamina and medial to the ilia, which are the equivalent of transverse processes fused together.

The sacral alae are bound by the intermediate and lateral sacral crests and are a key location for fixation. The upper sacral alae are the structures over which McCarthy rods are passed (**Fig. 23.2D**) and where Harrington sacral hooks were inserted, and are used for bone grafting up to the lumbar transverse processes. Also, Jackson's intrasacral rod technique for SPF involves having the lower portions of the rods inserted into the sacral ala below the S1 pedicle and lateral to the S1 dorsal foramina, with the rods directed inferiorly, laterally, and anteriorly toward the SI joint for a distance of ~30 mm (**Fig. 23.2B**).[9]

Fixation techniques for SPF often involve penetration of the anterior cortex of the sacrum and in some cases anterior approaches to the lumbosacral area are used for fusion. Therefore, the neurovascular anatomy of the lumbosacral region must be taken into account for both implant placement and surgical approaches to lumbosacral fusion (**Fig. 23.6**). The dominant motor-sensory nerve roots in this area exit through the anterior neuroforamina to form the lumbosacral plexus, with portions of L4, L5, and S1 nerve roots passing inferiorly and laterally across the anterior sacral alae. Typically, the bifurcation of the aorta and vena cava into the common iliac vessels occurs anterior to L4 or at the L4–L5 disc, whereas the bifurcation of the common

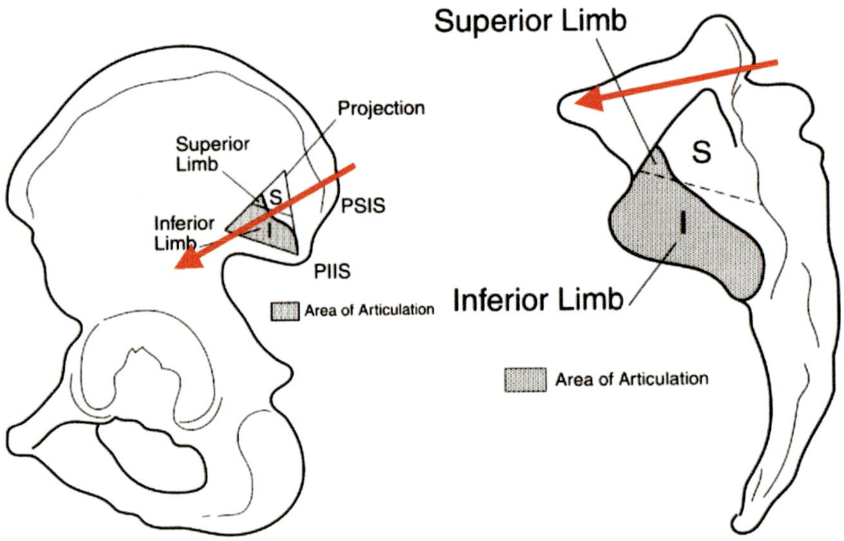


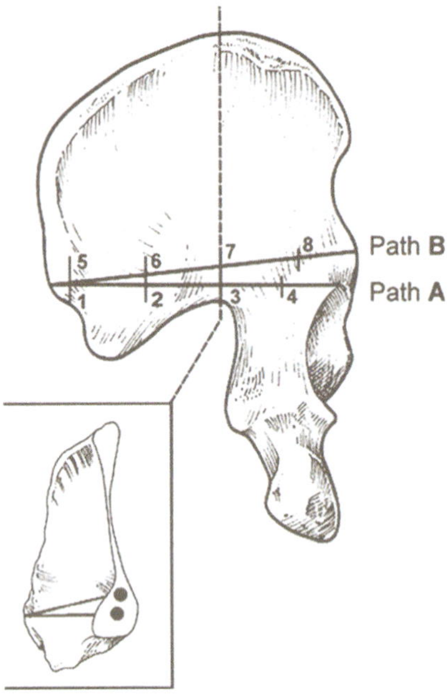


**Fig. 23.4** Lateral projection of the ilium and sacrum demonstrating the path of an iliac screw from the posterior–superior iliac spine along the roof of the ilium, and the sacroiliac joint with dorsal and superior area (labeled S) being the site for passage of iliosacral screws into the S1 body. The red arrow demonstrates the trajectory of an S1 pedicle screw towards the sacral promontory. The lower figure shows that two paths and potentially two screws can be inserted into the ilium (see text).

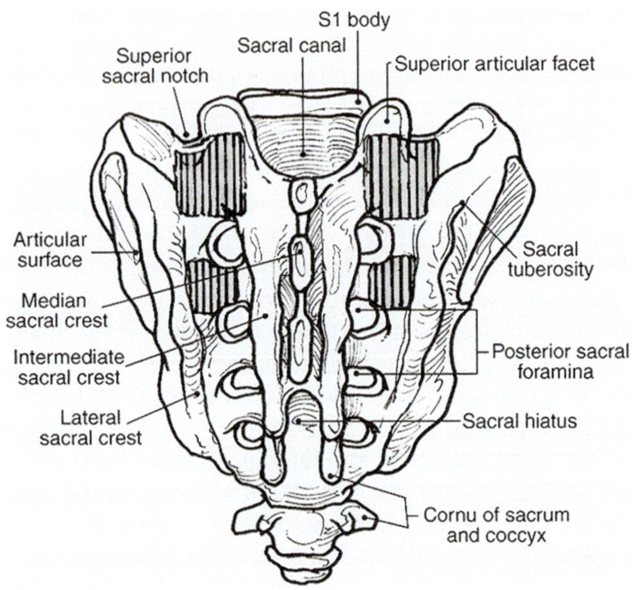


**Fig. 23.5** Posterior sacrum. The *shaded area* denotes the regions of the underlying S1 and S2 pedicles. Permission granted by Arlet V, *Surgical Anatomy of the Sacrum and Pelvis*. In Dewald RL (ed.), *Spinal Deformities: The Comprehensive Text*. New York: Thieme Medical Publishers, 2003.

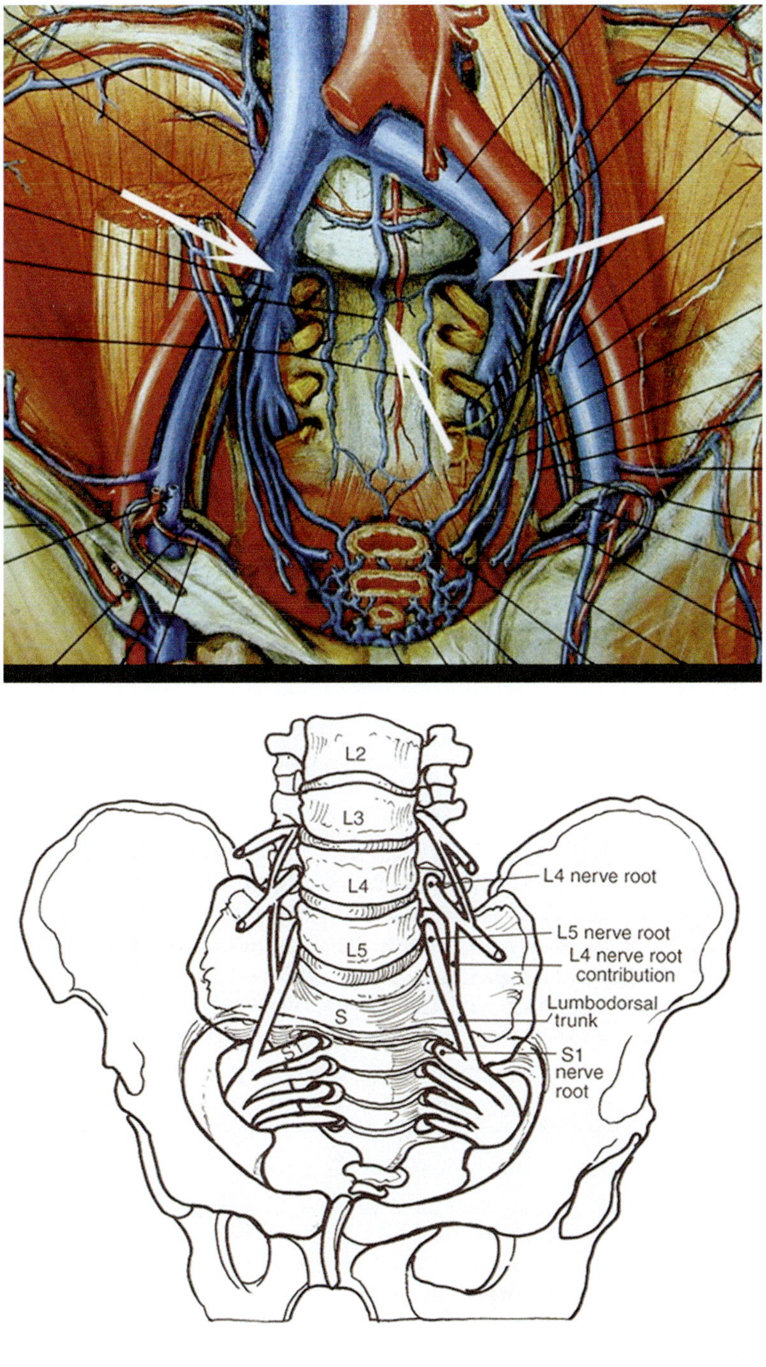


**Fig. 23.6** Vascular and neural structures are shown in relation to the anterior sacrum. The aortic bifurcation to form the common iliac arteries is at the L4–L5 level. The bifurcation of the internal and external iliac vessels is lateral to the L5–S1 disc. Beneath the bifurcation and lying on the sacral ala are parts of the lumbosacral plexus with components from L5 and L4.

iliac vessels into the internal and external iliac vessels is located over the lateral edge of S1, near the anterior SI joint.[20–22] The internal iliac vessels, after arising from the common iliac vessels, lie directly anterior to the ala. The middle sacral artery comes directly off the aorta to lie on the mid sacrum. Also over the midsacrum is the presacral parasympathetic plexus, which is important for sexual function. Damage to this plexus can result in male impotence and retrograde ejaculation.

Given this description of the anterior lumbosacral anatomy, one can see that the safest projection of screws and safest surgical approaches to lumbosacral fusion lie in the midline. For example, S1 pedicle screws should be directed toward the sacral promontory and midline approaches to L5–S1 are preferentially made between the common iliac vessels. If laterally directed screws are used (e.g., alar screws), they should be directed toward the anterior SI joint and not penetrate excessively through the anterior cortex, to avoid injury to the internal iliac veins and roots of the lumbosacral plexus.[23] Blunt self-tapping screws are preferred.

Another aspect of spinopelvic anatomy to keep in mind when approaching the anterior lumbosacral spine is that the left common iliac vein is medial to the artery, whereas the right common iliac artery is medial to the right common iliac vein. Theoretically, a right-of-midline approach to the L5–S1 disc is recommended for keeping away from the left common iliac vein.[22] However, the left paramedian retroperitoneal approach allows both midline access (between the vessels for L5–S1) and a left lateral approach to the L4–L5 disc through ligation of the L4 and L5 lumbar vessels. The surgeon must be aware that variations of this vascular anatomy exist.[21]

## Osteology

The shape and bone quality of the lumbosacral region provide challenges for secure fixation. The lumbar facets are large and sagittally oriented, although in cases of dysplasia the L5–S1 facet can be more horizontal. Under normal circumstances, the L5–S1 facet is quite large and facet screws were one of the first forms of local internal fixation used in the spine.[1,2,24] The screws are inserted at the base of the spinous process and directed laterally across the facet and into the base of the transverse process or ala. This technique has only been tested for short lumbosacral fusions, and is not strong enough as a main fixation method in the long constructs related to scoliosis and SPF.[24]

The junction of the superior S1 endplate with the anterior S1 cortex forms the sacral promontory and is the site of greatest bone density and the strongest fixation point in the sacrum.[25–27] Bone density in the midsacral ala is 30% less than in the S1 body, and within the substance of the ala there is a particular bone void that makes strong fixation at this location unlikely.[28,29] The best bone in the ala is found at the intersection of the lateral ala and anterior sacral trabeculae, anterolateral sacral cortex, and the anterior SI joint (**Fig. 23.7**). Lateral alar screws should therefore be directed to this bone.

For the average adult, the bone dimensions of the L4 and L5 pedicles are ~10 mm by 10 mm in the coronal plane, with L5 being wider than L4. The transverse angle increases caudally, being ~20 degrees for L4 and 30 degrees for L5 and S1.[30] The S1 pedicle is quite large, lying between the intermediate crest (neural canal) and lateral crest (the SI joint) in the region superior to the S1 neuroforamen. Two screw trajectories can be used in the region of the S1 pedicle: one medial and toward the promontory, and one lateral and toward the anterolateral cortex of the ala, as described above (**Fig. 23.7**). Because the S1 pedicles are large, pedicle screws will not necessarily achieve ideal purchase in the cortical bone of the pedicle. The medial S1 pedicle-screw trajectory enters lateral to the S1 articular process and is directed medially (by 20 to 30 degrees) and upward (by 10 to 20 degrees) toward the promontory, to engage the cortex and achieve tricortical purchase. The screws engage the junction of both the anterior cortex of the promontory and the S1 endplate (**Fig. 23.4**). The medial trajectory at S1 maximizes screw length, allows the triangulation of implants, and provides stronger fixation than the lateral S1 screw trajectory (**Fig. 23.7, 23.8**).[27,30,31,32,34,35]

The lateral trajectory involves an alar screw inserted over the S1 pedicle area and directed 30 to 40 degrees laterally, toward the junction of the ala with the SI joint in a dorsal-to-ventral direction (**Fig. 23.7**). As discussed, penetration of the ala endangers the lumbosacral plexus (L4 and L5 nerve roots) and the internal iliac veins, and should be done cautiously and with blunt screws.[20,23] The laterally directed screws are not as strong as those directed into the promontory, but triangulating these two screws will provide stronger fixation than using either one alone.[33]

The S2 pedicle is bounded superiorly and inferiorly by the S1 and S2 neuroforamina, medially by the spinal canal and the intermediate crest, and laterally by the lateral crest (**Fig. 23.5**). Because of the tapered shape of the sacrum, possible screw lengths for sacral fixation decrease rapidly from S1 to S3. Although 40- to 50-mm screws can often be placed in S1 when a medial trajectory is utilized, screws in S2 and S3 may be limited to a length of 25 to 30 mm. As described earlier, sacral bone density is greatest along surfaces where cortical and cancellous bone merge.[28] S2 screws are relatively safe, although penetrating the anterior cortex excessively, particularly on the left, has the potential to damage the sigmoid colon.[23]

The ilium of the pelvis extends posterior to the sacrum as the posterior-superior iliac spine (PSIS), and overhangs the SI joint medially (**Fig. 23.4** and **Fig. 23.7**). A dorsal midline incision is often used to expose the iliac crest, PSIS, and sciatic notch for instrumentation or bone grafting. Subperiosteal exposure of the outer ilium will help avoid injury to the superior gluteal nerve and vessel, located around the sciatic notch. The PSIS of the ilium has a thickness of up to 25 mm and is located inferior to the origin of the dorsal S1 pedicle, with the result that iliac screws will be caudal to the S1 pedicle screw. The PSIS serves as the entry point for the iliac screws, which are directed toward the anterior inferior iliac spine, tracking to within 1.5 cm above the sciatic notch, to capitalize on the thick, trabeculated bone in this region of the ilium (**Fig. 23.4**). When this track is followed, the screws can be up to 10 mm in diameter and 15 cm in length for adults, and at least 7 mm in diameter and 8 cm in length for most adolescents.[34,35] Screw fixation in this iliac column is more secure than is the smooth Galveston-rod technique,[35] but crossing the SI joint can lead to pain. As will be discussed, the mechanical advantages of this approach outweigh its disadvantages.

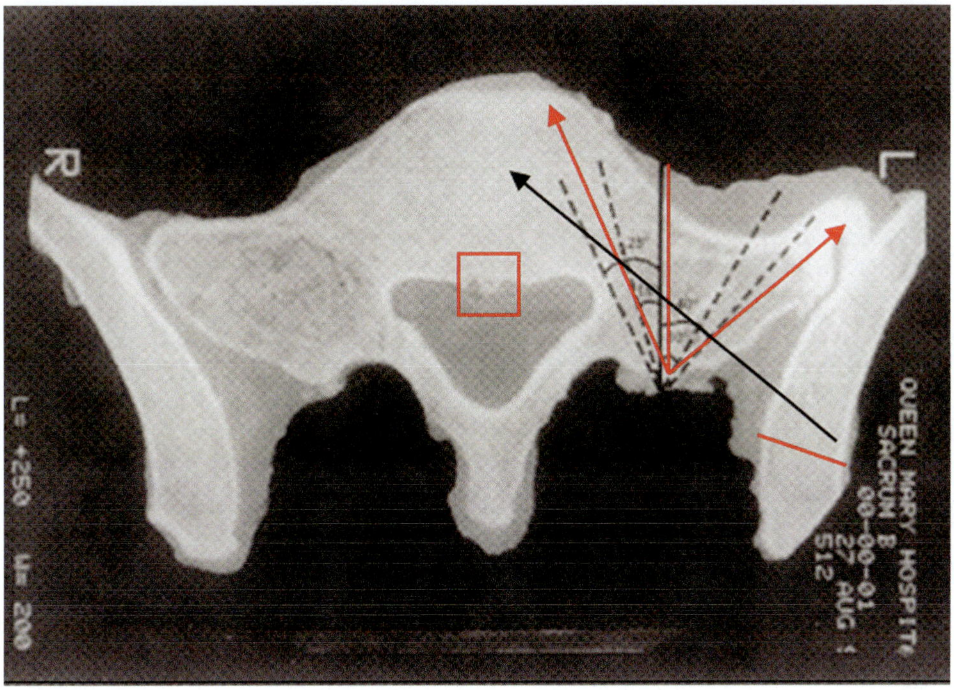


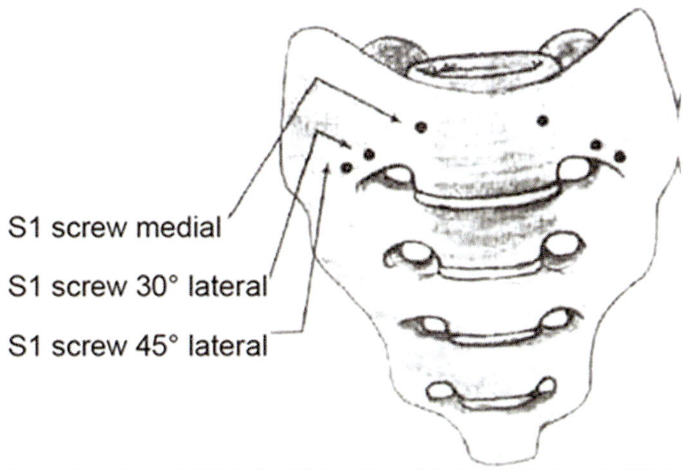


**Fig. 23.7** Cross-section of the iliosacral area at S1. The S1 pedicle screw entry is lateral to the facet and directed 20 to 30 degrees medially, toward the sacral promontory. The screw lengths are typically 45 to 55 mm. An alar screw can also be used and directed laterally at 30 to 40 degrees toward the anterior SI joint. Note also that the width of the iliac wing is ~20 mm and can easily accommodate an iliac screw of up to 8- to 10-mm diameter. The black *arrow shows* the trajectory of an iliosacral screw passing posterior to the SI joint toward the centrum. The *square* shows the IAR. The farther the screw implant extends out from the IAR, the greater the resistance to bending stress (see text).

## Biomechanical Studies

Several important biomechanical studies have been conducted to provide insights into the stability of instrumentation techniques used for SPF. McCord et al used bovine calf specimens instrumented from the sacrum to the thoracolumbar junction to study the load that could be borne before failure occurred in 10 different SPF techniques.[36] The study compared the older Harrington constructs, screw-and-rod constructs, constructs including iliac fixation, iliosacral screw constructs, and plate–block systems combining S1 and distal S2 fixation. One of the

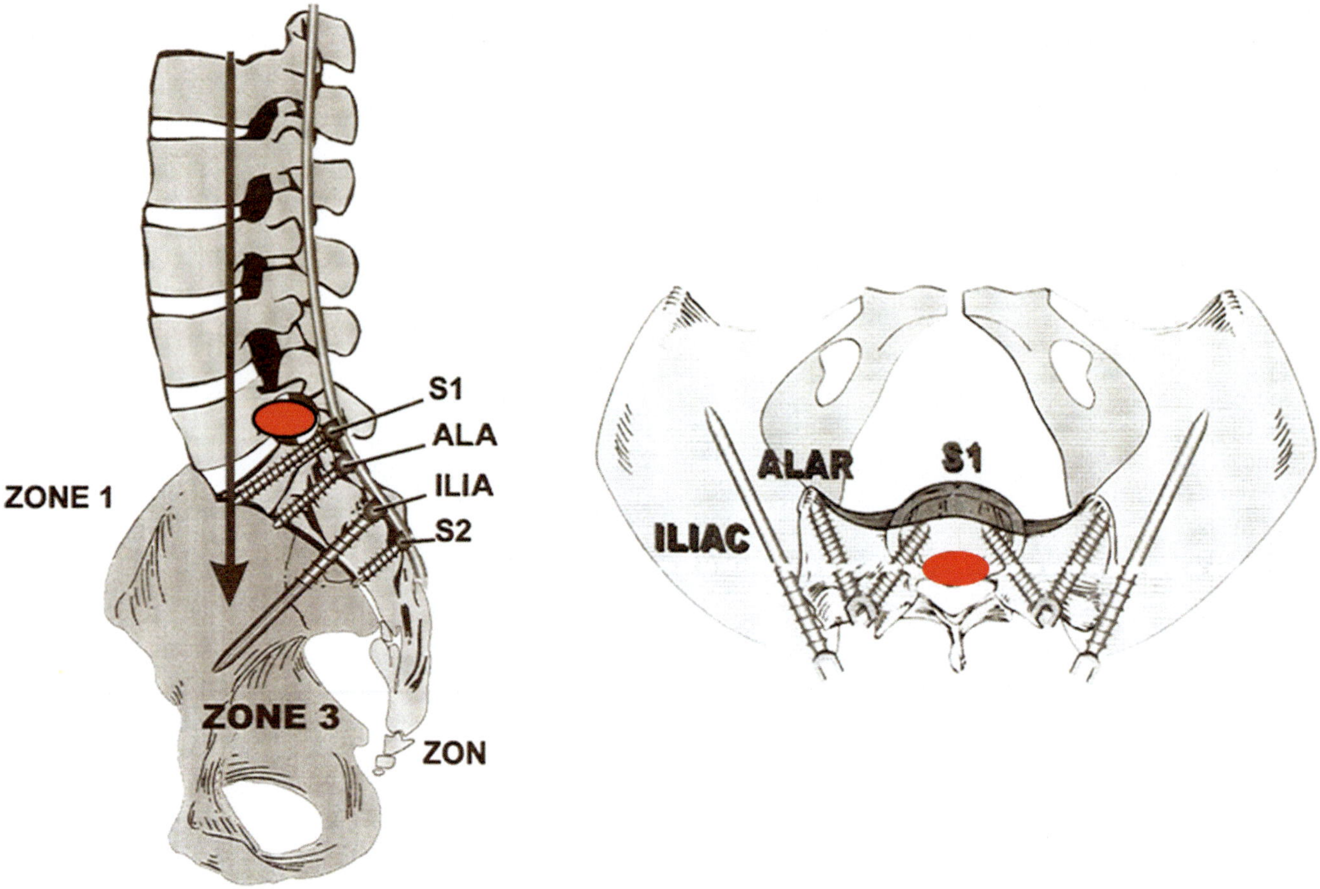


**Fig. 23.8** The *red dot* signifies the IAR. Fixation options in the lumbosacral region will resist bending in proportion to their extension outward from the IAR. Iliac screws extend anteriorly and laterally to a greater extent than do other anchors, and thus have a mechanical advantage over them. (From O'Brien MF. Sacropelvic fixation in spinal deformity. In: DeWald RL, ed. Spinal Deformities: The Comprehensive Text. New York: Thieme Medical Publishers; 2003:609. Reprinted with permission.)

most important points highlighted by the study was the relationship of the constructs to the IAR.[36] As previously described, the middle osteoligamentous column at the posterior L5–S1 disc is the IAR or pivot point for flexion and extension at the lumbosacral junction (**Fig. 23.8**). Therefore, the farther an implant extends outward from the IAR, the greater is its strength for resisting bending. Iliac-screw constructs show the greatest strength against flexion because they extend the farthest distance anterior from the IAR. Also, triangulation will increase the strength of constructs for lumbosacral fusion; therefore, by combining S1 screws with iliac screws, greater strength is achieved than with iliosacral screws alone. S2 screws are generally stronger than hooks, but the fixation strength of S2 is more variable and certainly lower than that of more proximal pedicles.

In a subsequent study, in which they used synthetic models to assess the strength of long (L2–sacrum) constructs, Alegre and colleagues confirmed the strain-reducing effect (70% reduction) of iliac screws on the S1 screw.[37] Because of their anterior position, interbody structural grafts augment SPF and more effectively counter flexion moments than do pedicle screws alone. Alegre and coworkers' study demonstrated that anterior interbody grafts substantially reduce the flexion moment of the S1 screw. However, anterior-column support may not be necessary at L5–S1 when iliac screws are used in constructs unless the anterior-column support is being used to restore sagittal balance. In contrast to other investigators, Alegre and co-workers felt that screw fixation in S2 obviated the need for anterior-column support. A major weakness of their study was that their synthetic model did not replicate the lower pullout strength of S2 screws in human bone, especially in elderly patients.

One must keep in mind that the necessary strength of a construct in the human biological system is not known with certainty. Some strain is necessary to avoid stress shielding, but too much strain will lead to pseudarthrosis. However, long SPF constructs are particularly at risk for implant failure, pseudarthrosis, or both. Cunningham et al used a porcine model to assess lumbosacral constructs and compared four constructs, having pedicle-screw fixation alone; pedicle screws plus an inter-vertebral-body mesh cage; pedicle screws plus iliac screws; and pedicle screws, a cage, and iliac screws.[38] They found that the stiffest construct was provided by the combination of an inter-vertebral-body cage, pedicle screws, and iliac screws. Constructs with iliac screws afforded the most resistance to axial rotation, lateral bending, and sagittal bending. Furthermore, iliac screws are biomechanically preferable to intrasacral rods. Even when mechanical tests are done with lateral bending and rotation, as in flexion–extension, iliac screws show the best performance. Therefore, for long SPF constructs, iliac screws provide the most reliably strong fixation, extending anteriorly, laterally, and some distance caudally to the IAR, and such fixation is certainly preferable to fixation solely at S2 as the distal level of fixation.[13] The added stability with iliac screws justifies crossing the SI joint. Should pain develop in the SI joints, the iliac screws may have to be removed.

The biomechanical success of any construct is particularly dependent on bone quality.[33,39] In cadaveric specimens of subjects <30 years of age, the load to failure of the S1 pedicle-and-alar combination was 1450 N; specimens of subjects >60 years of age showed failure at significantly lower loads (980 N). This documents a 32% lower load to failure in the specimens from older subjects. Studies of the bone mineral density of the lumbar vertebral body indicate that it peaks at ~25 years of age and falls at a rate of 0.46% per year.[28]

## Biomechanical Zones of Fixation

On the basis of the anatomical considerations presented above, the sacropelvic unit can be considered as having three zones for fixation.[1] Zone 1 consists of the S1 body and cephalic half of the ala (**Fig. 23.9**). Zone 2 includes the remaining sacrum including and remaining ala, and the S2 pedicle down to the tip of the coccyx. Zone 3 consists of the iliac wings. The relevance of this zonal classification stems from the fact that the more zones that are included in a construct, the greater the mechanical strength of the resulting SPF.

Fixation options for Zone 1 include S1 screws gaining purchase in the promontory (converging) at the junction of the superior endplate and anterior cortex. Alternatively, divergent sacral ala screws may be used. Anterior interbody structural support with fusion between L5–S1 or L4–L5–S1 allows incorporation of the lowest lumbar vertebrae into "Zone I," creating additional fixation points and more robust fixation options via multilevel posterior pedicle fixation. Bilateral L5–S1 transfacet screws may also be considered for Zone I fixation.[24] Alone, fixation at these sites is not adequate, but

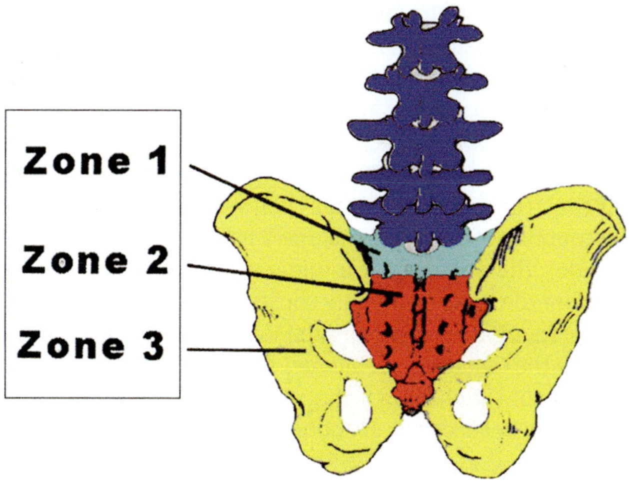


**Fig. 23.9** Fixation points for SPFs can be categorized by osseous zones of the iliosacral unit. Zone 1 includes the S1 vertebra and the upper half of the ala. Fixation options can include S1 pedicle screws and alar screws. Zone 2 comprises S2 and levels below this (the remainder of the sacrum), as well as the lower half of the ala. Fixation options can include intrasacral rods, S2 pedicle screws, alar screws, or hooks in the foramen. The strength of fixation is inferior to that in Zone1 (see text). Fixation in Zone 3 includes iliac screws. Up to two screws on each side can be used if necessary. (From O'Brien MF. Sacropelvic fixation in spinal deformity. In: DeWald RL, ed. Spinal Deformities: The Comprehensive Text. New York: Thieme Medical Publishers; 2003:602. Reprinted with permission.)

when coupled with fixation in other zones it can be a useful component of a multifaceted SPF construct.

Fixation in Zone 2 can improve the strength of a construct for SPF by extending the construct distal to the IAR. Coupling fixation between Zone 2 and Zone 1 is essential for stable fixation[33]; if iliac screws are not used, options for fixation in Zone 2 include S2 pedicle screws with or without laterally directed alar screws linked to S1 via rod or plate-rod constructs.[36] Alar screws take advantage of the significantly thicker bone present in the anterolateral margins of the sacral ala. When coupled with medially directed S1 screws, the diverging paths of the S1 and alar screws in a construct with multiple fixation points anterior to the IAR engage a broad cross-sectional area of the sacrum, providing resistance to flexion forces that is intermediate between that provided by S1 screws alone and S1 screws supplemented with iliac screws.[12,33,36] Leong and colleagues showed the advantage of divergent, triangulated fixation by comparing S1 pedicle screws alone with S1 pedicle screws and alar screws connected through a Chopin block.[33] Coupling of the S1 and alar screws through the Chopin block increased the compression, tension, and torsional stiffness of the resulting system by >100% over that with S1 screws alone. Similarly, an S2–S3 hook-claw construct can be used around the dorsal foramina and may be preferable to a construct using screws; ideally, the hook–claw connections must be linked to an S1 screw to increase the strength of the construct. Screws can also be safely placed in S2 and S3, but are short and generally have low pullout strength, as already mentioned.

The close spacing of anchors in Zone 1 and Zone 2 predisposes to problems such as sacral fractures and hardware prominence. Furthermore, attaching the anchors to the rods of a construct can be difficult even with polyaxial screws. The coupling of Zone 1 with Zone 3 is technically easier and provides the strongest combination for fixation, and is therefore the most commonly chosen option for fixation.

Iliac fixation was popularized for neuromuscular scoliosis with the Galveston technique; however, the smooth rods that are continuous with the spinal fixation in this technique have been largely abandoned in favor of the improved fixation and versatility provided by iliac screws.[40] The most commonly used Zone 3 fixation is with iliac screws, which extend anteriorly and laterally from the IAR to resist flexion, rotation, and lateral bending to a greater extent than do pedicle-screw options (**Fig. 23.8**).[36] Iliac screws have been shown to improve lumbosacral fusion, especially if combined with S1 screws.[13,14] To place an iliac screw, the cancellous bone between the iliac tables is bluntly probed with a pedicle probe to create a trajectory for the screw between the inner and outer iliac tables, just above the sciatic notch. Because of the wide intratabular thickness of the ilium, especially in adults, screws ranging from 7 to 10 mm in diameter can routinely be placed. When additional iliac fixation is required, two screws can be used in each ilium (**Fig. 23.4**).

The heads of iliac screws can be prominent and must be buried to prevent pain. To accomplish this, a notch is cut in the posterior–superior iliac spine at its most caudal extent. The "floor" of the notched area is made level with the posterior cortex of the sacrum to allow the screw head, with its rod connector, to be countersunk below the level of the posterior iliac crest. If a low-profile screw is used and seated as described, and if the rod is contoured along the posterior sacral cortex, the instrumentation will not be prominent. It is prudent to discuss with the patient before surgery the possibility of having to remove the iliac screws after fusion has been achieved if symptoms develop and are related to prominent screw heads or SI joint pain.

Other Zone 3 fixation techniques include the sacral or "Kostuik Bar" and the King modification of the Luque technique, in which the L-rod is placed directly through the ilium in a medial-to-lateral direction.[41,42] It suffices to say that these older techniques do not provide fixation as rigid as do iliac screws.

Iliosacral screws, popularized by Cotrel, pass through the ilium and posterior SI joint into the S1 body, as previously described, thus providing a combination of Zone 1 and Zone 3 fixation (**Fig. 23.2A**). Iliosacral screws resist torsion well, but do not perform as well in resisting bending as do iliac screws because they do not extend as far anteriorly to the IAR.[12,38] Furthermore, iliosacral screws cross the SI joint transversely and require more extensive dissection than does iliac fixation.[43] Iliosacral screws have been combined with iliac screws for cases of neuromuscular deformity, with some success.[44] Arlet and colleagues describe this as "MW" fixation on the basis of the appearance on the radiograph of the bilateral iliosacral screws linked to the bilateral iliac screws.[44]

Unique modes of failure have been identified for each type of fixation within each fixation zone of the spinopelvic unit (**Fig. 23.10**).[36] Facet screws have failed through fracture

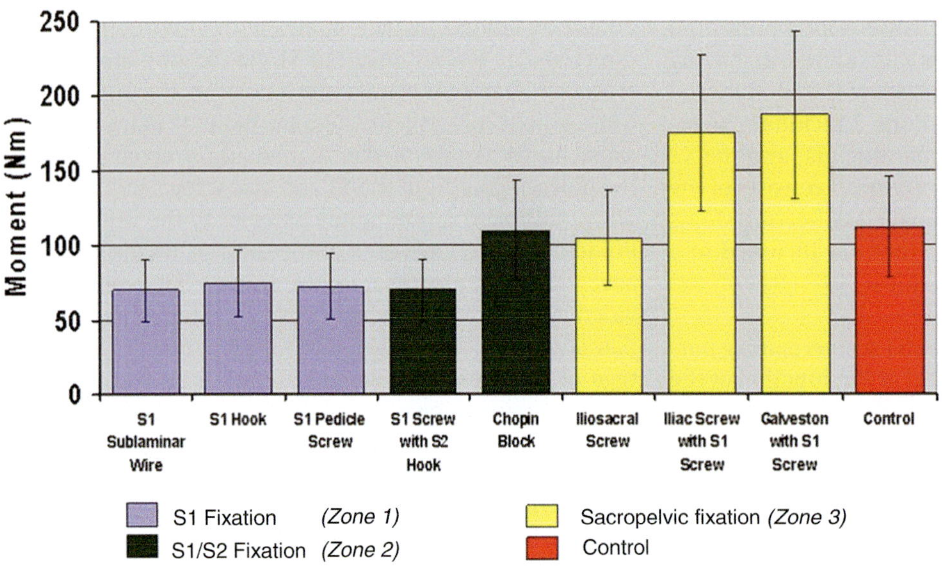


**Fig. 23.10** Data adapted from in vitro biomechanical testing relating lumbosacral fixation zones to the maximum moment at failure. Only iliac-screw constructs with S1 screws had a statistically significantly greater moment at failure. (From McCord DH, Cunningham BW, Shono Y, Myers JJ, McAfee PC. Biomechanical analysis of lumbosacral fixation. Spine 17: Suppl-43, 1992. Reprinted with permission.)

of the S1 facet, with screw pull-through posteriorly. S1 screws protected by S1 hooks begin to fail by hook pullout or lamina fracture followed by screw dislodgment from S1. Chopin blocks in Zone 2 have failed by loosening of the alar screws followed by dislodgment of the S1 screws. Kornblatt et al noted proximal migration of rods within the intrailiac tables as being the mode of failure for Galveston fixation in Zone 3.[24] McCord and colleagues identified delamination of the ilium, with the subsequent migration of iliac screws within the intrailiac tables, followed by fracture of the sacrum and the dislodgment of S1 screws.[36] These findings make it clear that failure begins at the most distal fixation point when a flexion force is applied to the model.

## Clinical Series Review

There is little doubt that adult scoliosis patients with fixed lumbosacral deformities and pain present a challenging problem. Indications for surgical reconstruction in such cases are usually unremitting pain with or without radiculopathy and significant deformity. As described by Kostuik et al, these adults have typically had previous fusions as adolescents, and then develop pain and/or radiculopathy in the unfused distal segment of the spine.[3] In reviewing 107 such cases treated between 1975 and 1996, Kostuik and colleagues demonstrated the evolution of techniques required to establish SPF. In the cases they reviewed, 91% of patients presented with back pain and 24% had associated sciatica. Fixation and fusion techniques changed from posterior fixation in the form of Harrington instrumentation to techniques with anterior and posterior approaches and segmental fixation. With this, the rate of pseudarthrosis reportedly dropped from 83 to 3%. Nineteen patients required spinal osteotomies to restore lordosis, for which the pedicle substraction technique was adopted.[45] The incidence of complications was high, with 18 intraoperative vascular tears, 15 neurological deficits (2 of which were permanent), and 10 instances of respiratory distress. In addition, one patient developed severe coagulopathy, another developed pancreatitis, two patients had delayed ureteral obstruction from pelvic fibrosis, and three patients reported postoperative SI joint pain. Although the techniques for SPF have improved, such fixation is still a challenging clinical problem.

In 1986, Balderston and coworkers reviewed 43 patients instrumented to the sacrum for fusion proximal to T11.[17] Of those treated with posterior instrumentation using Harrington distraction rods with sacral hooks, combined with Harrington compression rods over the convexity of their scoliotic curves, 72% experienced treatment failure, which included pseudarthrosis, decompensation into kyphosis, or loss of lordosis. However, when an anterior fusion was combined with a posterior fusion, or when a posterior fusion was augmented with bone graft in a second stage, the failure rate fell to 28% (5 of 18 cases). Failures again consisted of pseudarthrosis and collapse into kyphosis. Balderston et al concluded that anterior inter-vertebral-body fusion was an important step in attaining a stable lumbosacral fusion.

In a similar study, Emami and associates reviewed 54 adult patients with deformities treated with long instrumented anterior fusions (proximal to T11 from the sacrum).[40] The purpose of their review was to assess which fixation techniques—iliac screws, Galveston rods or sacral screws—were best at maintaining correction. These surgeons used several key procedures in their cohort, including structural anterior grafts to preserve lordosis at L4–L5 and L5–S1, posterior osteotomies to restore lordosis, and posterior instrumentation. They concluded that failures were more likely if sagittal balance was not restored. Emami and colleagues concluded that the Galveston technique was inferior to iliac screws in terms of achieving fusion. Ultimately, they recommended either an inter-vertebral-body graft or iliac screws to augment posterior instrumentation and fusion. If iliac screws are used, they may require removal after solid fusion is verified, and Emami et al suggested that this be discussed with patients in advance.[40]

In a similar series, Islam and colleagues reviewed the hospital and clinic charts of 41 patients (40 female, 1 male) at a mean of 41 months (range: 24 to 116 months) after surgery for extension to the pelvis of previous fusions for scoliosis. Thirty-nine of the 41 patients had combined anterior and posterior approaches; 2 had posterior extension only. Complications were seen in 30 of the 41 patients. The pseudarthrosis rate was 37% (15 of 41 patients ) and was significantly related to the method of distal posterior fixation. With sacral fixation only, the rate of pseudarthrosis was 53% (8 of 15 patients), with iliac fixation only it was 42% (3 of 7 patients), and with both iliac and sacral fixation it was 21% (4 of 19 patients).[15] This and other studies confirm that fixation including at least two zones is needed to achieve lumbosacral rigidity, and that the use of three zones is preferable.[13,16]

Kim and associates identified three risk factors for later implant failure including: (1) failure to correct sagittal balance (persistent forward sagittal balance); (2) inadequate sacropelvic fixation (not using both iliac screws and S1 screws); and (3) older age.[16] They also concluded that the direct access to the L5–S1 disc provided by a paramedian anterior approach led to a greater rate of fusion than does the lateral thoracoabdominal approach.

Most recently, Schwab et al, reporting for a multicenter spinal-deformity treatment group, analyzed the relationship between deformity, surgical approach, and outcome.[18] This study included 784 patients, of whom 268 underwent surgery, with the surgery in 192 patients (72%) involving fusion to the pelvis. Although the prime indicator for surgery was pain, the radiographic findings most closely associated with surgery included loss of lumbar lordosis (51%), positive global truncal balance (58%: >9.5 cm; 46%: 4 to 9.5 cm), and lateral listhesis or subluxation (52%). Circumferential procedures were done in 45 to 50% of all cases and in up to 65% of cases with severe subluxation. Osteotomies and posterior approaches were used to address the positive truncal balance and loss of lumbar lordosis. In this recent series, more than 80% of patients with positive global truncal balance (>4 cm) underwent fusion to the sacrum. In terms of outcome measures, including scores on the Oswestry Disability Index, Scoliosis Research Society (SRS-22) instrument, and Short Form (SF)-12, patients with loss of lordosis and positive balance had the greatest disability and the greatest improvement when their scoliotic curves were surgically corrected. When the group that had fusion to the sacrum was compared with the group that had fusion into the lumbar spine only, the former group had greater disability at baseline. The changes in SRS scores following surgery were not statistically different. Complications occurred in 35% of the patients who had fusion to the sacrum, compared with 20% of those who had fusion into the lumbar spine. Thus, as shown in older studies, complications are highest in patients with positive truncal balance.

## Complications of Spinopelvic Fixation

The surgical complications experienced with SPF techniques reflect the high stress on the implants used in them owing to the magnitude of the deformity being treated, the extent of the surgical procedures used for fusion, the advanced age and comorbidities of the population undergoing these procedures, and the poor quality of bone in this population. Perioperative complications include dural tears, pneumonia, urinary tract infections, deep venous thrombosis, radiculopathy from screw impingement, cauda equina from hematoma, and implant infections. Later complications come from mechanical failure. Perhaps the single greatest cause of screw pullout or rod fracture and pseudarthrosis in SPF is failure to restore sagittal balance. Bone grafting is essential, and the use of bone morphogenic protein is now common for reducing the risk of these mechanical complications. Also, fixation including at least two zones (if not three zones) of fixation, with augmented anterior-column support, is advised in modern techniques of SPF.

The insertion of any implant can be associated with technical errors. Alar screws that are too long can cause injury to the lumbosacral plexus or internal iliac vessels. S1 pedicle screws that violate the walls of the pedicle can irritate the nerve root or penetrate the dura. S2 screws that protrude anteriorly can injure the colon. Iliac screws that are too long can enter the acetabulum, and if inserted too medially can injure the internal iliac vessels or if inserted too low can injure the superior gluteal vessels. Bilateral iliac-wing fractures and sacral fractures have been reported with iliac fixation (Dwyer, O'Brien presentation at SRS in Cleveland 2001).[46,47] Fracture of the proximal sacrum at the level of S1 pedicle screws may be entirely overlooked if it is nondisplaced, but can progress to a traumatic spondylooptosis. Thin-slice computed tomography scanning with sagittal and coronal reconstructions may be necessary to confirm this condition.

## Conclusion

SPF is necessary to achieve frontal and sagittal balance in cases of multilevel lumbar deformity or deformity below long constructs. The fixation must include as many sites (zones) as necessary to overcome the weak bone stock in the pelvis and the anticipated mechanical stresses, thereby avoiding construct failure and pseudarthrosis. Fixation should extend out from the IAR in all directions, especially in the flexion and extension plane, because bending in this plane is the typical mode of clinical failure at the lumbosacral junction. Augmented anterior inter-vertebral-body fusions are recommended to increase the strength of the SPF construct. Familiarity with the anatomy of the lumbosacral region and surgical skill are needed to create the requisite constructs and avoid operative complications that can include damage to the SI joint, skin breakdown over prominent hardware, dural penetration, nerve-root impingement, vascular injury, and visceral injury.

### References


1. O'Brien MF. Sacropelvic fixation in spinal deformity. In: DeWald RL, ed. Spinal Deformities: The Comprehensive Text. New York: Thieme; 2003:601–614
2. Moshirfar A, Rand FF, Sponseller PD, et al. Pelvic fixation in spine surgery. Historical overview, indications, biomechanical relevance, and current techniques. [Review] [65 refs] J Bone Joint Surg Am 2005;87(suppl 2):89–106
3. Kostuik JP, Musha Y. Extension to the sacrum of previous adolescent scoliosis fusions in adult life. Clin Orthop Relat Res 1999; 364:53–60
4. Kostuik JP, Hall BB. Spinal fusions to the sacrum in adults with scoliosis. Spine 1983;8:489–500
5. Kostuik JP. Treatment of scoliosis in the adult thoracolumbar spine with special reference to fusion to the sacrum. Orthop Clin North Am 1988;19:371–381

6. Luque ER. The anatomic basis and development of segmental spinal instrumentation. Spine 1982;7:256–259
7. Luque ER. Segmental spinal instrumentation for correction of scoliosis. Clin Orthop Relat Res 1982;163:192–198
8. Ogilvie JW, Schendel M. Comparison of lumbosacral fixation devices. Clin Orthop Relat Res 1986;203:120–125
9. Jackson RP, McManus AC. The iliac buttress. A computed tomographic study of sacral anatomy. Spine 1993;18:1318–1328
10. McCarthy RE, Dunn HK, McCullough FL. Luque fixation to the sacral ala using the Dunn-McCarthy modification. Spine 1989;14:281–283
11. Allen BLJ Jr, Ferguson RL. The Galveston technique for L rod instrumentation of the scoliotic spine. Spine 1982;7:276–284
12. Farcy JP, Rawlins BA, Glassman SD. Technique and results of fixation to the sacrum with iliosacral screws. Spine 1992;17(6, suppl): S190–S195
13. Lebwohl NH, Cunningham BW, Dmitriev A, et al. Biomechanical comparison of lumbosacral fixation techniques in a calf spine model. Spine 2002;27:2312–2320
14. Tsuchiya K, Bridwell KH, Kuklo TR, Lenke LG, Baldus C. Minimum 5-year analysis of L5-S1 fusion using sacropelvic fixation (bilateral S1 and iliac screws) for spinal deformity. Spine 2006;31:303–308
15. Islam NC, Wood KB, Transfeldt EE, et al. Extension of fusions to the pelvis in idiopathic scoliosis. Spine 2001;26:166–173
16. Kim YJ, Birdwell KH, Lenke LG, Rhim S, Cheh G. Pseudoarthrosis in long adult spinal deformity instrumentation and fusion to the sacrum: Prevalence and risk factor analysis of 144 cases. Spine 2006;31:2329–2336
17. Balderston RA, Winter RB, Moe JH, Bradford DS, Lonstein JE. Fusion to the sacrum for nonparalytic scoliosis in the adult. Spine 1986;11:824–829
18. Schwab F, Lafage V, Farcy JP, et al. Surgical rates and operative outcome analysis in thoracolumbar and lumbar major adult scoliosis: Application of the new adult deformity classification. Spine 2007;32:2723–2730
19. Xu R, Ebraheim NA, Douglas K, Yeasting RA. The projection of the lateral sacral mass on the outer table of the posterior ilium. Spine 1996;21:790–794, discussion 795
20. Ebraheim NA, Xu R, Farooq A, Yeasting RA. The quantitative anatomy of the iliac vessels and their relation to anterior lumbosacral approach. J Spinal Disord 1996;9:414–417
21. Isaacs RC, Fessler RG. The lumbar and sacral spine: Anatomy and surgical approaches and exposures of the vertebral column. In: Benzel EC, ed. Spine Surgery: Techniques, Complications, Avoidance and Management, ed. 2. Philadelphia: Elsevier; 2005:294–315
22. Hoppenfeld S, deBoer P. The spine. In: Hannon BC, ed. Surgical Exposures in Orthopaedics: The Anatomic Approach, ed. 2. Philadelphia: Lippincott; 1994:215–302
23. Mirkovic S, Abitbol JJ, Steinman J, et al. Anatomic consideration for sacral screw placement. Spine 1991;16(6, suppl):S289–S294
24. Kornblatt MD, Casey MP, Jacobs RR. Internal fixation in lumbosacral spine fusion. A biomechanical and clinical study. Clin Orthop Relat Res 1986;203:141–150
25. Smith SA, Abitbol JJ, Carlson GD, Anderson DR, Taggart KW, Garfin SR. The effects of depth of penetration, screw orientation, and bone density on sacral screw fixation. Spine 1993;18:1006–1010
26. Ebraheim N, Sabry FF, Nadim Y, Xu R, Yeasting RA. Internal architecture of the sacrum in the elderly. An anatomic and radiographic study. Spine 2000;25:292–297
27. Luk KD, Chen L, Lu WW. A stronger bicortical sacral pedicle screw fixation through the s1 endplate: An in vitro cyclic loading and pull-out force evaluation. Spine 2005;30:525–529
28. Zheng Y, Lu WW, Zhu Q, Qin L, Zhong S, Leong JC. Variation in bone mineral density of the sacrum in young adults and its significance for sacral fixation. Spine 2000;25:353–357
29. Peretz AM, Hipp JA, Heggeness MH. The internal bony architecture of the sacrum. Spine 1998;23:971–974
30. Ebraheim NA, Xu R, Li J, Yeasting RA. Computed tomographic considerations of dorsal sacral screw placement. J Spinal Disord 1998;11:71–74
31. Lu J, Ebraheim NA, Yang H, Heck BE. Anatomic evaluation of the first three sacral vertebrae and dorsal screw placement. Am J Orthop 2000;29:376–379
32. Lehman RA Jr, Kuklo TR, Belmont PJ Jr, Andersen RC, Polly DW Jr. Advantage of pedicle screw fixation directed into the apex of the sacral promontory over bicortical fixation: A biomechanical analysis. Spine 2002;27:806–811
33. Leong JC, Lu WW, Zheng Y, Zhu Q, Zhong S. Comparison of the strengths of lumbosacral fixation achieved with techniques using one and two triangulated sacral screws. Spine 1998;23: 2289–2294
34. Berry JL, Stahurski T, Asher MA. Morphometry of the supra sciatic notch intrailiac implant anchor passage. Spine 2001;26: E143–E148
35. Schwend RM, Sluyters R, Najdzionek J. The pylon concept of pelvic anchorage for spinal instrumentation in the human cadaver. Spine 2003;28:542–547
36. McCord DH, Cunningham BW, Shono Y, Myers JJ, McAfee PC. Biomechanical analysis of lumbosacral fixation. Spine 1992;17(8, suppl): S235–S243
37. Alegre GM, Gupta MC, Bay BK, Smith TS, Laubach JE. S1 screw bending moment with posterior spinal instrumentation across the lumbosacral junction after unilateral iliac crest harvest. Spine 2001;26:1950–1955
38. Cunningham BW, Lewis SJ, Long J, Dmitriev AE, Linville DA, Bridwell KH. Biomechanical evaluation of lumbosacral reconstruction techniques for spondylolisthesis: an in vitro porcine model. Spine 2002;27:2321–2327
39. Carlson GD, Abitbol JJ, Anderson DR, et al. Screw fixation in the human sacrum. An in vitro study of the biomechanics of fixation. Spine 1992;17(6, suppl):S196–S203
40. Emami A, Deviren V, Berven S, Smith JA, Hu SS, Bradford DS. Outcome and complications of long fusions to the sacrum in adult spine deformity: Luque-Galveston, combined iliac and sacral screws, and sacral fixation. Spine 2002;27:776–786
41. King AG, Thomas KA, Eiserloh HL III, Mills TE, Pisciotta DN. Analysis of the STIF technique for spino-pelvic fixation: Clinical results in 19 patients with neuromuscular scoliosis. J Pediatr Orthop 2000; 20:667–676
42. Widmann RF, Hresko MT, Hall JE. Lumbosacral fusion in children and adolescents using the modified sacral bar technique. Clin Orthop Relat Res 1999;364:85–91
43. Ebraheim NA, Xu R, Biyani A, Nadaud MC. Morphologic considerations of the first sacral pedicle for iliosacral screw placement. Spine 1997;22:841–846
44. Arlet V, Marchesi D, Papin P, Aebi M. The "MW' sacropelvic construct: An enhanced fixation of the lumbosacral junction in neuromuscular pelvic obliquity. Eur Spine J 1999;8:229–231

45. Bridwell KH, Lewis SJ, Rinella A, Lenke LG, Baldus C, Blanke K. Pedicle subtraction osteotomy for the treatment of fixed sagittal imbalance. Surgical technique. J Bone Joint Surg Am 2004;86A(suppl 1):44–50
46. Koh YD, Kim JO, Lee JJ. Stress fracture of the pelvic wing-sacrum after long-level lumbosacral fusion: A case report. Spine 2005; 30:E161–E163
47. Dwyer, TF, O'Brien MF, Dewald C, Gelb DG, Flawn LB, Lowe TG, Donnelly RE. Traumatic sacral spondylolisthesis following instrumentation mentation for spinal deformity. Spine: Affiliated Society Meeting Abstracts 2001. Meeting Abstracts: Scoliosis Research Society, Paper 55, 2001

# 24 Untreated Late-onset Idiopathic Scoliosis and Revision Surgery in Adults

*Charles A. Sansur, Rod J. Oskouian Jr, Michael F. O'Brien, and Christopher I. Shaffrey*

The evaluation and management of late-onset adult idiopathic scoliosis (LIS) can present a significant challenge to the spine surgeon. With aging, many patients with untreated adolescent idiopathic scoliosis (AIS) have minimal or no symptoms related to scoliosis. In a subgroup of patients, however, aging is accompanied by degenerative changes at the facet joints and discs that can eventually result in the progression of scoliotic curvature, pain, or neural impingement. Unlike the treatment of AIS during adolescence, the management of LIS often requires the principles and techniques developed for treating degenerative scoliosis. Compared with the surgical management of AIS in the young patient, the greater likelihood of degeneration in the lower lumbar spine and at the lumbosacral junction with aging often results in the need for more extensive surgical procedures in LIS.[1] Special attention is required in the evaluation of adults with a known history of AIS who have coronal curves with Cobb angles >40 degrees, or who have developed coronal or sagittal imbalance, or both.[2,3]

This chapter discusses in detail the salient points in the evaluation and management of LIS. It also discusses the natural history and presenting symptoms of LIS, and the outcomes of its nonoperative management. The differences in the types of adult spinal deformity are reviewed, focusing mainly on the diagnosis and treatment of LIS and the differences in its evaluation and management, when compared to degenerative scoliosis. The effect of age and medical comorbidity on the risks of surgical intervention, surgical planning, and the outcomes and complications associated with surgical intervention in LIS are examined. Surgical strategies including the planning of instrumentation levels, the use of and indications for lumbosacral and spinopelvic fixation, and strategies to reduce pseudarthrosis and instrumentation failure are discussed in detail. Methods for reducing common complications and future directions in the surgical management of LIS are also explored.

## Natural History of Untreated Adolescent and Late-onset Idiopathic Scoliosis

Approximately half a million adults in the United States have spinal curves >30 degrees.[4,5] However, the decision to operate on patients with LIS should be based on the premise that the surgery will ease pain and improve function as compared with the natural history of the disease, and will have a relatively low incidence of adverse sequelae. To better understand the treatment of LIS, one must first understand the natural history of untreated idiopathic scoliosis, because many patients with LIS have had undiagnosed or untreated AIS. Another category of LIS comprises patients who have had surgical management of AIS but who have developed symptoms as a consequence of this or have developed degeneration or decompensation in unfused segments of the spine.

Many cases of untreated AIS are asymptomatic or minimally symptomatic throughout adulthood and never require any form of medical management. Several studies have disproved the notion that all types of idiopathic scoliosis inevitably end in disability. In 1969, Collis et al[6] reviewed a series of 215 untreated patients with LIS and 100 controls with more than 20 years of follow-up. In 71% of this group, spinal curvatures were >50 degrees. These patients were not treated and were found after more than 20 years of follow-up to have productive lives with minimal disability from their scoliosis.[6] Korovessis and co-workers[7] followed 91 patients with lumbar curvatures >10 degrees for more than 2 years, and were able to identify multiple risk factors for progression of their curvature. Patients at the greatest risk for progression had curves >30 degrees, >30% apical vertebral rotation, 6 mm or more of lateral listhesis, and degenerative disc disease at the lumbosacral junction.

In a recent landmark prospective study, Weinstein and co-workers[3] compared 117 patients who had had untreated

AIS with 62 age- and sex-matched volunteers at a 50-year follow-up. The mean age of the patients was 66 years. The main outcomes assessed were mortality, back pain, pulmonary symptoms, general function, depression, and body image. There was no significant difference in survival in the patient and volunteer groups. However, there was an increased likelihood of difficulty in breathing in the scoliosis group, which was statistically significant for patients with a Cobb angle >80 degrees and a thoracic apex of their curvature. Sixty-one percent of the scoliosis patients reported chronic back pain, as compared with 35% of the controls ($P$ = 0.003). There was no significant difference in clinical depression in the two groups, but body satisfaction in the scoliosis patient group was significantly poorer than in the control group.[3]

Additionally, Weinstein and coworkers' study showed that coronal curves progress longitudinally and that almost 70% of patients with untreated AIS have progression of their curves after skeletal maturity. Thoracic curves >50 degrees progressed on average by 1 degree per year; however, thoracic curves <30 degrees did not show a propensity to progress over time. Thoracolumbar (TL) curves progressed by ~0.5 degrees per year, whereas purely lumbar curves progressed by 0.24 degrees per year.[3]

Although many adult patients with LIS experience few symptoms, a subpopulation of patients develops significant chronic symptoms that respond poorly to nonsurgical measures. Dickson et al[8] described 81 patients with adult idiopathic scoliosis who underwent surgery, and compared them with 30 patients who refused surgery. The treated patients had "significantly reduced pain (and) fatigue and increased function." Eighty percent of these patients reported some pain relief with surgery, whereas only 10% reported some relief of pain without surgery. However, the relief of pain came at the cost of a 43% overall incidence of early and late complications with surgery.

## Late-onset Idiopathic versus Degenerative Scoliosis

Adult scoliosis can generally be divided into two major types.[5,9–12] LIS develops before skeletal maturity but may become symptomatic in adulthood. Degenerative scoliosis develops after skeletal maturity. The coronal curves in LIS often consist of a main thoracic (MT), proximal thoracic (PT), or TL curve, whereas the curves in degenerative scoliosis are primarily found in the TL or lumbar spine. As patients with LIS age, their pre-existing scoliosis may be complicated by facet-joint pain, disc degeneration, and curve progression.

LIS is an imprecise name for the condition to which it is applied. It can include cases of AIS that were never diagnosed during childhood or adolescence, or that were diagnosed but not treated or were managed with some form of bracing. LIS can also include surgically managed cases of scoliosis that have subsequently developed curve progression above or below the area of fusion, or cases in which symptoms develop as a result of poor sagittal alignment or degenerative changes.

Positive sagittal balance may develop in either LIS or degenerative scoliosis.[1,13] It can result from a loss of physiological lordosis in the lumbar spine as a consequence of degenerative changes or of the previous treatment of scoliosis. True flat back syndrome with severe sagittal imbalance traditionally results from the treatment of TL scoliosis, particularly in patients with Harrington distraction instrumentation. Less commonly, thoracic or TL junctional kyphosis may occur with a pseudarthrosis at the site of prior surgery, or proximal junctional kyphosis may occur after spinal instrumentation and fusion.[1]

Degenerative scoliosis usually presents during the sixth or seventh decades, with an equal incidence in men and women.[13,14] The degeneration is often widespread and associated with facet-joint arthropathy, osteophyte formation, and hypertrophy of the ligamentum flavum. The apex of this type of curve is usually between L3 and L4,[15] and the curve may have significant rotational translation of the apical vertebra, as well as lateral listhesis of the vertebral bodies at or near the apex of the curve.[16]

Although it is occasionally difficult to differentiate between LIS with extensive degenerative changes and degenerative scoliosis, and there are similarities in the treatment of both disease processes, this chapter will be restricted to the evaluation and management of LIS.

## Adult Scoliosis in Patients with Previous Spine Surgery

As the number of patients treated for AIS increases, it is more common for patients with symptomatic LIS who have undergone previous spine surgery to come to medical attention. A subgroup of patients present with recurrent or progressive scoliosis after prior intervention.[17] Some patients develop degeneration at adjacent vertebral levels, whereas others are found to have a symptomatic pseudarthrosis at the site of a prior fusion. Several recent publications have evaluated the long-term results of surgical intervention for AIS, and provide insight into the incidence of symptomatic LIS in patients with previously treated AIS. Danielsson and coworkers followed 283 patients, of whom 156 were treated with Harrington-rod instrumentation and fusion, and the remainder of whom were treated with a brace. The mean follow-up times were 23 years for the surgically treated group and 22 years for the brace-treated group. Surgical complications included pseudarthrosis in three patients and flat back syndrome with positive sagittal imbalance in four patients. Eight of the patients treated with fusion (5.1%) required additional surgery for complications related to fusion. Of the patients who had revision surgery, three had hook displacement caused by fracture of the vertebral arch within the first 2 months after surgery. One patient required surgery for treatment of pseudarthrosis. Two patients who developed flat back syndrome were treated with osteotomies. Two additional patients had a rod removed.[18]

Several studies have examined the effect of the extent of fusion on the natural history of patients who have undergone fusion for AIS. Poitras and coworkers reported the prevalence, nature, and consequences of back pain in patients who had undergone Harrington-rod instrumentation for AIS. This study sought to determine whether back pain was related to the number of vertebrae fused, the distal level of hook insertion, and the degree of correction. The distal level of fusion was not found to influence the occurrence of back pain during adulthood.[17] However, this finding is contradicted by several other studies that have described a relationship between the distal extent of fusion and the occurrence of symptoms later in life. In 1983, Cochran et al reported the results of Harrington-rod instrumentation and fusion in 95 patients. The proportion of patients with back pain increased significantly with lower levels of fusion. Thus, among patients who had fusion at L1, 25% had pain, rising to 30, 39, 62, and 82% of those who had undergone fusion at L2, L3, L4, and L5, respectively.[19] The extent of fusion was also found to correlate with back pain in several other series.[20,21]

It is difficult to set general guidelines for the treatment of LIS in patients who have previously undergone fusion because many factors affect their subsequent condition. Factors including the duration and severity of symptoms, curve progression, degenerative changes at the end of fusion constructs, spinal alignment, and pseudarthrosis can affect the the appropriate treatment, requiring its clinical correlation with specific symptoms. **Figure 24.1** shows radiographs of a 47-year-old woman who had undergone treatment of idiopathic scoliosis with a double major curve at the age of 13 years. The patient had a history of back pain with progressive worsening of radicular pain in her lower extremities that was worse on the left than on the right. The patient had undergone extensive trials of conservative therapy, and had a computed tomography (CT) myelogram that showed circumferential narrowing at the L4–L5 and L5–S1, with severe neural foraminal narrowing particularly on the left side at L4–L5.

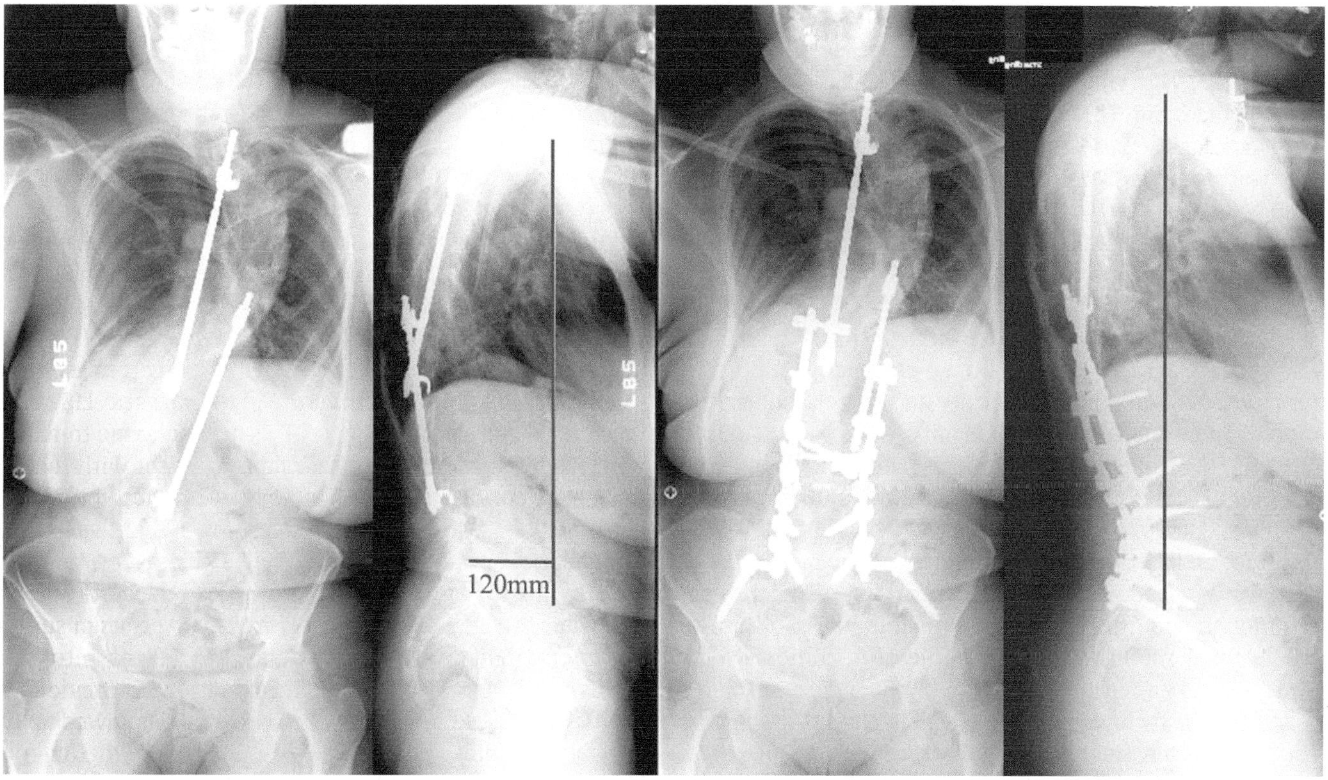


**Fig. 24.1** Standing AP and lateral films of a patient with severe and progressive LIS, and a history of fusion. **(A,B)** AP and lateral preoperative long-cassette plain films. **(C,D)** Postoperative view of construct with correction of sagittal imbalance and improvement of lumbar curve.

The patient underwent a two-stage operation, of which the first stage was an anterior retroperitoneal approach to the lumbar spine with radical diskectomies and correction of scoliosis at L4–L5 and L5–S1, and inter-vertebral-body instrumentation at these levels with the use of bone morphogenetic protein (BMP). Stage 2 was a posterior exposure of the thoracic and lumbar spine followed by partial removal of the previously inserted Harrington-rod instrumentation, inspection of the fusion mass and visualization of a known pseudarthrosis at the L3–L4 level, and transpedicular instrumentation of L1 through S1 on the left side and from L3 through S1 on the right side. Connection instrumentation was joined to the Harrington rods to provide instrumentation from T12 through S1 with bilateral iliac screws; bilateral bone grafts harvested from the iliac crest; laminectomies at L3, L4, and L5; and Smith–Petersen osteotomies at L3–L4, L4–L5, and L5–S1. An arthrodesis was done from T12 to S1 with a combination of local bone-graft material, BMP, and allograft. Postoperatively, the patient's radicular symptoms resolved and her back pain eased considerably.

## Clinical Symptoms and Radiographic Associations

Historically, it has been difficult to predict health status on the basis of radiographic measures of deformity. Recent studies of adult scoliosis have attempted to correlate radiographic appearances with clinical symptoms, but this correlation has been inconsistent. The ability to associate clinical symptoms with radiological measures of scoliosis has improved with the use of objective outcome measures.[13,22,23] More objective criteria have been used both to assess the risk of progression of symptoms before surgery and the likelihood of a satisfactory result after surgery.

Sagittal balance has been recognized as a critical factor in the assessment of adult patients with spinal deformity. Glassman et al reviewed data from a prospective multicenter study of adult spinal deformity and correlated various radiographic measures of deformity with patient-based outcome measures in adult scoliosis. The radiographic parameters studied were the type, location, and magnitude of spinal curves; coronal balance; sagittal balance; apical rotation; and rotatory subluxation. The study included 172 patients who had not undergone prior surgery and 126 patients who had undergone spinal fusion. Positive sagittal balance was the most reliable predictor of clinical symptoms in both patient groups. TL and lumbar coronal curves correlated with lower outcome scores than did thoracic curves in both patient groups. Coronal imbalance of >4 cm was associated with poorer pain and function scores for patients without prior surgery but not for those who had previously had surgery.[23] This study highlighted the strong relationship between sagittal balance and outcomes in adult scoliosis.

Schwab and colleagues were also able to demonstrate a correlation between radiographic parameters and pain in patients with adult scoliosis.[13] They prospectively studied 95 patients who completed a clinical questionnaire that included a self-reported visual analogue scale of pain and underwent full-length standing anteroposterior (AP) and lateral plain radiography. Radiographic analysis included measurement of the Cobb angle, the number of vertebrae in each curve, the plumbline offset from T1 to the midsacral line, the upper endplate obliquities of L3 and L4, and the maximal lateral olisthesis between two adjacent lumbar vertebrae. Measurements in the sagittal plane included lumbar lordosis, TL kyphosis, and the pelvic tilt index. Lateral vertebral olisthesis, endplate obliquity angles at L3 and L4, lumbar lordosis, and TL kyphosis were significantly correlated with pain. Surprisingly, Schwab and colleagues found that neither the Cobb angle nor age correlated with symptoms.

## Presurgical Planning

Most patients with symptomatic adult scoliosis have undergone numerous prior evaluations and treatments before having been referred to a spine surgeon. A careful review of a patient's past treatments and tests over time can give insight into the progression and response to treatment of the patient's disease. A correlation of the patient's symptoms with the clinical and radiological findings provides the clinician with important information toward finding the optimal treatment for the patient.

A thorough clinical and radiographic assessment of spinal deformity should be done in all patients at the time of their initial presentation to the surgeon, especially if any surgical intervention is anticipated. The radiographic analysis begins with full-length, upright 36 x 14-in. posteroanterior (PA) and lateral films that permit measurement of all coronal curves, the thoracic and lumbar curvature in the sagittal plane and the coronal and sagittal balance. This may be complemented with studies done for surgical planning, including supine, flexion, extension, and side-bending radiographs to evaluate curve flexibility. To optimize visualization of the entire spine on the lateral radiograph, the "clavicle position" should be used. In this position the patient fully flexes the elbows, with the hands in a relaxed fist, wrists flexed, and proximal interphalangeal joints placed comfortably into the supraclavicular fossa with passive forward flexion of the humerus. This position permits significantly better overall visualization of critical vertebral landmarks.[24–27] Ideally, on the lateral radiograph, one should be able to visualize the trunk from C7 to the pelvis, including the hip joints, to assess the global sagittal balance of the spinal column.

Similarly, on the PA view, the margins of the rib cage and the pelvis, along with the femoral heads, should be clearly visualized. Assessment of the hips and an evaluation for possible leg-length discrepancy, arthritis of the hip, and pelvic pathology is essential. Visualization of the ribs helps in determining deformity of the thoracic cage associated with a congenital deformity rather than with untreated AIS. Either a congenital fusion of the ribs or a significant chest wall deformity can be associated with rigid or fused spinal segments. After spinal balance is assessed in the sagittal and coronal planes, Cobb-angle measurements are made on each area of the spine including the cervical, PT, MT, TL, and lumbar areas. The vertebral-body rotation at the apex of the curve in the coronal plane is a factor determining the rigidity of the curve. The greater the vertebral-body rotation the more likely it is that there will be substantial rigidity of the coronal curve. Loss of disc space height, extensive degenerative changes of the facet joints, and bridging osteophytes are also associated with curve rigidity.

Sagittal balance is determined by examining the vertical axis constructed through the middle of the C7 vertebral body and projecting it inferiorly to intersect the horizontal line through the L5–S1 disc space.[22] In a balanced spine this line should ideally pass through the posterior third of the L5–S1 disc space. It is probably acceptable to have the C7 plumbline at least pass through or be posterior to the center of the acetabulum. The C7 plumbline may be acceptably located in elderly patients if it is up to 4 cm anterior to the L5–S1 disc space.

CT myelography is a frequently used diagnostic procedure in the evaluation of adults with scoliosis when surgery is planned. The CT myelogram provides intimate details of bone anatomy and is helpful in identifying areas of lateral recess and far-lateral stenosis. The diagnostic value of the CT myelogram is particularly relevant in patients with severe spinal deformity, substantial degenerative changes or a history of previous surgery. An evaluation of bone anatomy with this technique will dictate the specific instrumentation options available for the patient.

Magnetic resonance imaging (MRI) scans of the spine provide additional information about relevant soft tissues such as neural elements and vasculature, and the extent of disc hydration. The degenerative status of the discs in the lower lumbar spine is important in determining the lowest instrumented segment in a corrective construct, a topic discussed later in this chapter.

The determination of whether each sagittal and coronal component of a spinal deformity is fixed or fused and rigid or flexible contributes significantly to the surgical decision-making process. The characteristics of each portion of the spinal deformity should be evaluated in determining the overall flexibility of the deformity. Curve magnitudes may vary with the elimination of gravity; supine and standing films should be obtained for every patient who has a significant increase in symptoms when moving from a supine to a standing position. For certain cases in which large rigid scoliotic or kyphotic curves are found, push–prone, traction, or bolster radiographs help in the further assessment of flexibility.[22,28,29] A rigid or fixed deformity will dictate whether an anterior release and fusion, a posterior osteotomy, or a vertebral column resection should be done to successfully achieve the desired correction of a deformity and spinal balance. For instance, an isolated 35-degree idiopathic scoliotic lumbar curve in a young adult is usually flexible and is often substantially reduced on side-bending films. Improvements exceeding 70% in postoperatively measured Cobb angles in such patients are common with the use of modern surgical instrumentation and techniques for correcting posterior deformities. However, the treatment of an elderly patient with LIS and a curve of similar magnitude would rarely produce the same amount of correction. Hence, management plans for curves of a particular magnitude may differ according to the inherent flexibility of the curves.

It is also necessary to assess the flexibility of sagittal curves. A bolster placed under the apex of a kyphotic deformity to maximize postural correction is particularly useful. This technique permits a better assessment of sagittal curve flexibility than can be obtained by the patient's attempting maximal extension.

## Treatment Options

Nonsurgical treatments such as nonsteroidal anti-inflammatory drugs (NSAIDs), muscle relaxants, narcotic analgesics, muscle exercises, physical therapy, aquatics therapy, massage, and gentle traction are all options for treating LIS but have unproven long-term efficacy in its treatment.[30] Epidural and selective nerve-root blocks and facet-joint blocks are more invasive interventions but may temporarily help to control pain.[31,32] A well-fitted brace to support a painful area of the spine may occasionally be of some benefit, but braces are generally not well tolerated on a long-term basis and may lead to deconditioning of the trunk musculature if worn for long periods.

The decision to perform surgery on an adult patient with a spinal deformity depends on the patient's symptoms, the disability caused by the deformity, the degree of curvature of the deformity, and the patient's age at presentation and medical and surgical history. Indications for surgery differ for young adults, healthy and active elderly individuals, and debilitated elderly patients with numerous medical problems. Adults under 40 years of age who have relatively mild symptoms but curves >70 degrees are surgical candidates because of the high propensity for curve progression in such cases. Among adults over 65 years of age surgery is usually reserved for those with neurological

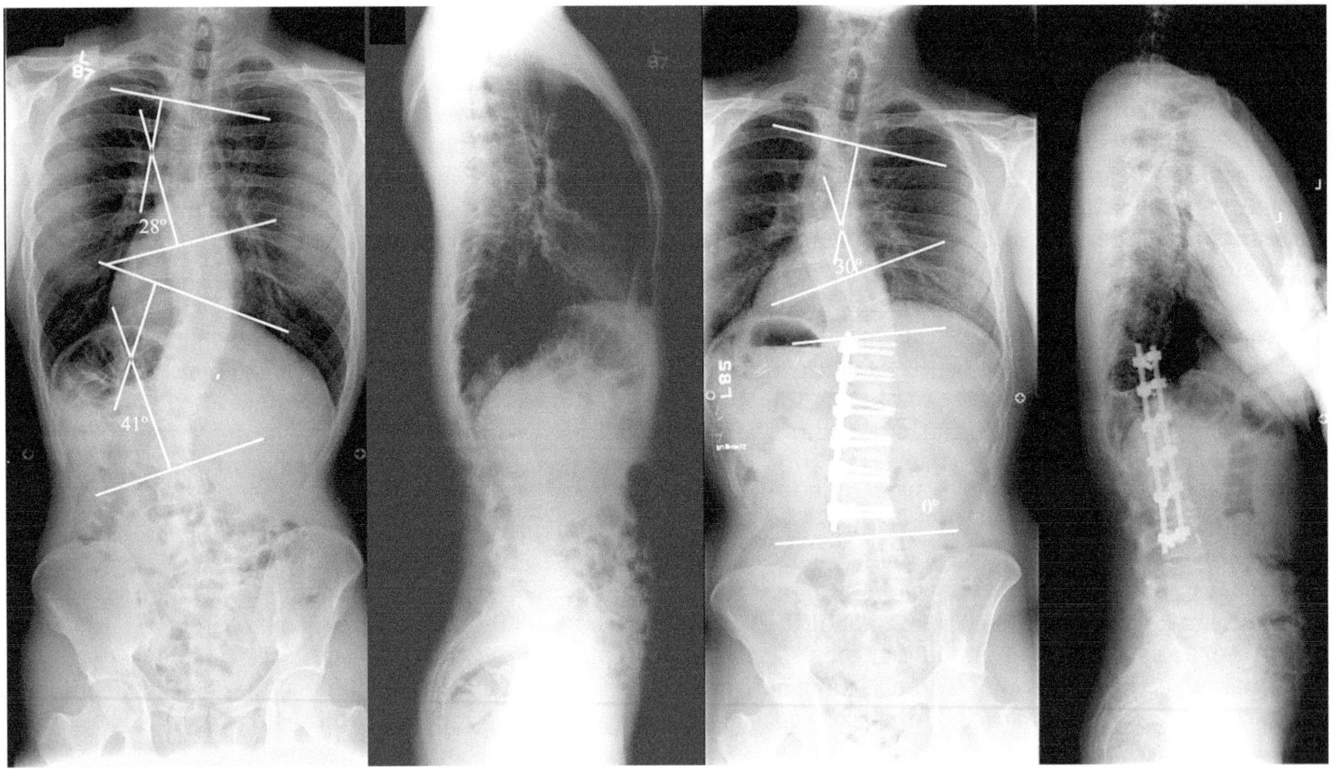


A–D

**Fig. 24.2 (A,B)** Preoperative long-cassette AP and lateral plain films. **(C,D)** Postoperative view of construct with correction of scoliotic curve. Note correction of 41-degree curve to zero degrees. The upper thoracic curve measured 28 degrees on the preoperative film and was essentially unchanged, with a measurement of 30 degrees, on the postoperative film.

symptoms or severe back pain unresponsive to nonsurgical treatment. Curve magnitude is only one factor in deciding upon surgical intervention; other factors include the risk of curve progression, spinal balance, and cosmetic effects of the deformity. The progression of scoliosis should be determined by comparing serial films of the patient's spine over time. **Figure 24.2** shows the AP and lateral radiographs of a 27-year-old man with a history of known idiopathic thoracolumbar scoliosis. The patient had a history of documented progression of his scoliotic curve, which was approaching 50 degrees. He had recently had progressive pain over the apex of his scoliotic curve that interfered with his work and leisure activities.

The patient underwent surgery through a left-sided thoracoabdominal approach to the thoracic and lumbar spine, followed by radical anterior diskectomies from T10–T11 through L2–L3 and release of his severe kyphoscoliosis. Inter-vertebral-body spacers were placed at the L2–L3, L1–L2, and T12–L1 levels, followed by anterior segmental instrumentation from T10 through L3. An arthrodesis was done from T10 through L3 using local bone graft (rib) and allograft bone. The patient's age and the flexibility of his curve allowed its nearly complete correction through an purely anterior approach. Two years postoperatively he reported marked resolution of pain and resumption of his activities of daily living.

The cosmetic effect of scoliosis in adults has been underestimated as a cause of their seeking medical attention.[33] Some patients present with concerns about back pain or radicular symptoms when cosmetic effects of their deformity are their main worry. Without a frank discussion of their expectations of cosmetic improvement, patients may be disappointed with the outcome of their surgical treatment. A review of psychosocial and support issues should be done before proceeding with surgical intervention. Because recovery from extensive surgery is prolonged, a frank discussion of the family or social support needed during the recovery period is essential to establish the foundation for a successful recovery. Many patients must undergo some of their recovery in a rehabilitation or skilled nursing facility. Multiple office visits with the patient are typically required to impart to the patient the numerous factors influencing the issues related to the patient's deformity.

The older patient with LIS can present with one or more complaints or findings including back pain, radicular pain or weakness, neurogenic claudication, radiographic curve progression, or worsening spinal imbalance. Any treatment should focus on addressing the specific presenting complaint(s) and improving associated radiographic abnormalities. Complaints of pain are evaluated and initially treated as would be any other back pain; mild to moderate pain is treated with appropriate weight loss, anti-inflammatory medications, general conditioning and spine-stabilization exercises including aquatics therapy. Unless there is a component of radicular pain or neurogenic claudication, epidural or foraminal steroid injections rarely give significant relief of symptoms. Occasionally, facet-joint injections of steroids can provide temporary relief of axial back pain, but their long-term efficacy has not been proven. A failure of other forms of nonoperative management of LIS may lead to consideration of an acute or chronic trial of narcotic analgesic medications. However, although narcotic analgesic medications can ease symptoms, the risks of their producing dependency, changes in mental status, nausea, and constipation must be balanced against the likelihood of significant, long-lasting improvement of symptoms.

Moderate-to-severe pain that is unresponsive to conservative therapy may lead to consideration of surgical intervention. The surgical plan must address the patient's complaints and maintain or restore spinal balance, particularly sagittal balance. The surgical management of deformity in an older patient can consist of correction of the deformity, decompression, stabilization, fusion procedures, or a combination of these. Decompression alone can provide relief of radicular symptoms in patients who have localized neural compression, mild scoliosis without signs of instability (e.g., rotatory subluxation, lateral listhesis, or spondylolisthesis), and good sagittal balance.

LIS is usually more rigid than typical AIS, and different treatment strategies are needed for it. Spinal curves of smaller magnitude and that are relatively flexible, with good coronal and sagittal balance, can usually be successfully managed with posterior pedicle-screw instrumentation alone. More fixed or fused deformities, especially those associated with coronal or sagittal imbalance, generally require a more aggressive and technically demanding surgical approach. Surgical options for rigid or decompensated curves include combined anterior and posterior releases or fusions, spinal osteotomy, or vertebral column resection procedures. There has been an increased tendency to attempt to treat complex curves through a posterior-only approach.[34,35] The length and complexity of these operations may require that they be performed in more than one stage. Rhee and associates[36] recently reported on the strategy of dividing a single prolonged, complex, posterior surgery into two smaller posterior procedures staged to be done during a single hospitalization. With this staged technique, Rhee and colleagues reported few surgical complications, no major medical complications, and an excellent outcome in a population known to be at high risk for adverse events. They stated that staging can be useful in performing complex posterior revision and osteotomy surgery while limiting hemodynamic stresses.

Patients with LIS who present with larger curves or significant imbalance will most often require a more extensive procedure than posterior pedicle screw fixation alone. Options for more predictably achieving adequate correction include anterior-release and posterior osteotomy procedures followed by posterior instrumentation. Performing an anterior operation not only increases the degree of correction but also increases the rate of fusion. In patients who have lost lumbar lordosis the anterior approach can restore this lordosis and may reduce the likelihood of having to extend fusion into the thoracic spine. However, anterior surgery can have consequences in older adults, including poor cosmesis caused by abdominal bulging. Anterior paramedian approaches cause fewer complications and produce better cosmetic appearance than do lateral retroperitoneal approaches.[37]

## Junctional Zones and Length of Fusion

It is unfavorable to stop a fusion at the apex of a coronal or kyphotic deformity. Until recently, it was generally thought that ending instrumentation at the TL junction would lead to proximal degeneration, kyphosis, and decompensation in a patient with scoliosis. To test this supposition, Kim et al[38] conducted a retrospective review of the postoperative influence of treatment at three different levels of the TL spine on the prevalence of revision in patients undergoing surgery for adult lumbar deformities with instrumented fusion from the distal thoracic or upper lumbar spine (T9 to L2) to L5 or S1. One hundred twenty-five adult patients (average age: 57.1 years) were compared and split into three groups according to whether the proximal level at which they had fusion was T9–T10 ($n = 37$), T11–T12 ($n = 49$), or L1–L2 ($n = 39$). The prevalence of revision and change in the sagittal Cobb angle at the proximal junction after surgery were compared. There were no significant differences in the prevalence of proximal junctional kyphosis in the three groups (T9–T10: 51%, vs. T11–12: 55%, vs. L1–2: 36%, $P = 0.20$). The rate of revision was ~25% and not significantly different among the three groups ($P = 0.99$). Subsequent changes in the proximal junctional angle and sagittal vertical axis from the preoperative to the ultimate follow-up evaluation were not significantly different in the three groups ($P = 0.10$ and $P = 0.46$, respectively). Because the three different levels of proximal fusion did not differ significantly with respect to the various outcomes assessed, including total scores on the Scoliosis Research Society (SRS)-24 instrument or its outcomes subscales, proximal fusion at a more distal, neutral, and stable vertebral level may be satisfactory.[38] However, because of the smaller pedicle size at L1 than in the lower thoracic spine, many surgeons intentionally end constructs at T10 or T11 rather than at T12 or L1, as dictated by the patient's anatomy.

Because of the risk of rapid failure, instrumentation should not be stopped at an area of rotatory subluxation, degenerative spondylolisthesis, isthmic spondylolisthesis; at an area of spinal stenosis; or at the level of posterior-column deficiency. This can lead to spinal instability, disease at the adjacent level above the fusion, segmental collapse, secondary kyphosis, progressive deformity, and spinal stenosis.[39–43]

A major controversy in the treatment of adult scoliosis is whether or not a fusion should extend across the lumbosacral junction.[44] Evaluation of the lumbosacral junction is critical in the preoperative planning for patients with LIS. Extending a fusion across the lumbosacral junction increases the length of the surgical procedure and removes a compensatory area that might accommodate residual spinal imbalance. Lumbar degenerative changes, spinal imbalance, or obliquity of the lower lumbar segments of the spine may require fusion across the lumbosacral junction for an optimal result. Long fusions extending across the lumbosacral junction, without anterior column support or supplemental sacral or spinopelvic fixation or both, have been associated with a high rate of pseudarthrosis. The increased risk of nonunion results from the high stress and unfavorable biomechanical loads at the junction between the two major lever arms of the fused spine and the rigid pelvis. The incidence of nonunion reported in the literature varies quite remarkably, ranging from 5 to 30%.[44–47] Anterior- column support at the lumbosacral junction has been recommended in TL instrumentation because posterior instrumentation and fusion alone carries a 15 to 30% rate of pseudarthrosis even with newer instrumentation systems.[45,46] Although anterior interbody lumbar fusion (ALIF) has often been used in treating adult scoliosis, inter-vertebral-body support provided by a posterior lumbar interbody fusion (PLIF) or tranforaminal lumbar interbody fusion (TLIF) is increasingly being used to allow a purely posterior approach to adult scoliosis.[48] Various types of sacral and pelvic instrumentation have been designed to enhance fusion, but to date none of these types of instrumentation alone has completely eliminated the problem of pseudarthrosis, even with anterior-column support. For long fusions to the sacrum, a combination of iliac screws and anterior-column support has been shown to be the most effective method of preventing pseudarthrosis at the lumbosacral junction. Although iliac screws may loosen or break under biomechanical loads and with movement at the SI joint, they have been successful in protecting sacral screws from breakage, pullout, or loosening.[45,46] If pseudarthrosis develops after an isolated posterior approach, the most effective approach to correcting it is a circumferential fusion with pelvic fixation.[45,46]

Ultimately, the decision to end a fusion at L5 or to go across the lumbosacral junction in patients with LIS is controversial.[49] An unacceptable failure rate has been found with fusions ending at L5 when there is L5–S1 disc-space narrowing, facet-joint arthropathy, vertebral obliquity and rotational deformity at L5, and positive sagittal balance.[50,51] Extending a fusion to L5 even in the case of a healthy L5–S1 segment may overload it and lead to secondary degeneration.[44,46,51] On the other hand, a fusion extended to the sacrum may not only have an effect on the sacroiliac joints but also on the hip joints, particularly in the presence of osteoarthritis of the hip. In cases of a painless, well-hydrated L5–S1 disc with good sagittal balance before surgery, ending a fusion at L5 can be considered. However, the possible eventual need to extend the fusion to the pelvis should be discussed with the patient before surgery.

## Correction Techniques

The correction strategy for achieving spinal balance in patients with LIS depends principally on the structural characteristics of their deformity curve(s) and their bone quality. Realignment of a deformity can be achieved by using its inherent flexibility and additional correction through the stress-relaxation characteristics of the surrounding connective tissue under continuous loading. In cases in which the deformity is too large or too stiff for stress relaxation to be the principal mode of correction, realignment can be accomplished by other techniques such as facet-joint resection, anterior release through annulectomy and diskectomy, osteotomy, or vertebral-column resection.[52–55] Suk and coworkers[52] recently reported a posterior-only approach with complete vertebrectomy to restore spinal balance in patients with rigid curves >80 degrees. With this technique they corrected a mean preoperative scoliosis of 109 degrees to 45.6 degrees, which corresponds to a 59% correction. A complete discussion of releases, osteotomies, and column resections is presented in Chapter 16.

## Pseudarthrosis

The mechanical enhancement of spinal fusion by applying rigid internal fixation has reduced the incidence of nonunion but has not eliminated it. Therefore, maximizing the osteogenic potential of spinal fusion has become increasingly important. There are limits in harvesting autologous bone, including donor-site morbidity, a limited amount of available bone, and unpredictable incorporation and resorption of bone. Reported donor-site complications of using iliac bone grafts include wound infection, hematoma, pelvic fracture, cutaneous nerve pain, and chronic donor-site pain. These problems of donor-site morbidity and pseudarthrosis have led to a search for a dependable bone-graft substitute that has both osteoconductive and osteoinductive properties. These challenges are accentuated in patients who have undergone prior surgical procedures or who have significant osteoporosis or documented pseudarthrosis, or are in disease states associated with poor bone healing. Patients who smoke, use steroids, have diabetes, or have metabolic bone disease are particularly challenging in terms of having these complications.

Morselized cancellous allograft bone has been a common choice as a bone-graft extender in the absence of sufficient autologous bone. The resulting allograft, when mixed with local autogenous graft or aspirated bone marrow, is used for many applications in adult spinal reconstructive surgery. Allograft bone is osteoconductive and can be combined with autologous bone-marrow stem cells to render the resulting graft osteogenic. New generations of allograft bone, such as a demineralized bone matrix, have been shown to have osteoinductive properties in animal studies, but their efficacy in patients with adult scoliosis has not been proven.[56,57]

The use of growth factors, such as members of the BMP family (BMP-2, BMP-7, and growth differentiation factor-5 [GDF-5]) to enhance spinal arthrodesis has decreased the morbidity associated with autologous bone harvesting and increased the overall rate of arthrodesis. These growth factors are proteins that induce the differentiation of undifferentiated stem cells into osteoblasts. They have a very short half-life and must be administered in high doses with a carrier (collagen sponge). Many animal studies have demonstrated the efficacy and superiority of these proteins over autologous bone-graft material in producing solid fusion. Studies have also demonstrated the ability of BMPs to reverse the inhibitory effect of nicotine on the formation of a fusion mass, as well as the efficacy and safety of BMP and the other morphogens name above in human patients, although not in patients with adult scoliosis. Recombinant human BMP-2 (rhBMP-2) has been primarily investigated in lumbar spinal fusion, in which it has significantly enhanced the rate of fusion and decreased the duration of surgery, blood loss, and hospital stay.[58] Its practical application is limited by the significant cost of its use, which can reach $7000 per fusion level. Additionally, and despite rsearchers' early enthusiasm for using rhBMP-2 to enhance spinal fudsion, the use of BMPs at supraphysiological doses is attended by significant risks, including inflammatory reactions, effusions, seromas, ectopic bone formation, and other untoward side effects not appreciated earlier in their use.[59]

In 2005, Luhmann and colleagues reported the results of a prospective, single-center, nonblinded clinical and radiographic analysis of rhBMP-2 without iliac or rib-bone graft supplementation in a consecutive series of adult patients with spinal deformities. Patients treated with rhBMP-2 in multilevel anterior and posterior fusions with a minimum follow-up of 1 year were evaluated prospectively. The study involved a total of 95 patient samples (70 patients, of whom 25 had both anterior and posterior fusions), divided into three groups consisting of: (1) 46 patients who had anterior fusions (group 1); (2) 41 patients who had posterior fusions (group 2); and (3) 8 patients who had "compassionate use" of rhBMP-2 (group 3). Luhman and colleagues called group 3 the "compassionate use" group because they had had prior surgery and were deemed to need a higher dose of BMP than the patients in the other two groups. In the anterior-fusion group, mean dose of rhBMP-2 per fused vertebral level was 10.8 mg, contained in titanium mesh cages without any bone graft or other substance. The posterior-fusion group was given only local bone graft material, without harvested rib or iliac bone graft, and with a mean dose of rhBMP-2 per fused vertebral level of 13.7 mg. The "compassionate use" group ($n = 8$ patients) was given a higher concentration of rhBMP-2 and a different carrier, without local or harvested bone graft. The mean dose of rhBMP-2 per fused level in group 3 was 28.6 mg, and the median dose was 40 mg per level. The anterior-fusion group had a 96% rate of fusion. The posterior-fusion group had 93% rate of fusion, and the "compassionate use" group had an overall rate of fusion of 100%. Thus, with the use of rhBMP-2, a very high rate of apparent fusion was observed in all groups, without the morbidity associated with the harvesting of bone-graft material.[60]

## Surgical Outcomes and Complications in LIS

When evaluating a patient preoperatively, it is essential that the patient understand that undergoing any deformity surgery is a major undertaking. Adult scoliosis surgery carries a high risk of morbidity and also has a documented risk of mortality. Furthermore, the surgical treatment of scoliosis seldom provides complete relief of pain in such patients. Radicular pain after complex spinal reconstructive surgery persists in from 5 to 15% of patients, and a significant number of these patients complain of back pain postoperatively. The mortality rate of spine surgery in adult patients remains low, but is not insignificant at less than 1%. Common complications include wound infection (1 to 8%), neurological complications (as high as 5%), and nonunion (up to 30%).[61,62]

In 2004, Rinella et al conducted a retrospective analysis of LIS patients treated with long instrumented fusions from the proximal thoracic spine to segments that ranged from T11 to L4. The 67 patients in the study had an average age of 38.8 years, and their follow-up averaged 7.8 years. Upright radiographs and postoperative SRS-24 questionnaires from the latest follow-up date were analyzed. Patients requiring revision surgery (a total of 10 patients) had significantly lower total scores (average: 72.0) than those who did not (total score = 94.2; $P = 0.01$). Patients with pseudarthrosis (6 patients) had lower total scores (average: 74.7) than those without pseudarthrosis (average total score: 93.5; $P = 0.02$). An age older than 40 years did not correlate with an increased rate of pseudarthrosis, but was associated with higher rates of disc degeneration adjacent to instrumented levels (two patients) and sagittal or coronal imbalance (one patient with each). Subsequent distal disc degeneration did not correlate significantly with a more distal lowest instrumented vertebra (LIV) or older patient age. Smokers did not have higher rates of major complications or revision surgery than did nonsmokers.[63] A reviewof the SRS-24 scores of the patients who did not have revision surgery (93.5) yields a reasonable impression that patients with LIS do quite well from the standpoints of pain and functional outcome if they do not develop pseudarthrosis or other complications that require revision surgery.

In 2003, Ali and coworkers conducted a retrospective radiographic and chart review of 28 LIS patients who underwent primary corrective surgery to L5 or above after the age of 20 years. Clinical and radiographic parameters were assessed before surgery, after surgery, and at a 2-year follow-up. A self-perceived outcome questionnaire was administered to the study patients at a minimum of 2 years of follow-up. The patients' average preoperative major curve measurement was 65 degrees and their average postoperative major curve measurement was 24 degrees, for a correction of 64%. The average curve measurement at follow-up was 27 degrees, for a correction of 61%. Whereas 71% of the patientss were treated with an anteroposterior approach, 29% were treated with a purely posterior approach. There was 1 intraoperative complication among the 28 patients in the study, and 4 postoperative complications. Definite or probable relief of symptoms was reported in 74% of the patients. Improved ability to sleep was reported in 61%; ability to return to the patient's usual job was reported in 57%, and satisfaction with the results of surgery was reported in 87%.[64] It is important to note that Ali and colleagues' study excluded patients who had fusions below L5, among whom higher rates of complication from pseudoarthrosis have customarily been reported.[48]

Schwab et al[65] conducted a large multicenter prospective study to assess rates of surgery and operative outcomes in adult patients with TL and lumbar scoliosis. Of the 784 patients who were followed (mean age: 53 years), 339 had been treated surgically by the time of the study. It is not clear what percent of these patients had LIS, but on the basis of their mean age, a significant portion of them must have had idiopathic scoliosis. The risk of a complication occurring at any point along the continuum of the patients' care from the perioperative period to the 1-year follow-up point was assessed for a multitude of variables. Among the 268 patients with complete baseline data who underwent surgical treatment, significant variation in rates of complication was found according to the lordosis modifier ($P = 0.04$) and fixation extending to the sacrum ($P = 0.02$). Patients with type C deformities (no lordosis) had a 52.4% rate of complication at some point along the continuum of care. Patients with type B deformities (moderate lordosis) had a 33% rate of complication, and those with type A deformities (marked lordosis) patients had a rate of complication of 25%. Patients whose fusions extended to the sacrum had a complication rate of 35% as compared with a rate of 20% for those whose procedures terminated above the sacrum. Among patients for whom complete 1-year follow-up data were available ($n = 111$), significant differences in complication rates were found by sagittal balance and fixation to the sacrum. Higher rates of complications were found in patients with excessive sagittal imbalance (40 to 95 mm) and in those whose fusions extended to the sacrum.[65] This study confirms the importance of the sagittal profile in determining outcomes of scoliosis surgery in adults and underscores the difficulties encountered with fusions crossing the lumbosacral junction.

## Avoiding Complications

Complications are frequent with the aggressive treatment of any spinal deformity. In one series, complications occurred in 140 of 447 patients with 11% having at least one major complication and 24% having at least one minor complication.[66] Similarly, Weis and colleagues[67] reported complications in 46% of patients treated surgically for spinal deformity. Risk factors for major intraoperative neurological injury in such patients include combined anterior and posterior surgery, severe spinal curvatures, rigid curves, and kyphosis. Intraoperative paraplegia is another devastating complication following extensive spinal reconstructive surgery. Although direct surgical trauma to the spinal cord can occur, indirect injury has been attributed to ischemia of the spinal cord from hypovolemia, mechanical tension on the blood supply to the cord in the concavity of a curve, and peripheral vascular disease. Vigorous volume replacement and blood pressure monitoring may reduce the incidence of complications from these sources.

Visual loss can also result from major spinal surgery as a consequence of ischemic optic neuropathy, retinal artery occlusion, or cerebral ischemia.[68] Avoiding direct pressure on the eyes and the use of reverse Trendelenburg positioning during prone positioning of the patient may reduce the frequency of this complication.

The incidence of deep venous thrombosis or pulmonary embolism in adults undergoing surgery for spinal deformity varies from 2 to 20% depending on the series being considered, because most patients become deconditioned postoperatively and have prolonged periods of bed rest. The prophylactic use of inferior vena cava filters in patients undergoing high-risk spinal surgery is a current topic of discussion.[69]

Whether an anterior or purely posterior approach is associated with a greater incidence of perioperative complications has been a subject of debate. Recently, Coe and associates[61] evaluated the incidence of surgeon-reported complications in a large series of spinal fusions with instrumentation for patients with a diagnosis of a single spinal deformity and belonging to a specific age group. The impact of surgical approach was evaluated with the morbidity and mortality database of the SRS. Coe and colleagues reviewed 58,197 surgical cases submitted by members of the SRS in the years 2001, 2002, and 2003, and identified 10.9% who had an anterior, posterior, or combined approach to spinal fusion with instrumentation for the diagnosis of idiopathic scoliosis. Among the 6334 patients in this series, the total incidence of complications was 5.7%. Among patients undergoing anterior fusion and instrumentation, 5.2% had complications; of the patients with posterior instrumentation and fusion, 5.1% had complications; and among those who underwent combined anterior and posterior instrumentation and fusion, 10.2% had complications. Two patients (0.03%) died from their complications. Coe et al demonstrated that there was no statistical difference in the overall complication rates with anterior and posterior procedures. However, the difference in both overall complication rates and in neurological complication rates with anterior or posterior procedures as compared with combined procedures was highly significant ($P < 0.0001$). Advances in surgical techniques and spinal instrumentation increasingly permit the correction of spinal deformity through a single (usually posterior) surgical approach in the vast majority of cases. In certain complex cases, challenges caused by aberrant anatomy, unusual pathology, or the consequences of prior surgical interventions make circumferential procedures preferable despite the added surgical morbidity that they incur.

## Conclusion

The evaluation and management of LIS in the adult population has evolved significantly during the past decade. The goal of any surgery for spinal deformity is to achieve a stable, well-balanced spine centered over the pelvis, by fusing as few motion segments as possible while achieving results superior to those of the natural history of the deformity. A balanced spine is created by a close interplay of the patient's spinal anatomy, the biomechanical properties of the spine and its surrounding structures, and the corrective capabilities of surgical techniques and instrumentation.

The most important aspect of the surgical correction of any deformity is patient selection and matching of the surgical approach and method of instrumentation and fusion to the specific deformity. The goals of surgery for LIS should be to: (1) restore sagittal balance; (2) optimize coronal balance; (3) decompress compromised neural elements when needed; (4) minimize complications, pain, and discomfort; and (5) ease pain and improve functional outcome and cosmesis. Correction of the coronal curve in scoliosis is much less important than the other surgical goals listed here. In well-selected patients, the results of corrective surgery can be very rewarding for both the patient and the surgeon.

### References


1. Kuklo TR. Principles for selecting fusion levels in adult spinal deformity with particular attention to lumbar curves and double major curves. Spine 2006;31(19, suppl):S132–S138
2. Lonstein JE. Scoliosis: Surgical versus nonsurgical treatment. Clin Orthop Relat Res 2006;443:248–259
3. Weinstein SL, Dolan LA, Spratt KF, Peterson KK, Spoonamore MJ, Ponseti IV. Health and function of patients with untreated idiopathic scoliosis: A 50-year natural history study. JAMA 2003;289:559–567
4. Schwab F, Dubey A, Pagala M, Gamez L, Farcy JP. Adult scoliosis: A health assessment analysis by SF-36. Spine 2003;28:602–606
5. Schwab F, Dubey A, Gamez L, et al. Adult scoliosis: Prevalence, SF-36, and nutritional parameters in an elderly volunteer population. Spine 2005;30:1082–1085
6. Collis DK, Ponseti IV. Long-term follow-up of patients with idiopathic scoliosis not treated surgically. J Bone Joint Surg Am 1969;51:425–445
7. Korovessis P, Piperos G, Sidiropoulos P, Dimas A. Adult idiopathic lumbar scoliosis. A formula for prediction of progression and review of the literature. Spine 1994;19:1926–1932
8. Dickson JH, Mirkovic S, Noble PC, Nalty T, Erwin WD. Results of operative treatment of idiopathic scoliosis in adults. J Bone Joint Surg Am 1995;77:513–523
9. Aebi M. [Adult scoliosis]. Ther Umsch 1987;44:757–763
10. Aebi M. Correction of degenerative scoliosis of the lumbar spine. A preliminary report. Clin Orthop Relat Res 1988;232:80–86
11. Aebi M. The adult scoliosis. Eur Spine J 2005;14:925–948
12. Arlet V, Papin P, Marchesi D, Aebi M. Adolescent idiopathic thoracic scoliosis: Apical correction with specialized pedicle hooks. Eur Spine J 1999;8:266–271
13. Schwab FJ, Smith VA, Biserni M, Gamez L, Farcy JP, Pagala M. Adult scoliosis: A quantitative radiographic and clinical analysis. Spine 2002;27:387–392

14. Oskouian RJ Jr, Shaffrey CI. Degenerative lumbar scoliosis. Neurosurg Clin N Am 2006;17:299–315, vii
15. Pérennou D, Marcelli C, Hérisson C, Simon L. Adult lumbar scoliosis. Epidemiologic aspects in a low-back pain population. Spine 1994; 19:123–128
16. Schwab F, el-Fegoun AB, Gamez L, Goodman H, Farcy JP. A lumbar classification of scoliosis in the adult patient: Preliminary approach. Spine 2005;30:1670–1673
17. Poitras B, Mayo NE, Goldberg MS, Scott S, Hanley J. The Ste-Justine Adolescent Idiopathic Scoliosis Cohort Study. Part IV: Surgical correction and back pain. Spine 1994;19:1582–1588
18. Danielsson AJ, Nachemson AL. Radiologic findings and curve progression 22 years after treatment for adolescent idiopathic scoliosis: Comparison of brace and surgical treatment with matching control group of straight individuals. Spine 2001;26:516–525
19. Cochran T, Irstam L, Nachemson A. Long-term anatomic and functional changes in patients with adolescent idiopathic scoliosis treated by Harrington rod fusion. Spine 1983;8:576–584
20. Edgar MA, Mehta MH. Long-term follow-up of fused and unfused idiopathic scoliosis. J Bone Joint Surg Br 1988;70:712–716
21. Hayes MA, Tompkins SF, Herndon WA, Gruel CR, Kopta JA, Howard TC. Clinical and radiological evaluation of lumbosacral motion below fusion levels in idiopathic scoliosis. Spine 1988;13:1161–1167
22. Glassman SD, Bridwell K, Dimar JR, Horton W, Berven S, Schwab F. The impact of positive sagittal balance in adult spinal deformity. Spine 2005;30:2024–2029
23. Glassman SD, Berven S, Bridwell K, Horton W, Dimar JR. Correlation of radiographic parameters and clinical symptoms in adult scoliosis. Spine 2005;30:682–688
24. Vedantam R, Lenke LG, Bridwell KH, Linville DL. Comparison of push-prone and lateral-bending radiographs for predicting postoperative coronal alignment in thoracolumbar and lumbar scoliotic curves. Spine 2000;25:76–81
25. Vedantam R, Lenke LG, Bridwell KH, Linville DL, Blanke K. The effect of variation in arm position on sagittal spinal alignment. Spine 2000;25:2204–2209
26. Kuklo TR, Lenke LG, Graham EJ, et al. Correlation of radiographic, clinical, and patient assessment of shoulder balance following fusion versus nonfusion of the proximal thoracic curve in adolescent idiopathic scoliosis. Spine 2002;27:2013–2020
27. Horton WC, Brown CW, Bridwell KH, Glassman SD, Suk SI, Cha CW. Is there an optimal patient stance for obtaining a lateral 36″ radiograph? A critical comparison of three techniques. Spine 2005; 30:427–433
28. Engsberg JR, Lenke LG, Hollander KW, et al. Methods to locate center of gravity in scoliosis. Spine 2003;28:E483–E489
29. Duval-Beaupére G, Lespargot A, Grossiord A. Flexibility of scoliosis. What does it mean? Is this terminology appropriate? Spine 1985;10:428–432
30. Glassman SD, Schwab FJ, Bridwell KH, Ondra SL, Berven S, Lenke LG. The selection of operative versus nonoperative treatment in patients with adult scoliosis. Spine 2007;32:93–97
31. Cooper G, Lutz GE, Boachie-Adjei O, Lin J. Effectiveness of transforaminal epidural steroid injections in patients with degenerative lumbar scoliotic stenosis and radiculopathy. Pain Physician 2004;7:311–317
32. Boswell MV, Trescot AM, Datta S, et al; American Society of Interventional Pain Physicians. Interventional techniques: Evidence-based practice guidelines in the management of chronic spinal pain. Pain Physician 2007;10:7–111
33. Watanabe K, Hasegawa K, Hirano T, Uchiyama S, Endo N. Use of the scoliosis research society outcomes instrument to evaluate patient outcome in untreated idiopathic scoliosis patients in Japan: Part II: relation between spinal deformity and patient outcomes. Spine 2005;30:1202–1205
34. Lehman RA Jr, Lenke LG, Keeler KA, et al. Operative treatment of adolescent idiopathic scoliosis with posterior pedicle screw-only constructs: Minimum three-year follow-up of one hundred fourteen cases. Spine 2008;33:1598–1604
35. Dobbs MB, Lenke LG, Kim YJ, Luhmann SJ, Bridwell KH. Anterior/posterior spinal instrumentation versus posterior instrumentation alone for the treatment of adolescent idiopathic scoliotic curves more than 90 degrees. Spine 2006;31:2386–2391
36. Rhee JM, Bridwell KH, Won DS, Lenke LG, Chotigavanichaya C, Hanson DS. Sagittal plane analysis of adolescent idiopathic scoliosis: The effect of anterior versus posterior instrumentation. Spine 2002;27:2350–2356
37. Jagannathan J, Chankaew E, Urban P, et al. Cosmetic and functional outcomes following paramedian and anterolateral retroperitoneal access in anterior lumbar spine surgery. J Neurosurg Spine 2008;9:454–465
38. Kim YJ, Bridwell KH, Lenke LG, Rhim S, Kim YW. Is the T9, T11, or L1 the more reliable proximal level after adult lumbar or lumbosacral instrumented fusion to L5 or S1? Spine 2007;32:2653–2661
39. McMaster MJ, Singh H. Natural history of congenital kyphosis and kyphoscoliosis. A study of one hundred and twelve patients. J Bone Joint Surg Am 1999;81:1367–1383
40. Lenke LG. Lenke classification system of adolescent idiopathic scoliosis: Treatment recommendations. Instr Course Lect 2005;54: 537–542
41. Lenke LG, Edwards CC II, Bridwell KH. The Lenke classification of adolescent idiopathic scoliosis: How it organizes curve patterns as a template to perform selective fusions of the spine. Spine 2003; 28:S199–S207
42. Duval-Beaupére G, Robain G. Visualization on full spine radiographs of the anatomical connections of the centres of the segmental body mass supported by each vertebra and measured in vivo. Int Orthop 1987;11:261–269
43. Burton DC, Asher MA, Lai SM. The selection of fusion levels using torsional correction techniques in the surgical treatment of idiopathic scoliosis. Spine 1999;24:1728–1739
44. Eck KR, Bridwell KH, Ungacta FF, et al. Complications and results of long adult deformity fusions down to l4, l5, and the sacrum. Spine 2001;26:E182–E192
45. Kuklo TR, Bridwell KH, Lewis SJ, et al. Minimum 2-year analysis of sacropelvic fixation and L5-S1 fusion using S1 and iliac screws. Spine 2001;26:1976–1983
46. Tsuchiya K, Bridwell KH, Kuklo TR, Lenke LG, Baldus C. Minimum 5-year analysis of L5-S1 fusion using sacropelvic fixation (bilateral S1 and iliac screws) for spinal deformity. Spine 2006;31:303–308
47. Bridwell KH. Where to stop the fusion distally in adult scoliosis: L4, L5, or the sacrum? Instr Course Lect 1996;45:101–107

48. Weistroffer JK, Perra JH, Lonstein JE, et al. Complications in long fusions to the sacrum for adult scoliosis: minimum five-year analysis of fifty patients. Spine 2008;33:1478–1483
49. Swamy G, Berven SH, Bradford DS. The selection of L5 versus S1 in long fusions for adult idiopathic scoliosis. Neurosurg Clin N Am 2007;18:281–288
50. Bridwell KH, Edwards CC II, Lenke LG. The pros and cons to saving the L5-S1 motion segment in a long scoliosis fusion construct. Spine 2003;28:S234–S242
51. Edwards CC II, Bridwell KH, Patel A, et al. Thoracolumbar deformity arthrodesis to L5 in adults: The fate of the L5-S1 disc. Spine 2003;28:2122–2131
52. Suk SI, Chung ER, Kim JH, Kim SS, Lee JS, Choi WK. Posterior vertebral column resection for severe rigid scoliosis. Spine 2005;30: 1682–1687
53. Bullmann V, Halm HF, Schulte T, Lerner T, Weber TP, Liljenqvist UR. Combined anterior and posterior instrumentation in severe and rigid idiopathic scoliosis. Eur Spine J 2006;15:440–448
54. Berven SH, Deviren V, Smith JA, Hu SH, Bradford DS. Management of fixed sagittal plane deformity: Outcome of combined anterior and posterior surgery. Spine 2003;28:1710–1715, discussion 6
55. Berven SH, Deviren V, Smith JA, Emami A, Hu SS, Bradford DS. Management of fixed sagittal plane deformity: Results of the transpedicular wedge resection osteotomy. Spine 2001;26:2036–2043
56. Epstein NE. Efficacy of different bone volume expanders for augmenting lumbar fusions. Surg Neurol 2008;69:16–19, discussion 19
57. Buttermann GR, Glazer PA, Hu SS, Bradford DS. Anterior and posterior allografts in symptomatic thoracolumbar deformity. J Spinal Disord 2001;14:54–66
58. Boden SD, Kang J, Sandhu H, Heller JG. Use of recombinant human bone morphogenetic protein-2 to achieve posterolateral lumbar spine fusion in humans: A prospective, randomized clinical pilot trial: 2002 Volvo Award in clinical studies. Spine 2002;27: 2662–2673
59. Shields LB, Raque GH, Glassman SD, et al. Adverse effects associated with high-dose recombinant human bone morphogenetic protein-2 use in anterior cervical spine fusion. Spine 2006;31: 542–547
60. Luhmann SJ, Bridwell KH, Cheng I, Imamura T, Lenke LG, Schootman M. Use of bone morphogenetic protein-2 for adult spinal deformity. Spine 2005;30(17, Suppl):S110–S117
61. Coe JD, Arlet V, Donaldson W, et al. Complications in spinal fusion for adolescent idiopathic scoliosis in the new millennium. A report of the Scoliosis Research Society Morbidity and Mortality Committee. Spine 2006;31:345–349
62. Carreon LY, Puno RM, Dimar JR II, Glassman SD, Johnson JR. Perioperative complications of posterior lumbar decompression and arthrodesis in older adults. J Bone Joint Surg Am 2003;85A: 2089–2092
63. Rinella A, Bridwell K, Kim Y, et al. Late complications of adult idiopathic scoliosis primary fusions to L4 and above: the effect of age and distal fusion level. Spine 2004;29:318–325
64. Ali RM, Boachie-Adjei O, Rawlins BA. Functional and radiographic outcomes after surgery for adult scoliosis using third-generation instrumentation techniques. Spine 2003;28:1163–1169, discussion 1169–1170
65. Schwab F, Lafage V, Farcy JP, et al. Surgical rates and operative outcome analysis in thoracolumbar and lumbar major adult scoliosis: Application of the new adult deformity classification. Spine 2007;32:2723–2730
66. McDonnell MF, Glassman SD, Dimar JR II, Puno RM, Johnson JR. Perioperative complications of anterior procedures on the spine. J Bone Joint Surg Am 1996;78:839–847
67. Weis JC, Betz RR, Clements DH III, Balsara RK. Prevalence of perioperative complications after anterior spinal fusion for patients with idiopathic scoliosis. J Spinal Disord 1997;10:371–375
68. Myers MA, Hamilton SR, Bogosian AJ, Smith CH, Wagner TA. Visual loss as a complication of spine surgery. A review of 37 cases. Spine 1997;22:1325–1329
69. Leon L, Rodriguez H, Tawk RG, Ondra SL, Labropoulos N, Morasch MD. The prophylactic use of inferior vena cava filters in patients undergoing high-risk spinal surgery. Ann Vasc Surg 2005;19:442–447

# 25 Osteobiological Agents for Spinal Fusion

*Safdar N. Khan, William F. Lavelle, and Munish C. Gupta*

Complications in harvesting autogenous iliac crest bone-graft material, including pain at the donor site, has led to the investigation of potential alternatives to such grafts, including various allograft sources, demineralized bone-graft material, and bone morphogenetic protein (BMP). This chapter will review both alternative options and the biology involved in spinal fusion.

## Fracture Healing

For the treating surgeon to understand the process of spinal fusion, it is necessary to understand the process of healing of a bone fracture. Such healing involves the interaction with one another, in a well-orchestrated sequence of events, of four major types of tissue: cortical bone, periosteum, external soft-tissue sleeve, and bone marrow. Rigid internal fixation leads to primary cortical healing, which involves a biological response with remodeling units of cutting cones consisting of osteoclasts, followed by an influx of osteoblasts.[1] This type of healing is typified by an absence of bony callus. When rigid internal fixation is not provided to support healing, micromotion occurs at the fracture site. In this latter case, healing involves a combination of intramembranous and endochondral bone formation, in which both the periosteum and the external soft tissues are involved. This type of healing is typified by the formation of bony callus.

### Intramembranous Ossification

Intramembranous bone formation occurs without a cartilaginous intermediate. In the fracture callus, new bone is formed by osteoblasts located adjacent to the fracture site and deep to the proliferating periosteal cells. Immediately after injury, positive staining for BMP is evident in the cambium-cell layer of periosteum proximal and distal to the fracture site. As healing of the fracture progresses, the number of these periosteal cells increases. By 1 week after fracture there is evidence of new woven bone formation, with abundant staining of osteoblasts lining this primitive bone. As the amount of intramembranous bone increases over the course of the next few days, there is a corresponding increase in the number of osteoblasts lining the woven bone. As the process of lamellar bone formation progresses, the overall numbers of periosteal cells decrease as do the percentage of cells staining positively for BMP (**Figs. 25.1, 25.2, 25.3, 25.4, 25.5, 25.6**). As the process of intramembranous bone formation proceeds and the number of more mature cell types increases, the presence of BMP decreases.[2,3]

### Endochondral Ossification

To study the endochondral healing of a fracture, a closed transverse femoral fracture has been established in a rat model.[4] This type of fracture is associated with minimal soft-tissue damage, and is characterized by several different fracture-healing responses. The first 7 to 10 days of fracture

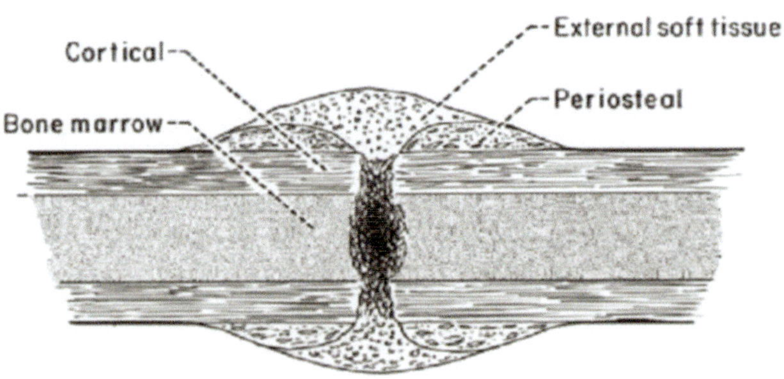


**Fig. 25.1** Fracture-healing responses. Fracture healing involves a response by four major types of tissue. (From Einhorn. J Orthop Trauma, Volume 19(10) Supplement. November/December 2005:S4–S6. Reprinted with permission.)

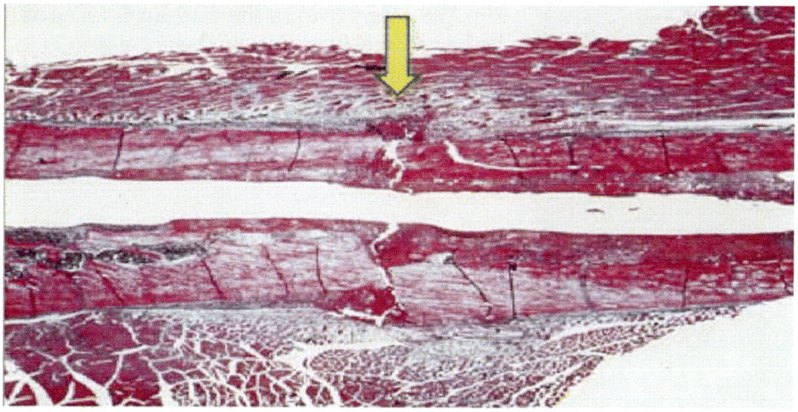

**Fig. 25.2** A closed transverse femoral fracture in a rat model on day 1. (From Einhorn. J Orthop Trauma, Volume 19(10) Supplement. November/December 2005:S4–S6. Reprinted with permission.)

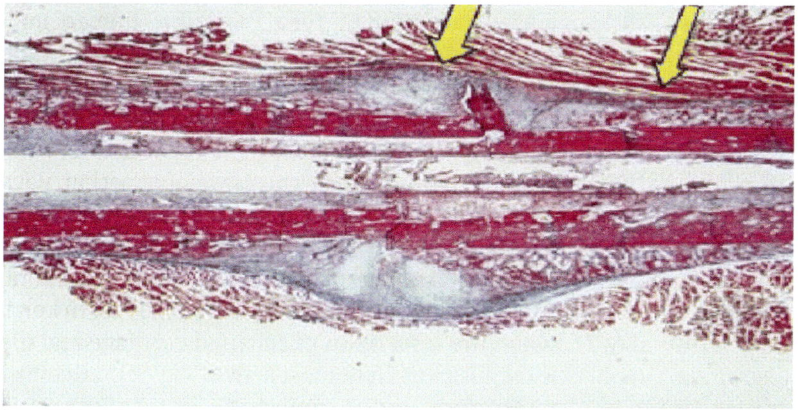

**Fig. 25.3** Chondrogenesis and inflammatory response at the fracture site in Fig. 25.2 are shown on day 7 after fracture. The *thick arrow* shows the chondrogenic response. The *thin arrow* indicates bone formation from the periosteum. (From Einhorn. J Orthop Trauma, Volume 19(10) Supplement. November/December 2005:S4–S6. Reprinted with permission.)

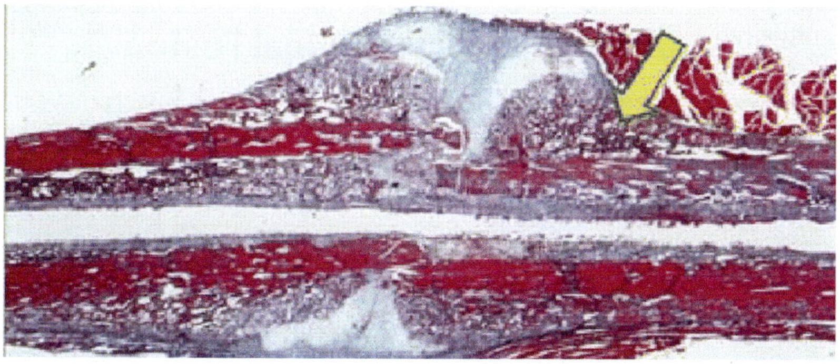

**Fig. 25.4** Day 14 after fracture. Calcification is shown in cartilage at the fracture site. The *arrow* shows calcified cartilage at the interface between cartilaginous callus and periosteal bone formation. (From Einhorn. J Orthop Trauma, Volume 19(10) Supplement. November/December 2005:S4–S6. Reprinted with permission.)

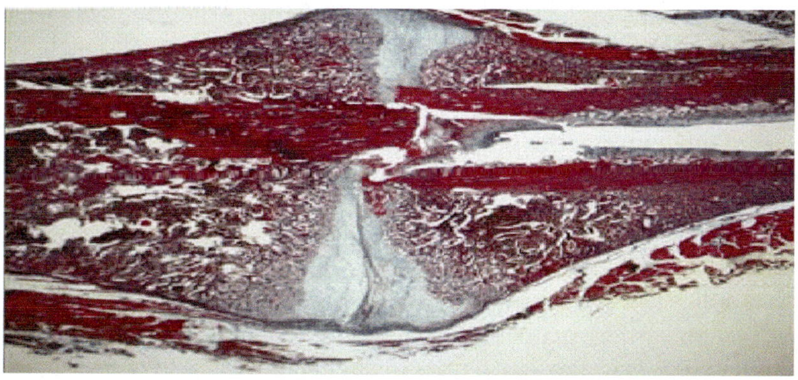

**Fig. 25.5** Day 21 after fracture. Most of the callus is composed of calcified cartilage. (From Einhorn. J Orthop Trauma, Volume 19(10) Supplement. November/December 2005:S4–S6. Reprinted with permission.)

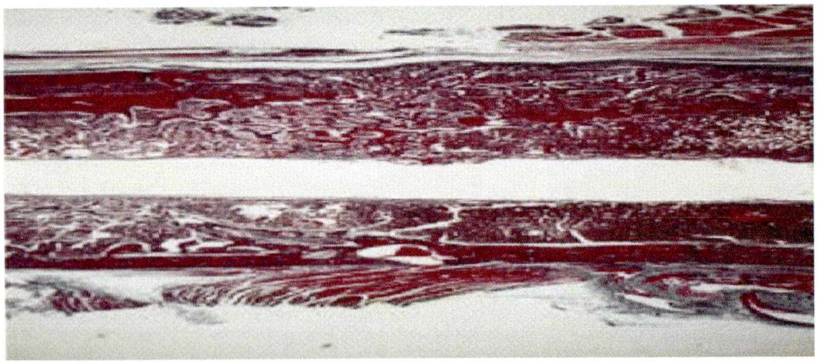

**Fig. 25.6** Days 28 to 35 after fracture. Calcified cartilage and newly formed woven bone are seen. (From Einhorn. J Orthop Trauma, Volume 19(10) Supplement. November/December 2005:S4–S6. Reprinted with permission.)

healing involve the process of *chondrogenesis*, which leads to cartilage formation adjacent to the fracture site and the formation of bone directly from osteoprogenitor cells under the periosteum. An inflammatory response occurs at the fracture site, heralded by the presence of macrophages, polymorphonuclear leukocytes, and lymphocytes, which secrete proinflammatory mediators. By 14 days after fracture, discrete areas within the cartilage anlage begin to calcify. In preparation for calcification, the chondrocytes release phosphatases and proteases. The phosphatases provide phosphate ions that combine with and precipitate with the calcium delivered from the mitochondria to form calcified cartilage. The proteases work by degrading inhibitory proteoglycans, allowing the chondrocytes to control the rate of the mineralization process.[4] In this model, the mid-diaphyseal fracture is well on its way to being united by 3 weeks after fracture. The callus is composed mainly of calcified cartilage, which is ultimately removed and replaced by bone. This process is initiated by chondroclasts, which are multinucleated cells specialized in the resorption of calcified tissues. The chondroclasts mediate vascularization and allow the arrival of mesenchymal stem cells that differentiate into osteoprogenitor cells and, ultimately, into bone-forming osteoblasts. The removal of calcified cartilage includes not only resorption of the mineralized matrix but also removal of the chondrocytes themselves. By 4 to 5 weeks after fracture, a combination of calcified cartilage and newly formed woven bone is present at the site of injury. At this time, large numbers of osteoclasts populate the tissue and begin to remodel the callus, converting it to a lamellar bone structure capable of supporting mechanical loads. This transition from cartilage to bone after injury involves a highly organized series of cell and molecular events leading to cell removal and matrix modification.[4]

Although the exact molecular basis for fracture healing is still unclear, several protein growth factors and cytokines are known to play an important role in the process of skeletal tissue repair.[5–8] Members of the transforming growth factor-β (TGF-β) supergene family, which include the BMP genes, have been shown to control several processes during skeletogenesis and repair. Cho et al[9] described the temporal expression of members of the TGF-β supergene family during fracture healing in a mouse-tibia model over a 28-day period. Within 24 hours after the fracture was sustained, there was an increase and a peak in activity of BMP-2. By the day 7 there was maximal expression of other cartilage genes: growth and differentiation factor (GDF)-5, TGF-β2, and TGF-β3. In contrast, BMP-3, BMP-4, BMP-7, and BMP-8 showed a restricted period of expression during the central period of the fracture-healing process from day 14 through day 21, when the resorption of calcified cartilage and osteoblastic recruitment were most active.

## The Biology of Spinal Fusion

The osterolateral arthrodesis of lumbar intertransverse processes is the most common spinal-fusion procedure, yet failure to achieve a solid bony union occurs in as many as 10 to 40% of patients with single-level uninstrumented fusions of this type. The percentage of such failure is even higher when multilevel fusions are attempted.[10] This high rate of nonunion indicates that the success of any fusion operation depends on a complex interplay of numerous physiological, biological, and molecular events. The most common recent clinical approach to preventing nonunion in the posterolateral spine has been the use of internal fixation with a pedicle-screw–rod construct. Although the use of internal fixation has decreased the number of nonunions, it has not eliminated the problem. Nonunions still occur in 10 to 15% of patients with instrumented fusions. Therefore, studying the biological sequence of events in spinal fusion provides key insights into devising biological products and bone-graft substitutes to enhance fusion rates.[10]

The biology of spinal fusion is a multifactorial process, which makes it difficult to study in the clinical setting. In the past, the fusion rates in animal models used to investigate the biological events in the healing of a fusion approached 100%, a figure much higher than is seen clinically. These models were skeletally immature organisms, and the fusion done in them was either an interfacet or an interlaminar fusion rather than a truly intertransverse fusion. In contrast to spinal fusions in humans, these fusions in animal models were usually unsuccessful only if the model involved a destabilized spine. These limitations led to the development by Boden et al of a rabbit model of intertransverse-process arthrodesis that was more clinically applicable to the human situation.[11] The major benefit of this type of model was that in it, nonunions occurred spontaneously at a rate comparable with that reported in humans who had fusion without internal fixation.

The rabbit model of lumbar intertransverse-process arthrodesis has been well characterized with the use of autogenous iliac crest as the graft material. Mechanically solid fusions in the model generally occur by 4 to 6 weeks, with an overall rate of nonunion of 30 to 40%. Radiographic analysis has shown progressive remodeling of bone graft material with time, usually by 10 to 12 weeks, but as in humans, radiographs were accurate in assessing success or failure to attain solid fusion only 70% of the time. Control animals showed that surgical exposure alone did not automatically result in spinal fusion, as has also been seen in other species.[11] Vascular injection studies indicated that the primary blood supply to the fusion mass originated from the decorticated transverse processes. The failure to achieve spinal fusion in the absence of decortication emphasizes the importance of careful fusion-bed preparation of the posterolateral elements of the spine for successful fusion. Proper preparation of the fusion bed is required to provide critical bone marrow, vascularization, and cellular elements to the fusion mass.[11]

Three distinct and reproducible temporal phases of healing in spinal fusion have been histologically identified, including an inflammatory phase, an endochondral phase, and a remodeling phase.[12] Histological analysis indicated that the maturation of a fusion occurs from the periphery and progresses centrally. The maturation of a spinal fusion was most advanced at the ends of the fusion mass, near the transverse processes (outer zone). A similar histological progression occurred in the central zone, but was delayed relative to the series of events in the outer zones. A similar lag has been noted in osteoblast-related gene expression, with the peak expression of all genes occurring 1 to 2 weeks later in the central zone than in the two outer zones. This is consistent with the peripheral-to-central healing pattern observed histologically in fusions done with autogenous bone-graft material. This central lag effect, with a transient cartilaginous area, was hypothesized as the reason for many nonunions in the central zones of fusion masses.

Variations were also seen in the temporal and spatial expression of the mRNA for BMP. In the peripheral zones, expression of the mRNA for BMP-2 was increased during weeks 2 through 6, with peak expression at weeks 3 and 4. BMP-6 in the outer zones had a first peak on day 2 and a second peak during week 5. BMP-6 in the central zone showed an initial peak on day 2, but did not demonstrate a later peak. This lower level of expression of BMP-6 observed in the central zone of the fusion mass may be correlated with the delayed timing and smaller amount of bone formation in the central zone (**Figs. 25.7, 25.8, 25.9**).[12]

The use of electrocautery in the healing of spinal fusion is controversial. Some spine surgeons use electrocautery (Bovie dissection) sparingly or avoid it completely through fear of increasing the chances of postoperative infection and delaying wound healing. They prefer to ligate bleeding vessels and mechanically elevate the muscles from the bone subperiosteally. However, most surgeons use Bovie dissection extensively. They feel that it is is quicker and produces much less bleeding during surgery. There is no evidence in the literature that extensive use of electrocautery alters cytokine expression or impairs the progression of fusion. We do not feel that extensive electrocautery in any way contributes to psuedarthrosis after spine surgery.

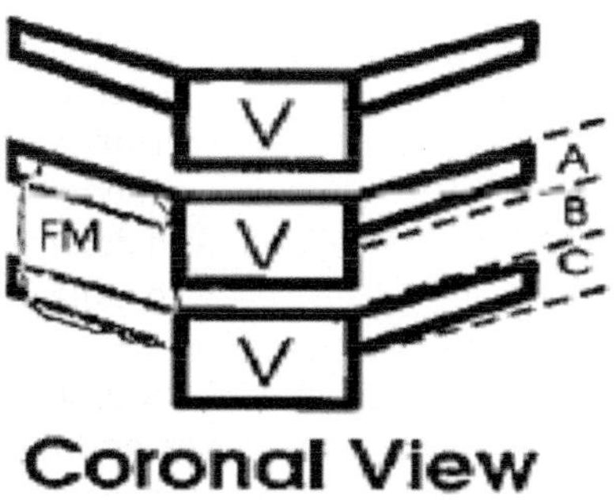


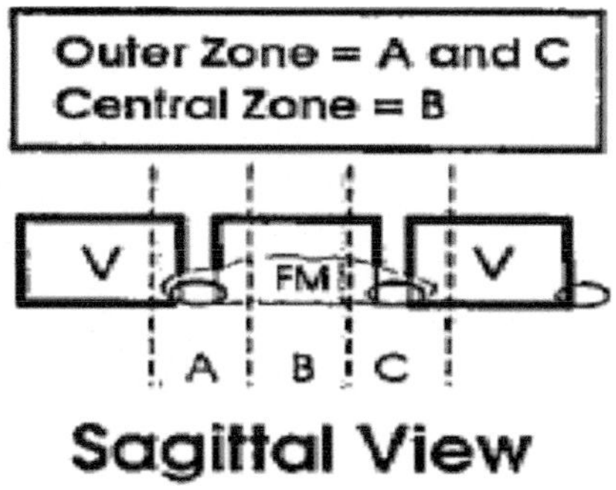


**Fig. 25.7** Schematic diagram of a lumbar spinal-fusion mass (FM) divided into thirds in the coronal and sagittal views, and the relationship of each third to the vertebral bodies (V). **(A,C)** The outer zones are distinguished from **(B)** the single central zone. (From Morone M. Clin Orthop Related Res, 351:252-265, 1998. Reprinted with permission.)

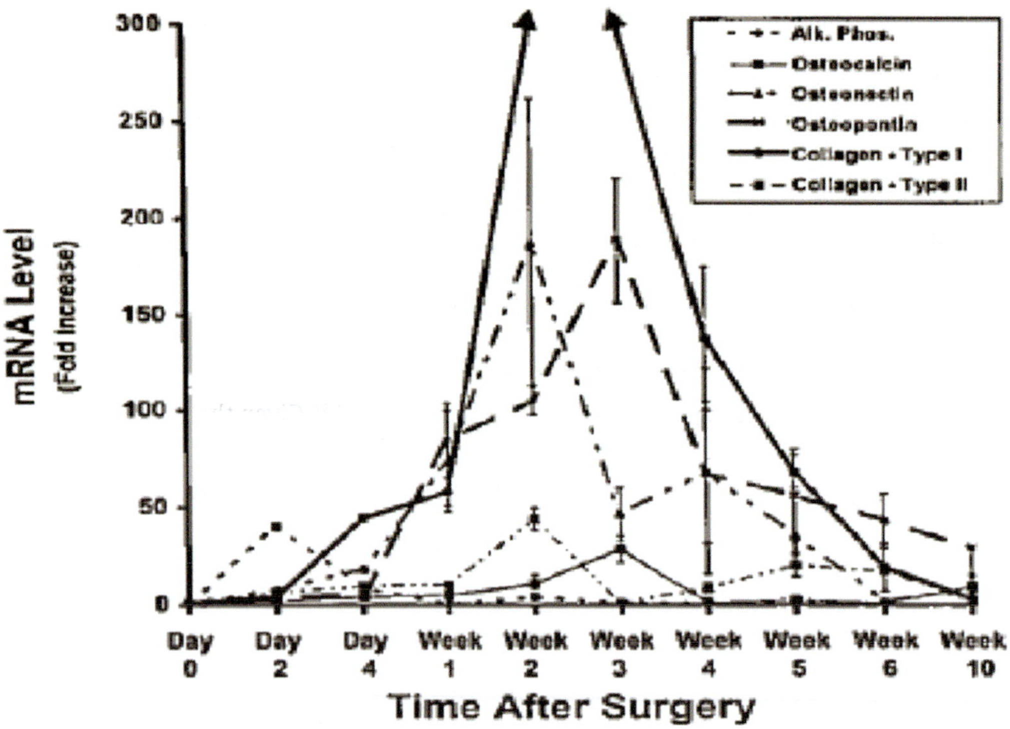


**Fig. 25.8** Osteoblast-related gene expression in the outer zone of a spinal-fusion mass at specific times after surgery. The values of mRNA levels are given as multiples of the level present in iliac-crest bone (day 0). A reproducible sequence of gene expression was seen and was paralleled in the central zone (not shown) but delayed by 1 to 3 weeks. (From Morone M. Clin Orthop Related Res, 351:252-265, 1998. Reprinted with permission.)

## Osteobiological Products and Spinal Fusion

Nearly half a million bone-graft procedures are performed in the United States annually. Of these, the vast majority are spinal fusions, potentially representing up to $2 billion spent per year on agents for enhancing bone repair and bone-graft substitutes (**Table 25.1**).[13,14] Because of the distinct biological conditions and biomechanical forces specific to the anterior spinal column and the posterior elements, it is likely that the efficacy of each bone-graft material in promoting successful fusion will also depend on the particular clinical application for which it is being used (e.g., interbody fusion versus posterolateral fusion) (**Table 25.2**).[15–17]

The processes of bone regeneration and formation during spinal fusion require three critical elements: (1) osteogenic

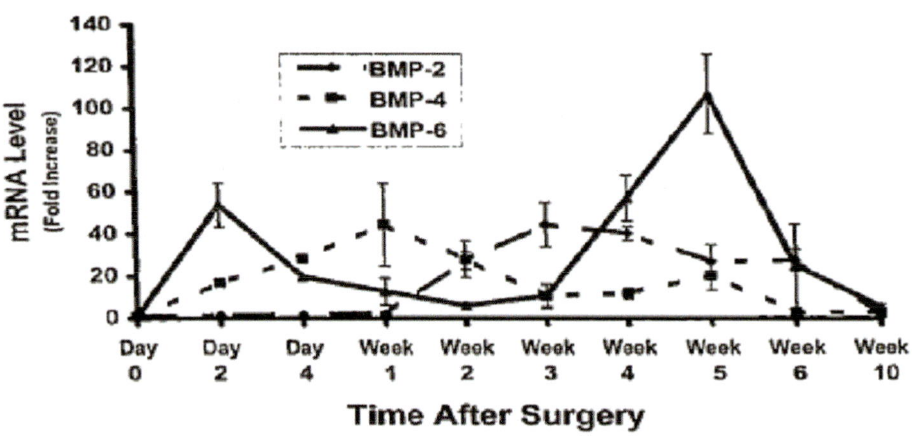


**Fig. 25.9** Expression of BMP in the outer zone of a spinal-fusion mass at specific times after surgery. The mRNA levels are given as multiples of the levels present in iliac-crest bone (day 0). A reproducible sequence of gene expression was seen with BMP-6 mRNA peaking earliest, on day 2, followed by BMP-4 mRNA, BMP-2 mRNA, and a second peak of BMP-6 mRNA. (From Morone M. Clin Orthop Related Res, 351:252-265, 1998. Reprinted with permission.)

**Table 25.1 Classification of Osteobiologics for Enhancement of Spinal Fusion**

| Class | Description | Examples |
|---|---|---|
| Allograft based | Allograft bone | OrthoBlast, Opteform, Grafton |
| Factor based | Recombinant growth factors used with appropriate carriers | BMP, GDF-5 |
| Cell based | Cells used to generate new tissue alone or seeded onto a support scaffold | Mesenchymal stem cells |
| Ceramic based | Includes calcium phosphate and calcium sulfate | Norian SRS, ProOsteon, Osteoset |
| Polymer based | Both degradable and nondegradable polymers | Cortoss, OPLA |

cells that have the capacity to make new bone; (2) osteoinductive factors (i.e., growth factors and cytokines) that promote the differentiation of stem cells into an osteoblastic phenotype; (3) and an osteoconductive scaffold that facilitates neovascularization and supports the ingrowth of bone. Autogenous bone is believed to have all three of these essential properties for bone formation. It is therefore considered the "gold-standard" graft material for spinal fusion. Autograft bone for use in the spinal column is most often taken from the iliac crest, but may also be obtained from other sources, such as a resected rib or from local bone harvested at the fusion site, depending on the location and extent of the surgical procedure (**Table 25.3**). Procurement of autogenous bone often necessitates a separate operative incision, thus involving additional iatrogenically induced surgical trauma. Besides increasing the operative time and blood loss, the harvesting of bone-graft material from a separate site is also associated with considerable donor site morbidity. Nearly 30% of patients who undergo such procedures experience some kind of complication postoperatively. The complications include infection, hematoma, nerve or vascular injury, fracture, persistent pain, abdominal herniation, and pelvic instability. The amount of bone available for grafting may also be insufficient in children as well as in adults requiring revision surgery or fusion of multiple spinal segments.[18–20] Given the limitations of autogenous bone grafts, significant research has been done to find and improve graft-extending materials and other sources of grafts.

A *bone-graft extender* is a substance that adds bulk to a given amount of autogenous bone that is to be used over a greater surface area with the same rate of success. A *bone-graft enhancer* is a substance that when added to autograft bone increases its healing potential with either the usual or a smaller amount of graft material. A *bone-graft substitute* is a substance that may entirely replace autogenous bone-graft material with the same or a better rate of successful fusion.[21]

## Allograft Bone

Allograft bone obtained from cadaveric sources has been the most widely used substitute for autogenous bone-graft material.[22] Allografts are osteoconductive, with minimal or no osteoinductive potential, primarily because the donor's cells are eradicated during tissue processing. Allografts are prepared either by freezing or lyophilization (i.e., freeze-drying) to decrease their antigenicity and permit their storage for

**Table 25.2 Bone Graft Activity by Type**

| | Osteogenesis | Osteoconduction | Osteoinduction | Mechanical Properties | Vascularity |
|---|---|---|---|---|---|
| Autograft | | | | | |
| Bone marrow | ++ | +/− | + | − | − |
| Cancellous | ++ | ++ | + | + | − |
| Cortical | + | + | +/− | ++ | − |
| Vascularized | ++ | ++ | + | ++ | ++ |
| Allograft | | | | | |
| Cancellous | − | ++ | + | + | − |
| Cortical | − | +/− | +/− | ++ | − |
| Demineralized | − | ++ | + | − | − |

*Note*: −, +, ++, +++ = extent of activity (− = no activity to +++ = maximal activity)

**Table 25.3 Local and Systemic Factors Influencing Spinal-Fusion Biology**

| Factor | Positive | Negative |
|---|---|---|
| Local | Good vascular supply at the graft site | Radiation |
| | Large surface area | Tumor |
| | Mechanical stability | Mechanical instability |
| | Mechanical loading | Local bone disease |
| | Growth factors | Infection |
| | Electrical stimulation | Corticosteroids |
| Systemic | Growth hormone | Nonsteroidal anti-inflammatory drugs |
| | Thyroid hormone | Chemotherapy |
| | Somatomedins | Smoking |
| | Vitamins A and D | Sepsis |
| | Insulin | Diabetes |
| | Parathyroid hormone | Malnutrition |
| | Metabolic bone disease | |

extended periods. Frozen allografts may be kept for up to 1 year at −20°C without a change in their structural properties. Lyophilized allografts are dehydrated and vacuum packed, which allows their storage at room temperature. Freeze-drying reduces the immunogenicity of allografts more than does freezing, but upon rehydration and reconstitution, freeze-dried grafts may lose up to 50% of their mechanical strength. Allografts may also be treated with ethylene oxide or radiation, although these methods may further compromise their material properties and reduce their osteoinductive capacity.[22]

A common patient concern with the use of cadaveric allografts is the possible spread of infectious diseases, such as hepatitis and human immunodeficiency virus (HIV) infection. To date, only two cases of transmission of HIV in allograft bone have been documented, both of which involved unprocessed grafts. Only one of these cases involved allograft bone used for a spinal fusion. The combination of meticulous donor screening and tissue processing has reduced the risk of infection from allograft bone to less than one per million transplants.[23]

Cortical allografts offer substantial structural stability and are well suited for inter-vertebral-body arthrodesis. Threaded cylinders (of cortical allogratft) may serve as a source of bone-graft material while stabilizing the spinal column. Hollow centers allow the insertion of carrier soaked in growth factors or autograft material to aid anterior fusions. Fusion with these techniques occurs slowly, by means of periosteal new-bone formation around the allograft. Cortical allografts never fully incorporate at their site of engrafting, and remain a mixture of necrotic and viable bone. On the other hand, corticocancellous allograft material initially imparts very little mechanical support, but because of its relatively large surface area is integrated more rapidly and fully than a purely cortical bone graft.

Both autogenous bone and allograft bone are incorporated into the fusion mass according to a well-defined cascade of biological events, consisting of hemorrhage, inflammation, and vascular invasion, culminating in the replacement of graft material with new bone. With bone allograft this remodeling process occurs more slowly and there is greater resorption of the graft than with autograft bone. This may manifest itself in the inter-vertebral-body milieu by cortical lucencies that indicate resorption and vascular invasion. Genetic incompatibility of the donor and recipient has been found to be associated with increased resorption of allograft bone and histological evidence of rejection; however, routine screening for genetic compatibility may be impractical.[24]

The differing mechanical and biological properties of the various types of allografts make each type suitable for differing applications. Predominantly cortical allografts, such as femoral rings or fibular struts, can be useful in applications in which there is a need for structural support under compression (e.g., inter-vertebral-body applications). Allografts of cancellous bone, such as cancellous-bone chips, are best suited in areas that require little mechanical strength and greater osteopromotion such as posterolateral fusions. In these applications there is a need for more rapid bone incorporation, remodeling, and revascularization.

Zdeblick and Ducker[25] obtained equivalent results when using allograft or autograft bone for single-level fusions, but the incidence of nonunion was 62% among patients receiving allograft bone for two-level anterior cervical fusion, as compared with only 17% among patients receiving autologous bone. It must be noted, however, that these results were acieved before the advent of routine anterior cervical plating. In another retrospective review of patients treated with multilevel uninstrumented arthrodeses of the cervical spine,[26] An and colleagues found that fusion occurred in 85% of those implanted with autograft bone, whereas successful healing occurred in only 50% of a group treated with allografts. These results were contested by Samartzis et al,[27] who reviewed the fusion and clinical outcome data for 80 consecutive patients who underwent anterior cervical discectomy and fusion (ACDF) with either allograft or autograft bone and anterior plate fixation involving two and three vertebral levels. Of these 80 patients, 45 received autogenous tricortical grafts from the iliac crest and 35 received tricortical allograft bone and were treated with multilevel ACDF with anterior plate fixation at a single institution. The overall rate of fusion was 97.5%, with no significant difference in the rates of fusion with allograft and autografts. Excellent and good clinical outcomes were noted in 88.8% of the patients.

The literature appears to support the success of single-level noninstrumented fusions with autograft bone, but in biomechanically challenging multilevel fusions, the results with the use of rigid instrumentation are the same with allograft or autograft bone.

In two studies, patients treated with autograft were found to have solid posterolateral fusion more often than those receiving allograft bone.[28,29] Interestingly, Dodd et al[30] reported a 100% fusion rate in adolescent patients with idiopathic scoliosis who had implants of femoral head allograft and local autograft bone. Betz and colleagues[31] compared the clinical results of posterior spinal fusion (PSF) with allograft-bone augmentation and those without grafting in patients with adolescent idiopathic scoliosis (AIS). Ninety-one patients with AIS were randomized into two treatment groups. Seventy-six patients had more than 2-years of follow-up and were included in this review. In the group treated with allograft bone alone, 37 patients underwent a standard PSF with multisegmented hook–screw-and-rod instrumentation with the use of corticocancellous bone allografts for augmentation. The study group included 39 patients with AIS who underwent the same procedure without any bone graft (no graft group). The treatment groups were similar with respect to age, preoperative deformity, and degree of postoperative correction. The overall pseudarthrosis rate was 1.3%. Pseudarthrosis was identified in a single patient in the study. This pseudarthrosis occurred in the allograft group, whereas none of 39 patients in the no-graft group experienced pseudarthrosis. Betz and colleagues concluded that PSF with newer-generation multisegmented hook–screw-and-rod systems could be successful with allograft or local bone graft or both without the use of supplemental autogenous bone graft in patients with AIS. In summary, these studies suggest that corticocancellous allografts may be used as either graft extenders or as alternatives to autogenous bone grafts in many spinal-fusion procedures.

## Ceramics

Ceramics are synthetic bone-graft substitutes that consist of an inorganic material that acts as scaffolding for growing bone. Ceramics are commonly made of hydroxyapatite (HA), tricalcium phosphate (TCP), or a combination of these two materials, such as coralline HA, which is derived from sea coral (Pro Osteon, Interpore Cross, Irvine, CA). In these bone-graft substitutes the calcium carbonate originally present in the exoskeleton of coral is replaced with HA through a specialized hydrothermal chemical exchange technique, generating a synthetic matrix whose microscopic architecture mimics that of human cancellous bone. Ceramics are exclusively osteoconductive and contain a pore structure that allows the ingrowth of new bone.[32] Ceramics are nontoxic, nonimmunogenic, easy to sterilize, and available in virtually unlimited supply. However, they have the disadvantages of being brittle and having little shear strength or fracture resistance.[33] Ceramics are commonly used in conjunction with internal fixation, owing to their poorer mechanical strength; they must be protected from loading until they are incorporated into host bone.

HA is an inert substance that is retained in vivo for a prolonged period, whereas the more porous TCP typically undergoes osseo-integration within 6 weeks of implantation. Ransford and co-workers[34] evaluated the use of a synthetic porous biphasic calcium phosphate ceramic consisting 60% HA and 40% β-TCP (Triosite; Zimmer Ltd., Swindon, UK) as a substitute for bone graft in PSF for idiopathic scoliosis in a prospective, randomized study of 341 patients. Patients were randomly allocated to receive either autograft from the iliac crest or rib segments or to receive Triosite blocks alone. The rates of maintenance of correction were similar in the two patient groups, suggesting a similar efficacy of autograft and Triosite in fusion. Histological findings on biopsy indicated that Triosite provided a favorable scaffolding for the formation of new bone and was gradually incorporated into the fusion mass. There were more problems with wound healing in the autograft group than in the Triosite group. There was also significant donor-site morbidity in the autograft group, including infection ($n = 7$), hematoma, and delayed healing. In addition, 6% of patients in the autograft group had persistent donor-site pain at 18 months after surgery. These results suggested that Triosite synthetic porous ceramic was a safe and effective substitute for autograft bone in these patients. Other clinical studies of ceramics have also demonstrated their efficacy as osteoconductive graft materials in scoliosis surgery.[35]

Ceramics do not exhibit osteogenic or osteoinductive properties; as a result, they depend on the local environment for osteoprogenitor cells and signals. However, ceramic scaffolds facilitate cellular adhesion, support vascular ingrowth, and promote new bone formation when used with autogenous bone graft or bone-marrow aspirate. An additional benefit of ceramics as components of composite graft substitutes is that they act as viscous matrices that limit the diffusion of osteogenic cells and signals away from the fusion site.[36]

## Demineralized Bone Matrix

Demineralized bone matrices (DBMs) are generated by the acid extraction of processed allograft bone, giving rise to a demineralized matrix consisting of type I collagen and noncollagenous proteins, as well as numerous signaling cytokines. Removal of the mineral phase of the bone releases these biologically active cytokines, making them more accessible to osteogenic or inflammatory cells. BMPs constitute less than 0.1% by weight of all bone proteins found in DBMs. However, these growth factors are essential to osteoinduction and ultimately to bone formation.[37]

After being extracted from bone, DBM exists as a particulate powder. Its effectiveness in grafting depends on its localization and retention at a graft such, such as a site of spinal fusion. Human DBM is often combined with other components (carriers) intended to make DBM easier to handle by turning it into a putty or paste. These carriers must be biocompatible with bone, not reduce the osteoconductivity of DBM, maintain graft containment during wound irrigation and closure, and maintain graft localization until the graft site is stabilized.

When DBM, with its small amounts of osteoinductive proteins, is combined with a carrier, a significant portion of the complex is the carrier (~85% carrier and 15% DBM). The first DBM–carrier products were introduced clinically in 1991, and such products have since become among the most widely used alternative graft products in spinal-fusion surgery. Today, at least eight manufacturers market more than six types of carriers and 25 products. DBM is commercially available in several different forms (e.g., powder, chips, crushed granules, putty, and gel-filled syringes).

As noted above, the carriers used in current DBM formulations are varied. DBM carriers include glycerol, gelatin, calcium sulfate, lecithin, and hyaluronic acid. Glycerol is the primary carrier found in Grafton™ (Osteotech; Eatontown, NJ). Osteofil™ (Regeneration Technologies Inc.; Alachua, FL) is a DBM product that utilizes a porcine-derived gelatin that is stored in frozen form and needs to be heated and hydrated before surgical implantation. Accell™ (IsoTis Orthobiologics Inc.; Irvine, CA) utilizes a gelatin derived from human DBM that can be stored at room temperature. Allomatrix™ (Wright Medical Technologies; Arlington, TN) uses a calcium sulfate hemihydrate mixed with carboxymethylcellulose. Water is added at the time of fusion-bed preparation. Lecithin, a phospholipid derived from soybeans, is found in InterGro™ (Interpore Cross Inc.; Irvine, CA). DBX™ (Synthes; West Chester, PA) utilizes hyaluronic acid produced in a recombinant manner as its carrier.

Although DBMs are generally deemed safe for implantation, DBM carriers must also be scrutinized. Ultrahigh doses of glycerol containing DBMs (Grafton™) have proven toxic when administered to athymic rats, eventually leading to death from renal failure in a dose-dependent manner.[38] However, there have been no reported cases of glycerol toxicity related to the implantation of these DBM products in humans. Preparations containing hyaluronic acid (DBX™) have a more neutral pH and thus may be less harmful to host tissues. Other products, such as Allomatrix™, which utilize a physiologically inert calcium sulfate carrier, may also be less toxic to the fusion bed.

Cost-effective and readily available from human tissue banks, DBM formulations are attractive graft enhancers and extenders. The demineralization process eradicates the antigenic epitopes in bone, making DBM considerably less immunogenic than mineralized bone allograft material. In addition, when bone marrow is combined with DBM, the instant source of osteogenic precursor cells may provide an additional biological contribution to osteogenesis, with the DBM acting primarily as a carrier.

The osteoinductive capability of commercially available DBMs varies from one product to another, and may even vary from lot to lot of a specific product. This variability is thought to come from differences in BMP content, as noted by Bae et al.[39] However, the absolute concentration of BMP in a particular DBM preparation may not correlate with its clinical efficacy. The demineralization process and method of sterilization may alter intrinsic BMP activity and therefore indirectly modify the osteoinductive capability of the DBM.[40,41] In addition, the donor source affects the osteoinductive properties of a DBM product, with bone from younger donors having greater osteoconductive potential.[42] As a result, the amount of DBM used does not correlate with the efficacy of a DBM product because the different methods of processing and sterilization, as well as the carrier used in the product, can affect its osteoinductivity. Despite these discrepancies, DBM products are not closely regulated by the U.S. Food and Drug Administration (FDA), because they are considered to be minimally manipulated tissues for transplantation.

As with ceramics, DBMs appear to be most effective in fusion environments that allow unimpeded angiogenesis and a steady passage of osteoprogenitor cells. Autograft or bone marrow aspirates may be added to DBMs to increase the osteoinductive index. However, in preclinical models, DBMs have been found to promote successful arthrodesis of the spine when used alone or in conjunction with autograft, bone marrow, or ceramics.[43–45] These results may be a direct indication of the species-specific nature of DBMs for spinal fusion.

Initial studies of the efficacy of DBM in human spinal fusion focused on its application to anterior cervical spinal fusion. In a prospective study of 77 patients undergoing such fusion for cervical disc disease, the fusion rates with freeze-dried allograft bone augmented with DBM (Grafton™) were compared with those of autograft bone from the anterior iliac crest.[46] This study demonstrated a trend toward an increased rate of pseudarthrosis for the allograft-DBM group (46.2%) as compared with the autograft group (26.3%). The investigators who conducted the study also compared the rate of graft collapse $>3$ mm, and as in the case of psuedarthrosis found a greater rate of such collapse in the allograft–DBM group (19%) than in the autograft group (11%). Although the findings were remarkable, they did not reach statistical significance in either comparison. The study investigators concluded that allograft bone and DBM could not effectively replace autograft bone in this clinical scenario, although the percentage of smokers in the trial was a confounding factor.

Sassard and associates[47] compared the fusion rates with a local autograft–DBM composite and those with iliac-crest autograft bone alone in 108 patients with lumbar posterolateral spinal fusions. The fusion rates in the two groups did not differ at 2-year follow-up. Cammisa et al[48] performed a prospective randomized study of 120 patients undergoing posterolateral spinal fusions of up to three vertebral levels. They compared the fusion rates with autogenous iliac-crest bone alone and those with a combination of DBM (Grafton™) and autogenous iliac-crest bone in a 3:1 mixture. At a 2-year follow-up, fusion rates achieved with the DBM–autograft composite were similar to those with the traditional iliac-crest autograft with respect to mineralization and integrity of the developing fusion mass. It must be noted, however, that this was not a true group-to-group randomized trial but a side-to-side comparison in the same patients. The results of this study indicated that fusion rates were the same with the DBM–iliac-crest mixture as with iliac-crest autograft when one-third of the normal amount of autograft was combined with DBM. This suggests that DBM may serve as a graft extender in human posterolateral spinal fusion. Price et al[49] conducted a retrospective study of posterior fusions augmented by bone graft in patients with AIS and found no difference in fusion rates with autograft and allograft bone combined with DBM.

Not all clinical trials of DBM have been favorable to it. In a retrospective study in which 40 patients who underwent instrumented posterolateral fusion were followed for an average of 53 months, the fusion site was augmented with coralline HA with or without Grafton DBM™ gel. Patients who received the Grafton DBM™ gel had a higher rate of pseudarthrosis.[50]

In summary, current data suggest that DBMs may have limited efficacy as graft substitutes, but may be indicated for use as bone-graft extenders and enhancers when used in combination with autograft bone, bone marrow, or other graft materials, such as ceramics, especially in situations in which there is a decreased amount of available autograft bone.

## Osteoinductive Proteins

The most extensively studied osteopromotive factors in the processes of osteoinduction and bone formation are the BMPs, which have been shown to initiate and encourage the osteoblastic differentiation of pluripotential mesenchymal stem cells in vitro (**Table 25.4**). They are also the only protein signaling molecules capable of inducing ectopic bone production in vivo. The BMPs are soluble, low-molecular-weight glycoproteins that share extensive homology with TGF-β. By binding to specific receptors on the surfaces of receptive mesenchymal stem cells, these extracellular factors activate intracellular signal-transduction pathways responsible for osteoblastic differentiation and function.

The genes encoding the BMPs have been sequenced and subsequently cloned, allowing the mass production of a single specific BMP including BMP-2 and BMP-7 (also known as osteogenic protein-1).[51–53] Recombinant human BMP-2 (rhBMP-2; INFUSE; Medtronic Sofamor Danek, Memphis, TN) has been approved by the FDA specifically for applications in anterior spinal fusion (**Fig. 25.10**) as well as for open tibial fractures. Osteogenic protein (OP)-1 has been approved by the FDA under the Humanitarian Device Exemption (HDE) program as an alternative to autograft bone in cases of recalcitrant long-bone nonunion in which the use of autograft bone is unfeasible and alternative treatments have failed.

An important feature in relating these protein factors to the enhancement of fusion is that they tend to diffuse away from the fusion site when used without an appropriate carrier, thus diluting their osteoinductive ability. As a result, these factors need to be combined with an inert carrier that serves to restrict their elution, keeping them in the fusion bed without having an adverse affect on the osteoinductive properties of the particular protein factor being used. The carrier may also act as an osteoconductive scaffold that supports new bone formation by promoting cellular adhesion and angiogenesis. Autogenous bone graft, DBMs, collagen, ceramics, and polylactic acid have all been used to deliver

**Table 25.4 Influence of Growth Factors on Graft Incorporation and Bone Healing**

| Growth Factor | Cell Origin | Function |
|---|---|---|
| Tumor necrosis factor | Macrophages | Increases bone resorption |
| Fibroblast growth factor | Inflammatory cells, osteoblasts, chondrocytes | Increases cell replication and collagen formation. Angiogenic |
| Platelet-derived growth factor | Platelets, monocytes, endothelial cells | Increases cellular proliferation and collagen formation |
| Insulin-like growth factor | Osteoblasts, chondrocytes | Stimulates chondrocyte formation |
| Transforming growth factor-β | Platelets, osteoblasts, chondrocytes | Increases proteoglycan synthesis, decreases collagen synthesis |
| Bone morphogenetic proteins 2, -4, -7 | Mesenchymal stem cells, osteoblasts | Induces progenitor cells to become bone-forming cells |

A

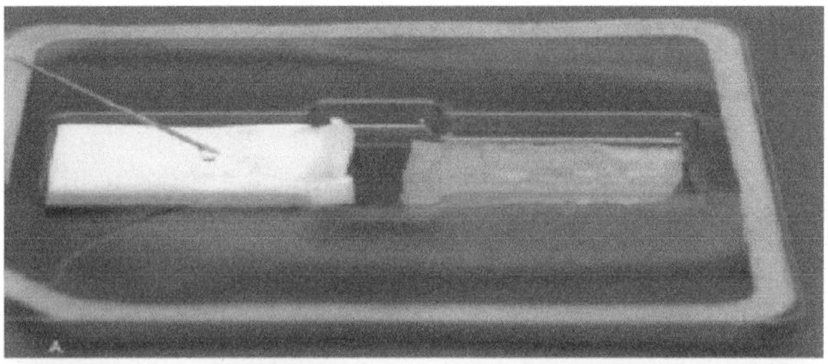

B

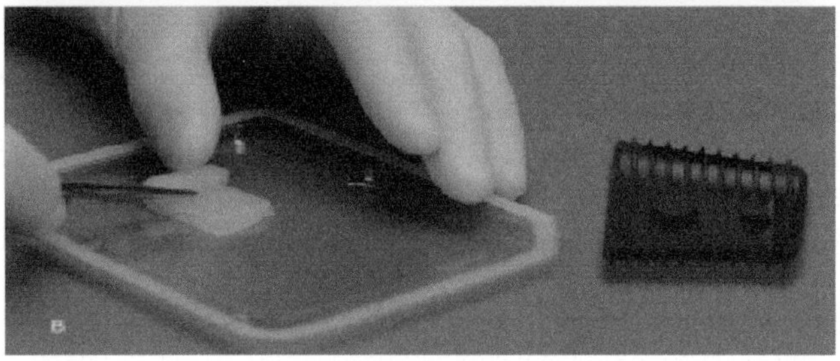

**Fig. 25.10** **(A)** A collagen sponge carrier is soaked with rhBMP-2 at the time of surgery and **(B)** then rolled and placed within an inter-vertebral-body fusion cage. (From McKay B. Spine 2002 27(16 Suppl):S66. Reprinted with permission.)

rhBMPs, but the ideal carrier for these recombinant proteins remains elusive. Although the osteopromotive potential of the growth factor will not change, the indication for its use, such as in anterior spinal fusion as compared with posterolateral intertransverse fusion, will make site-specific mechanical and biological demands. As a result, a carrier that works well in one environment may not be adaptable to another environment.

## Recombinant Human Bone Morphogenetic Protein-2/INFUSE

rhBMP-2 has been tested clinically for use in spinal fusion in several prospective, randomized, multicenter clinical trials conducted since 1997.[54] Subsequently, a scientific advisory panel of the FDA advised in 2002 that rhBMP-2 be approved as the first complete bone-graft substitute for anterior inter-vertebral-body spinal fusion. Currently, rhBMP-2 carried on a type I collagen sponge is approved for use in conjunction with a tapered, threaded intervertebral cage (LT-Cage; Medtronic Sofamor Danek, Minneapolis, MN) for the treatment of degenerative lumbar disc disease.

### *Animal Studies*

The first animal study of the use of an inter-vertebral-body cage filled with rhBMP-2 was conducted by Sandhu et al.[55] The study groups consisted of single-level anterior lumbar inter-vertebral-body fusions in a sheep model. Cylindrical threaded fusion cages were filled with either autologous iliac crest bone graft or rhBMP-2 on a type I bovine absorbable collagen sponge carrier (**Fig. 25.11**). At 6 months after surgery, radiographically observed fusion had occurred in all of the animals, but only 37% of the animals treated with autograft-filled cages had a histological union, as compared with 100% of those treated with rhBMP-2 in collagen-filled cages. Boden et al[56] used rhBMP-2 on a collagen carrier contained in a titanium lumbar inter-vertebral-body fusion cage in rhesus monkeys (**Fig. 25.12**). They inserted two different concentrations of rhBMP-2 (0.75 and 1.5 mg/mL) on the carrier into cylindrical, tapered titanium cages. All animals treated with either concentration of rhBMP-2 achieved radiographically and histologically demonstrated fusion. However, through a more detailed review of the histology of the fusion sites, this study revealed an important dose–response phenomenon. The bone formed in association with the higher concentration of rhBMP-2 was more dense and developed more rapidly than that associated with the lower concentration.

Hecht and associates[57] studied the use of an rhBMP-2 on a collagen sponge that was loaded into threaded cortical allograft dowels in a rhesus monkey model of inter-vertebral-body fusion (**Fig. 25.13**). All animals treated with allograft bone dowels filled with rhBMP-2 had solid fusions at 6 months, whereas only one of three animals treated with allograft bone dowels filled with autologous bone graft alone achieved arthrodesis. Radiographs and histological analysis revealed that the allograft dowels containing rhBMP-2 had undergone complete resorptive remodeling. It was surmised that rhBMP-2 upregulated not only osteoblastic bone formation but also osteoclastic activity. No bone remodeling was observed in the control group of animals. These findings were a key point in the literature about rhBMP-2 because subsequent human clinical trials used them to define the 1.5 mg/mL dose for inter-vertebral-body fusion. In a canine model of fusion in the posterolateral spine, Sandhu et al[58] reported a 100% rate of fusion within 12 weeks after the implantation of rhBMP-2 on a collagen sponge. Later studies of the same model found decortication to be unnecessary for fusion in the presence of rhBMP-2.[59]

In an important dose–response study, Martin and co-workers[60] found that a concentration of rhBMP-2 (0.43 mg/mL) that was effective in posterolateral fusions in lower animals (0.43 mg/mL) was not effective in primates. The overlying paraspinal muscles caused compression of the collagen-sponge carrier and hastened elution of the protein into surrounding tissues. As a result, a porous polyethylene shield was designed to be placed over the collagen-sponge carrier across the transverse processes, for protection against muscle compression. This intervention led to successful fusion with a lower rhBMP-2 concentration. Boden et al[61] developed a porous, biphasic calcium phosphate ceramic carrier consisting of 60% HA and 40% TCP for use in posterolateral fusions in primates. This carrier composition allowed resorption of the TCP while maintaining the residual scaffold

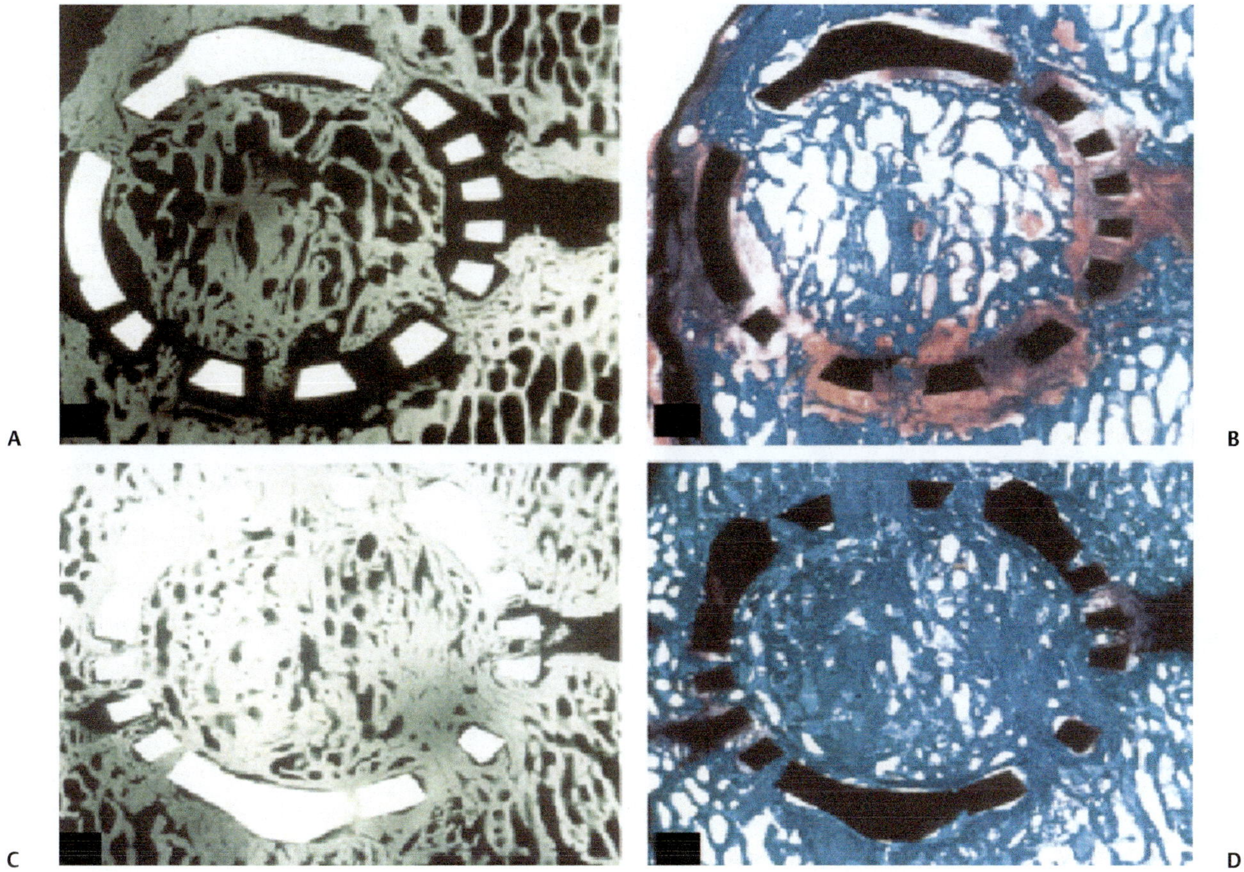


**Fig. 25.11** **(A,C)** Microradiographs and **(B,D)** corresponding histological sections of **(A,B)** inter-vertebral-body cages filled with iliac-crest autograft or **(C,D)** rhBMP-2 on a collagen sponge. Fibrous tissue (*pink*) was present around the perimeter of autograft-filled cages to a greater extent than around rhBMP-2–filled cages. (From McKay B. Spine 2002 27(16 Suppl):S66. Reprinted with permission.)

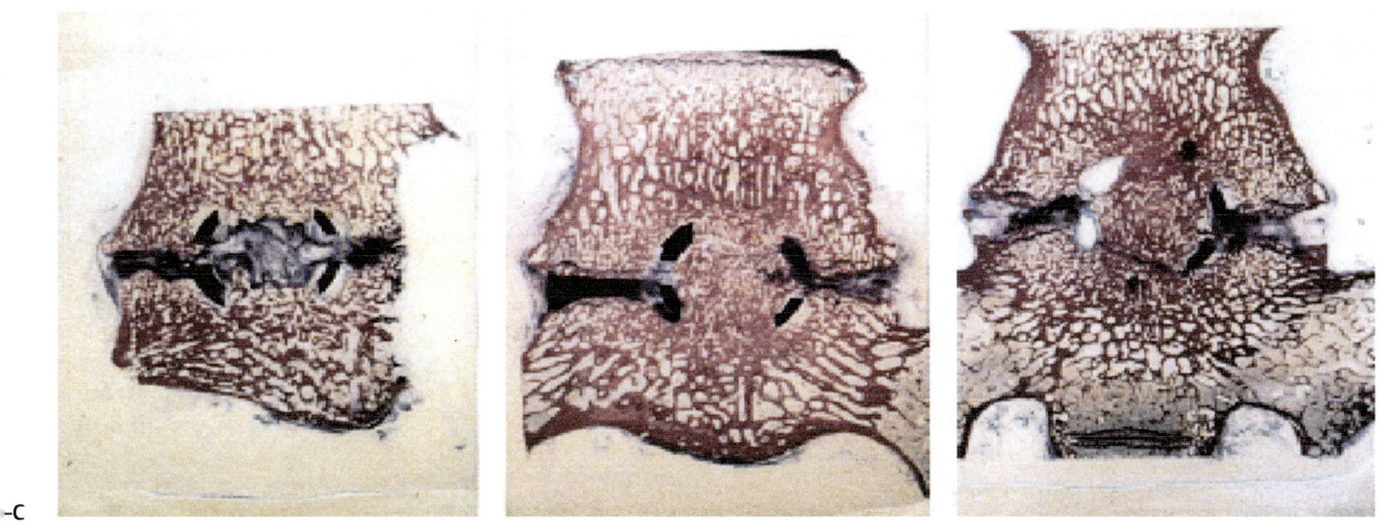


**Fig. 25.12** **(A)** Histology of a control group treated with collagen sponge alone, **(B)** 0.75 mg/mL of rhBMP-2, and **(C)** 1.50 mg/mL of rhBMP-2. (From McKay B. Spine 2002 27[16 Suppl]S66. Reprinted with permission.)

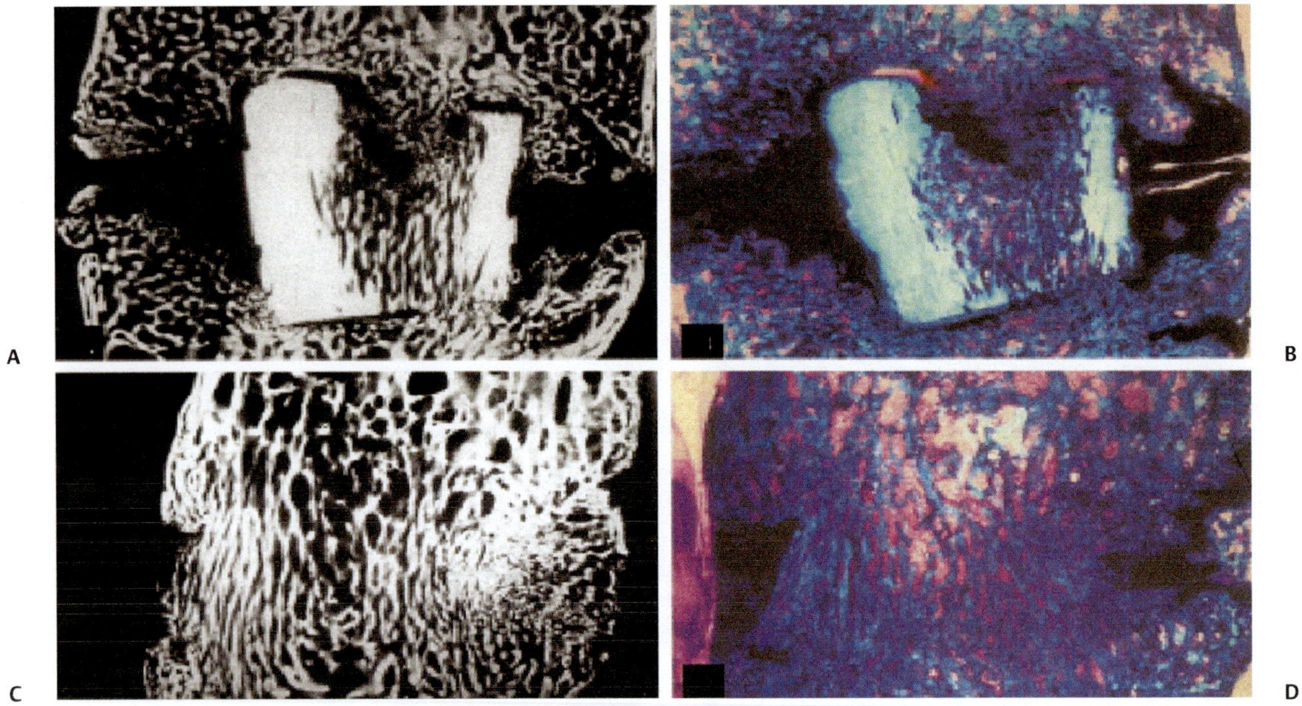


**Fig. 25.13** **(A,C)** Microradiographs and **(B,D)** corresponding histological sections of **(A,B)** allograft bone dowels filled with iliac-crest autograft or **(C,D)** rhBMP-2 on a collagen sponge. (From McKay B. Spine 2002 27(16 Suppl):S66. Reprinted with permission.)

of HA on which new bone could be deposited. All three concentrations of rhBMP-2 (1.4, 2.1, and 2.8 mg/mL) resulted in solid fusions; whereas fusion was not achieved in animals in which autograft alone had been implanted (**Fig. 25.14**).

### Clinical Trials

The first human study of rhBMP-2 was a small pilot study by Boden and colleagues of 11 patients undergoing lumbar fusions with a tapered lumbar inter-vertebral-body device

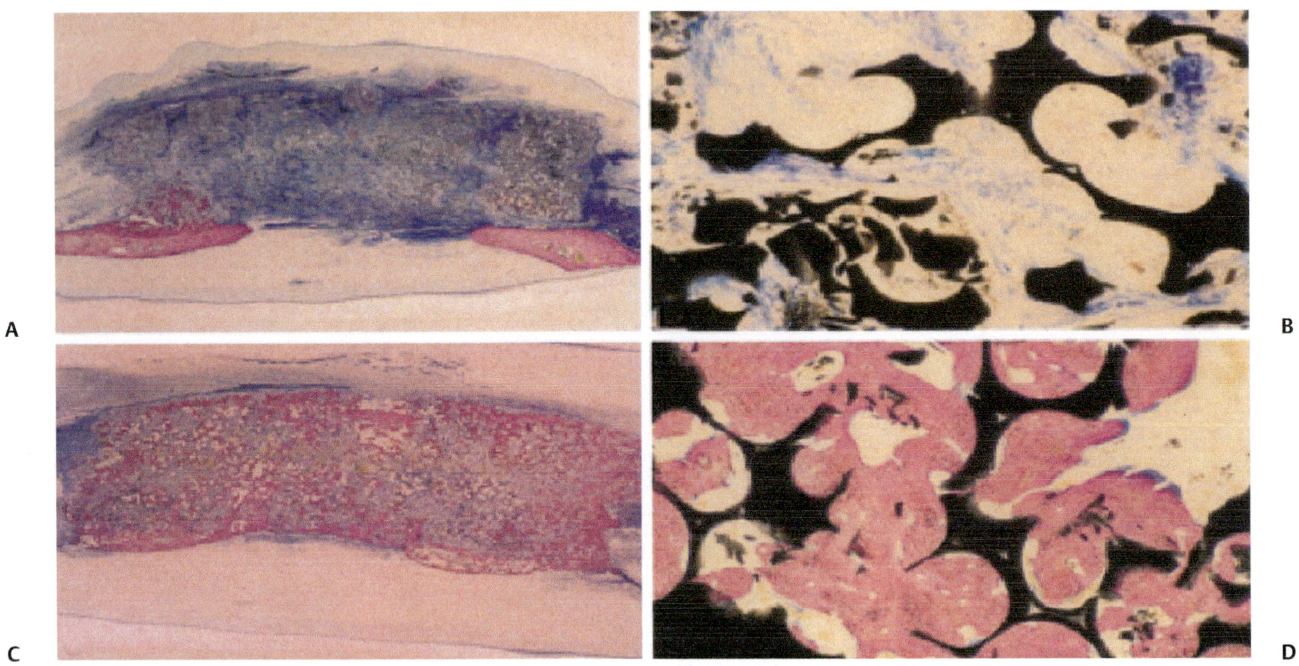


**Fig. 25.14** Low- and high-power histological sections of fusion masses from monkeys 24 weeks after arthrodesis with HA and TCP alone **(A** and **B**, respectively**)** and HA–TCP with rhBMP-2 **(C** and **D**, respectively**)**. Minimal bone (*pink*) ingrowth and primarily fibrous tissue (*blue*) are observed in the fusion masses with HA–TCP alone (no rhBMP-2). Extensive new bone ingrowth occurred in the fusion masses with the combination of HA–TCP and rhBMP-2. (From McKay B. Spine 2002 27[16 Suppl]S66. Reprinted with permission.)

(LT Cage) containing rhBMP-2 on a collagen sponge. All 11 patients had superior Oswestry scores and solid fusions by 6 months, as confirmed by thin-section computed tomographic (CT) scans. None of the study patients developed measurable titrs of antibody to rhBMP-2. Three patients had increased titers of anti-bovine type I collagen antibody, but no clinical sequelae were noted in these patients, and all three of the patients had successful spinal fusions.

This pilot clinical trial was used as the basis for initiating a larger trial.[62] In this larger study, 143 patients were treated with rhBMP-2 in the LT-Cage for a single-level anterior lumbar inter-vertebral-body fusion and 136 control patients were treated with the LT-Cage filled with iliac-crest autograft. The operative time and blood loss were significantly less in the rhBMP-2-treated than in the control group. Donor-site pain was noted by more than one-third of the patients in the autograft group at up to 2 years after surgery. No significant differences were observed with regard to Oswestry outcome scores, back pain, or number of patients returning to work in the two study groups. Successful fusion was seen radiographically in 99.2% in the rh-BMP-2-treated group as compared with 96.7% of the autograft group at 6 months, with corresponding figures of 100% versus 95.7% respectively at 2 years. Overall clinical success was achieved in 94.5% of the rhBMP-2-treated group and 88.7% of the autograft group.

Boden and colleagues evaluated the clinical use of rhBMP-2 with a biphasic calcium phosphate carrier in single-level posterolateral lumbar fusion.[63] This small study compared rhBMP-2 in the biphasic carrier with or without instrumentation and iliac-crest bone grafting with instrumentation in the treatment of symptomatic grade I spondylolisthesis. At 17 months, only two of five patients receiving iliac crest bone grafts exhibited fusion, as compared with all of the patients treated with rhBMP-2, regardless of whether or not instrumentation was used. Oswestry scores for pain and function were equivalent among the three groups at final follow-up. Excluded from the final analysis because of their high grade of spondylolisthesis were two patients with grade II spondylolisthesis who were treated with rhBMP-2 and the biphasic calcium phosphate carrier without instrumentation. Only one of these patients experienced fusion. This indicated the essential role of mechanical stability in promoting fusion even when BMP is used.

Although the FDA has approved INFUSE for use in anterior lumbar inter-vertebral-body fusion, only limited clinical data exist about dose and carrier recommendations for its use in the posterior lumbar spine and anterior cervical spine. There have been reports of bone formation adjacent to neural elements when INFUSE is introduced into the disc space through a transforaminal–posterior lumbar inter-vertebral-body approach.[64] This unintended bone formation is likely to be the result of technical factors directly related to the surgical procedure and improper placement of the INFUSE-soaked sponge.

Baskin et al have studied the clinical results of implantation of machined fibular-ring grafts (Cornerstone; Medtronic Sofamor Danek) filled with autograft or INFUSE for ACDF.[65] The experimental group in this trial consisted of 18 patients treated with a machined fibular ring filled with INFUSE. Ten members of this experimental group underwent a single-level fusion and 8 underwent a two-level fusion. Fifteen patients were enrolled in the control group and were treated with a machined fibular ring filled with autograft bone obtained from the iliac crest. Eight of the 15 patients in this latter group underwent single-level fusion and 7 underwent two-level fusion. Blood loss was significantly smaller in the group treated with INFUSE and having single-level cervical fusions than in the control group. All patients had radiographic evidence of fusion at 6 months after surgery.

The concentration of BMP needed to bring about osteogenesis in all of the applications described above is several magnitudes of order greater than its normal physiological levels. This is an observation that has raised concerns about the potential safety of BMP. Several instances of postoperative soft-tissue swelling adjacent to sites of use of INFUSE in cervival fusions have been reported to the FDA. Smucker and co-workers[66] reported a retrospective series of ACDF procedures done with and without rhBMP-2 and noted a higher incidence of events involving swelling, such as difficulty in breathing, difficulty in swallowing, or visible swelling og the anterior neck in fusions done with rhBMP-2 than in those done with autograft (28% vs. 4%; $P < 0.001$). The cause of the generalized “edema” remains unknown, but it may have come from hyperconcentration of the product or placement of an INFUSE-soaked sponge adjacent to anterior cervical soft tissues. Surgeons should therefore be cautious about the use of this product for off-label indications, especially in the anterior cervical spine. Further clinical studies are under way to determine the appropriate concentration and carrier for these off-label indications.

### Recombinant Human Bone Morphogenetic Protein-7/Osteogenic Protein-1

Recombinant human OP-1 (rhOP-1, rhBMP-7) was isolated through cloning techniques and introduced into a Chinese hamster ovarian cell line that was able to express rhOP-1. Commercially available rhOP-1 is marketed by Stryker Biotech (Hopkinton, MA). A carrier that contains 1 g of type I bovine bone collagen is combined with 3.5 mg of lyophilized rhOP-1 for a final rhOP-1 concentration of 0.875 mg/mL in an OP-1 implant currently approved by the FDA for treating nonunions in long-bone fractures. The addition of 230 mg of carboxymethylcellulose (CMC) to the rhOP-1 implant yields rhOP-1 putty.

### Animal Studies

Cook and associates[67] compared autograft bone with rhOP-1 in a canine model of posterolateral fusion. Their study was done with 12 dogs divided into four groups of three dogs each. The first group was treated with OP-1 with a collagen carrier, the second group with bovine collagen (type I) carrier alone, the third group with autologous iliac crest bone, and the fourth group without any implant material. The implants were randomly assigned to be made at various vertebral locations such that each animal received all four types of implant. The animals were killed at 6, 12, and 26 weeks. All rhOP-1-treated vertebral levels showed stable fusion by 6 weeks and complete fusion by 12 weeks. Vertebral levels treated with autologous bone graft showed slower progression to fusion by 26 weeks. No fusion was noted at levels treated with either collagen carrier alone or no implant. Histological findings were consistent with radiographic results, showing that rhOP-1 induced bone formation more rapidly than did autograft.

Magin et al[68] compared rhOP-1 at 3.5 mg in combination with 1 g of bovine bone collagen with an osteoconductive HA bone-graft substitute or autograft bone in a sheep model. Thirty sheep underwent inter-vertebral-body fusion through a posterolateral approach and supplemental transpedicular instrumentation. At 4 months, bone formation was greater in the rhOP-1-treated animals than in either the autograft- or HA-treated animals. Mechanical testing and histological examination confirmed the superior maturity and stiffness of the fusion masses in the rhOP-1 treated animals than in the HA-treated group, in which fusion failed to occur, or in the autograft-treated group, in which fusion occurred at a much slower rate.

Grauer and co-workers[69] used a rabbit model of posterolateral fusion to compare rhOP-1 with autograft and with collagen–CMC carrier alone in a total of 31 animals. By manual palpation they found that all eight rabbits (100%) in the rhOP-1 group achieved solid fusions, as compared with five (63%) of eight rabbits in the autograft group and none (0%) of eight rabbits in the carrier group. Histological examination showed that rhOP-1-treated sites had mature trabecular bone surrounded by a cortical shell, as compared with a predominance of fibrocartilage at the autograft-treated fusion sites.

Cunningham et al[70] studied skip-level posterolateral fusion in a dog model with autograft alone, autograft and rhOP-1, or rhOP-1 alone. At 8 weeks, 22% of the sites treated with autograft alone, 88% of those treated with autograft and rhOP-1, and 66% of those treated with rhOP-1 alone showed fusion. At 3 months 83% of the autograft- and rhOP-1-treated sites were considered to be fused, as compared with 72% of the sites treated with rhOP-1 alone. Mechanical testing at the 8- and 12-week time points showed significantly greater stiffness at the OP-1-treated sites than at the sites treated with autograft alone.

The efficacy of rhOP-1 in single-level fusions may not apply in the case of multilevel fusions. Mermer and Gupta[71] compared the influence of rhOP-1 with that of autograft and that of collagen carrier in multilevel fusions ending at S1 in sheep spines. Manual palpation failed to show fusion at all three treated levels in any of the specimens, or fusion at the lumbosacral junction. No statistically significant difference was found in the rates of fusion in the rhOP-1-treated and autograft groups on the basis of radiographic grading or biomechanical testing. Histological analysis showed no qualitative difference in bone morphology or cellularity of fusion masses in the autograft and rhOP-1-treated spines. Mermer and Gupta concluded that the extrapolation of data from both single-level preclinical and clinical studies of BMPs for use in multilevel fusion requires careful review.

Paramore et al studied the toxicity profile of rhOP-1[72] by intentionally placing it into the subarachnoid space during lumbar laminectomy and fusion in a canine model. They noted bone formation adjacent to the spinal cord and causing mild cord compression; however, they found no histological evidence of spinal cord inflammation or neuronal cell death.

### Clinical Trials

Vaccaro and colleagues[73] evaluated the safety and efficacy of rhOP-1 by using it in combination with autograft in a putty implant in 12 patients undergoing lumbar decompression with uninstrumented inter-transverse-process fusions. Successful fusion, defined according to stringent criteria, was observed in slightly more than half the patients in their study. There was a significant improvement in Oswestry scores postoperatively, and no observed systemic toxicity, ectopic bone formation, recurrent stenosis, or other adverse event related to the rhOP-1 implant. Vaccaro and co-workers[74] also conducted a prospective, randomized, controlled, multicenter clinical trial comparing the safety and clinical and radiographic outcomes of rhOP-1 putty with autogenous iliac-crest bone graft in a population of patients undergoing decompression and posterolateral fusion for symptomatic lumbar stenosis associated with degenerative spondylolisthesis. Thirty-six patients with degenerative lumbar spondylolisthesis and symptoms of neurogenic claudication underwent decompression and posterolateral fusion using either iliac-crest autograft or rhOP-1 putty. Data were available for 27 patients at the 2-year time point and for an additional 4 patients (without evaluable 24-month results) at 36-months postoperatively. Clinical success, defined as a 20% improvement over the preoperative Oswestry score, occurred in 17 of 20 (85%) of the rhOP-1 putty-treated patients and 7 of 11 (64%) of the autograft-treated patients. Successful posterolateral fusion was achieved in 11 of 20 (55%) of the rhOP-1 putty-treated patients and 4 of 10 (40%) of the autograft-treated patients. Scores on the Short Form (SF)-36 showed similar clinical improvement in both groups. In this larger study, no adverse events were observed in relation to use of the rhOP-1 putty implant. Vaccaro and coworkers concluded that their results compared favorably with the historical fusion rates reported for uninstrumented arthrodesis with autograft bone (45%) in this challenging clinical scenario.

Kanayama et al[75] using radiographic examination, surgical exploration, and histological assessment, conducted a prospective, randomized, and controlled study of fusion rates in instrumented posterolateral lumbar fusions treated with rhOP-1 putty ($n = 9$) or autograft with HA–TCP granules ($n = 10$). Fusion status was evaluated with plain radiography and CT scanning. After a minimum follow-up of 1-year, patients who showed radiographic evidence of fusion had their instrumentation removed and underwent surgical exploration of the fusion site. Radiographically observed fusion was found in 7 of the 9 rhOP-1-treated patients and 9 of the 10 control patients given autograft with HA–TCP. Surgical exploration of these 16 patients revealed macroscopic new bone formation in the posterolateral lumbar region in all of them; however, solid fusion was observed in only 4 of 7 patients treated with rhOP-1 putty and 7 of the 9 patients treated with autograft and HA–TCP. Histological assessment demonstrated viable bone in 6 of 7 rhOP-1-treated patients. All specimens from the control group treated with autograft and HA–TCP contained viable bone and fibrous tissue surrounding ceramic granules, suggesting slow incorporation of the graft material. Kanayama and associates concluded that in a human trial of posterolateral lumbar spinal fusion, rhOP-1 reliably induced viable new bone formation, but the rate of success of fusion as evaluated by surgical exploration was only slightly better than 50%. This study does not support the efficacy of rhOP-1 over autograft for use in spinal fusion, but may support its equivalency with autograft, especially when weighed against the morbidity of harvesting bone graft if local bone is insufficient for grafting.

### Growth and Differentiation Factor-5

GDF-5 is a member of the TGF-β/BMP superfamily that is required for proper skeletal patterning and development of the vertebrate limb. The inductive activity of a recombinant form of human GDF-5 (rhGDF-5) was evaluated in a series of in vitro assays and in vivo bone-formation models.[76] The in vitro response to rhGDF-5 was the formation of chondrogenic nodules in fetal rat calvarial cells cultured with extracellular matrices of collagen or collagen–hyaluronate. Matrices loaded with rhGDF-5 induced ectopic growth of cartilaginous and osseous tissue when implanted in subcutaneous or intramuscular sites.

Spiro and co-workers[77] evaluated the bone-forming activity of a mineralized collagen matrix combined with rhGDF-5 in a rabbit model of posterolateral spinal fusion. They found that the radiographic density, histological quality, and mechanical strength of fusion at 12 weeks after treatment were similar in all animals in the treatment group. These results demonstrated that the combination of a mineralized collagen matrix with rhGDF-5 maximized the inherent conductive and inductive properties of each component to provide an effective alternative to autograft for bone-grafting procedures.

Magit et al[77] performed single-level, intertransverse process fusions [78] in 67 rabbits, using iliac-crest autograft bone ($n = 13$); Healos (a type I collagen–HA matrix) alone ($n = 13$); or 0.5, 1.0, or 1.5 mg/mL of rhGDF-5 lyophilized to Healos ($n = 13$ per group). The rabbits were euthanized at 8 weeks. Manual palpation revealed fusion rates of 38% with iliac-crest autograft, 0% with Healos alone, and 100% with each of the doses of rhGDF-5 lyophilized to Healos. In this rabbit model of fusion, histological analyses confirmed that the combination of Healos with rhGDF-5 induced fusion in 100% of the rabbits studied, a rate significantly higher than the rate of fusion induced by iliac-crest autograft bone (38%). Overall, these results support continued research on the combination of Healos with rhGDF-5 as a potential bone-graft alternative.

Gupta and colleagues[79] recently presented data from an evaluation of rhGDF-5 at concentrations of 0.5 or 1.0 mg/mL as a bone-graft substitute in and around carbon fiber-reinforced polymeric (CFRP) cages (Leopard™ Cage; DePuy Spine, Raynham, MA) to facilitate single-level, anterior inter-vertebral-body fusion in a sheep model, and compared the results of this with those of autograft-filled and empty-cage controls. At 3 months, radiodensity was observed in axial CT slices through the center of all cages implanted with either autograft or rhGDF-5. Four of the six sheep in which empty cages were implanted also showed progression of radiodensity. At 6 months, histological evaluation revealed complete fusion in all six of the animals treated with Healos and rhGDF-5 at 1.0 mg/mL, in five of six of the animals treated with Healos and rhGDF-5 at 0.5mg/mL, five of six of the animals treated with autograft alone, and four of six of the animals in which empty cages were used. This study demonstrated that the combination of Healos with rhGDF-5 at 1.0 mg/mL could successfully produce inter-vertebral-body fusion in large animal models. Although no clinical data are yet available for rhGDF-5, it may prove to be another useful tool in promoting fusion in the human spine.

## Platelet Concentrates

Platelets release several growth factors that may function in concert to enhance bone formation by promoting pluripotent stem cell chemotaxis, proliferation, and differentiation. This collection of signaling factors does not include any of the BMPs. In making the autologous platelet-gel systems currently in use, plasma rich in platelets is separated from the patient's blood and concentrated in a fibrinogen matrix. This fibrinogen preparation is combined with thrombin, forming a fibrin clot that can be administered with an osteoconductive matrix or a source of osteogenic cells to form a composite bone graft. Siebrecht et al[80] used a platelet-growth-factor concentrate in a rat mode of a bone chamber and found an increase in bone ingrowth into porous coralline hydroxyapatite. Lowery and colleagues[81] retrospectively examined 39 patients undergoing anterior or posterior fusion of the lumbar spine who were treated with autologous platelet concentrate, autogenous bone graft, and coralline HA in conjunction with stable internal fixation. After an average follow-up of 13 months, no pseudarthroses were noted clinically or radiographically.

Weiner and colleagues[82] compared 27 consecutive patients who underwent a single-level intertransverse lumbar fusion with iliac-crest bone graft and 32 patients undergoing an identical procedure for the same indications with iliac crest bone graft augmented with autologous-growth-factor concentrate (AGF). At 2 years of follow-up fusion had occurred in 24 of 27 patients (91%) in the control group as compared with 18 of 32 patients (62%) in the AGF group. On the basis of these results, Weiner at al cautioned against the routine use of AGF. Similarly, Carreon et al[83] used AGF in combination with autograft in posterolateral lumbar fusions. With a nonunion rate approaching 25% in their study cohort, they concluded that AGF failed to enhance fusion when added to autograft in patients undergoing instrumented posterolateral spinal fusion, and did not recommend the use of AGF to supplement autologous bone graft.

However, Jenis et al[84] found that their clinical and radiographic results with AGF combined with allograft in lumbar inter-vertebral-body fusions were equivalent to those with autograft. Their 12- and 24-month radiographic results confirmed an 85% rate of arthrodesis in the autograft-treated patients and an 89% rate of fusion in the AGF-treated patients. The clinical outcomes in the two groups were similar, and no significant differences were noted on pain or improvement in functional outcome. Janis and colleagues concluded that AGF combined with an appropriate carrier was a reasonable alternative to autograft for inter-vertebral-body applications.

A lack of consistency in the processing techniques and carriers used in the studies described here appears to preclude appropriate comparisons of their results. It is important to point out that BMPs are osteoinductive differentiation factors, whereas AGFs are predominantly growth factors. Various platelet concentrates may have different levels of cytokines and differences in platelet survival after the concentration process. Indeed, several animal studies have shown that a combination of AGF and BMP may reduce bone formation.[85,86]

We believe that further research, with emphasis on optimum carriers, preparation, and formulation, is needed before the widespread use of these platelet concentrate products is attempted.

## Conclusion

Clinically available osteobiological products have differing cellular, biochemical, and structural properties that determine their specific clinical indications. None of these products now provides all three of the components (osteogenic cells, osteogenic signals, and osteoconductive scaffolds) required for bone regeneration. Consequently, the future may show that it is more efficacious in terms of safety, patient satisfaction, and cost-effectiveness to combine several techniques to construct a composite graft. In the future, osteobiological products may be tailored intraoperatively to overcome specific biological deficits and biomechanical challenges at the sites of fusion. Randomized controlled clinical trials should be conducted to confirm the efficacy, safety, and cost-effectiveness of any strategy for this before it is introduced into clinical practice.

### References


1. Einhorn TA. The cell and molecular biology of fracture healing. Clin Orthop Relat Res 1998;355(suppl):S7–S21
2. Bostrom MP. Expression of bone morphogenetic proteins in fracture healing. Clin Orthop Relat Res 1998;355(suppl):S116–S123
3. Campbell JT, Kaplan FS. The role of morphogens in endochondral ossification. Calcif Tissue Int 1992;50:283–289
4. Einhorn TA. The science of fracture healing. J Orthop Trauma 2005; 19(10, suppl):S4–S6
5. Lee FY, Choi YW, Behrens FF, DeFouw DO, Einhorn TA. Programmed removal of chondrocytes during endochondral fracture healing. J Orthop Res 1998;16:144–150
6. Aspenberg P, Lohmander LS, Thorngren KG. Failure of bone induction by bone matrix in adult monkeys. J Bone Joint Surg Br 1988; 70:625–627
7. Aspenberg P, Turek T. BMP-2 for intramuscular bone induction: Effect in squirrel monkeys is dependent on implantation site. Acta Orthop Scand 1996;67:3–6
8. Aspenberg P, Lohmander LS, Thorngren KG. Failure of bone induction by bone matrix in adult monkeys. J Bone Joint Surg Br 1988;70:625–627
9. Cho TJ, Gerstenfeld LC, Einhorn TA. Differential temporal expression of members of the transforming growth factor beta superfamily during murine fracture healing. J Bone Miner Res 2002;17: 513–520
10. Boden SD, Sumner DR. Biologic factors affecting spinal fusion and bone regeneration. Spine 1995; 20(24, suppl):102S–112S
11. Boden SD, Schimandle JH, Hutton WC. An experimental lumbar intertransverse process spinal fusion model. Radiographic, histo-

logic, and biomechanical healing characteristics. Spine 1995;20: 412–420
12. Boden SD. Biology of lumbar spine fusion and use of bone graft substitutes: Present, future, and next generation. Tissue Eng 2000;6:383–399
13. Arrington ED, Smith WJ, Chambers HG, Bucknell AL, Davino NA. Complications of iliac crest bone graft harvesting. Clin Orthop Relat Res 1996;329:300–309
14. Ludwig SC, Boden SD. Osteoinductive bone graft substitutes for spinal fusion: A basic science summary. Orthop Clin North Am 1999;30:635–645
15. Boden SD. Bioactive factors for bone tissue engineering. Clin Orthop Relat Res 1999;367(suppl):S84–S94
16. Schimandle JH, Boden SD. Spine update. The use of animal models to study spinal fusion. Spine 1994;19:1998–2006
17. Boden SD, Schimandle JH. Biologic enhancement of spinal fusion. Spine 1995;20(suppl):113S–123S
18. Laurie SWS, Kaban LB, Mulliken JB, Murray JE. Donor-site morbidity after harvesting rib and iliac bone. Plast Reconstr Surg 1984;73: 933–938
19. Fernyhough JC, Schimandle JJ, Weigel MC, Edwards CC, Levine AM. Chronic donor site pain complicating bone graft harvesting from the posterior iliac crest for spinal fusion. Spine 1992;17: 1474–1480
20. Banwart JC, Asher MA, Hassanein RS. Iliac crest bone graft harvest donor site morbidity. A statistical evaluation. Spine 1995;20: 1055–1060
21. Boden SD. Clinical application of the BMPs. J Bone Joint Surg Am 2001;83A(Pt 2, suppl 1):S161
22. Hamer AJ, Strachan JR, Black MM, Ibbotson CJ, Stockley I, Elson RA. Biochemical properties of cortical allograft bone using a new method of bone strength measurement. A comparison of fresh, fresh-frozen and irradiated bone. J Bone Joint Surg Br 1996;78: 363–368
23. Tomford WW. Transmission of disease through transplantation of musculoskeletal allografts. J Bone Joint Surg Am 1995;77:1742–1754
24. Stevenson S, Horowitz M. The response to bone allografts. J Bone Joint Surg Am 1992;74:939–950
25. Zdeblick TA, Ducker TB. The use of freeze-dried allograft bone for anterior cervical fusions. Spine 1991;16:726–729
26. An HS, Simpson JM, Glover JM, Stephany J. Comparison between allograft plus demineralized bone matrix versus autograft in anterior cervical fusion. A prospective multicenter study. Spine 1995; 20:2211–2216
27. Samartzis D, Shen FH, Matthews DK, Yoon ST, Goldberg EJ, An HS. Comparison of allograft to autograft in multilevel anterior cervical discectomy and fusion with rigid plate fixation. Spine J 2003;3: 451–459
28. Jorgenson SS, Lowe TG, France J, Sabin J. A prospective analysis of autograft versus allograft in posterolateral lumbar fusion in the same patient. A minimum of 1-year follow-up in 144 patients. Spine 1994;19:2048–2053
29. An HS, Lynch K, Toth J. Prospective comparison of autograft vs. allograft for adult posterolateral lumbar spine fusion: Differences among freeze-dried, frozen, and mixed grafts. J Spinal Disord 1995;8:131–135
30. Dodd CA, Fergusson CM, Freedman L, Houghton GR, Thomas D. Allograft versus autograft bone in scoliosis surgery. J Bone Joint Surg Br 1988;70:431–434
31. Betz R, Petrizzo AM, Kerner PJ, et al. Allograft versus no graft with a posterior multisegmented hook system for the treatment of idiopathic scoliosis. Spine 2006 15;31:121–127
32. Jarcho M. Calcium phosphate ceramics as hard tissue prosthetics. Clin Orthop Relat Res 1981;157:259–278
33. Tay BK, Patel VV, Bradford DS. Calcium sulfate- and calcium phosphate-based bone substitutes. Mimicry of the mineral phase of bone. Orthop Clin North Am 1999;30:615–623
34. Ransford AO, Morley T, Edgar MA, et al. Synthetic porous ceramic compared with autograft in scoliosis surgery. A prospective, randomized study of 341 patients. J Bone Joint Surg Br 1998;80:13–18
35. Passuti N, Daculsi G, Rogez JM, Martin S, Bainvel JV. Macroporous calcium phosphate ceramic performance in human spine fusion. Clin Orthop Relat Res 1989;248:169–176
36. Ohgushi H, Goldberg VM, Caplan AI. Heterotopic osteogenesis in porous ceramics induced by marrow cells. J Orthop Res 1989;7: 568–578
37. Urist MR. Bone: Formation by autoinduction. Science 1965;150: 893–899
38. Martin GJ Jr, Boden SD, Titus L, Scarborough NL. New formulations of demineralized bone matrix as a more effective graft alternative in experimental posterolateral lumbar spine arthrodesis. Spine 1999;24:637–645
39. Bae HW, Zhao L, Kanim LE, Wong P, Delamarter RB, Dawson EG. Intervariability and intravariability of bone morphogenetic proteins in commercially available demineralized bone matrix products. Spine 2006;31:1299–1306, discussion 1307–1308
40. Schwartz Z, Mellonig JT, Carnes DL Jr, et al. Ability of commercial demineralized freeze-dried bone allograft to induce new bone formation. J Periodontol 1996;67:918–926
41. Buring K, Urist MR. Effects of ionizing radiation on the bone induction principle in the matrix of bone implants. Clin Orthop Relat Res 1967;55:225–234
42. Schwartz Z, Somers A, Mellonig JT, et al. Ability of commercial demineralized freeze-dried bone allograft to induce new bone formation is dependent on donor age but not gender. J Periodontol 1998;69:470–478
43. Bostrom MP, Yang X, Kennan M, Sandhu H, Dicarlo E, Lane JM. An unexpected outcome during testing of commercially available demineralized bone graft materials: how safe are the nonallograft components? Spine 2001;26:1425–1428
44. Frenkel SR, Moskovich R, Spivak JM, Zhang ZH, Prewett AB. Demineralized bone matrix. Enhancement of spinal fusion. Spine 1993;18:1634–1639
45. Morone MA, Boden SD. Experimental posterolateral lumbar spinal fusion with a demineralized bone matrix gel. Spine 1998;23: 159–167
46. An HS, Simpson JM, Glover JM, Stephany J. Comparison between allograft plus demineralized bone matrix versus autograft in anterior cervical fusion. A prospective multicenter study. Spine 1995;20: 2211–2216
47. Sassard WR, Eidman DK, Gray PM, et al. Augmenting local bone with Grafton demineralized bone matrix for posterolateral lumbar spine fusion: Avoiding second site autologous bone harvest. Orthopedics 2000;23:1059–1064, discussion 1064–1065
48. Cammisa FP Jr, Lowery G, Garfin SR, et al. Two-year fusion rate equivalency between Grafton DBM gel and autograft in posterolateral spine fusion: A prospective controlled trial employing a side-by-side comparison in the same patient. Spine 2004;29:660–666

49. Price CT, Connolly JF, Carantzas AC, Ilyas I. Comparison of bone grafts for posterior spinal fusion in adolescent idiopathic scoliosis. Spine 2003;28:793–798
50. Thalgott JS, Giuffre JM, Fritts K, Timlin M, Klezl Z. Instrumented posterolateral lumbar fusion using coralline hydroxyapatite with or without demineralized bone matrix, as an adjunct to autologous bone. Spine J 2001;1:131–137
51. Wang EA, Israel DI, Kelly S, Luxenberg DP. Bone morphogenetic protein-2 causes commitment and differentiation in C3H10T1/2 and 3T3 cells. Growth Factors 1993;9:57–71
52. Wang EA, Rosen V, Cordes P, et al. Purification and characterization of other distinct bone-inducing factors. Proc Natl Acad Sci U S A 1988;85:9484–9488
53. Wang EA, Rosen V, D'Alessandro JS, et al. Recombinant human bone morphogenetic protein induces bone formation. Proc Natl Acad Sci U S A 1990;87:2220–2224
54. Boden SD, Zdeblick TA, Sandhu HS, Heim SE. The use of rhBMP-2 in interbody fusion cages. Definitive evidence of osteoinduction in humans: A preliminary report. Spine 2000;25:376–381
55. Sandhu HS, Toth JM, Diwan AD, et al. Histologic evaluation of the efficacy of rhBMP-2 compared with autograft bone in sheep spinal anterior interbody fusion. Spine 2002;27:567–575
56. Boden SD, Martin GJ Jr, Horton WC, Truss TL, Sandhu HS. Laparoscopic anterior spinal arthrodesis with rhBMP-2 in a titanium interbody threaded cage. J Spinal Disord 1998;11:95–101
57. Hecht BP, Fischgrund JS, Herkowitz HN, Penman L, Toth JM, Shirkhoda A. The use of recombinant human bone morphogenetic protein 2 (rhBMP-2) to promote spinal fusion in a nonhuman primate anterior interbody fusion model. Spine 1999;24:629–636
58. Sandhu HS, Kanim LE, Kabo JM, et al. Effective doses of recombinant human bone morphogenetic protein-2 in experimental spinal fusion. Spine 1996;21:2115–2122
59. Sandhu HS, Kanim LE, Toth JM, et al. Experimental spinal fusion with recombinant human bone morphogenetic protein-2 without decortication of osseous elements. Spine 1997;22:1171–1180
60. Martin GJ Jr, Boden SD, Marone MA, Marone MA, Moskovitz PA. Posterolateral intertransverse process spinal arthrodesis with rhBMP-2 in a nonhuman primate: important lessons learned regarding dose, carrier, and safety. J Spinal Disord 1999;12: 179–186
61. Boden SD, Martin GJ Jr, Morone MA, Ugbo JL, Moskovitz PA. Posterolateral lumbar intertransverse process spine arthrodesis with recombinant human bone morphogenetic protein 2/hydroxyapatite-tricalcium phosphate after laminectomy in the nonhuman primate. Spine 1999;24:1179–1185
62. Burkus JK, Gornet MF, Dickman CA, Zdeblick TA. Anterior lumbar interbody fusion using rhBMP-2 with tapered interbody cages. J Spinal Disord Tech 2002;15:337–349
63. Boden SD, Kang J, Sandhu HS, Heller JG. Use of recombinant human bone morphogenetic protein-2 to achieve posterolateral lumbar spine fusion in humans: a prospective, randomized clinical pilot trial: 2002 Volvo Award in clinical studies. Spine 2002;27: 2662–2673
64. Chen NF, Smith ZA, Stiner E, Armin S, Sheikh H, Khoo LT. Symptomatic ectopic bone formation after off-label use of recombinant human bone morphogenetic protein-2 in transforaminal lumbar interbody fusion. J Neurosurg Spine 2010;12(1):40–46
65. Baskin DS, Ryan P, Sonntag V, Westmark R, Widmayer MA. A prospective, randomized, controlled cervical fusion study using recombinant human bone morphogenetic protein-2 with the CORNERSTONE-SR allograft ring and the ATLANTIS anterior cervical plate. Spine 2003;28:1219–1224, discussion 1225
66. Smucker JD, Rhee JM, Singh K, Yoon ST, Heller JG. Increased swelling complications associated with off-label usage of rhBMP-2 in the anterior cervical spine. Spine 2006;31:2813–2819
67. Cook SD, Dalton JE, Tan EH, Whitecloud TS III, Rueger DC. In vivo evaluation of recombinant human osteogenic protein (rhOP-1) implants as a bone graft substitute for spinal fusions. Spine 1994;19:1655–1663
68. Magin MN, Delling G. Improved lumbar vertebral interbody fusion using rhOP-1: a comparison of autogenous bone graft, bovine hydroxylapatite (Bio-Oss), and BMP-7 (rhOP-1) in sheep. Spine 2001;26:469–478
69. Grauer JN, Patel TC, Erulkar JS, Troiano NW, Panjabi MM, Friedlaender GE. 2000 Young Investigator Research Award winner. Evaluation of OP-1 as a graft substitute for intertransverse process lumbar fusion. Spine 2001;26:127–133
70. Cunningham BW, Shimanoto I, Sefter JC, et al. Posterolateral spinal arthrodesis using osteogenic protein-1: an in vivo time-course study using a canine model. Paper presented at: 15th Annual Meeting of the North American Spine Society, New Orleans, LA, October 25–28, 2000
71. Mermer MJ, Gupta MC, Wheeler DL, et al. Efficacy of osteogenic protein-1 in a challenging multilevel fusion model. Spine 2004;29:249–256
72. Paramore CG, Lauryssen C, Rauzzino MJ, et al. The safety of OP-1 for lumbar fusion with decompression: A canine study. Neurosurgery 1999;44:1151–1155, discussion 1155–1156
73. Vaccaro AR, Patel TC, Fischgrund J, et al. A pilot safety and efficacy study of OP-1 putty (rhBMP-7) as an adjunct to iliac crest autograft in posterolateral lumbar fusions. Eur Spine J 2003;12:495–500
74. Vaccaro AR, Anderson DG, Patel T, et al. Comparison of OP-1 Putty (rhBMP-7) to iliac crest autograft for posterolateral lumbar arthrodesis: A minimum 2-year follow-up pilot study. Spine 2005; 30:2709–2716
75. Kanayama M, Hashimoto T, Shigenobu K, Yamane S, Bauer TW, Togawa D. A prospective randomized study of posterolateral lumbar fusion using osteogenic protein-1 (OP-1) versus local autograft with ceramic bone substitute: Emphasis of surgical exploration and histologic assessment. Spine 2006;31(10):1067–1074
76. Buxton P, Edwards C, Archer CW, Francis-West P. Growth/differentiation factor-5 (GDF-5) and skeletal development. J Bone Joint Surg Am 2001; 83A(Pt 1, suppl 1):S23–S30
77. Spiro RC, Thompson AY, Poser JW. Spinal fusion with recombinant human growth and differentiation factor-5 combined with a mineralized collagen matrix. Anat Rec 2001;263:388–395
78. Magit DP, Maak T, Trioano N, et al. Healos/recombinant human growth and differentiation factor-5 induces posterolateral lumbar fusion in a New Zealand white rabbit model. Spine 2006;31: 2180–2188
79. Gupta MC, Jayaraman V, Turner A, et al. Growth and differentiation factor-5 combined with a novel flowable graft material indices fusion in an ovine interbody spine fusion model. Paper presented at: 53rd Annual Meeting of the Orthopaedic Research Society, San Deigo CA, February 11–14, 2007
80. Siebrecht MA, De Rooij PP, Arm DM, Olsson ML, Aspenberg P. Platelet concentrate increases bone ingrowth into porous hydroxyapatite. Orthopedics 2002;25:169–172

81. Lowery GL, Kulkarni S, Pennisi AE. Use of autologous growth factors in lumbar spinal fusion. Bone 1999;25(2, suppl):47S–50S
82. Weiner BK, Walker M. Efficacy of autologous growth factors in lumbar intertransverse fusions. Spine 2003;28:1968–1970, discussion 1971
83. Carreon LY, Glassman SD, Anekstein Y, Puno RM. Platelet gel (AGF) fails to increase fusion rates in instrumented posterolateral fusions. Spine 2005;30:E243–E246, discussion E247
84. Jenis LG, Banco RJ, Kwon B. A prospective study of autologous growth factors (AGF) in lumbar interbody fusion. Spine J 2006;6:14–20
85. Marden LJ, Fan RS, Pierce GF, Reddi AH, Hollinger JO. Platelet-derived growth factor inhibits bone regeneration induced by osteogenin, a bone morphogenetic protein, in rat craniotomy defects. J Clin Invest 1993;92:2897–2905
86. Harris SE, Bonewald LF, Harris MA, et al. Effects of transforming growth factor beta on bone nodule formation and expression of bone morphogenetic protein 2, osteocalcin, osteopontin, alkaline phosphatase, and type I collagen mRNA in long-term cultures of fetal rat calvarial osteoblasts. J Bone Miner Res 1994; 9:855–863

# 26 Electrophysiological Monitoring

*Joshua D. Auerbach, Amer F. Samdani, and John P. Dormans*

Progress in operative techniques has allowed the spine surgeon to treat patients with increasingly complex spinal deformities. Correcting more complex deformities requires sophisticated intraoperative neuromonitoring (IONM) techniques, which facilitate the detection and prevention of potentially devastating iatrogenic neurological injury. This chapter discusses the advantages and limitations of the various IONM tools available to the deformity surgeon.

The reported incidence of spinal-cord injury in scoliosis surgery varies from 0.3 to 1.4%.[1–3] Surveying the Scoliosis Research Society (SRS) database, MacEwen et al reported an incidence of spinal-cord injury of 0.72%, with complete paraplegia occurring in 55% of these cases.[3] A variety of mechanisms may account for spinal-cord injury during corrective scoliosis surgery. Misdirected wires, hooks, or pedicle screws may cause direct trauma to the cord. The correction of scoliosis may distract the spinal cord and compromise the local blood supply.[4] Similarly, occlusion of segmental vessels during anterior procedures may cause ischemia of the cord.[5,6] A decreased mean arterial blood pressure (MABP <60 mm Hg) and a low hemoglobin concentration exacerbate these tenuous situations.[7]

## ■ Clinical Tests of Global Spinal Function

Since its description in 1973 by Vauzelle and colleagues, the Stagnara wake-up test has been a widely used tool for assessing neurological function intraoperatively.[8] The test involves a temporary reduction in anesthesia during which the patient is instructed by verbal command to move the extremities, starting with the upper extremities and progressing to the lower extremities. Failure to move the lower extremities symmetrically indicates a neurological injury. The benefit of the test is that it is a simple, cost-effective procedure that can be performed in any operating room, and does not require the participation of a specialized team of trained neurophysiologists. Furthermore, it provides a direct measure of global motor function. Although some still consider the wake-up test the "gold standard" for the intraoperative assessment of neurological function, it has significant shortcomings. Potential complications related to the wake-up test include patient recall, accidental extubation, air embolism, pain, construct-rod dislocation, disruption of intravenous and intra-arterial lines, added surgical time (between 30 and 45 minutes), and false-negative and false-positive results.[9,10]

Hoppenfeld and colleagues described the ankle clonus test in 1997 as a predictor of neurological compromise following scoliosis surgery.[11] They reported that the absence of bilateral ankle clonus on emergence of the patient from anesthesia is abnormal and indicates neurological injury. The ankle clonus test is predicated on the normal presence of bilateral ankle clonus upon recovery from general anesthesia as a result of the return of lower-motor-neuron function before the return of inhibitory upper-motor-neuron impulses, leading to a temporary excitatory state. In Hoppenfeld's review of 1006 patients who underwent spinal arthrodesis and instrumentation for scoliosis, 6 patients had new neurological deficits postoperatively, all of whom had a "positive" ankle clonus test. There were three false-positive findings but no false negatives.[9,11] Although this method of monitoring spinal-cord function is cheap, sensitive, and easily performed, some have questioned its specificity in the setting of inhalational anesthesia.[12]

The major drawback of both the wake-up test and ankle clonus test, however, is their failure to provide a real-time and continuous assessment of spinal-cord integrity. Both tests reflect global spinal integrity and cannot provide a real-time assessment of dorsal sensory or ventral motor cord tracts. This lag between injury and its detection (between 30 and 45 minutes in the wake-up test) may jeopardize the small window of opportunity for intervention, resulting in a transient deficit becoming permanent. Such limitations have served as the impetus for the development of IONM, which provides a real-time (and sometimes instantaneous) indication of spinal-cord integrity in patients undergoing corrective scoliosis surgery. Advances in neurophysiological monitoring of the spinal cord have complemented improvements in corrective spinal instrumentation and design, and together the two facilitate the improved care that can be offered to patients with more complex spinal deformities.

## ■ Monitoring of Somatosensory Evoked Potentials

Although the monitoring of somatosensory evoked potentials (SSEPs) was first described almost 70 years ago, its use in clinical practice was first reported by Nash and colleagues in 1977 for detecting impending neurological injury

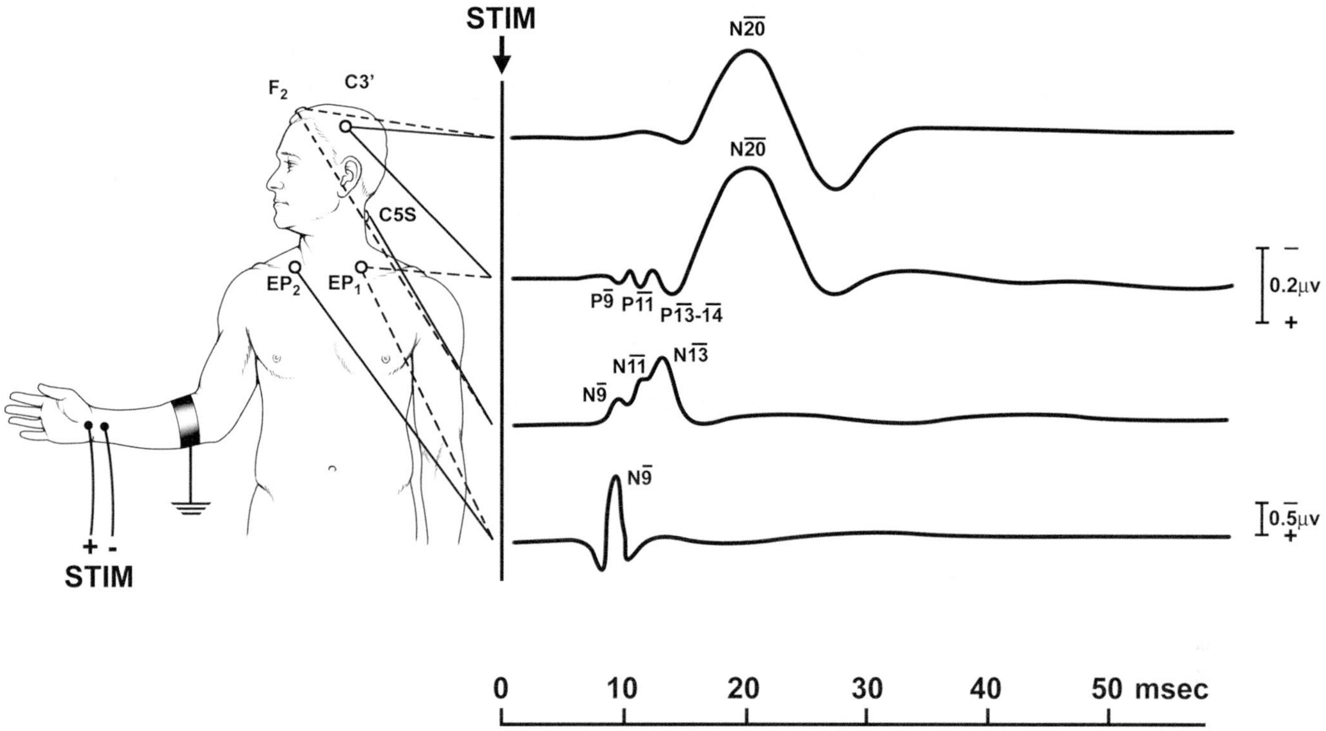


**Fig. 26.1** SSEP recording with ulnar-nerve stimulation.

during scoliosis surgery.[13,14] Despite the advent of more sophisticated monitoring modalities, monitoring of SSEPs is still considered by some to be the "gold standard" against which all other IONM techniques should be compared.

SSEP monitoring represents the averaging of electrical responses to repetitive electrical or mechanical stimulation of a peripheral nerve, most commonly the posterior tibial or peroneal nerves. The spinal cord is the conduit through which the afferent volley travels, largely reflecting the integrity of the dorsal sensory columns of the cord. Signal transduction is mediated by large-diameter myelinated sensory fibers that traverse the peripheral nerve and then enter the spinal cord and ascend through the dorsal columns (**Fig. 26.1**). After synapsing in the medullary nuclei of the brainstem, the neural signal then crosses the brainstem and enters into the medial lemniscal pathway. After another synapse in the thalamic nuclei, the signal proceeds to the parietal (sensorimotor) cortex. The afferent signal is then recorded either at the level of the spinal cord or, more commonly, the scalp (**Fig. 26.2**). Monitoring of the upper extremities at the brachial plexus is best done by stimulating SSEPs in the ulnar nerve (**Fig. 26.3**).[15,16] Monitoring of SSEPs in the lower extremities is done by stimulating the posterior tibial nerves or peroneal nerves (**Fig. 26.4**).[17,18]

SSEP monitoring has several distinct advantages over the ankle clonus and wake-up tests for spinal-cord integrity. It is highly effective in reducing the rate of neurological injuries below the rate found without IONM; it can detect injuries at the time of their occurrence rather than after the fact; and it can be performed on patients who are neurologically intact and those who are compromised.[3,19,20] Although still commonly done in conjunction with the wake-up test, SSEP monitoring can prevent the well-known complications of the wake-up test. Numerous studies have shown the efficacy of SSEP monitoring in reducing the rate of new neurological deficits in surgery for scoliosis.[21–23] As compared with the results obtained by MacEwen et al, without intraoperative monitoring was utilized, Nuwer and associates found that SSEP monitoring was effective at reducing the rate of major deficits of new-onset by ~60%.[3,20] In their survey of 51,263 scoliosis procedures, the latter investigators reported that SSEP monitoring had a sensitivity of 92%, although it also had a tendency toward giving a relatively high rate of false-positive results. In this large series, the primary predictors of deficits of new-onset were the experience of the neurophysiology team followed by that of the surgeon. Overall, the rate of false-positive results with the use of SSEP monitoring averages 2%, with a reported range of 0 to 7%.[24–27] In 1992, the SRS issued a position statement advocating SSEP monitoring as the standard of care for scoliosis surgery.[28] A recent survey of 37 members of the Spinal Deformity Study Group of the SRS revealed that the mode of neuromonitoring in surgery for adolescent idiopathic scoliosis (AIS) varied on a case-by-case basis, with SSEP monitoring alone being used in 10% of

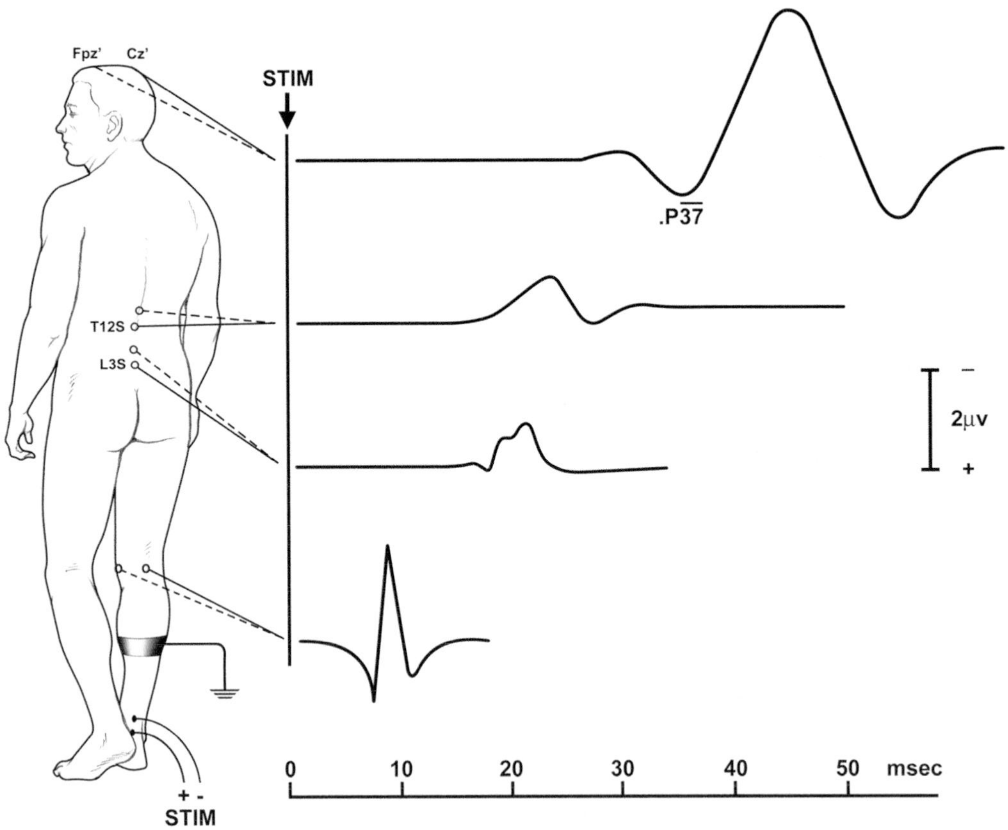


**Fig. 26.2** SSEP recording with posterior-tibial-nerve stimulation.

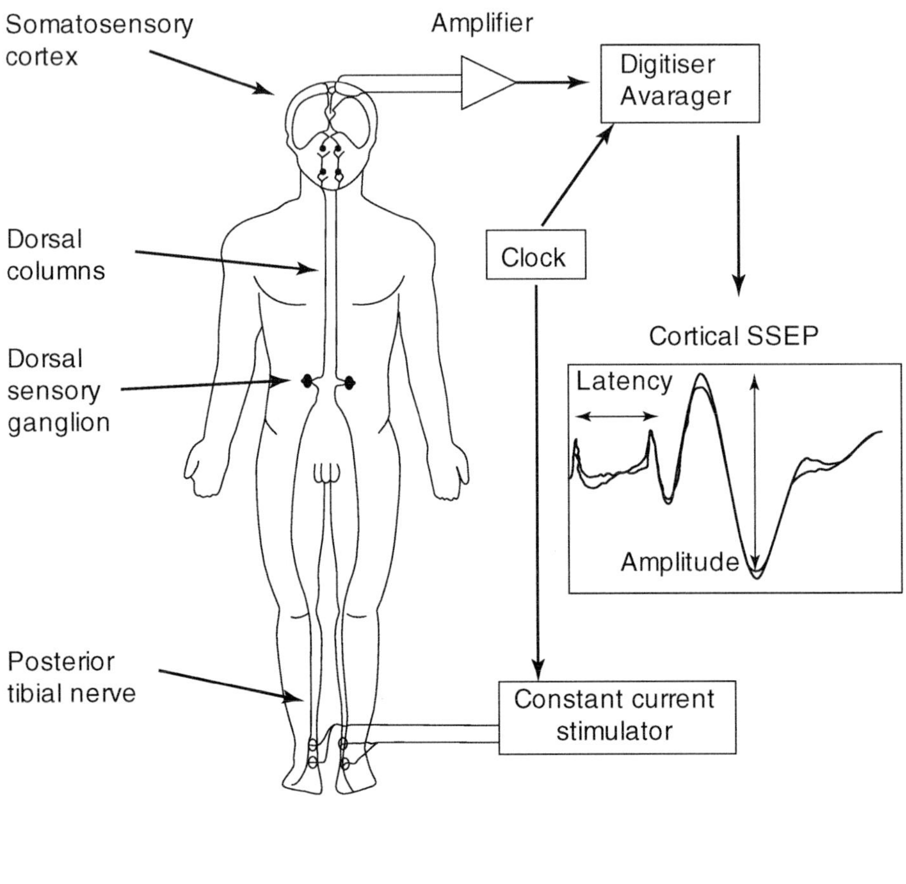


**Fig. 26.3** Cortical SSEP. Constant-current stimulation of the posterior tibial nerves at the ankle, with recording of the responses from the somatosensory cortex. (From de HP, Kalkman CJ. Spinal cord monitoring: Somatosensory- and motor-evoked potentials. Anesthesiol. Clin North America. 2001;19:923-45. Reprinted with permission.)

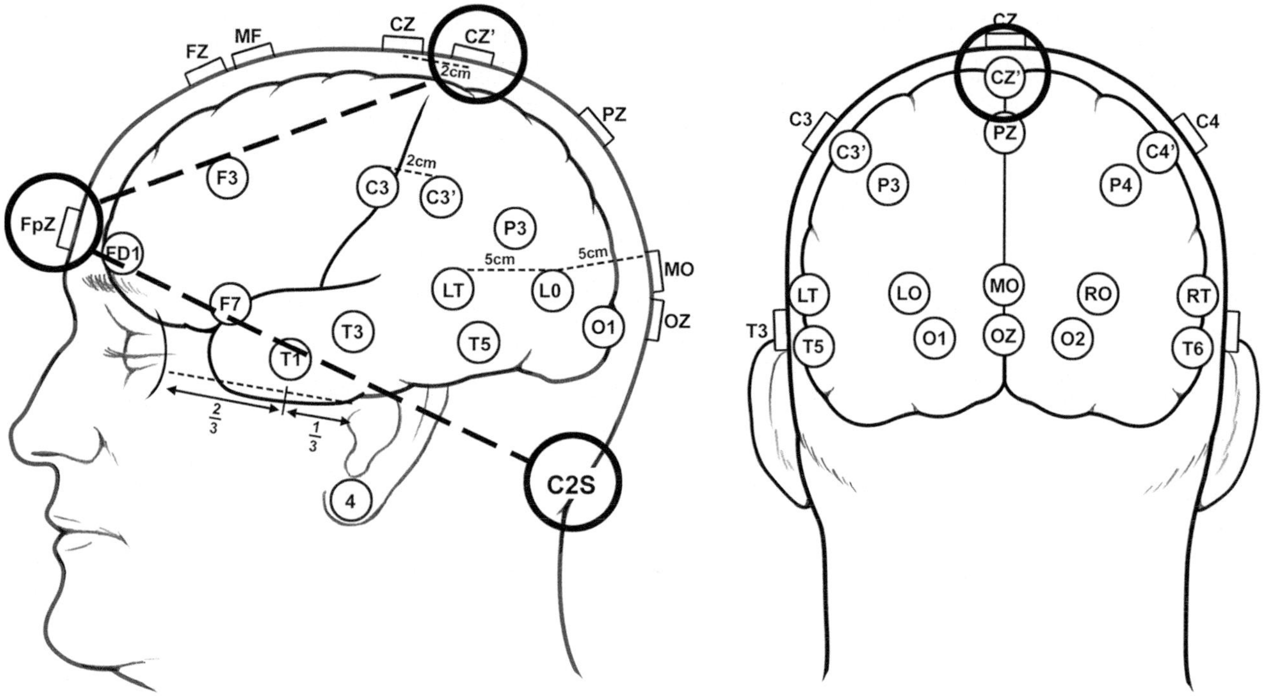


**Fig. 26.4** Lower-extremity SSEP (scalp recording sites).

cases, the wake-up test in 1.1%, and no IONM in 0.6%.[29] These results confirm the persistence of wide variation in IONM practice patterns in AIS surgery (**Table 26.1**).

Despite its excellent clinical track record, SSEP monitoring has limitations that have recently become of growing concern among spinal-deformity surgeons.[21,30–34] Because

**Table 26.1 Variability of Practice Patterns of Intraoperative Neuromonitoring in Surgery for Adolescent Idiopathic Scoliosis**

| Type of IONM Utilized | No. of Cases (%) |
|---|---|
| No form of IONM | 6 (0.6) |
| Wake-up test only | 11 (1.1) |
| SSEP only | 100 (10) |
| tcMEP only | 6 (0.6) |
| Combined SSEP and tcMEP | 436 (44) |
| Combined SSEP, tcMEP, and wake-up test | 196 (20) |
| SSEP, MEP, and EMG | 233 (24) |
| Total | 988 |

*Source*: Auerbach JD, Diab M, Sanders JO et al. Variability in spinal cord monitoring practice patterns in adolescent idiopathic scoliosis. Proceedings of the 14th Annual International Meeting on Advanced Spine Techniques, Paradise Island, Bahamas, July 2007. Adapted with permission.

*Abbreviations:* IONM, intraoperative neuromonitoring; EMG, electromyography; SSEP, somatosensory evoked potential; tcMEP, transcranial electrical motor evoked potential

SSEP monitoring primarily assesses the integrity of the dorsal sensory columns of the spinal cord, primary motor injuries, usually reflecting ischemia of the ventral motor tracts of the cord from hypotension, distraction, or derotation, may go undetected. Pelosi and co-workers reported a false-negative rate of 2.4% in monitoring of SSEPs, as compared with no false-negatives in monitoring of transcranial electrical motor evoked potentials (tcMEPs).[33] Others have similarly reported a failure to detect deficits of new onset with SSEP monitoring.[10,21,30–38] In the largest series to date to compare SSEP monitoring with tcMEP monitoring in AIS, Schwartz et al found that SSEP monitoring failed to detect four of seven cases (57%) of new-onset motor deficits, whereas tcMEP monitoring detected all seven cases.[34]

Besides its weaker sensitivity in detecting impending neurological injury, monitoring of SSEPs shows a well-documented delay in detecting ischemic injury as compared with monitoring of tcMEPs. Schwartz and associates showed that the average time to detection of an intraoperative insult with SSEP monitoring lagged behind that with tcMEP monitoring by an average of 5 minutes, with the lag ranging from instantaneous to 10 minutes.[34] This relative delay in detecting ischemia with SSEP monitoring has also been reported in the literature on thoracoabdominal aneurysm (TAA), and as a result, the technique has been abandoned for the prevention of neurological injury in surgery for TAA.[35,37] There are two potential explanations for the delay in detecting ischemia with SSEP monitoring: (1) monitoring primarily of the dorsal sensory columns allows ischemia of the ventral cord and motor tract only to be inferred rather than measured directly, in contrast to monitoring of tcMEPs, which correlates directly with the blood supply to the ventral cord; and (2) unlike tcMEP impulses, SSEP impulses relay afferent sensory signals nonsynaptically, which, because of the relative resistance of axonal conduction to ischemia, may result in a lag between the onset of an ischemic injury and detection of the causative ischemic event.[35,39] When these factors are taken together, they show that SSEP monitoring alone is incapable of direct monitoring of vascular blood flow to the ventral cord in real time, and therefore at best serves as an indirect measure of the global ventral-cord blood supply.

With the improved sensitivity afforded by the monitoring of tcMEPs, a residual role of SSEP monitoring of the spinal cord during AIS surgery may be to confirm the integrity of the cord in the setting of unchanged tcMEPs.[33,34] One critical and unique contribution of SSEP monitoring, however, is in monitoring of blood flow to the brachial plexus during the prone positioning of patients.[40] Prolonged or inappropriate prone positioning is an increasingly recognized source of iatrogenic neurological injury to both extremities in scoliosis surgery. With the arm in abduction and with increasing axillary pressure, brachial plexopathy can occur. Typically, ulnar-nerve SSEPs are recorded immediately after positioning of the arm in the flexed, abducted position. The point prevalence of positional brachial plexopathy reported in recent studies has ranged from 3.6 to 15%, depending on the criteria used for a significant change.[15,16,40] A reduction in SSEP amplitude of 30% indicates an impending injury and should prompt the surgical team to reposition the patient's arm.[15,16,41] In 18 arms for which there was an intraoperative SSEP alert, repositioning resulted in a nearly immediate return of ulnar-nerve SSEP tracings to baseline and in normal neurological function upon awakening of the patient (**Fig. 26.1**).[16] Another study demonstrated that SSEP monitoring was 78% sensitive in detecting sensory deficits in the upper extremity, 100% sensitive in detecting combined sensory and motor deficits, and 98.5% specific in predicting a normal neurological status postoperatively.[40] For routine AIS surgery, the continued use of SSEP monitoring is recommended because of its confirmatory role in the setting of negative tcMEPs, for providing information on the dorsal sensory cord, and for its ability to monitor the brachial plexus during prone positioning of the patient.

## Monitoring of Transcranial Electrical Motor Evoked Potentials

Transcranial electrical stimulation of the motor cortex generates an electrical impulse that descends the corticospinal tract (CST) and, at the distal end of the signal volley, enters the peripheral muscle in which this electrical impulse, or tcMEP, is ultimately recorded. Beginning with a transcranial electrical stimulus that delivers a brief (50 μsec), high-voltage (250 to 500 V) train of anodal pulses (two to seven pulses, with an interstimulus interval of 1 to 5 msec), a neuroelectric signal is generated (**Fig. 26.5**). Axons in the CST mediate the electrical impulse, which travels from the cortex through the internal capsule to the caudal medulla, where the fibers of the CST decussate and form the lateral CST. The signal then descends the CST in the lateral and anterior funiculi of the spinal cord. Upon entering the gray matter of the spinal cord, the axons of the CST interact with the interneurons of the spinal cord and synapse with α– motor neurons. The subsequent electrical responses are recorded at peripheral muscles, most commonly the anterior tibialis, although recording at the abductor hallucis, iliopsoas, quadriceps, and foot flexors has been described (**Fig. 26.6**).[42] The first dorsal interosseous muscle is also monitored as a control, to assess whether or not an intraoperative tcMEP alert represents global spinal-cord dysfunction (reflected by reductions in the amplitude of tcMEPs in both the upper and lower extremities) or localized injury (in which only tcMEPs in the lower extremity are affected). Once baseline signals are obtained, there are no absolute standards about what constitutes an alert. Some authors advocate ≥50% decrease in unilateral or bilateral tcMEP amplitude as the criterion for an alert, whereas others use an 80% decrease in amplitude.[2,33] In our institution, a tcMEP alert is defined as a sustainable decrease in tcMEP amplitude of 65%.

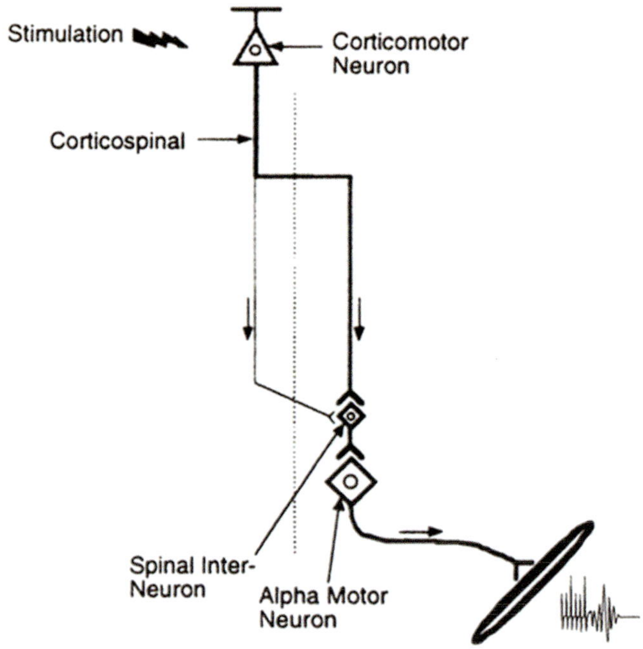


**Fig. 26.5** The pathway for signal transduction in tcMEP monitoring. See text for details.

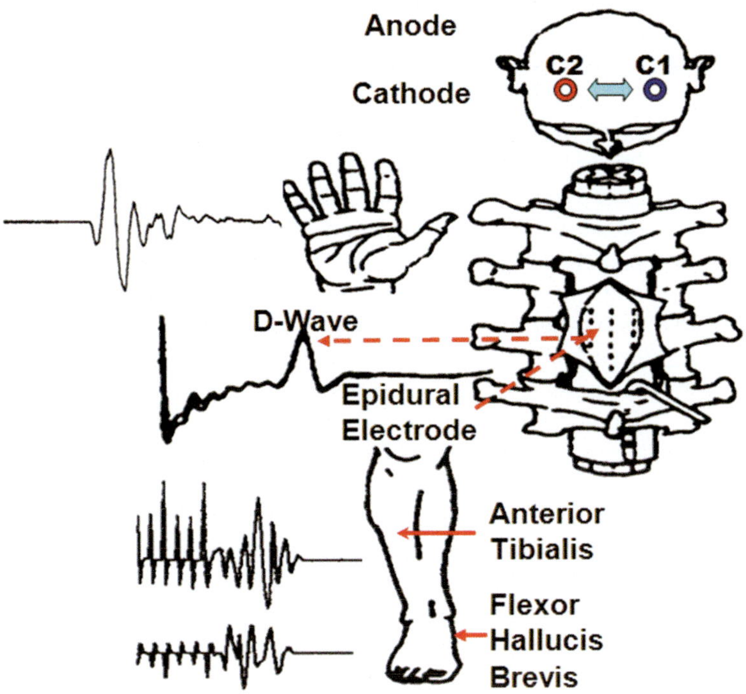


**Fig. 26.6** Direct activation of the pyramidal axons produces the D-wave, which is measured by an epidural recording catheter. This signal is another monitor of the functional integrity of the corticospinal tract.

The neurophysiological mechanism of signal transduction is probably responsible for the preferential sensitivity of tcMEP over SSEP monitoring in the detection of motor deficits during scoliosis surgery. Although SSEPs in the lower extremity provide information about the sensory dorsal columns, they do not reflect the integrity of the CSTs. The sensory dorsal columns consist of nonsynaptic axonal white matter, which is inherently more resistant to ischemia than is gray matter.[39,43] On the other hand, motor neurons in the anterior horn of the gray matter of the spinal cord have a high metabolic rate and are exquisitely vulnerable to ischemic changes.[35,39] TcMEPs, which are mediated by synapses in the ventral spinal cord, are thus highly sensitive to localized ischemic changes affecting the motor cells and interneurons of the anterior horn of the spinal cord. This is of particular clinical relevance because the vascular supply to the ventral motor pathways is less redundant than that to the posterior sensory columns, making the ventral motor tracts highly vulnerable to cord ischemia. During scoliosis surgery, hypotension and corrective maneuvers such as distraction and derotation may further compromise the local blood supply to the spinal cord.[10,30,33] On the basis of its sensitivity to ischemic changes affecting the ventral cord, tcMEP monitoring serves as a real-time neurophysiological indicator of impending injury to the ventral motor tract (**Table 26.2**).[31,34,35,38]

Numerous studies document the efficacy of tcMEP monitoring for detecting impending neurological injury during scoliosis surgery.[2,33–36,38,41,44] Schwartz et al reported the largest series of scoliosis surgeries in which tcMEP monitoring was used.[34] They retrospectively reviewed the intraoperative records of 1121 patients with AIS. All four participating pediatric spine centers adhered strictly to optimal anesthesia protocols and used the same team of highly trained, experienced neurophysiologists. Seventeen patients experienced depression of tcMEPs >65% (alert level) without any changes in SSEPs. Seven patients (0.6%) in the 1121-patient cohort experienced transient motor deficits, all of which were identified during surgery and were met with appropriate and timely

**Table 26.2 Cause of Intraoperative Neuromonitoring Alert in 1121 Consecutive Cases of Surgery for Adolescent Idiopathic Scoliosis**

| | Cause of Intraoperative Alert ($n$ = 38) |
|---|---|
| Distraction/derotation | 16/38 (42%) |
| Hypotension only (MABP <60 mm Hg) | 9/38 (24%) |
| Passing/tightening of sublaminar wires | 5/38 (13%) |
| Thoracic hook | 4/38 (11%) |
| Segmental vessel clamping | 3/38 (8%) |
| Thoracic pedicle screw | 1/38 (3%) |

*Source*: Schwartz DM, Auerbach JD, Dormans JP et al. Neurophysiological detection of impending spinal cord injury during scoliosis surgery. J Bone Joint Surg Am 2007;89:2440–9. Adapted with permission.

*Abbreviation:* MABP, mean arterial blood pressure

intervention. No patient sustained a permanent neurological deficit, possibly because of the rapid detection of neurological compromise and subsequent appropriate intervention at a point when the impending injury was still reversible. All neurological deficits resolved within 90 days, and most (six of nine cases) resolved within 7 days.[34] Other studies have confirmed the efficacy of tcMEP monitoring during scoliosis surgery.[2,33,38]

The issue of false-positives in IONM deserves special mention. A perceived limitation of spinal-cord monitoring is the relatively high rate of false-positive readings in some series. As a result of an IONM alert, the team response (i.e., a pause in surgery, raising of the patient's systemic blood pressure, reduction in the degree of spinal correction, administration of steroids, or removal of hardware) when the postoperative neurological examination is normal can be frustrating and perhaps perceived as unwarranted, and may be a source of significant risk to the patient. Traditionally, the outcome variable that is assessed in evaluating the efficacy of spinal-cord monitoring is whether or not the patient awakens with a neurological deficit of new onset (a true positive). According to these criteria, a false-positive alert is therefore defined as an intraoperative alert in which a patient has a normal neurological examination upon awakening. We would argue, however, that an intraoperative neurophysiological alert, especially in tcMEP monitoring, indicates a true physiological event affecting the spinal cord (i.e., ischemia), and has the potential to become a neurological deficit if not addressed acutely. The bases for this are numerous animal and clinical studies demonstrating the relationship between spinal-cord ischemia (a true physiological event), a significant tcMEP alert, and the onset of new neurological injuries.[35,45,46] A recent study showed that up to 74% of tcMEP alerts may be attributable to a mechanism of spinal-cord ischemia arising from systemic hypotension, distraction, or derotation maneuvers, in 32% of which patients awakened with a neurological injury of new onset.[34] It can therefore be concluded that the ischemic cord is "at risk" for permanent injury and that a tcMEP alert provides an opportunity to correct a threatening neurological deficit.[31,33,34,38] Although it is difficult to prove in a controlled study, false-positive tcMEP readings are likely to represent a true positive made "false" by appropriate and timely intervention.

## Electromyography

Intraoperative evaluation of the integrity of the pedicle and pedicle-screw position before and after screw placement is a three-step procedure, involving: (1) manual palpation of the ventral, medial, lateral, superior, and inferior pedicle walls with a pedicle probe or feeler; (2) intraoperative imaging[47]; and (3) electromyographic (EMG) stimulation.

In more traditional hook or hybrid constructs, EMG monitoring is used only during lumbar or lower-thoracic pedicle-screw placement. More recently, however, thoracic pedicle-screw constructs have become more common as numerous clinical and biomechanical studies have shown improved rotational correction, improved fixation, and reduced loss of correction with their use as compared with hook or sublaminar wire constructs.[48–51] Given the smaller pedicle diameter in the thoracic spine, the variable pedicle angle, and the proximity of the great vessels, thoracic spinal nerve roots, and spinal cord, the risk of a pedicle breach and injury of adjacent structures is greater than in the lumbar spine.[52–55] Consequently, there is growing interest in studying the capabilities of EMG monitoring as a means of improving patient safety during the placement of both lumbar and thoracic pedicle screws.[52,53]

Earlier cadaveric studies revealed a rate of 12.5 to 54.7% of thoracic cortical violation with thoracic pedicle-screw placement[56–60] More recently, a cadaveric study in which the freehand technique was used to place thoracic pedicle screws along the anatomic axis demonstrated a 97% rate of success in screw placement with less than 1 mm of pedicle-wall violation. In addition, 87.5% of the screws inserted were fully contained within the pedicle.[57] In the largest clinical study of its kind to date, Lehman and coworkers used postoperative computed tomography (CT) to evaluate the thoracic positioning of of 1023 pedicle screws placed in 60 patients with spinal deformity through the freehand technique. They reported a 91.2% rate of success, without any neurological, vascular, or visceral complications.[61] Reported clinical sequelae of erroneous pedicle-screw placement include incidental durotomies, nerve-root irritation, pedicle fracture, and leakage of cerebrospinal fluid (CSF).[52,53,62]

EMG monitoring is done by placing subdermal needle electrodes into the muscle groups innervated by the spinal nerves relevant to a surgical procedure. For the cervical and lumbar spine, well-established EMG recording sites that correspond with the nerve roots at risk have been described (**Table 26.3**). For monitoring thoracic pedicle-screw placement in the upper spine (T2 to T6), electrodes are placed at the corresponding intercostal spaces at the nipple line, and compound muscle action potentials (CMAPs; electrical potentials evoked by stimulation of the motor nerve innervating a specific group of muscles) in the intercostal musculature are assessed. For monitoring the placement of screws in the lower thoracic spine (T7 to T12) according to the method described by Shi and coworkers, paired electrodes are placed along the nipple line at evenly spaced intervals between the lower margin of the 10th rib and the iliac ridge (**Fig. 26.7**).[53] In most instances of monitoring of lower thoracic screw placement, CMAP activity is assessed in the rectus abdominus musculature.[52,63]

**Table 26.3 Cervical and Lumbar Recording Sites for Intraoperative Electromyography**

| Spinal Level | Muscle Group |
|---|---|
| C5 | Deltoid, biceps |
| C6 | Biceps, wrist extensors |
| C7 | Triceps, wrist extensors, wrist flexors |
| C8 | Hand intrinsics, finger extensors |
| L2 | Adductor longus, adductor magnus |
| L3 | Adductors, vastus medialis |
| L4 | Vastus medilais, vastus lateralis |
| L5 | Anterior tibialis, extensor hallucis longus, medial gastrocnemius, peroneus longus |
| S1 | Perianal musculature |
| S2–4 | |

*Source*: Padberg AM. Electrophysiology. In: DeWald RL, Arlet V, Carl A et al, eds. Spinal Deformities: The Comprehensive Text. New York: Thieme, 2004:135–48. Adapted with permission.

The regimen in EMG monitoring consists of two components: (1) monitroring of spontaneous EMGs (spEMGs); and (2) monitoring of stimulated EMGs (stEMGs). Monitoring of spEMGs involves the continuous acquisition of data from spontaneous muscle activitys at rest. With chronic nerve-root compression, impulse-train activity is the most common pattern seen in spEMG recordings. More acute changes in spEMG activity may manifest in the form of burst or train activity resulting from mechanical stretching, retraction, or sudden compression of a nerve root. The major contribution of spEMG monitoring is its ability to instantly notify the surgical team about a nerve-root insult. It does not, however, provide information about the conductive capacity of the nerve root after insult or injury. The frequency of postoperative neurological injuries following spEMG alerts is low, indicating a low specificity for this technique.[63,64]

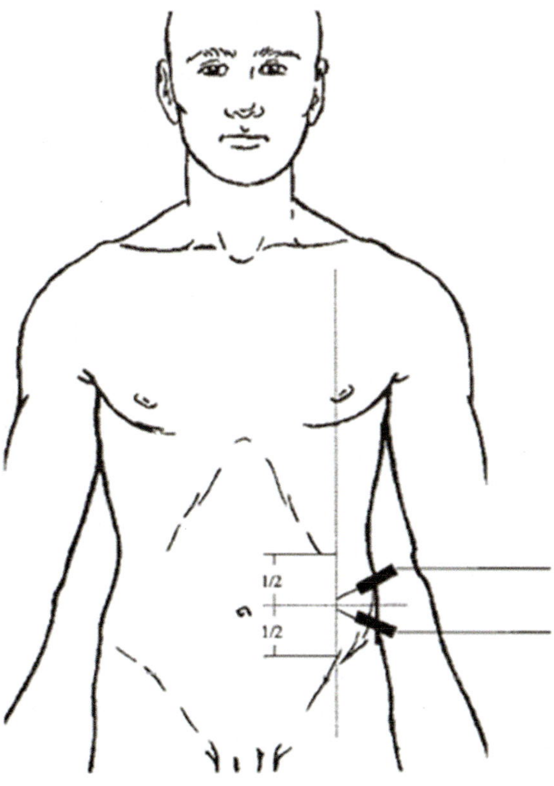


**Fig. 26.7** Placement of subdermal needle electrodes into the rectus abdominus musculature for EMG monitoring of lower thoracic pedicle screws (T7 to T12).

stEMG monitoring involves the electrical stimulation of a pedicle channel or screw and the recording of the stimulation threshold needed to trigger a CMAP.[63] The stimulating probe is placed into the pedicle-screw channel or on the surface of the pedicle screw, and a threshold potential for stimulation of a CMAP is recorded. The rationale behind stEMG monitoring is that the electrical stimulus required to activate the neighboring nerve root is proportional to the electrical impedance characteristics of the pedicular bone. If the pedicle is intact, the greater resistance to current flow would result in a high threshold for screw stimulation (i.e., >15 mA). If there is violation of the pedicle, however, the resistance to current flow is reduced and the screw-stimulation threshold will be lower (i.e., <3mA), indicating damage.[41,52,53,65] Studies have confirmed a significant correlation between low pedicle-screw stimulation thresholds and misdirected placement of lumbar pedicle screws.[52,53,62,66,67]

It is important to maintain proper technique when performing stEMG to avoid false recorded values. Steps should be taken in every case to: (1) ensure that no soft tissue is in contact with the EMG probe, which can artificially increase the stimulation threshold (i.e., give a false-negative result); and (2) stimulate circumferentially inside the pedicle and vertebral body, being aware that in patients with osteoporosis or poor bone quality a low impedance value (from diminished resistance to the applied electrical current) can be seen despite the pedicle being intact (i.e., a false-positive result)[68]; (3) apply the cathode stimulator probe to the hexagonal screw port or directly to the shank of the pedicle screw, and not to the mobile crown, to avoid a false-negative EMG result (**Figs. 26.8, 26.9**).[69] Anderson et al recently reported that polyaxial pedicle screws can have high electrical resistances between their mobile crowns and shanks, and may therefore fail to produce a response during stEMG testing despite the presence of a pedicle breach.

The clinical results with triggered EMG for monitoring the placement of lumbosacral pedicle screws have been excellent.[41,52,66,70] Overall, the negative predictive value of lumbar pedicle-screw monitoring with stEMG has been

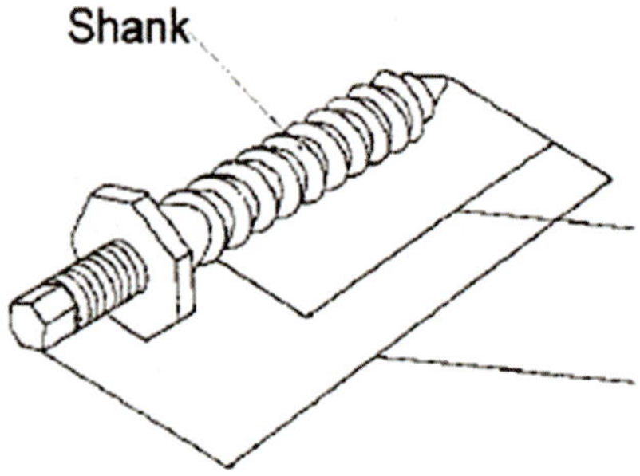


**Fig. 26.8** Diagram of a monoaxial pedicle screw showing the location of electrode placement during electrical-resistance testing. (From Anderson DG, Wierzbowski LR, Schwartz DM et al. Pedicle screws with high electrical resistance: A potential source of error with stimulus-evoked EMG. Spine 2002;27:1577-81. Reprinted with permission.)

98% when the impedance values have been ≥11 mA.[53] If the threshold of stimulation is low (<6 to 7 mA), a pedicle breach is more likely. Impedance values between 7 and 11 mA represent a possible pedicle breach.[66,67] In results resembling those in the lumbar spine, Shi et al recently reported that stEMG for monitoring pedicle-screw placement in the thoracic spine had a negative predictive value of 98% when stimulation thresholds were >11 mA.[53] Raynor and associates reported that all screws with stimulation thresholds >6 mA were safely implanted, without breaching of the medial pedicle wall. For screws with a stimulation threshold of <6 mA, however, Raynor et al recommend concomitant evaluation of the "average" of all other screw-stimulation thresholds in a given patient, and suspicion of a pedicle-wall breach only if the threshold is 60 to 65% below the patient's average threshold.[52] In a later study, Raynor et al analyzed the EMG results for the placement of 4857 lumbar pedicle screws, and established 8.0 mA as a threshold above which the stimulated screw was very likely to be present in an intact pedicle (a 0.33% false-negative rate). At lower thresholds of stimulation, Raynor and colleagues recommended removal of the relevant screw and repeated palpation to evaluate for a pedicle breach.[71] Certainly the higher the threshold of EMG stimulation the less likely a pedicle is to have been breached, but using a higher threshold of stimulation as the criterion for repeat palpation carries the risk of increaseing the frequency of false-positive results and unnecessary repeat palpations.

## H-Reflex Monitoring

The H-reflex is a monosynaptic reflex produced by stimulation of the afferent fibers of the S1 nerve root (tibial nerve) in the popliteal fossa. This segmental reflex provides a measure of the excitability of the motor-neuron pool within the gray matter, and can be used to assess the integrity of both afferent and efferent neural connections. The afferent volley traverses the mixed peripheral nerve via group Ia fibers and exits via motor neurons that transmit the efferent signal to the muscle (gastrocnemius or soleus), where the signal is detected. Defects in this reflex pattern classically correlate with S1 radiculopathies. Because spinal shock suppresses stretch reflexes, however, H-reflexes have been shown to reflect the integrity of the motor pathways of the more rostral spinal cord.[72] The H-reflex is mediated over a long course (peripheral nerve, spinal cord, sacral plexus, and tibial and sciatic nerves), and injury at any point along this pathway can therefore cause an abnormal H-reflex. Animal and clinical studies in humans also suggest that the H-reflex can provide immediate feedback about the status of the descending motor tracts of the ventral spinal cord.[73-76] A transient change in the H-reflex warns of an impending neurological injury, and permanent suppression of the H-reflex predicts postoperative neurological deficits.[75]

Leis and associates, investigating a group of 31 patients undergoing spinal cord surgery, found that 4 of 6 patients who had temporary changes in H-reflex amplitude of <50% (which resolved with intraoperative measures) were neurologically normal upon awakening from anesthesia. For the two patients in whom the amplitude of the H-reflex was permanently suppressed by >90%, severe postoperative neurological deficits were observed.[75] Mechanical perturbation of the spinal cord produced nearly instantaneous changes in the H-reflex, corroborating the findings in animal studies of rapid changes in the H-reflex with spinal-cord insults.[73,74,76] Some authors have proposed that by providing almost instantaneous warning of potential motor-tract injury in the spinal cord, and with changes in

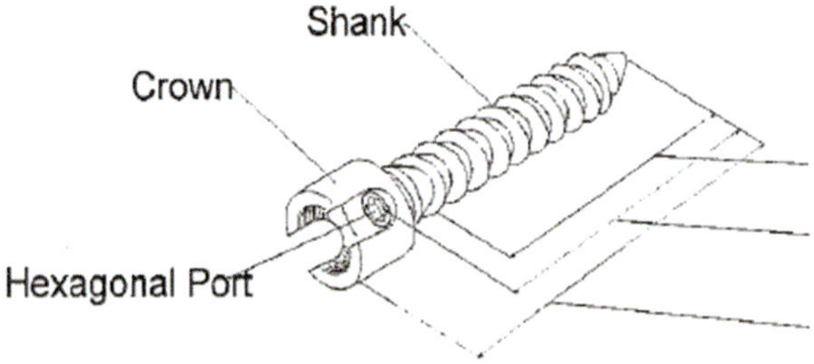


**Fig. 26.9** Diagram of a polyaxial pedicle screw showing the location of electrode placement during electrical-resistance testing. (From Anderson DG, Wierzbowski LR, Schwartz DM et al. Pedicle screws with high electrical resistance: A potential source of error with stimulus-evoked EMG. Spine 2002;27:1577-81. Reprinted with permission.)

amplitude corresponding with neurological outcome, changes in the H-reflex reflect the severity of spinal-cord injury. Other potential advantages of H-reflex monitoring include a relative resistance of H-reflex wave recording to suppression by general anesthesia, and the ability to detect subtle sensory deficits in the S1 nerve root.[72]

Although there have been reports of the successful use of H-reflex monitoring in scoliosis surgery,[77–80] several limitations have precluded its use in common practice in such surgery. H-reflexes are commonly absent in patients over 60 years of age or who have had a prior laminectomy. In a patient with a baseline deficit of the S1 nerve root that renders the H-reflex immeasurable, monitoring of the reflex will not be capable of detecting spinal-cord injury of new onset. As with other monitoring techniques, the use and interpretation of the H-reflex monitoring is highly operator- and technique-dependent, and its results may therefore be ambiguous in inexperienced hands. Consequently, monitoring of the H-reflex is currently limited to a role complementary to that of EMG monitoring and the use of other, more established modalities for spinal-cord monitoring in AIS surgery.

## ■ D-Wave Monitoring

The D-wave is evoked by direct activation of the pyramidal axons and measured with an epidural recording catheter, and has been considered another means of monitoring the functional integrity of the corticospinal tract (**Fig. 26.6**). Variations >20% in D-wave amplitude are evidence of impending neurological injury.[81] In patients undergoing surgery for intramedullary spinal-cord tumors, variations >50% in D-wave amplitude correlate with poor outcome. Reports of the efficacy of D-wave monitoring of the spinal cord in scoliosis surgery have described mixed results.[82] Ulkatan and colleagues recently reported that 27% of 93 patients with scoliosis who underwent D-wave and tcMEP monitoring showed significant alterations in D-wave activity without any changes in tcMEP or SSEP tracings or changes on postoperative neurological examination. The changes in D-wave activity occurred immediately after correction of the scoliosis. On the basis of findings with magnetic resonance imaging (MRI) that revealed displacement of the spinal cord toward the curve concavity in scoliosis, Ulkatan and colleagues postulated that the reason for D-wave variability in scoliosis surgery is the new spatial relationship between the spinal cord and spinal canal that occurs with curve correction.[81] In addition to the difficulty in perfectly achieving the requisite midline position of the epidural recording catheter used in D-wave monitoring, the technique also carries the risk of causing epidural complications because placement of the catheter is usually done via a laminectomy or laminotomy. Continued research will further define the role, if any, of D-wave monitoring in monitoring spinal-cord function during surgery for scoliosis.

## ■ Team Response to an Intraoperative Alert

Although a detailed description of the treatment algorithms used in response to an IONM alert is beyond the scope of this chapter, we present herein several guidelines used in our institution. **Figure 26.10** depicts the IONM protocol used for AIS patients instrumented with pedicle-screw systems. In our institution, the team response to an

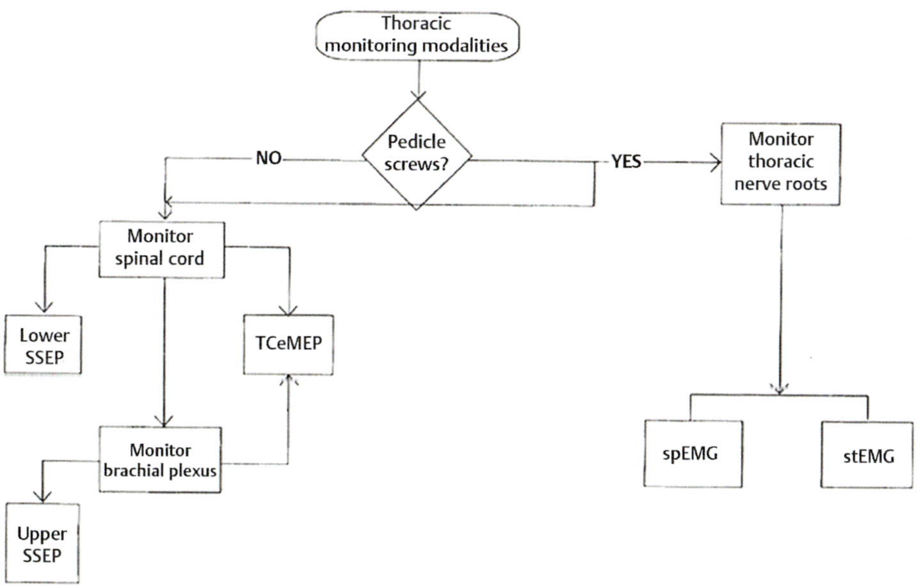


**Fig. 26.10** Recommended guidelines for IONM modalities to be used in thoracic surgery for AIS.

alert is initially a surgical pause and confirmation that the reduced IONM amplitude is not being caused by an anesthetic agent or technical factors in monitoring. Simultaneously, the patient's MABP is raised to at least 90 mm Hg through volume repletion, possibly accompanied by packed red blood cell transfusion to raise the hematocrit and if necessary, by pharmacological modulation. The decision to administer steroids according to the protocol for spinal-cord injury, as well as the threshold required to initiate the protocol, are determined on a case-by-case basis. The institutional protocol and practitioner response to an IONM alert may vary if the amplitude of the signal continues to be decreased after 15 minutes. If the alert coincided with curve correction or with the placement of a wire, screw, or hook, the relevant anchor is removed or some of the surgically imposed curve correction is released. Should the IONM tracings still suggest an impending neurological injury after 25 to 30 minutes of team response, all instrumentation is removed and surgery is stopped. Although debate continues to surround the absolute threshold of amplitude reduction that defines a "significant" alert, our institutional guidelines allow a procedure to continue with caution upon a return of 50% in the amplitude of the IONM signal. Traditionally, a loss of 75% in signal amplitude suggests a transient injury that in most cases will resolve.[41] Should removal of instrumentation be indicated, introducing the potential for spinal instability, the patient is put in a brace postoperatively. Return to the operating room for reinstrumentation is based on the results of the postoperative neurological examination, and may be delayed for as long as 2 or 3 weeks. The case examples given at the end of the chapter are useful for discussing the management of several of the more commonly encountered situations in which IONM alerts can occur.

A recent review of 38 intraoperative IONM alerts revealed that the most common team response was to correct hypotension to at least 85 mm Hg. The next most common team response was a pause in surgery, which occurred in 45% of cases and averaged 8.7 minutes in duration. This was followed in frequency by steroid administration, the removal of spinal instrumentation, reduction of a spinal correction, and the wake-up test (**Table 26.4**).[34]

**Table 26.4 Team Response to an Intraoperative Neuromonitoring Alert in 1121 Consecutive Cases of Adolescent Idiopathic Scoliosis**

| | Team Response to Alert ($n = 38$) |
|---|---|
| Surgical pause | 17/38 (45%) |
| Hypotension correction | 22/38 (58%) |
| Steroid administration | 11/38 (29%) |
| Instrumentation removed | 11/38 (29%) |
| Correction reduced | 10/38 (26%) |
| Intraoperative wake-up test performed | 3/38 (8%) |

*Source*: Schwartz DM, Auerbach JD, Dormans JP, et al. Neurophysiological detection of impending spinal cord injury during scoliosis surgery. J Bone Joint Surg Am 2007;89:2440–9. Adapted with permission.

## Limitations of IONM

The ability to use IONM to reliably monitor the integrity of the spinal cord during surgery for AIS has dramatically improved patient safety and made it possible to safely treat more complex spinal deformities. However, IONM has the following three limitations, which will be described below: (1) effects of anesthesia and the operating-room envionment; ( 2) delayed postoperative neurological deficits; and (3) complications of tcMEP monitoring.

### Considerations Relating to Anesthesia and the Operating-room Environment

Several significant considerations relating to the operating-room environment and anesthesia can affect the stability and clarity of both SSEP and tcMEP monitoring. One is that inhalational anesthetic agents (i.e., desflurane, sevoflurane, isoflurane, and nitrous oxide) have a dose–response effect on SSEP monitoring.[83–85] The depressant effect of inhalational anesthetic agents is manifested both by a reduction in the latency of SSEP signals and, more importantly, by degradation of the cortical SSEP wave.[35,86] One study reported a 50% reduction in SSEP amplitude with nitrous oxide.[87] Similarly, tcMEP signals are highly suppressed by inhalational anesthetics.[35,88] Volatile inhalational anesthetics decrease the excitability of both cortical and spinal-cord motor neurons in tcMEP monitoring. With increased variability and reduced reliability in both SSEP and tcMEP signal tracing, the risk of ambiguity in signal interpretation is significantly increased. Efforts to reduce the risk of false-positive alerts and unreliable signal baselines in surgery for AIS commonly consist of using total intravenous anesthesia and avoiding the use of paralytic agents. In our institution, a standardized anesthesia protocol is strictly followed. After induction and intubation with nitrous oxide and a low concentration of a potent agent such as sevoflurane, all inhalational agents and muscle relaxants are discontinued. Throughout surgery, general anesthesia is maintained by the pump-controlled intravenous infusion of propofol and remifentanyl and the maintenance of an MABP ≥65 mmHg. Remifentanyl has an extremely short half-life, and when infused at a constant rate produces constant plasma concentrations and minimal variability in the tcMEP response.[88] Occasional boluses of narcotic agents are provided as needed. Although the specifics of an anesthesia regimen for AIS surgery may vary, adhering to these principles will minimize signal variability and maximize the neurophysiologist's ability to provide reliable information to the surgical and anesthesia teams.

Elements of the operating-room environment and physiological considerations that might influence the intraoperative quality of IONM signals include external 60-Hz noise and artifacts from electronic beds, warming blanket, poor electrical grounding, surgical headlights, microscopes, blood warmers, and electric drills.[89] Additionally, hypothermia has been shown to delay the rate of synaptic transmission in SSEP monitoring, which may affect SSEP latency but not amplitude. As discussed above, hypotension may have an additive effect on iatrogenic spinal-cord ischemia produced by distraction, compression, derotation, or vessel ligation.[35,45]

## Delayed Postoperative Neurological Deficit

A delayed postoperative neurological deficit (DPND) is one of the most feared complications following surgery for AIS. Despite an uneventful surgery, unremarkable intraoperative monitoring profile, and normal postoperative neurological examination, a DPND is characterized by the development of postoperative paresis within hours or days after a surgical procedure.[90–92] Among possible reasons for a DPND are postoperative spinal-cord swelling and vascular spasm with resultant ischemia. In such cases IONM shows no changes in tcMEPs. Progressive neurological decline often prompts emergent return of the patient to the operating room for exploration and the removal of corrective hardware. In such situations a loss of tcMEP signals commonly corroborates the change in neurological status. A second potential mechanism for DPND is delayed ischemia of the spinal cord following distractive and derotational forces applied to the spine hours earlier. Similarly, prolonged intraoperative hypotension during instrumentation and curve correction can predispose to a later ischemic event. For these reasons, we routinely recommend that the patient's MABP never dip below 65 mm Hg. Patients who are dehydrated should be aggressively volume-resuscitated prior to surgery.[34] A further mechanism for DPND is an epidural hematoma that creates tension in the epidural space and mechanical compression of the cord or nerve roots, resulting in neural ischemia.[90]

Management of a suspected DPND should begin with a careful physical examination of the patient. This should include a detailed motor and sensorineural examination of the lower extremities and evaluation of bowel and bladder function, peroneal and perirectal sensation, and reflex function. If implants containing titanium alloys are used, MRI is a feasible imaging option for detecting problems because the decreased ferromagnetic properties of titanium reduce the scatter distortion of the MRI image.[93] Alternatively, CT myelography can be used to evaluate whether or not an epidural hematoma is present or if there is compression of neurological structures adjacent to a hardware component. In some instances the treatment plan may warrant urgent return to the operating room for implant removal, reduction of a correction before imaging is done, or both. The treatment plan must be individualized and devised on a case-by-case basis.[90,94] Treatment by partial removal of hardware and staged correction has in many cases been shown to be effective for facilitating full neurological recovery.[90,95,96] When DPND is attributable to an epidural hematoma, we recommend re-instrumentation with pedicle screws instead of sublaminar wires or hooks, to minimize the risk of recurrent bleeding.

Measures that can be taken to maximize postoperative spinal-cord perfusion and reduce the risk fof DPND include: (1) aggressive preoperative hydration and volume repletion of the patient to keep the MABP >65 mm Hg during instrumentation; (2) transfusion with packed red blood cells to maintain the hematocrit at a physiological level; (3) a stay in the intensive care unit stay with monitoring through an arterial line for maintenance of the MABP at 80 to 90 mm Hg, especially in the case of an intraoperative IONM alert denoting a potential risk of cord ischemia; (4) regular neurological examination; and (5) limiting the use of patient-controlled analgesia to optimize patient cooperation with the neurological examination.[34,90]

## Complications of Monitoring Transcranial Electrical Muscle Evoked Potentials

Because it involves repetitive electrical stimulation of the brain, tcMEP monitoring raises several unique safety concerns. Some of the potential complications of tcMEP monitoring include brain damage, seizure activity, bite injuries, scalp burns, adverse cognitive or affective disorders, cardiac arrhythmia, and intraoperative awareness. In a recent analysis of the safety profile of tcMEP monitoring in more than 15,000 cases of its use, Macdonald[97] reported an exceedingly low complication rate (**Table 26.5**). The most common complication encountered (tongue or lip laceration) can be prevented with a properly inserted bite block.[97] To the best of our

**Table 26.5 Summary of Identified Adverse Events in More Than 15,000 Cases of Monitoring of Transcranial Electrical Motor Evoked Potentials**

| Complication | Published | Unpublished | Total |
|---|---|---|---|
| Tongue or lip laceration | 3 | 26 | 29 |
| Mandibular fracture | 1 | 0 | 1 |
| Seizure | 0 | 5 | 5 |
| Cardiac arrhythmia | 0 | 5 | 5 |
| Scalp burn | 0 | 2 | 2 |
| Intraoperative awareness | 0 | 1 | 1 |

*Source*: MacDonald DB. Safety of intraoperative transcranial electrical stimulation motor evoked potential monitoring. J Clin Neurophysiol 2002;19:416–29. Adapted with permission.

knowledge, the few reports of seizure as a consequence of tcMEP monitoring have involved unanesthetized patients with predisposing brain lesions.[97,98] Although no published study has reported cardiac arrhythmia during tcMEP monitoring, five unpublished cases of premature ventricular contraction and bradycardia of sudden but reversible onset have occurred. Relative contraindications to tcMEP monitoring include epilepsy, cortical lesions, cardiac disease, vascular clips or shunts, and implanted cardiac pacemakers.[97] The remaining complications are reported in **Table 26.5**.

## Conclusion

The evolution of spinal-cord monitoring in contemporary surgery for AIS continues to evolve. Although clinical tests of global spinal function are still commonly used during such surgery, it is safe to say that these tests should be used as supplements to some form of electrophysiological monitoring. The limitations of monitoring SSEPs, which include its failure to provide a real-time assessment of ventral motor pathways in the spinal cord and in some series an unacceptable false-negative rate, have been the impetus for the development of more sensitive, instantaneous markers of spinal-cord integrity. Monitoring of tcMEPs represents the most advanced method for assessing cord integrity during surgery for AIS, but the search continues for improvements in understanding of the physiological events that cause detectable intraoperative electrophysiological changes. Such understanding will facilitate further refinements in clinically meaningful electrophysiological thresholds, better sensitivity and specificity of monitoring, and ultimately, better patient care.

Future work will also need to be done on the ever-changing nature of the "standard of care" for spinal cord monitoring. As evidenced by a recent review, ~10% of AIS surgery is still done without the use of combined motor and SSEP monitoring techniques, despite ample evidence of the relatively poor sensitivity of SSEP monitoring alone.[29] Given this continued variability in the practice patterns of spinal-cord monitoring, one of the goals of continued research should be to refine the protocols for spinal-cord monitoring with the understanding that these protocols will continue to evolve to reflect progress in understanding the meaning of monitoring signals and technological advances in their use. The driving forces behind the evolution of such guidelines will include the findings in ongoing and future research, as well as patients', families', and other societal demands. Another goal should be the active dissemination of developments and findings in current research to all groups involved in spine surgery, including surgeons, hospitals, physician societies, and neuromonitoring groups, to improve education, training, certification, and the standardization of qualifications for spinal-cord monitoring. Also needed will be protocols for routine spinal-cord monitoring developed by interdisciplinary research efforts and treatment algorithms for interpreting intraoperative neurophysiological changes. Ultimately, the potential benefits of the scientific gains in spinal-cord monitoring can be realized only if high-quality neuromonitoring, delivered in a cost-effective manner, is accepted and available.

## Case Examples*

### Case Example 1

A 14-year-old girl who underwent a posterior spinal fusion (PSF) from T4 to L1 for a 54-degree Lenke type 1 curve. During positioning of the patient for surgery, her baseline ulnar-nerve SSEP recording demonstrated a 50% loss in amplitude with the patient's right arm in excessive abduction (**Fig. 26.11**). The surgical team was notified and the arm was repositioned in less abduction. With this, the SSEP amplitude was restored, there were no further SSEP alerts throughout the remainder of the patient's surgery, and the patient awoke with normal neurological function.[16,40]

Impending brachial plexopathy resulting from prone patient positioning can be reliably detected with SSEP monitoring. Repositioning of the arm following an SSEP restores baseline SSEP values.

### Case Example 2

A 16-year-old girl with AIS underwent a PSF with a hybrid construct (hooks and sublaminar wires in the thoracic spine and segmental pedicle fixation in the lumbar spine) from T3 to T12. The patient underwent multimodal IONM consisting of tcMEP, SSEP, and EMG, because pedicle-screw fixation was anticipated. There were no intraoperative alerts during positioning of the patient or during exposure of her spine. Total intravenous anesthesia was utilized throughout the surgery after exposure of the patient's spine. Thoracic hooks were placed in the upper thoracic spine without any difficulty. However, the placement of the hooks at T8 caused a sudden complete loss of the tcMEP signal. There was no accompanying SSEP alert. The patient's MABP was raised to 85 mm Hg and the hook at T8 was removed. However, the amplitude of the tcMEP did not return to within 75% of its preoperative baseline value, and the steroid protocol for treating spinal-cord injury was therefore initiated. The decision was made to stop surgery and remove all instrumentation from the patient. tcMEP tracings recorded before a wake-up test revealed minimal recovery of the tcMEP amplitude throughout the remainder

*Courtesy of Daniel M. Schwartz, PhD

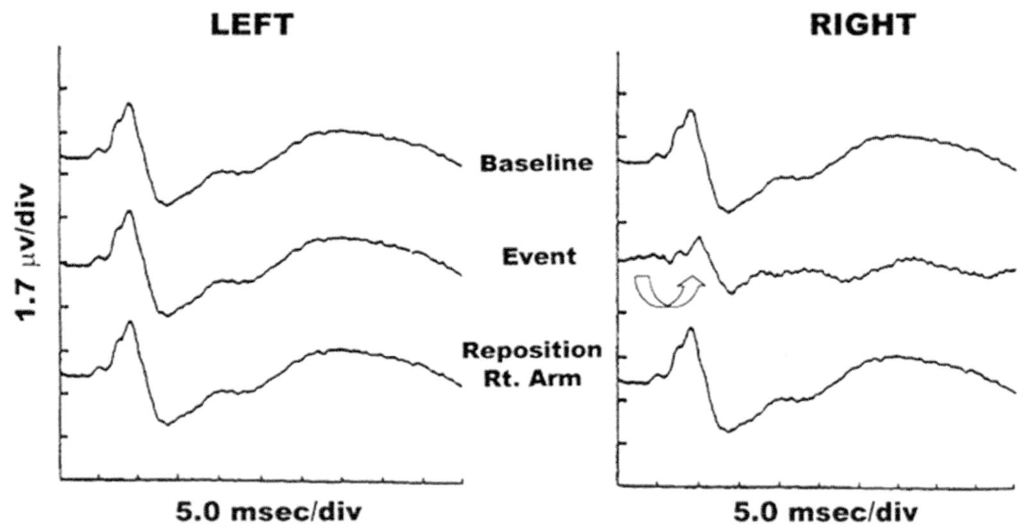


**Fig. 26.11** Loss of SSEP amplitude with excessive arm abduction as seen in the right arm. SSEP signals returned to baseline after repositioning of the arm.

of the procedure. Upon awakening, the patient had extreme weakness in her right leg (2/5), indicating that a true positive IONM alert had occurred. The SSEP amplitude was unchanged throughout the course of the treatment procedure (**Fig. 26.12**).

In this case the encroachment of the hook at T8 on the spinal canal is likely to have caused the loss of tcMEP amplitude. The failure of SSEP monitoring to detect the patient's motor deficit highlights the dangers of using SSEP alone in surgery for spinal deformity.

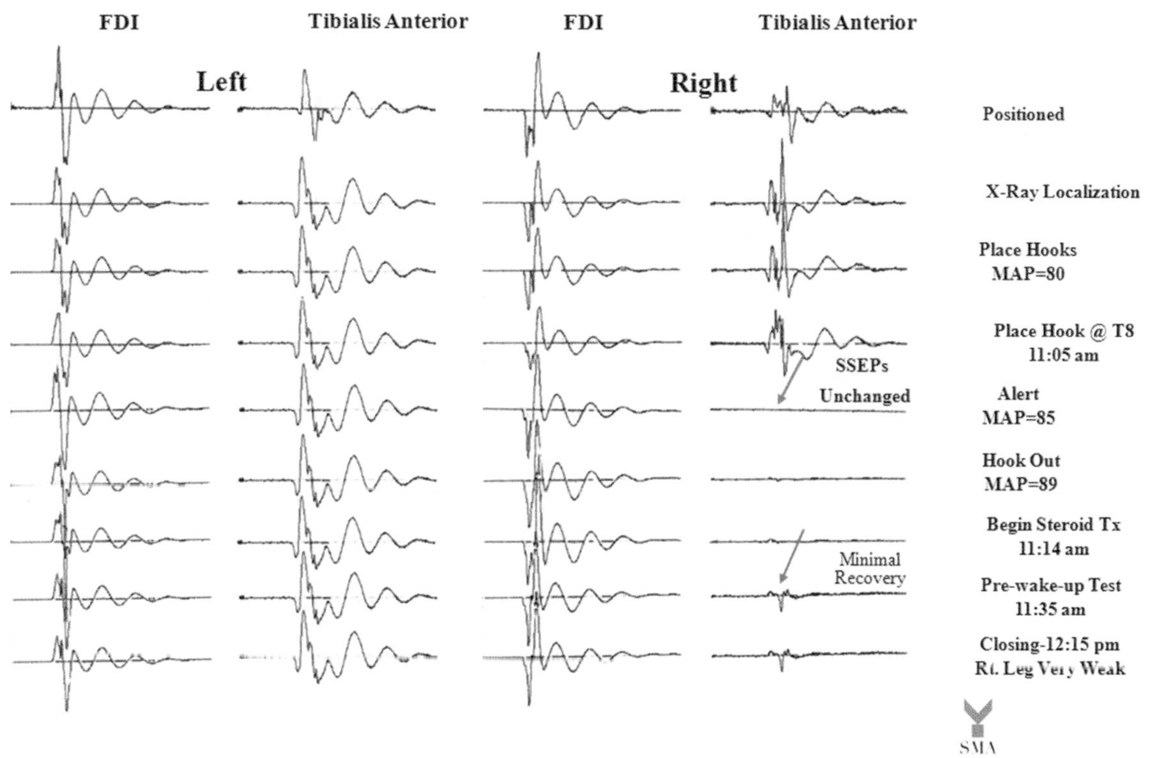


A

**Fig. 26.12** **(A)** tcMEP data from the right tibialis anterior muscle show a sudden alert following hook placement at T8. Following hook removal and initiation of the steroid protocol for treating a spinal-cord injury, tcMEP signals began to recover but did not reach baseline values. The patient awoke with a weak tibialis anterior muscle (2/5) on neurological examination. (*Continued on page 286*)

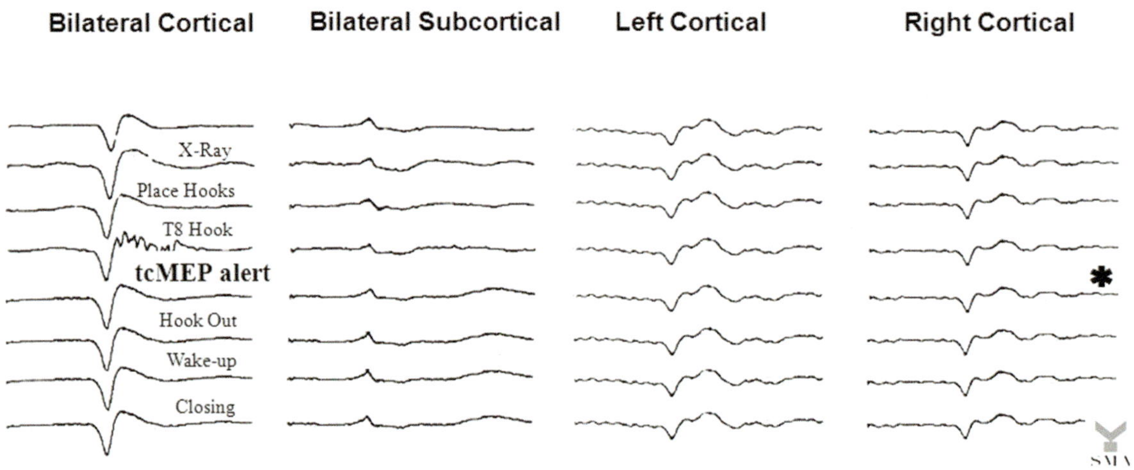


B

**Fig. 26.12** (*Continued*) **(B)** SSEP monitoring did not produce any alerts tduring the procedure, and failed to detect the motor deficit.

## Case Example 3

During PSF, a patient undergoing derotation suddenly experienced an acute loss (100% loss of amplitude) of the tcMEP signal. Nine minutes later, the patient's SSEP amplitude fell by 50%, thus signifying an SSEP alert (**Fig. 26.13**).

Derotation maneuvers in scoliosis surgery have a lordosing effect and essentially lengthen the anterior column, and may thus predispose to spinal-cord ischemia, as detected in this instance by tcMEP monitoring.

## Case Example 4

A 50% loss of tcMEP amplitude was noted during a PSF from T1 to T12 for the treatment of AIS. Following notification of the surgical team, the correction was released, the patient's

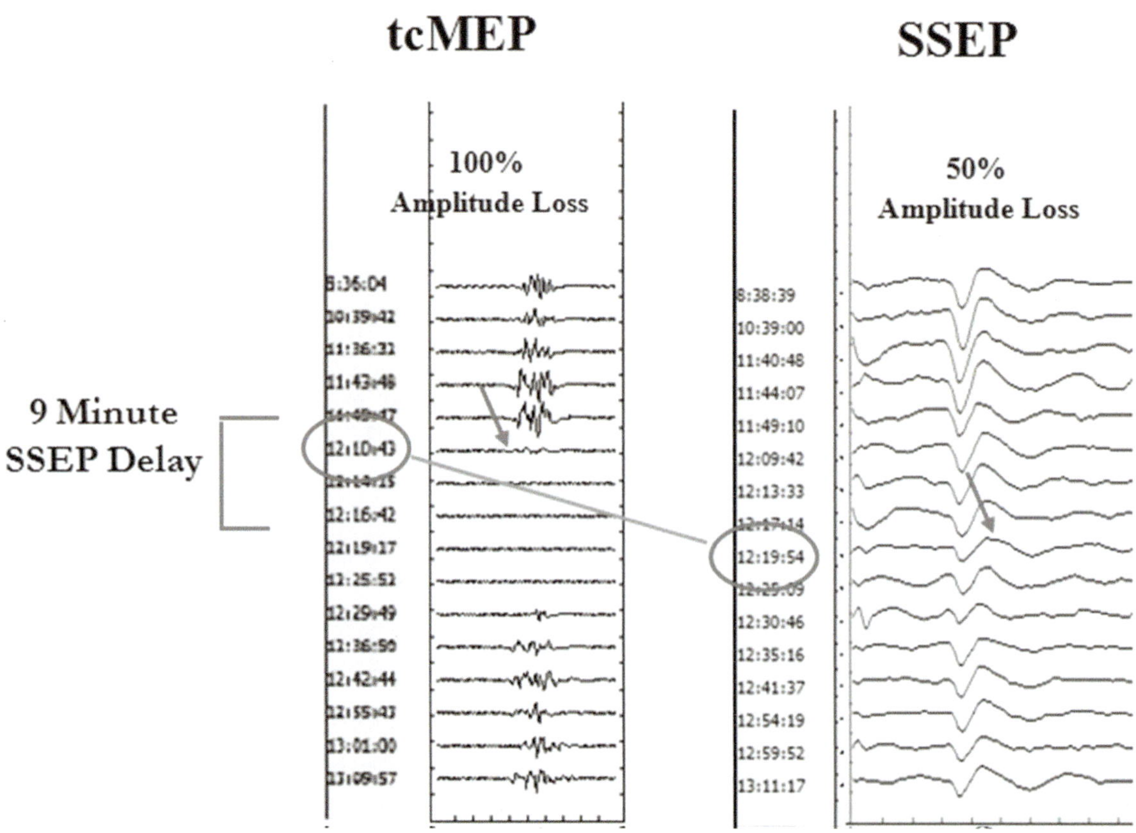


**Fig. 26.13** tcMEP monitoring immediately detected an impending neurological deficit during a derotation maneuver. Although SSEP monitoring also detected an impending injury, the SSEP alert for this occurred 9 minutes after the tcMEP alert.

MABP was raised to 90 mm Hg, and the patient's surgery was paused for 10 minutes. This resulted in a return to baseline of the tcMEP amplitude (no changes were noted in the SSEP amplitude). A less ambitious correction of the patient's spinal curve was then undertaken and final tightening was done of the patient's instrumentation. With this, however, a 50% reduction in tcMEP amplitude was again noted. Another surgical pause was taken and the steroid protocol for spinal-cord injury was begun, with a complete return to baseline of the tcMEP amplitude. The decision was made to leave the patient's instrumentation in place, complete the remainder of the surgical procedure, and perform a wake-up test, which revealed 5/5 motor strength. Following wound closure, the patient was transferred to the intensive care unit for maintenance of the MABP in the 90-mm Hg range and continuation of the methylprednisolone drip begun in the steroid protocol. At 6 hours after a normal initial postoperative examination, the results of a second neurological examination had fallen to 0/5 motor in the right lower extremity, with intact sensation. The patient was emergently taken back to the operating room, where a baseline preoperative tcMEP recording showed a 100% loss of amplitude in the right lower extremity, corroborating the 0/5 motor result in the neurological examination on that side. The patient's spinal rods and sublaminar cables were removed, the pedicle screws were left in place (**Fig. 26.14**), and the spine was allowed to return to its resting position. A postoperative CT scan did not show malpositioning of the pedicle screws. No new changes or improvements in the tcMEP were detected during removal of the patient's instrumentation.

One week later the results of the patient's neurological examination had improved to 5/5 and the patient was therefore designated as stable and was taken back to the operating room for re-instrumentation. At baseline the tcMEP had been restored to 80% of its normal amplitude. The rods initially used in the patient's construct were replaced, with a smaller correction of kyphosis. There were no new changes in the tcMEP or SSEP tracings, and the patient awoke neurologically intact with a stable construct (**Fig. 26.15**).

This patient developed a delayed postoperative neurological deficit. The etiology in this case was most likely ischemic, with the specific cause of the ischemia most probably being cord swelling, a stretch injury, vasospasm, or epidural hematoma.

## Case Example 5

During anterior spinal fusion for a Lenke type 5 curve, segmental vessel clamping at T9 was done to determine the safety of vessel ligation before the insertion of vertebral-body screws. During a 2-minute test vessel clamping, a tcMEP alert occurred, without an accompanying change in SSEP. The tcMEP amplitude was restored by unclamping of the vessel. Reclamping for 1 minute again produced an alert. Following unclamping for 5 minutes, the baseline tcMEP amplitude was again restored. It was decided not to clip or ligate the T9 segmental vessel. Vertebral-body screws were inserted without difficulty and without any further changes in the patient's status throughout the fusion procedure (**Fig. 26.16**).

This case highlights the exquisite sensitivity of tcMEP to spinal cord ischemia, and the relative lack of sensitivity of SSEP monitoring to ischemic changes.

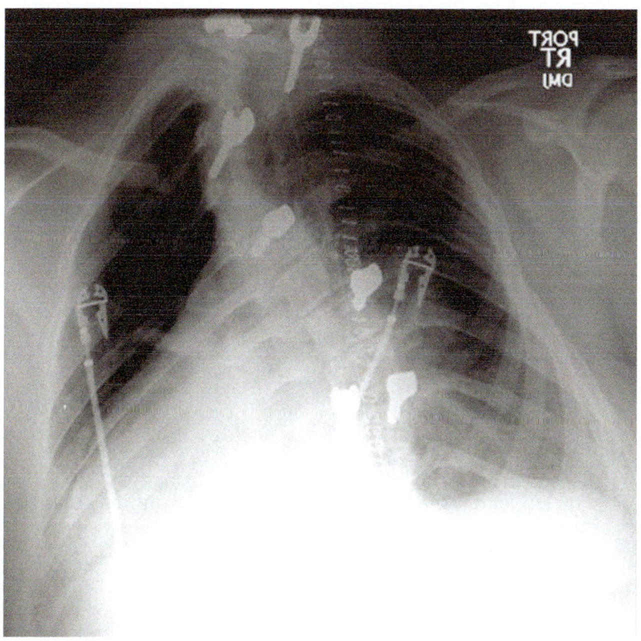


**Fig. 26.14** This patient developed a delayed postoperative neurological deficit (DPND) at 6 hours after surgical correction of AIS. She was then immediately taken back to the operating room for the removal of rods for correcting her deformity, although her spinal implants, which X-ray and CT scanning showed as being in good position, were retained.

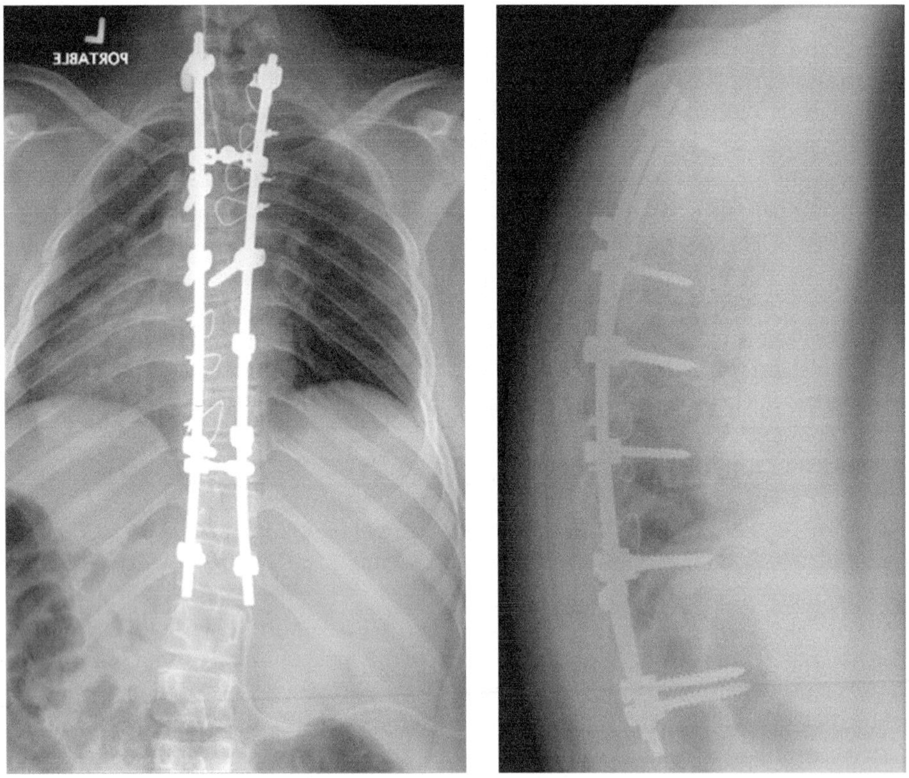


**Fig. 26.15 (A,B)** One week after the development of a delayed postoperative neurological deficit (DPND), this patient's neurological status had completely recovered and she was taken back to the operating room for re-instrumentation and completion of her corrective procedure. She awoke neurologically intact with excellent correction.

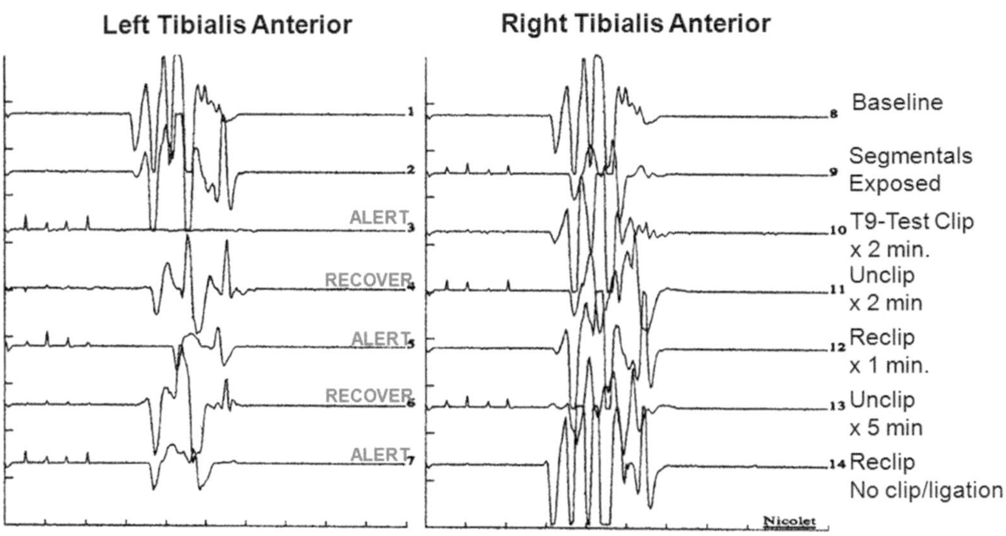


**Fig. 26.16** Repeated test clipping of segmental vessels during anterior spinal fusion for a thoracolumbar curve produced immediate tcMEP alerts, without any changes in the SSEP tracing.

## References


1. Coe JD, Arlet V, Donaldson W, et al. Complications in spinal fusion for adolescent idiopathic scoliosis in the new millennium. A report of the Scoliosis Research Society Morbidity and Mortality Committee. Spine 2006;31:345–349
2. Langeloo DD, Lelivelt A, Louis Journée H, Slappendel R, de Kleuver M. Transcranial electrical motor-evoked potential monitoring during surgery for spinal deformity: A study of 145 patients. Spine 2003;28:1043–1050
3. MacEwen GD, Bunnell WP, Sriram K. Acute neurological complications in the treatment of scoliosis. A report of the Scoliosis Research Society. J Bone Joint Surg Am 1975;57:404–408
4. Seyal M, Mull B. Mechanisms of signal change during intraoperative somatosensory evoked potential monitoring of the spinal cord. J Clin Neurophysiol 2002;19:409–415
5. Bandi S, Davis BJ, Ahmed NB. Segmental vessel sparing during convex growth arrest surgery: A modified technique. Spine J 2007;7: 349-352
6. Wu L, Qiu Y, Ling W, Shen Q. Change pattern of somatosensory-evoked potentials after occlusion of segmental vessels: Possible indicator for spinal cord ischemia. Eur Spine J 2006;15:335–340
7. Noonan KJ, Walker T, Feinberg JR, Nagel M, Didelot W, Lindseth R. Factors related to false- versus true-positive neuromonitoring changes in adolescent idiopathic scoliosis surgery. Spine 2002; 27:825–830
8. Vauzelle C, Stagnara P, Jouvinroux P. Functional monitoring of spinal cord activity during spinal surgery. Clin Orthop Relat Res 1973; (93):173–178
9. Banit DM, Darden BV. The wake-up test. In: Clark CR, ed. The Cervical Spine, ed. 4. Philadelphia: Lippincottm Williams & Wilkins; 2005:245–247
10. Ben-David B, Taylor PD, Haller GS. Posterior spinal fusion complicated by posterior column injury. A case report of a false-negative wake-up test. Spine 1987;12(6):540–543
11. Hoppenfeld S, Gross A, Andrews C, Lonner B. The ankle clonus test for assessment of the integrity of the spinal cord during operations for scoliosis. J Bone Joint Surg Am 1997;79:208–212
12. Ewen A, Cox RG, Davies SA, et al. The ankle clonus test is not a clinically useful measure of spinal cord integrity in children. Can J Anaesth 2005;52:524–529
13. Dawson GD. Cerebral responses to electrical stimulation of peripheral nerve in man. J Neurol Neurosurg Psychiatry 1947;10:134–140
14. Nash CL Jr, Lorig RA, Schatzinger LA, Brown RH. Spinal cord monitoring during operative treatment of the spine. Clin Orthop Relat Res 1977; (126):100–105
15. Labrom RD, Hoskins M, Reilly CW, Tredwell SJ, Wong PK. Clinical usefulness of somatosensory evoked potentials for detection of brachial plexopathy secondary to malpositioning in scoliosis surgery. Spine 2005;30:2089–2093
16. Schwartz DM, Drummond DS, Hahn M, Ecker ML, Dormans JP. Prevention of positional brachial plexopathy during surgical correction of scoliosis. J Spinal Disord 2000;13:178–182
17. Dvorak J, Vohanka S, Sutter M. Diagnosis of cervical spine disorders: Neurophysiologic tests. In: Clark CR, ed. The Cervical Spine, ed. 4. Philadelphia: Lippincott, Williams & Wilkins; 2005:220–223
18. Sutter M, Dvorak J. Multimodal intraoperative monitoring during cervical spine surgery. In: Clark CR, ed. The Cervical Spine, ed. 4. Philadelphia: Lippincott, Williams & Wilkins; 2005:224–237
19. Dawson EG, Sherman JE, Kanim LE, Nuwer MR. Spinal cord monitoring. Results of the Scoliosis Research Society and the European Spinal Deformity Society survey. Spine 1991;16(8, suppl):S361–S364
20. Nuwer MR, Dawson EG, Carlson LG, Kanim LE, Sherman JE. Somatosensory evoked potential spinal cord monitoring reduces neurologic deficits after scoliosis surgery: results of a large multicenter survey. Electroencephalogr Clin Neurophysiol 1995;96:6–11
21. Dinner DS, Lüders H, Lesser RP, Morris HH, Barnett G, Klem G. Intraoperative spinal somatosensory evoked potential monitoring. J Neurosurg 1986;65:807–814
22. Forbes HJ, Allen PW, Waller CS, et al. Spinal cord monitoring in scoliosis surgery. Experience with 1168 cases. J Bone Joint Surg Br 1991;73:487–491
23. Lubicky JP, Spadaro JA, Yuan HA, Fredrickson BE, Henderson N. Variability of somatosensory cortical evoked potential monitoring during spinal surgery. Spine 1989;14:790–798
24. Chatrian GE, Berger MS, Wirch AL. Discrepancy between intraoperative SSEP's and postoperative function. Case report. J Neurosurg 1988;69:450–454
25. Hermanns H, Lipfert P, Meier S, Jetzek-Zader M, Krauspe R, Stevens MF. Cortical somatosensory-evoked potentials during spine surgery in patients with neuromuscular and idiopathic scoliosis under propofol-remifentanil anaesthesia. Br J Anaesth 2007;98:362–365
26. Ryzhova OE, Tikhodeev SA, Vishnevski AA, Zhulev SN, Beliakov NA. [Evaluation of the capacities of neurophysiological intraoperative monitoring in reconstructive surgery on the vertebral column]. Vopr Neirokhir 2003;1:27–31, discussion 31–32
27. Tsai TM, Tsai CL, Lin TS, Lin CC, Jou IM. Value of dermatomal somatosensory evoked potentials in detecting acute nerve root injury: An experimental study with special emphasis on stimulus intensity. Spine 2005;30:E540–E546
28. Scoliosis Research Society Position Statement. Somatosensory evoked potential monitoring of neurologic spinal cord function during spinal surgery. Scoliosis Research Society, Milwaukee, WI, September. 1992
29. Auerbach JD, Diab M, Sanders JO, et al. Variability in spinal cord monitoring practice patterns in adolescent idiopathic scoliosis. Proceedings of the 14th Annual International Meeting on Advanced Spine Techniques, Paradise Island, Bahamas, July 2007
30. Ginsburg HH, Shetter AG, Raudzens PA. Postoperative paraplegia with preserved intraoperative somatosensory evoked potentials. Case report. J Neurosurg 1985;63:296–300
31. Hilibrand AS, Schwartz DM, Sethuraman V, Vaccaro AR, Albert TJ. Comparison of transcranial electric motor and somatosensory evoked potential monitoring during cervical spine surgery. J Bone Joint Surg Am 2004;86A:1248–1253
32. Lesser RP, Raudzens P, Lüders H, et al. Postoperative neurological deficits may occur despite unchanged intraoperative somatosensory evoked potentials. Ann Neurol 1986;19:22–25
33. Pelosi L, Lamb J, Grevitt M, Mehdian SM, Webb JK, Blumhardt LD. Combined monitoring of motor and somatosensory evoked potentials in orthopaedic spinal surgery. Clin Neurophysiol 2002;113:1082–1091
34. Schwartz DM, Auerbach JD, Dormans JP, et al. Neurophysiological detection of impending spinal cord injury during scoliosis surgery. J Bone Joint Surg Am 2007;89:2440–2449
35. de Haan P, Kalkman CJ ; de HP. Spinal cord monitoring: somatosensory- and motor-evoked potentials. Anesthesiol Clin North America 2001;19:923–945

36. Drummond DS, Schwartz DM, Johnston DR, et al. Neurologic injury complicating surgery. In: DeWald RL, Arlet V, Carl A, et al, eds. Spinal Deformities: The Comprehensive Text. New York: Thieme; 2004:615–625
37. Griepp RB, Ergin MA, Galla JD, et al. Looking for the artery of Adamkiewicz: A quest to minimize paraplegia after operations for aneurysms of the descending thoracic and thoracoabdominal aorta. J Thorac Cardiovasc Surg 1996;112:1202–1213, discussion 1213–1215
38. MacDonald DB, Al Zayed Z, Khoudeir I, Stigsby B. Monitoring scoliosis surgery with combined multiple pulse transcranial electric motor and cortical somatosensory-evoked potentials from the lower and upper extremities. Spine 2003;28:194–203
39. Follis F, Scremin OU, Blisard KS, et al. Selective vulnerability of white matter during spinal cord ischemia. J Cereb Blood Flow Metab 1993;13:170–178
40. O'Brien MF, Lenke LG, Bridwell KH, Padberg A, Stokes M. Evoked potential monitoring of the upper extremities during thoracic and lumbar spinal deformity surgery: A prospective study. J Spinal Disord 1994;7:277–284
41. Schwartz DM, Sestokas AKA. Systems-based algorithmic approach to intraoperative neurophysiological monitoring during spinal surgery. Semin Spine Surg 2002;14:136–145
42. Vaccaro AR, Schwartz DM. Neurophysiologic monitoring during cervical spine surgery. In: Clark CR, ed. The Cervical Spine, ed. 4. Philadelphia: Lippincott, Williams & Wilkins, 2005:238–244
43. Falcao AL, Reutens DC, Markus R, et al. The resistance to ischemia of white and gray matter after stroke. Ann Neurol 2004;56:695–701
44. Schwartz DM, Drummond DS, Schwartz JA, et al. Neurophysiological monitoring during scoliosis surgery: A mulitimodality approach. Semin Spine Surg 1997;9:97–111
45. Kalkman CJ, Boezeman EH, Ribberink AA, Oosting J, Deen L, Bovill JG. Influence of changes in arterial carbon dioxide tension on the electroencephalogram and posterior tibial nerve somatosensory cortical evoked potentials during alfentanil/nitrous oxide anesthesia. Anesthesiology 1991;75:68–74
46. Reuter DG, Tacker WA Jr, Badylak SF, Voorhees WD III, Konrad PE. Correlation of motor-evoked potential response to ischemic spinal cord damage. J Thorac Cardiovasc Surg 1992;104:262–272
47. Kothe R, Matthias Strauss J, Deuretzbacher G, Hemmi T, Lorenzen M, Wiesner L. Computer navigation of parapedicular screw fixation in the thoracic spine: A cadaver study. Spine 2001; 26:E496–E501
48. Dobbs MB, Lenke LG, Kim YJ, Kamath G, Peelle MW, Bridwell KH. Selective posterior thoracic fusions for adolescent idiopathic scoliosis: Comparison of hooks versus pedicle screws. Spine 2006; 31:2400–2404
49. Kim YJ, Lenke LG, Kim J, et al. Comparative analysis of pedicle screw versus hybrid instrumentation in posterior spinal fusion of adolescent idiopathic scoliosis. Spine 2006;31:291–298
50. Lee SS, Lenke LG, Kuklo TR, et al. Comparison of Scheuermann kyphosis correction by posterior-only thoracic pedicle screw fixation versus combined anterior/posterior fusion. Spine 2006;31: 2316–2321
51. Luhmann SJ, Lenke LG, Kim YJ, Bridwell KH, Schootman M. Thoracic adolescent idiopathic scoliosis curves between 70 degrees and 100 degrees: Is anterior release necessary? Spine 2005;30:2061–2067
52. Raynor BL, Lenke LG, Kim Y, et al. Can triggered electromyograph thresholds predict safe thoracic pedicle screw placement? Spine 2002;27:2030–2035
53. Shi YB, Binette M, Martin WH, Pearson JM, Hart RA. Electrical stimulation for intraoperative evaluation of thoracic pedicle screw placement. Spine 2003;28:595–601
54. Vaccaro AR, Rizzolo SJ, Balderston RA, et al. Placement of pedicle screws in the thoracic spine. Part II: An anatomical and radiographic assessment. J Bone Joint Surg Am 1995;77:1200–1206
55. Vaccaro AR, Rizzolo SJ, Allardyce TJ, et al. Placement of pedicle screws in the thoracic spine. Part I: Morphometric analysis of the thoracic vertebrae. J Bone Joint Surg Am 1995;77:1193–1199
56. Cinotti G, Gumina S, Ripani M, Postacchini F. Pedicle instrumentation in the thoracic spine. A morphometric and cadaveric study for placement of screws. Spine 1999;24:114–119
57. Elliott MJ, Slakey CJ. Thoracic pedicle screw placement: Analysis using anatomical landmarks without image guidance. J Pediatr Orthop 2007;27:582–586
58. Kim KD, Johnson JP, Babbitz JD. Image-guided thoracic pedicle screw placement: A technical study in cadavers and preliminary clinical experience. Neurosurg Focus 2001;10:E2
59. Kim KD, Patrick Johnson J, Bloch BS O, Masciopinto JE. Computer-assisted thoracic pedicle screw placement: An in vitro feasibility study. Spine 2001;26:360–364
60. Xu R, Ebraheim NA, Ou Y, Yeasting RA. Anatomic considerations of pedicle screw placement in the thoracic spine. Roy-Camille technique versus open-lamina technique. Spine 1998; 23:1065–1068
61. Lehman RA, Lenke LG, Kim YH, et al. Computed tomography (CT) evaluation of pedicle screws placed into deformed spines over an 8 year period. Proceedings of the 41st Annual Meeting of the Scoliosis Research Society, Monterey, CA, September. 2006
62. Lenke LG, Padberg AM, Russo MH, Bridwell KH, Gelb DE. Triggered electromyographic threshold for accuracy of pedicle screw placement. An animal model and clinical correlation. Spine 1995;20: 1585–1591
63. Padberg AM. Electrophysiology. In: DeWald RL, Arlet V, Carl A et al, eds. Spinal Deformities: The Comprehensive Text. New York: Thieme; 2004:135–148
64. Dimopoulos VG, Feltes CH, Fountas KN, et al. Does intraoperative electromyographic monitoring in lumbar microdiscectomy correlate with postoperative pain? South Med J 2004;97:724–728
65. Darden BV II, Owen JH, Hatley MK, Kostuik J, Tooke SM. A comparison of impedance and electromyogram measurements in detecting the presence of pedicle wall breakthrough. Spine 1998;23: 256–262
66. Calancie B, Madsen P, Lebwohl N. Stimulus-evoked EMG monitoring during transpedicular lumbosacral spine instrumentation. Initial clinical results. Spine 1994;19:2780–2786
67. Clements DH, Morledge DE, Martin WH, Betz RR. Evoked and spontaneous electromyography to evaluate lumbosacral pedicle screw placement. Spine 1996;21:600–604
68. Dickerman RD, Guyer R. Intraoperative electromyography for pedicle screws: technique is the key! J Spinal Disord Tech 2006;19:463
69. Anderson DG, Wierzbowski LR, Schwartz DM, Hilibrand AS, Vaccaro AR, Albert TJ. Pedicle screws with high electrical resistance: A potential source of error with stimulus-evoked EMG. Spine 2002;27:1577–1581
70. Danesh-Clough T, Taylor P, Hodgson B, Walton M. The use of evoked EMG in detecting misplaced thoracolumbar pedicle screws. Spine 2001;26:1313–1316
71. Raynor BL, Lenke LG, Bridwell KH, Taylor BA, Padberg AM. Correlation between low triggered electromyographic thresholds and

lumbar pedicle screw malposition: Analysis of 4857 screws. Spine 2007;32:2673–2678
72. Slimp JC. Intraoperative neurophysiological monitoring of the spinal cord and nerve roots. Spineline September/October, 6–15. 2006. North American Spine Society
73. Cope TC, Nelson SG, Mendell LM. Factors outside neuraxis mediate "acute" increase in EPSP amplitude caudal to spinal cord transection. J Neurophysiol 1980;44:174–183
74. Cope TC, Hickman KR, Botterman BR. Acute effects of spinal transection on EPSPs produced by single homonymous Ia-fibers in soleus alpha-motoneurons in the cat. J Neurophysiol 1988;60: 1678–1694
75. Leis AA, Zhou HH, Mehta M, Harkey HL III, Paske WC. Behavior of the H-reflex in humans following mechanical perturbation or injury to rostral spinal cord. Muscle Nerve 1996;19:1373–1382
76. Schadt JC, Barnes CD. Motoneuron membrane changes associated with spinal shock and the Schiff-Sherrington phenomenon. Brain Res 1980;201:373–383
77. Massei R. [Results of surgical treatment of scoliosis by Harrington's procedure: neurological complications and reliability of intraoperative monitoring of the H-reflex]. Agressologie 1994;34 Spec No. 1:47
78. Merzagora AC, Bracchi F, Cerutti S, Rossi L, Gaggiani A, Bianchi AM. Evaluation and application of a RBF neural network for online single-sweep extraction of SEPs during scoliosis surgery. IEEE Trans Biomed Eng 2007;54:1300–1308
79. Rossi L, Bianchi AM, Merzagora A, Gaggiani A, Cerutti S, Bracchi F. Single trial somatosensory evoked potential extraction with ARX filtering for a combined spinal cord intraoperative neuromonitoring technique. Biomed Eng Online 2007;6:2
80. Schieppati M, Viganò P. [The H reflex during the Harrington operation (author's transl)]. Chir Ital 1979;31:245–248
81. Ulkatan S, Neuwirth M, Bitan F, Minardi C, Kokoszka A, Deletis V. Monitoring of scoliosis surgery with epidurally recorded motor evoked potentials (D wave) revealed false results. Clin Neurophysiol 2006;117:2093–2101
82. Burke D, Hicks R, Stephen J, Woodforth I, Crawford M. Trial-to-trial variability of corticospinal volleys in human subjects. Electroencephalogr Clin Neurophysiol 1995;97:231–237
83. Koht A, Schütz W, Schmidt G, Schramm J, Watanabe E. Effects of etomidate, midazolam, and thiopental on median nerve somatosensory evoked potentials and the additive effects of fentanyl and nitrous oxide. Anesth Analg 1988;67:435–441
84. Koht A. Anesthesia and evoked potentials: Overview. Int J Clin Monit Comput 1988;5:167–173
85. Sloan TB, Ronai AK, Toleikis JR, Koht A. Improvement of intraoperative somatosensory evoked potentials by etomidate. Anesth Analg 1988;67:582–585
86. Peterson DO, Drummond JC, Todd MM. Effects of halothane, enflurane, isoflurane, and nitrous oxide on somatosensory evoked potentials in humans. Anesthesiology 1986;65:35–40
87. Sebel PS, Flynn PJ, Ingram DA. Effect of nitrous oxide on visual, auditory and somatosensory evoked potentials. Br J Anaesth 1984;56: 1403–1407
88. Scheufler KM, Zentner J. Total intravenous anesthesia for intraoperative monitoring of the motor pathways: An integral view combining clinical and experimental data. J Neurosurg 2002;96:571–579
89. Mitchell W, Buono L, Benzel E. Nonparalytic anesthesia and realtime monitoring. In: Clark CR, ed. The Cervical Spine, ed. 4. Philadelphia: Lippincott, Williams & Wilkins, 2005:248–54
90. Chang JH, Hoernschemeyer DG, Sponseller PD. Delayed postoperative paralysis in adolescent idiopathic scoliosis: management with partial removal of hardware and staged correction. J Spinal Disord Tech 2006;19:222–225
91. Wilber RG, Thompson GH, Shaffer JW, Brown RH, Nash CL Jr. Postoperative neurological deficits in segmental spinal instrumentation. A study using spinal cord monitoring. J Bone Joint Surg Am 1984;66:1178–1187
92. Winter RB. Neurologic safety in spinal deformity surgery. Spine 1997;22:1527–1533
93. Torpey BM, Dormans JP, Drummond DS. The use of MRI-compatible titanium segmental spinal instrumentation in pediatric patients with intraspinal tumor. J Spinal Disord 1995;8:76–81
94. Hales DD, Dawson EG, Delamarter R. Late neurological complications of Harrington-rod instrumentation. J Bone Joint Surg Am 1989;71:1053–1057
95. Letts RM, Hollenberg C. Delayed paresis following spinal fusion with Harrington instrumentation. Clin Orthop Relat Res 1977; (125):45–48
96. Mineiro J, Weinstein SL. Delayed postoperative paraparesis in scoliosis surgery. A case report. Spine 1997;22:1668–1672
97. MacDonald DB. Safety of intraoperative transcranial electrical stimulation motor evoked potential monitoring. J Clin Neurophysiol 2002;19:416–429
98. Wassermann EM. Risk and safety of repetitive transcranial magnetic stimulation: Report and suggested guidelines from the International Workshop on the Safety of Repetitive Transcranial Magnetic Stimulation, June 5–7, 1996. Electroencephalogr Clin Neurophysiol 1998;108:1–16

# 27 Correction Without Fusion

*Randal R. Betz, William F. Lavelle, and Peter O. Newton*

Motion-sparing techniques are appealing to spine surgeons who treat growing children with spinal deformities. For patients with adolescent idiopathic scoliosis (AIS), there is a widely held belief that postoperatively, truncal range of motion is limited by spinal fusion and that this limitation is related to the most distal fused segment. With videographic techniques similar to those reported by Engsberg and colleagues,[1] it has been documented that long spinal fusions result in a global loss of motion. There is also evidence that disc degeneration occurs adjacent to the fused segments.[2] The prevalence of adjacent-level disc degeneration in patients who have undergone fusions for degenerative lumbar spinal disorders has reportedly been as high as 15% within 7 years after fusion.[2] Although selected thoracic fusion has been promoted by many surgeons,[3] this often leaves significant residual deformity in the lumbar spine. Scoliosis surgeons constantly debate the virtues of a stiff but straight lumbar spine against the flexibility of a residual lumbar deformity. In the future, the driving concept in surgery for spinal deformity will be correcting the deformity without fusing mobile segments or with fusion of fewer segments.

In the patient with early-onset idiopathic scoliosis (infantile and juvenile), the concept of correction without fusion, to allow continued spinal growth, is an extremely important one. Although growing rods have become popular,[4–6] spontaneous fusion typically occurs after three to four years of treatment, with surgeons noting a limited ability of treatment to produce any additional correction or extension of spinal length.[7,8] The vertical expandable prosthetic titanium rib (VEPTR) device developed by Dr. Robert Campbell is an appealing alternative to growing rods because of its ability to correct chest-wall deformity while indirectly allowing the spine to continue growing without fusion. Although the early results with the VEPTR device have been very encouraging, it is not yet known whether this technique will prevent spontaneous spinal fusion. Dr. John Smith has developed a technique for using the VEPTR device as a spinal growth modulation instrument with dual titanium ribs connected to the pelvic construct, leaving the spine itself unexposed.[9] Because there is no direct fixation to the spine in this technique, spontaneous fusion should theoretically not occur. The results of this technique are still preliminary, and it is unknown whether this theory will prove valid and the technique will prevent the spontaneous spinal fusion that limits the continued correction, which occurs during serial lengthening of the spine or during the definitive spinal fusion typically performed after adequate chest growth.

This chapter will review the currently available techniques for growth modulation, as well as additional techniques now on the horizon. Discussions will revolve around biological approaches to growth modulation, anterior and posterior growth-modulating devices, and techniques to consider in treating deformity after spinal and chest-wall growth have ended.

## ■ Biological Growth Modulation

### Growth Modulation Secondary to Manipulation of the Ribs

Carrier et al developed a biomechanical model for evaluating the long-term correction resulting from rib shortening or lengthening in AIS.[10] A finite element model of the trunk, customized to the geometry of a scoliotic patient, was used to simulate rib surgery. Simulations were done in an iterative fashion over 24 months. Testing was done or rib shortening on the concave side of a scoliotic curve, inducing load patterns on the vertebral endplates that could act against progression of the scoliotic curve. Wedging of the apical vertebra in the frontal plane decreased from 5.2 degrees to a mean value of 3.8 degrees after 24 months. The decrease in wedging observed in the thoracic apical region was reflected by changes in the global curvature of the spine, with a decrease in the Cobb angle from 46 degrees to 44 degrees occurring immediately after the surgery. The model predicted a correction of deformity to a mean of 41 degrees after 24 months. These preliminary results showed the potential for long-term correction of spinal curvature from rib shortening on the concave side of a scoliotic curve. Xiong and Sevastik reported a successful case of treatment by the shortening of three concave-side ribs in a 7-year-old girl with a right thoracolumbar scoliosis treated by a shortening of three concave ribs.[11] The patient's curve decreased from 46 degrees to 21 degrees over a period of 27 months. It is surprising that the finite element model predicted a more modest curve correction, while another case report described a 50% reduction in curvature within the same time frame. This discrepancy may be explained by the limitations of the model used in the finite element analysis. In particular, the model was limited by its inability to accurately represent the adaptive ability of the patient's soft tissues. Specifically, the finite-element model neglected the long-term effects of muscle activity, the stress relaxation of ligaments in the spine and chest wall, and the adaptation of intervertebral discs caused by mechanical loads. On the other hand, the case report demonstrated the result of rib shortening only for a single patient. In view of this it is difficult to reach generalized conclusions about the ability of rib shortening to modify spinal growth.

### Growth Plate Asymmetry in the Neurocentral Junction

The neurocentral junction has been identified as a hypothetical cause of AIS. Disparate growth at this site has been thought to lead to pedicle asymmetry, which may in turn lead to vertebral rotation and ultimately to the development of scoliotic curves.[12] However, a finite element model integrating vertebral body growth and growth modulation in the thoracic and lumbar spine showed that asymmetric rates of pedicle growth do not independently cause scoliosis. Nor did other underlying deformations, such as changes in vertebral rotation or vertebral wedging, amplify the scoliotic deformity.[13] Despite this finding, unilateral pedicle epiphysiodesis has been shown to produce scoliosis in animal models.[12] The investigators who found this also demonstrated developmental asymmetry of the neurocentral synchondrosis, the pedicle, and the vertebral body in a cohort of patients with infantile and juvenile idiopathic scoliosis examined with magnetic resonance imaging (MRI).[14]

## Mechanical Growth Modulation and Motion-sparing Techniques for the Anterior Spine

Orthopedic surgeons have had their greatest experience in growth modulation for long-bone deformities. The growth-modulating concepts learned from long-bone stapling for genu and varus[15] have been extrapolated to the spine in animal models.[16–20] Because the bracing as a form of growth modulation in children who are developing spinal deformities has shown only modest success[21] and can have adverse psychosocial consequences,[22–24] we have pursued surgical options for growth modulation.

### Vertebral Body Stapling

Vertebral-body stapling (VBS) is a technique for modulating vertebral growth that has been studied in animal models and is now being actively studied in human clinical trials. Nachlas and Borden[25] first reported the effect of VBS in 1951 after inserting staples across the physeal endplates in a canine model of scoliosis. Six dogs underwent VBS in their study. At the conclusion of their study trial, Nachlas and Borden noted that two of their canine subjects had completely straight spines, two others had appreciable improvements in their scoliosis, one subject had an overcorrection of scoliosis, and one subject had correction only in the stapled segment. A number of the staples used in the study failed. It has been suggested that this failure occurred because the staples spanned two interspaces instead of one, and because the mechanical design of the staples was relatively poor as compared with that of modern staples. Early reports of human VBS were disappointing. In an early human study reported in 1954 by Smith et al,[26] three children who underwent VBS for congenital scoliosis had progression of their scoliosis despite stapling, but no progression of their curvature at the stapled levels. However, these children already had severe curves at the time of stapling, and were relatively mature as compared with children who currently undergo stapling.

Although there have been anecdotal reports of long-bone staples loosening and dislodging from the spine as a consequence of motion. This occurred with old-type staples, but not with the new Nitinol staples. We feel that the security of our staples, along with our ability to successfully control a progressing scoliotic curve with stapling in human subjects, may be at least partly attributable to staple design. The extent to which the rigidity of a growth-modulating device affects growth has been reported. Akyuz et al[27] examined a variety of implant strategies in a rat-tail model. Their study utilized both rigid and flexible implants for modulating vertebral-body growth, and showed that dynamic loading of the vertebrae provides the greatest growth modulation potential, although Akyuz et al offered little speculation about the reason for this effect. Aronsson and associates[28] showed that both a compressive force and a distractive force applied to a growing vertebra in the calf tail could respectively increase or decrease its growth, suggesting that growth modulation involved more than mere growth arrest. It has been proposed that a dynamically loading implant provides a more physiological pattern of growth modulation. On this basis, Braun and associates tested a newly developed Nitinol staple in an immature goat model of scoliosis[29,30] and found it to be both safe and useful for treating iatrogenic curves of <70 degrees. With a similar concept but different staple design, Wall et al[20] demonstrated the ability to create a scoliotic curve in a porcine model, and documented that growth-plate modulation occurred histologically.

Staples have been shown in goat studies to undergo micromotion within bone.[30] It is our hypothesis that this apparent motion is the reason for a low breakage rate of the staples used in our patients. Betz and coworkers began using Nitinol staples in surgery in March 2000.

## Surgical Procedure for Stapling

In the surgical procedure for stapling, a patient under general anesthesia is put in the lateral decubitus position, with the convexity of the patient's scoliotic curve facing upward. The curve is then visualized with fluoroscopic imaging. All vertebrae within the measured Cobb-angle curve are then stapled. For thoracic curves, a thoracoscopically assisted approach is preferable. Portals are made in the posterior axillary line for insertion of the staples. As an alternative to such posterolateral portals, two mini-thoracotomy incisions (<5 cm each) may be used (e.g., one centered at T4–T5 and the other at T9–T10). A radiopaque trial instrument is used to determine the dimension of each staple (3 to 12 mm) and to create pilot holes for the staples. The smallest staple that spans the disc and growth plates is used. The staple, which has been cooled in sterile iced water, is then inserted into the pilot holes. Two single staples (two-prong) or a double staple (four-prong) are placed laterally, spanning each disc within the measured Cobb-angle curve from the superior to the inferior end-vertebrae (**Fig. 27.1**). In most cases the parietal pleura is not excised and the segmental vessels are preserved. If there is significant hypokyphosis (kyphosis <10 degrees) at the apex of the thoracic curve, the staples are placed anterior to the midbody of the apical vertebra, or a third single staple is placed along the anterolateral aspect of the vertebral body (**Fig. 27.2**).[31,32] All of the staples are placed under fluoroscopic guidance (**Fig. 27.3**). Occasionally, the vertebrae at T4 and T5 the vertebrae are too small and can accommodate only a single two-prong staple. Staples that cross the thoracolumbar junction require a small partial anterior reflection of the diaphragm from the spine, so that the staples can be applied in their proper positions. The diaphragm is then repaired. A mini-open retroperitoneal approach is used for stapling lumbar vertebrae. The sequential vessels of one or two vertebral levels occasionally need to be ligated to allow posterior retraction of the psoas muscle. Staples must be placed in the posterior third of the vertebral body to allow normal lordosis with growth.

Betz and co-workers[33] retrospectively reviewed the 2-year follow-up results of VBS with proportional staples in patients with idiopathic scoliosis. Twenty-eight of 29 patients (96%) met the inclusion criteria of having a Risser grade of 0 or 1 and a coronal curve measuring 20 to 45 degrees. There were 26 thoracic and 15 lumbar curves that fulfilled these criteria. The average follow-up was 3.2 years. The procedure was considered successful if curves corrected to within 10 degrees of their measured preoperative values or decreased by >10 degrees. The success rate with thoracic curves measuring <35 degrees was 77.7%. The success rate with curves that measured ≤20 degrees on a first standing radiograph was 85.7%. The success rate in achieving >50% correction of flexible curves on a bending film was 71.4%. Four of 26 curves (15%) showed a correction of >10 degrees. Kyphosis improved in seven patients with hypokyphosis (<10 degrees of kyphosis T5 to T12). A normal thoracic kyphosis of 10 to 40 degrees was achieved in 83.5% of the patients. A success rate of 86.7% was achieved with lumbar curves, of which 4 of 15 (27%) showed a correction of >10 degrees.

Complications were divided into three categories of major, minor, and insignificant, as outlined by Weiss et al.[34] Major complications included the rupture of an unrecognized congenital diaphragmatic hernia (in one patient) and a curve overcorrection (in one patient). Two minor complications included a superior mesenteric artery syndrome and atelectasis from a mucous plug. There were no instances of staple dislodgement or neurovascular injury. The study found that patients with scoliosis who had high-risk idiopathic curves and remaining growth can be

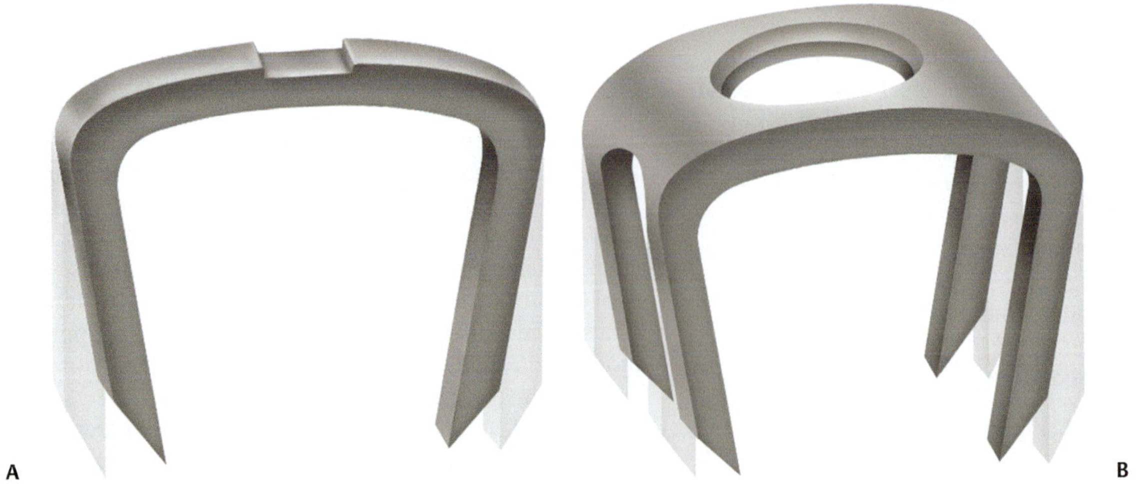


**Fig. 27.1** **(A)** Two-prong staple. **(B)** Four-prong staple.

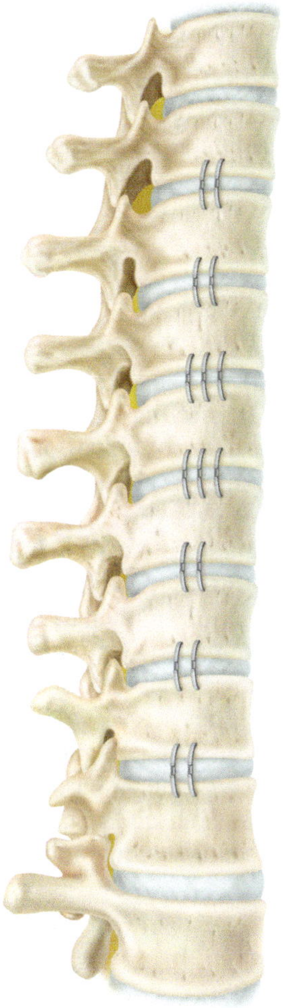

**Fig. 27.2** Schematic diagram of the spine showing a system utilizing two-prong staples and a third staple placed anterolaterally to the spine to correct the hypokyphosis or lordotic apical segment.

treated successfully with VBS. The best results were seen with flexible deformities in which the scoliotic curve was entirely lumbar or with thoracic curves <35 degrees, and in patients whose curve on a first erect radiograph measured <20 degrees.

In this study, thoracic and lumbar curves were analyzed separately because each type of curve responds differently to bracing. There were not enough curves to subanalyze the data by curve pattern (thoracic versus thoracolumbar/ lumbar versus double major).

In this group of patients, three broken staples were noticed, none of which had to be removed, and none of the staples dislodged. Subsequent to this study, with the placement of more than 1400 staples, we have seen only two cases in which a staple has moved (not dislodged). A major complication consisting of overcorrection was noticed in one patient. A 6-year-old girl underwent VBS for a double curve (thoracic curve: 21 degrees; lumbar curve: 25 degrees). Her thoracic curve remained stable and her lumbar curve corrected. At 29 months' follow-up, it was noticed that her lumbar curve had overcorrected and that she had developed a 12-degree lumbar scoliosis in the opposite direction by 12 degrees. She was followed closely with serial radiographs. At 4 years postoperatively her lumbar curve measured −33 degrees. Following discussion with the patient's family, the decision was made to remove the staples from the lowermost three vertebral levels in which they had been inserted. Following their removal, some improvement was seen and the patient's lumbar curve measured −25 degrees. At her most recent visit, her thoracic curve measured −12 degrees. We continue to monitor both of the patient's curves closely. On the basis of our experience in this case, we will remove staples from a spine that overcorrects by 10 degrees or more. Also, we generally

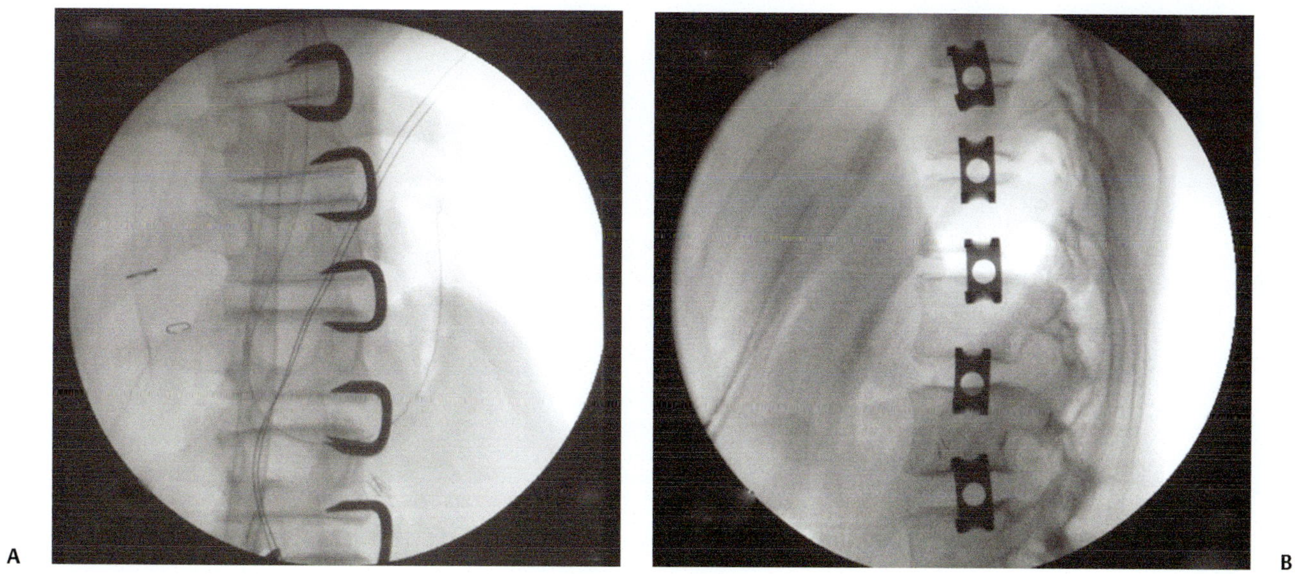


**Fig. 27.3** **(A,B)** Posterolateral (PA) and lateral images taken from a fluoroscopic image intensifier, showing proper placement of staples in the spine.

recommend waiting until the patient is at least 8 years old before considering VBS. In patients younger than 8 years old, VBS may be considered for a curve that has reached >30 degrees. However, we do not have enough clinical data to provide more specific recommendations.

On the basis of this review, the senior author of this chapter (R.R.B.) currently uses the following indications for recommending stapling to patients: (1) age <13 years in girls and <15 years in boys; (2) skeletal maturity of Risser grade 0 or 1, with 1 year of growth remaining by wrist radiography; (3) both thoracic and lumbar coronal curves < 45 degrees with minimal rotation, and flexible to <20 degrees; and (4) sagittal thoracic curve <40 degrees. If the thoracic curve measures 35 to 45 degrees and does not bend below 20 degrees, consideration is given to adding a posterior rib-to-spine hybrid construct at the same time. If the curve on a first erect film does not measure <20 degrees, the patient should wear a corrective brace until the curve measures <20 degrees.

In patients whose surgeries have failed and require an instrumented fusion, we have seen no evidence of spontaneous fusion, nor has there been any inhibition of correction of the spine with the use of pedicle screws. There has been no evidence of disc degeneration on MRI scans done before a posterior spinal fusion. The senior author (R.R.B.) has been able to demonstrate case examples of growth modulation of the vertebral bodies in cases that show correction (**Figs. 27.4 and 27.5**).

Although the preliminary results of VBS have been encouraging, rigorous scientific studies need to be undertaken with available genetic markers, braced patients as controls, and measures of bracing compliance.

## Vertebral Body Tethering

Anterior vertebral body tethering provides an alternative approach for modulating spinal growth. As do vertebral staples, the tether creates a compressive load on the anterior vertebral body, and works through the Heuter–Volkmann principle to correct the asymmetric anterior spinal overgrowth described by Guo and coworkers.[35] The theoretical advantage of verterbral body tethering over vertebral stapling is that it may provide a more rigid construct and may therefore be more effective for larger curves (>45 degrees), as demonstrated clinically by Braun et al.[36] Other uses of tethering would be the achievement of more definitive and powerful curve correction, including potential rotational correction. However, inserting a vertebral body screw is a much more difficult surgical procedure than inserting a staple, and in most cases will require sacrificing segmental vessels.

In 2002, Newton and colleagues evaluated the effects of flexible mechanical tethering of a single spinal motion

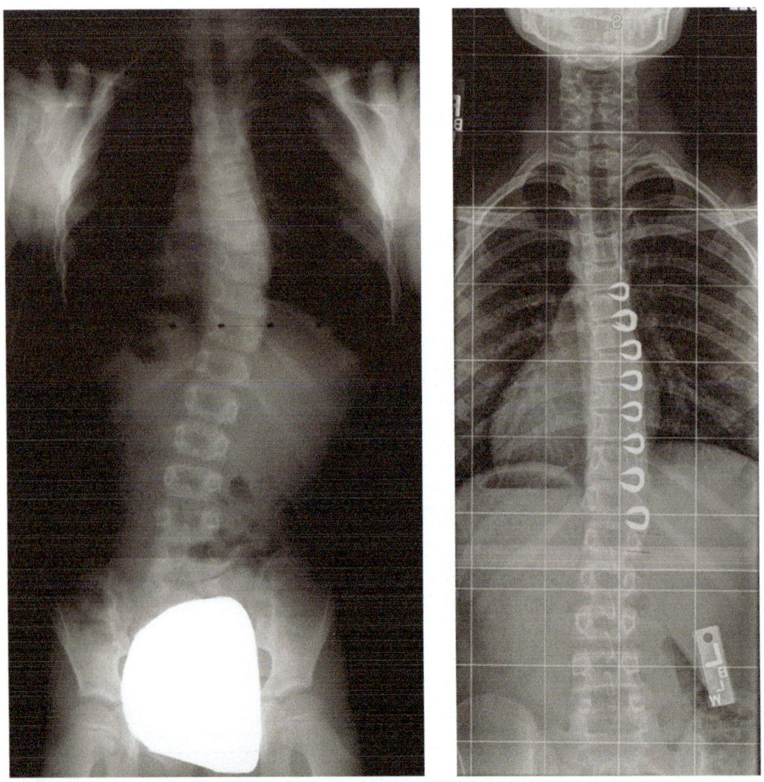

A B

**Fig. 27.4 (A,B)** Pre- and postoperative PA radiographs showing the spine of a 7-year-old boy with a 30-degree right thoracic curve and 8 degrees of thoracic kyphosis. At 4 years after surgery, the thoracic curve measured 15 degrees.

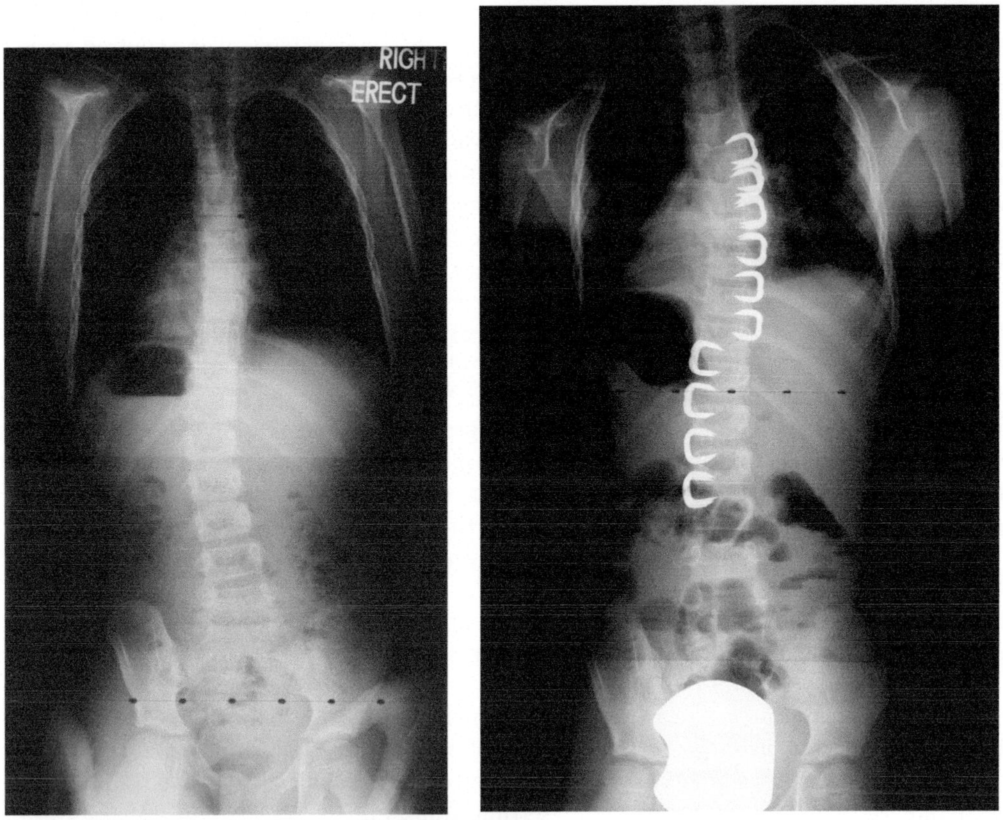


A B

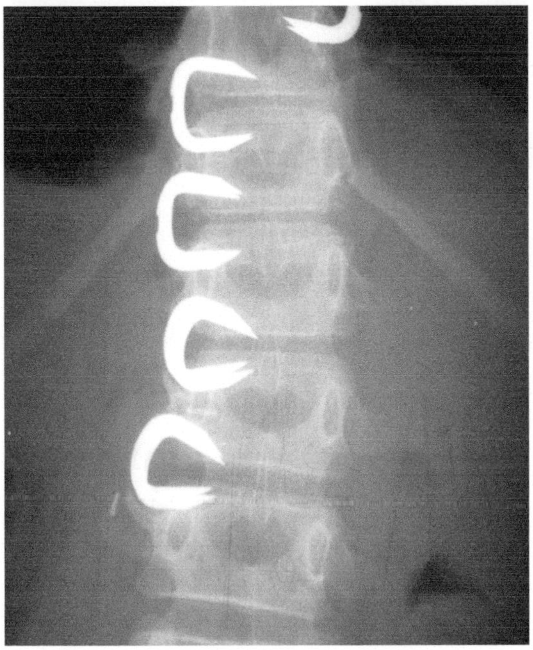

C

**Fig. 27.5** **(A–C)** Growth modulation. **(A)** AP radiograph of a 5-year-old girl with progression of her thoracic curve from 17 degrees to 22 degrees and of her lumbar curve from 20 degrees to 25 degrees over a 6-month period. **(B)** On the basis of that progression and the patient's age, both curves were stapled. **(C)** At three years postoperatively, a close-up of the lumbar curve shows that at the apical disc, the trapezoidal wedging has actually reversed from being compressed on the concave side of the original curve to being compressed on the staple side.

segment.[37] Eight immature calves were instrumented with anterior vertebral body screws inserted into four consecutive thoracic vertebrae. Two of the screws were connected by a stainless steel tether and two were left unconnected. After 12 weeks of growth, the tethering consistently created coronal and sagittal plane deformities over the tethered motion segments that did not occur in untethered control segments of the spine. In addition, vertebral-body wedging was observed, indicating that physeal growth had decreased on the side of the tether. Biomechanical analysis revealed that the tether restricted the lateral bending range of motion, but this motion returned to control levels when the tether was removed. This study suggested that the spine could be modulated by a tether without permanently affecting spinal motion.

In 2005, Braun et al compared the ability of shape memory alloy staples and bone-anchored ligament tethers for correcting experimentally induced scoliosis in 24 Spanish Cross-X goats.[36] The flexible ligament tethers were found to stabilize the progression of scoliosis, with an average 69.9-degree deformity after treatment versus a 73.4-degree deformity before treatment ($P = 0.34$). By comparison, scoliosis in the untethered goats progressed from 79.5 degrees to 96.8 degrees ($P < 0.05$), and from 77.3 degrees to 94.3 degrees ($P < 0.05$) in the goats treated with staples. Pullout testing demonstrated that the bone anchors had improved integration into the vertebral bodies, whereas the staples were found to loosen, with histological evidence of a halo of fibrous tissue around the staple tines. This study showed that an anterolateral tether could control the progression of scoliosis of the magnitude present in the study animals, but could not correct it.

The next step in the development of safe and effective vertebral tethering was to critically evaluate intervertebral disc health. If they are to be successful in the long term, fusionless treatment strategies require preservation of the intervertebral discs. Newton and coworkers[38] have reported histologically and biochemically evaluating intervertebral discs after the modulation of spinal growth. Intervertebral discs from 17 bovine spines instrumented with a multilevel flexible steel cable were compared with discs from 19 bovine controls that underwent sham instrumentation (screw only). A double-screw–double-tether construct was required to achieve adequate bone fixation in this rapidly growing model. No change in disc water content or gross morphological grading was observed in either of the two groups. However, decreased disc thickness, increased proteoglycan synthesis, and a change in collagen distribution between the concave and convex sides of the disc were found in the tethered discs. Further studies of disc health with noninvasive imaging modalities are required for detection early disc degeneration and after long-term growth modulation.

Lenke et al have applied anterior vertebral tethering in two patients.[39] The curve in the first case was reduced from 50 to 25 degrees and the correction was maintained over a 2-year follow-up period without complications. The second case was that of an 8-year-old girl with a 34-degree left thoracic curve that corrected to 6 degrees in the coronal plane during a 4-year postoperative follow-up period (**Fig. 27.6**).

Although long-term clinical data for vertebral stapling or other types of tethering are not yet available, modulation of anterior spinal growth provides an exciting alternative to controlling progressive scoliosis while maintaining spinal motion. The ideal application of such modulation is likely to be in the treatment of preadolescent idiopathic scoliosis with curves of 20 to 60 degrees that have a high likelihood of progression. In this setting, staples or a tether would act like an internal brace and limit curve progression, or possibly even reduce the degree of curvature during the patient's growth spurt.

A–D

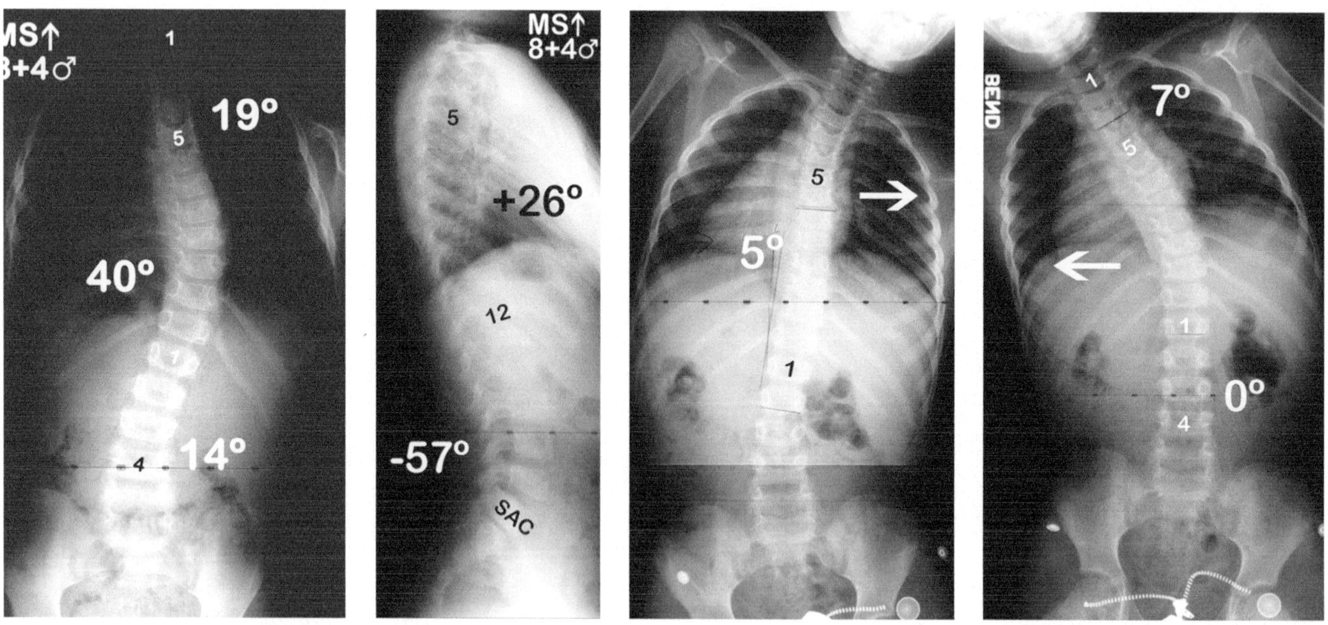


**Fig. 27.6** **(A)** This 8-year-old patient has a preoperative thoracic curve of 40 degrees despite bracing. An MRI scan of the spine was normal. **(B)** The patient has a normal sagittal profile, but the apical segment is hypokyphotic. **(C)** A right-bending film shows the thoracic curve to be extremely flexible, reducing to 5 degrees. **(D)** A left-bending film shows that the lumbar and upper thoracic curves are extremely flexible and still compensatory.

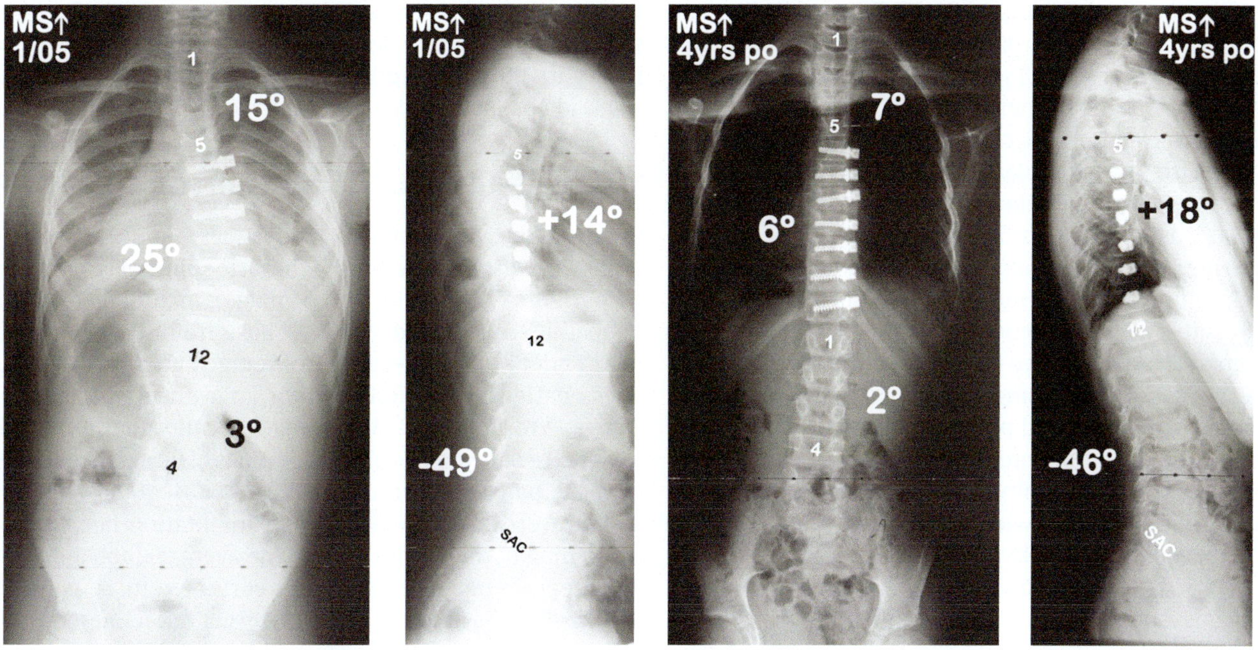


**Fig. 27.6** *(Continued)* **(E,F)** Postoperative films show evidence of anterior screws that closely resemble those in standard anterior-instrumented systems. There is no rod, but there is a flexible cable connecting all of the vertebral screws. The curve has been purposely reduced only to 25 degrees in anticipation of growth modulation and to avoid overcorrection of the thoracic spine. **(G,H)** Four-year postoperative images. The patient was 12 years old at the time, with a 6-degree thoracic curve and kyphosis of 18 degrees. (Courtesy of Lawrence G. Lenke, MD.)

## Correction of Existing Deformity After Growth Is Completed

### Wedge Osteotomy Technology

The concept of vertebral body wedging as a key component of scoliotic deformity was confirmed in a study in which Parent et al[40] measured the dimensions of 471 vertebrae from scoliotic spines and 510 vertebrae from normal specimens. Vertebral wedging increased progressively toward the apex of the spinal curve and was maximal at the apex.

In an existing deformity of moderate size (40 to 70 degrees), it would be appealing to correct the vertebral deformity at the apex of the curve without fusing the surrounding facet joints or disc spaces. Betz developed a conceptual idea for such correction that involves a partial opening wedge osteotomy on the concave side of the apical vertebral body and a partial closing wedge osteotomy on the convex side, thereby correcting the deformity caused by the residual wedging. Preclinical work on this concept, using intact calf spines, has been completed.[36] The wedge osteotomies were completed and held open either with a metallic wedge spacer alone or with a metallic wedge spacer secured with rod reconstruction. The data collected in this work suggest that the wedge–rod construct was as stiff as an intact spine, but that the wedge alone did not provide adequate stiffness to promote healing.[36] Preclinical work that has been completed in a porcine model of residual post-growth deformity has shown that wedge osteotomy and instrumentation could be undertaken without causing paralysis. If the temporary rod used in this work was not removed soon enough there was evidence of facet arthritis. It is therefore necessary to remove the temporary rod at an appropriate time (12 weeks) to prevent facet-joint fusion or arthritic changes.

Between 1992 and 1996, Lindseth and Kling[41] studied the concept of osteotomy for correcting lumbar scoliosis in humans. They performed wedge osteotomies between T12 and L3 in 17 patients. Five patients had four-level osteotomies and 12 patients had three-level osteotomies. Many of these patients had a thoracic fusion with a lumbar wedge osteotomy in the upper lumbar spine, whereas some had osteotomies for isolated thoracolumbar/lumbar curves. Preoperative curves averaged 58 degrees (range: 40 to 66 degrees), and the average correction obtained was 8.1 degrees per osteotomy. Range of motion at the osteotomy site was preserved, with 29 degrees of motion preoperatively and 30 degrees postoperatively. Two patients lost their corrections, and one patient developed foot drop. The major problem with wedge osteotomy without an implant was the kyphosing effect that occurred across the lumbar spine where the osteotomies were completed. It is for this reason that the senior author of this chapter (R.R.B.) considers an implant to be necessary when completing a vertebral osteotomy.

The senior author (R.R.B.) subsequently performed wedge osteotomies with instrumentation in 14 patients with myelodysplasia and spinal cord injury (SCI) with spastic paralysis. With this particular technique, osteotomies were done at three to six vertebral levels with vertebral body screws (at least one or two) inserted above and below the instrumented section. A temporary rod was left in place for 12 weeks and was then removed. The reported result[42,43] of this was that a 50% correction was maintained in 11 of the 14 patients (**Fig. 27.7**). Three patients' conditions worsened with curves actually reversing direction in two of the three. This clinical study included patients with SCI because they had the most to gain from preserved motion. They also provided an excellent opportunity for assessing outcome in neurological injury. Patients with neurological injury to the spinal cord would become flaccid for 6 weeks but would later return to a spastic state. This did not occur, and no patient with myelodysplasia lost function at a motor level. The results of this preliminary clinical series indicated that wedge osteotomy with instrumentation was safe for use in this clinical population. Healing of the patients' osteotomies occurred by 12 weeks, and the patients' spines remained flexible according to side-bending radiographs. The efficacy outcome measure of maintenance of curve correction in the paralytic model is difficult to sustain. However, the results of wedge osteotomy with instrumentation are encouraging enough to justify its pursuit in future work with patients who have single idiopathic thoracolumbar and lumbar curves.

## Wedge Osteotomy of the Thoracic Spine

In a study by Maruyama and colleagues,[44] multiple vertebral wedge osteotomies of the thoracic spine were done on 20 patients (17 females and 3 males), including 19 with idiopathic scoliosis and 1 with scoliosis from syringomyelia, who underwent surgery at an average age of 16.4 years. These patients were followed for an average of 8.9 years (range: 2 to 17 years). Maruyama and colleagues reported an absence of neurological complications of wedge osteotomy in these patients. Two patients had subsequent surgery and conversion to posterior instrumentation because of worsening of their deformities. The average Cobb angle of 64.0 degrees before surgery was corrected to an average of 48.2 degrees at 8.9 years after surgery. Declines in pulmonary function after surgery were not statistically significant. Although the average correction per level was only 16 degrees, a seemingly minimal correction for the magnitude of the surgery done on these patients, the progression of their curves was arrested. The effect of the surgery on spinal motion was not reported.

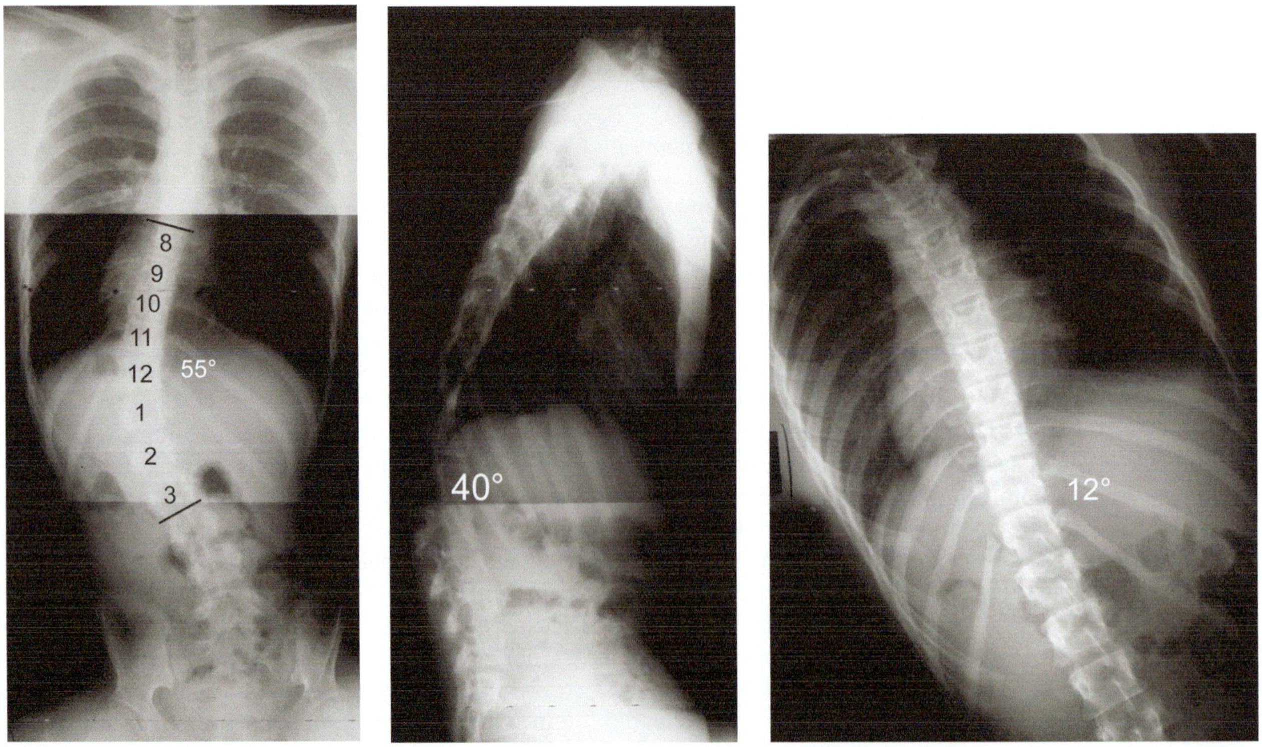


A–C

**Fig. 27.7 (A,B)** This 15-year-old girl has a left paralytic thoracolumbar curve of 55 degrees as a result of spinal cord injury. Her radiographs show a thoracolumbar kyphosis of 40 degrees. **(C)** The left-bending film shows a flexible curve reducing to 12 degrees.

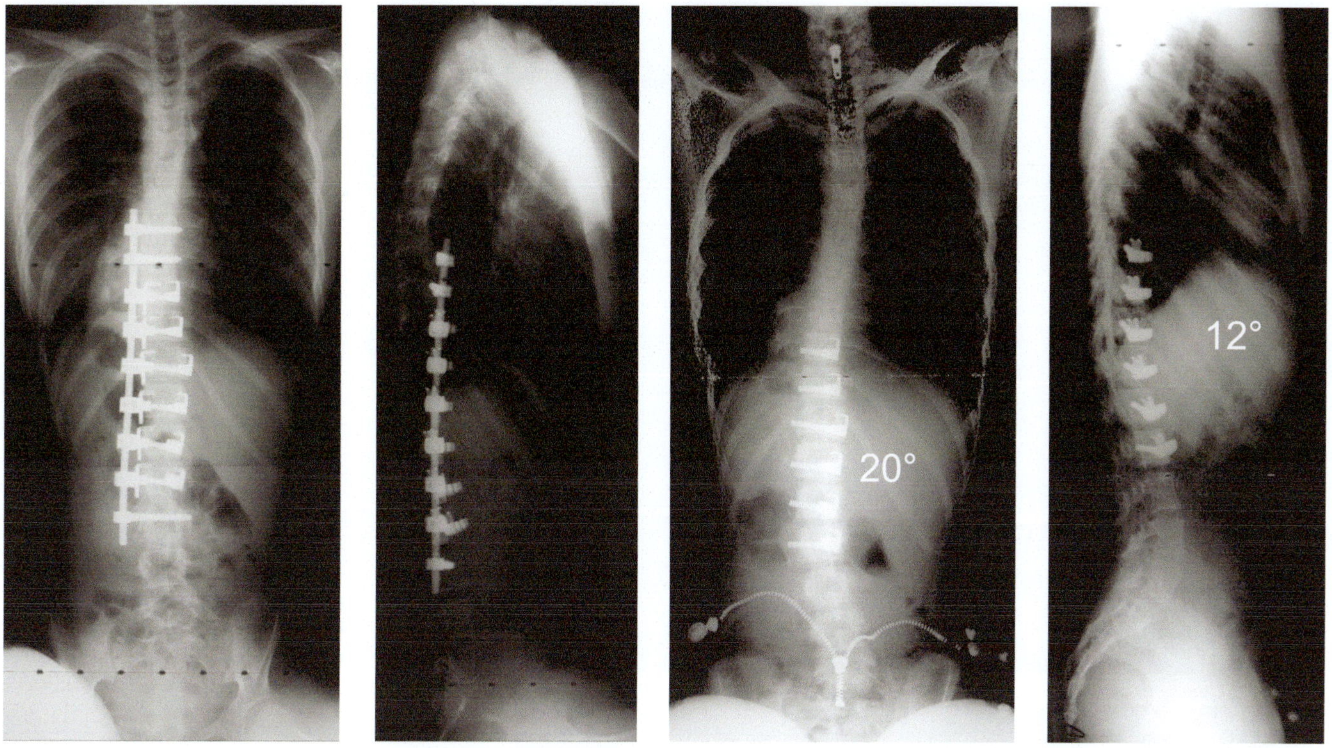


**Fig. 27.7** *(Continued)* **(D,E)** The patient underwent a wedge osteotomy from T10 to L3 with vertebral body screws in T8–T9 and L4 (she has six lumbar vertebrae). The lateral radiograph shows that the paralytic kyphosis is partly straightened but that some kyphosis is left to accommodate sitting. **(F,G)** The rod, screw heads, and staples were removed at 12 weeks. All of the osteotomies were healed at that time. These radiographs, taken 4 years postoperatively, show a residual scoliosis of 20 degrees and 12 degrees of kyphosis (normal kyphosis for a patient with SCI is 19 degrees).

## Mechanical Motion-sparing Techniques: Posterior

### Tethering

Lowe and associates investigated the application of a minimally invasive posterior tethering system in an immature sheep model to determine whether fusionless modulation of spinal growth in the sagittal plane can be successful.[45] They theorized that the procedure could potentially play a role in treating Scheuermann's kyphosis in instances in which bracing is not effective. Nine immature sheep were posteriorly tethered with polyethylene cords and compared with five control animals. At 13 months after surgery, the tethered groups had significantly less kyphosis and vertebral body wedging than the control group. Lowe and colleagues concluded that fusionless modulation of spinal growth in the sagittal plane could be successful and that the procedure may be a potential treatment for adolescents with Scheuermann's disease.

### Growing Rod Systems

Thompson et al reported a study of the use of growing rods in the management of early-onset scoliosis.[46] The three growing rod systems currently in use (single growing rod, dual growing rods, and the VEPTR [titanium rib] device) were compared with regard to efficacy and their advantages and disadvantages.

#### Single Growing Rod

A single growing rod uses a claw foundation proximally or distally or both.[47,48] The distal foundation may consist either of hooks or pedicle screws. Limited fusion can be achieved around the foundation sites. One technique for this is to leave a section of overlapping rod above or below the proximal or distal foundation and use this excess length for periodic lengthenings of the rod construct. Two rods that overlap in the middle and are connected either with side-by-side or end-to-end connectors may also be used. Side-to-side connectors are preferred by the senior author of this chapter (R.R.B.) (**Fig. 27.8**). Occasionally, a short apical anterior disc release or fusion may be performed. Alternatively, anterior staples may be used at the apex of the scoliotic curve. The worst results with this technique, reported by Thompson et al,[46] were in patients with anterior fusions. The rods are lengthened periodically, typically biannually, regardless of whether or not there is curve progression. When the patient has grown to sufficient adult height, fusion is recommended.

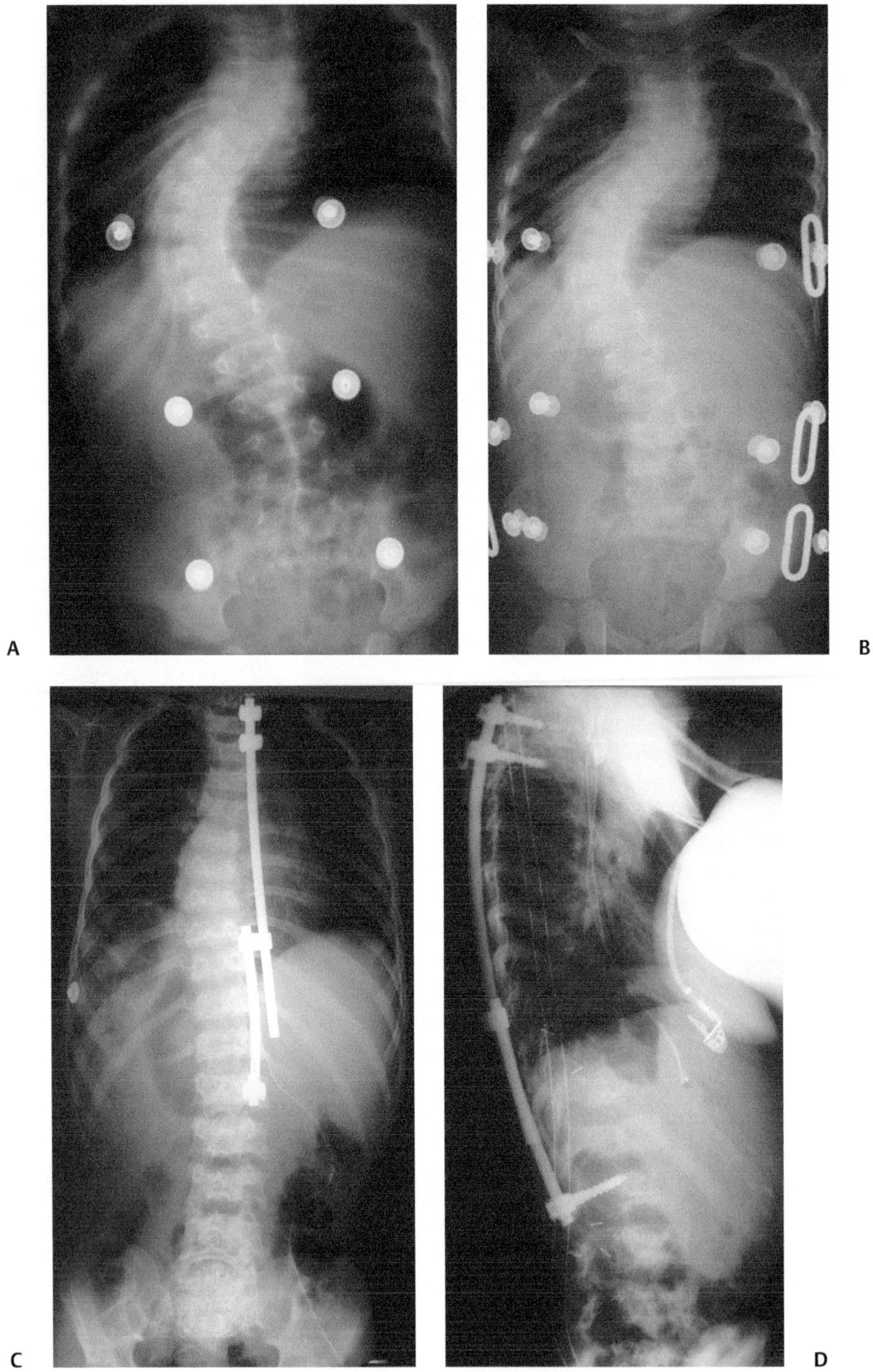

**Fig. 27.8** **(A)** An 18-month-old boy with early-onset scoliosis thought to be idiopathic. The patient's MRI was normal. **(B)** Despite bracing, the patient's scoliotic curve has continued to progress to 70 degrees. **(C,D)** AP and lateral films made after insertion of a unilateral curve correction system using a crossover technique with a domino. The curve was successfully managed until the patient was 11 years of age, at which time no further correction could be obtained. The patient had broken the single rod twice, fortunately near the time of anticipated rod exchange. Conversion to a fusion was to be scheduled within the next 2 years.

## Dual Growing Rods

Several authors[47,49–52] have recently popularized the use of dual growing rods. In this technique, each rod is composed of two sections that are connected by an end-to-end tandem connector or side-to-side connectors through which the system is lengthened (**Fig. 27.9**). Thompson and coworkers[46] reported the clinical and radiographic outcomes of 28 patients who had been treated with either single (21 patients) or dual (7 patients) growing rods and had undergone definitive spinal fusions with at least 2 years of follow-up. The percent final curve correction was greatest in the dual-rod group (**Table 27.1**). The senior author of this chapter (R.R.B.) has shifted to using more rib-to-spine or rib-to-pelvis constructs (described below) because of the high rate of extensive spontaneous fusion found with growing rods.[8]

**Table 27.1 Results of Thompson and Colleagues'[46] Study of the Results of Single versus Dual Rods**

| | Group 1 Single Rod with Anterior Spinal Fusion | Group 2 Single Rod Without Fusion | Group 3 Dual rods |
|---|---|---|---|
| Percent scoliosis correction | 23 ± 21% | 36 ± 23% | 71 ± 22% |
| Total T1 to S1 spinal growth | 6.4 ± 1.4 cm | 7.6 ± 4.7 cm | 12.1 ± 1.9 cm |

*Source*: Data from Thompson GH, Akbarnia BA, Campbell RM, Jr. Growing rod techniques in early-onset scoliosis. J Pediatr Orthop 2007;27: 354–61.

## Vertical Expandable Prosthetic Titanium Rib

As described earlier, the VEPTR device developed by Dr. Robert Campbell is a very appealing alternative to growing rods because of its ability to correct a scoliotic deformity, allow continued spinal growth, and potentially prevent the spontaneous fusion that typically occurs with growing rods. Thompson and coworkers reported the treatment results with the VEPTR device in 16 patients with noncongenital scoliosis without rib anomalies.[46] The mean curve in the group was 77 degrees preoperatively, 40 degrees immediately after placement of the implants, and 39 degrees at last follow-up, for an average correction of 34 degrees (49%). It is important to note that the patients in this series underwent expansion thoracoplasty. The senior author (R.R.B.) chooses not to perform an expansion thoracoplasty when the rib spaces open on the curve concavity on preoperative bending films. A comparison series is needed of patients undergoing thoracoplasty and those not having it.

Currently, the senior author of this chapter (R.R.B.) prefers the bilateral ribs-to-pelvis VEPTR technique developed by Dr. John Smith (**Fig. 27.10**).[53] Long-term results of this technique are pending; but hypothetically, it should not promote premature spontaneous fusion because the

A

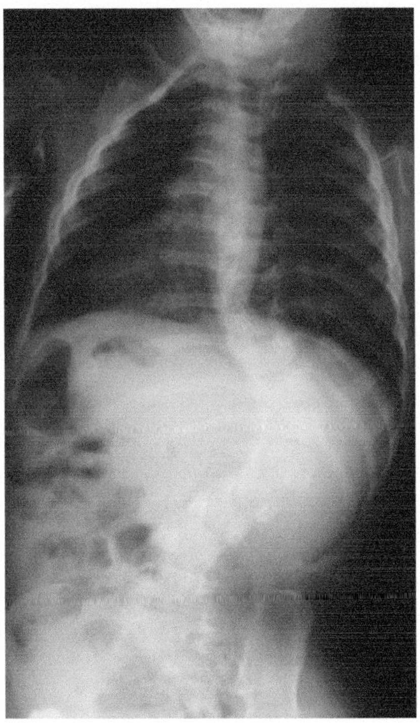

B

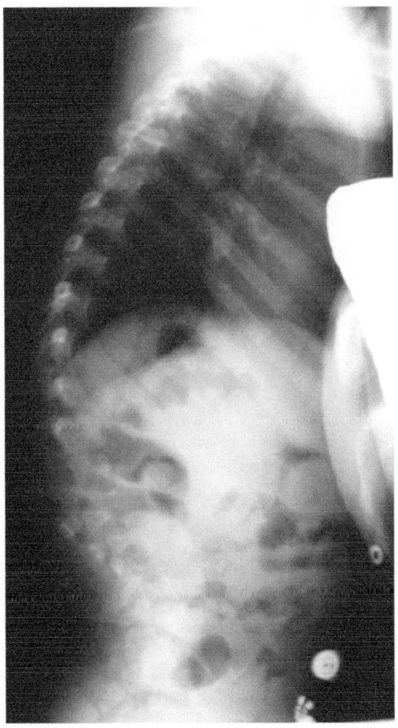

**Fig. 27.9 (A,B)** A 19-month-old girl with idiopathic infantile scoliosis. At the age of 12 months her curve measured 21 degrees; it had progressed to 76 degrees in 7 months. *(Continued on page 404)*

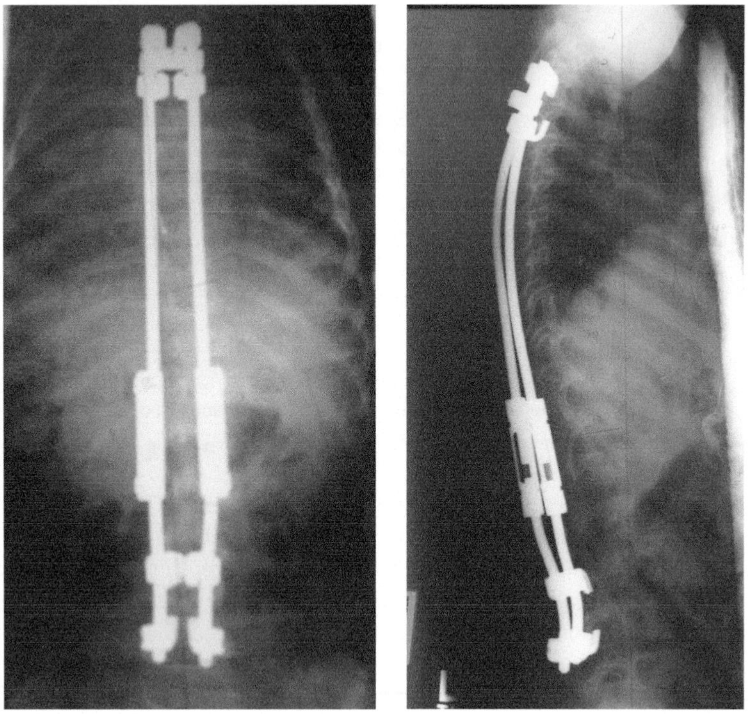

C D

**Fig. 27.9** *(Continued)* **(C,D)** At the age of 19 months, the patient underwent dual growing-rod instrumentation. Following insertion of the instrumentation, the patient's curve measured 35 degrees. (Courtesy of Behrooz Akbarnia, MD.)

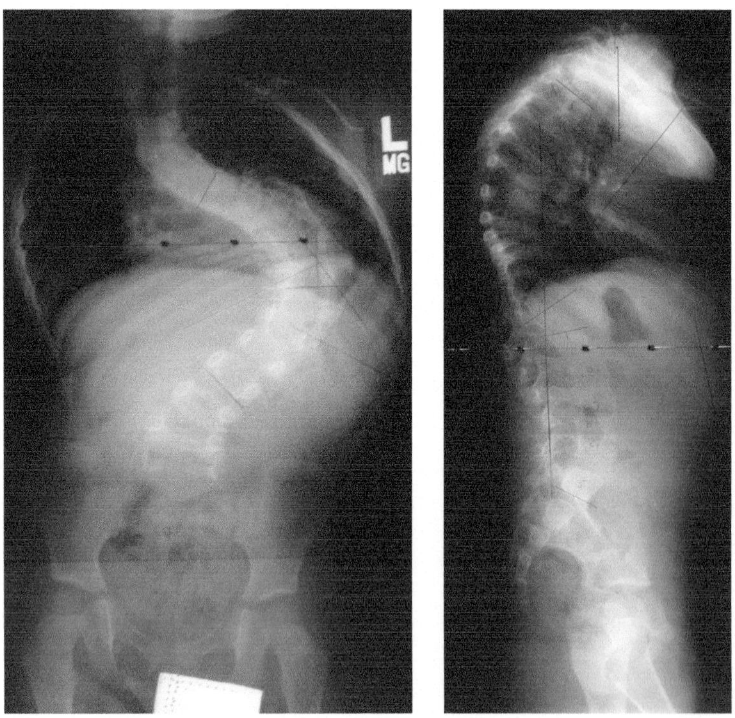


A B

**Fig. 27.10** **(A–D)** A 4-year-old girl with a 109-degree early-onset scoliosis that bent to 68 degrees with a flexible kyphosis. She was treated with a bilateral VEPTR device from T2–T3 to the pelvis.

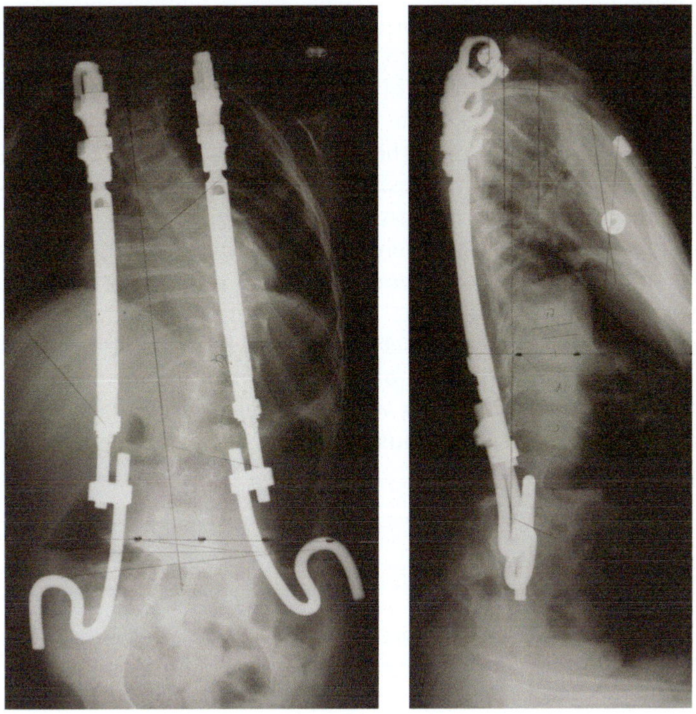

C D

**Fig. 27.10** *(Continued)* **(A–D)** A 4-year-old girl with a 109-degree early-onset scoliosis that bent to 68 degrees with a flexible kyphosis. She was treated with a bilateral VEPTR device from T2–T3 to the pelvis.

spine is not rigidly immobilized as it is with dual rods fixed to pedicle screws. The other advantage of the VEPTR technique is the ability to control rotation with the more lateral attachment sites on the iliac wings, applying derotation forces directly to the convex side of the spine. The senior author (R.R.B.) uses the 6-mm McCarthy rod for iliac fixation. In ambulatory patients, it is especially important to bend adequate lordosis into the rod in the L4-to-S1 region so as to preserve erect posture. Smith and Smart reported problems with ambulation in a series of patients treated with bilateral ribs-to-pelvis constructs.[9] However, patients within that series had an earlier construct design utilized for iliac fixation that did not allow for adequate distal lumbar lordosis.

## Complications with Posterior Growing Systems

High rates of complications are associated with each of these growing support systems, whether growing rods or titanium ribs are used. Most of the complications are anticipated, and the patient's family should be prepared for their occurrence. The risk of soft-tissue sloughing and subsequent infection is partly within the surgeon's control. Perioperative nutrition, careful planning and location of skin incisions, and meticulous wound care can reduce the incidence of skin and wound problems with the systems described here. A comparison of complications in Dr. Campbell's series with that of two growing-rod series is shown in **Table 27.2**.

**Table 27.2 Comparison of Campbell and Smith's Series[54] of Complications Associated with Growing Systems with Two Other Published Reports**

| | Campbell and Smith[54] | Klemme et al[5] | Tello[55] |
|---|---|---|---|
| Number of patients | 201 | 67 | 44 |
| Procedures per patient | 7.02 | 6.1 | 3.4 |
| Follow-up (years) | 6 | 3.1 | 4.75 |
| Infection rate per procedure | 3.3% | 1.5% | 5.3% |
| Skin sloughing | 8.5% | 4.5% | 13.6% |
| Migration/year | 0.09 | 0.1 | 0.029 |
| Percentage of patients | 27% | 31% | 14% |
| Time | 3.2 Years | Not reported | Not reported |
| Device breakage | 6% | 18% | 27% |

*Source*: Data from Campbell & Smith, Klemme et al, and Tello.

## Conclusion

Preliminary clinical results of stapling in patients with idiopathic scoliosis are encouraging, but additional clinical studies with controls are needed. It appears that residual growth is important for curve correction. Tethering appears promising in preclinical studies, and clinical trials under an investigational device exemption (IDE) will begin in the near future. Wedge osteotomy can potentially be used to treat residual wedging in some patients with thoracolumbar or lumbar curves, but the fate of the intervening disc space and its role in deformity must be further studied. Current results indicate that expandable posterior spinal instrumentation techniques, such as with single or dual growing rods and VEPTR, can be beneficial in controlling severe spinal deformities and allowing spinal growth. Dual growing rods with more frequent lengthenings seem to offer better results (in percent correction and spine length) than does a single growing rod because of their greater ability to control the spine. However, a high rate of spontaneous fusion necessitates a more complex final procedure with numerous osteotomies. The VEPTR with a ribs-to-spine or ribs-to-pelvis construct may offer the potential of avoiding spontaneous fusion, but this remains unknown. A short apical spinal fusion should be avoided because it appears to adversely affect long-term results with respect to the correction of spinal deformity and spinal growth. Anterior stapling with a posterior growing system may be more efficacious in allowing additional modulation of spinal growth.

### References


1. Engsberg JR, Lenke LG, Reitenbach AK, Hollander KW, Bridwell KH, Blanke K. Prospective evaluation of trunk range of motion in adolescents with idiopathic scoliosis undergoing spinal fusion surgery. Spine 2002;27:1346–1354
2. Hilibrand AS, Robbins M. Adjacent segment degeneration and adjacent segment disease: The consequences of spinal fusion? Spine J 2004; 4(6, suppl):190S–194S
3. Edwards CC II, Lenke LG, Peelle M, Sides B, Rinella A, Bridwell KH. Selective thoracic fusion for adolescent idiopathic scoliosis with C modifier lumbar curves: 2- to 16-year radiographic and clinical results. Spine 2004;29:536–546
4. Gillespie R, O'Brien J. Harrington instrumentation without fusion. J Bone Joint Surg Br 1981;62:461
5. Klemme WR, Denis F, Winter RB, Lonstein JW, Koop SE. Spinal instrumentation without fusion for progressive scoliosis in young children. J Pediatr Orthop 1997;17:734–742
6. McCarthy RE, McCullough FL. Growing instrumentation for scoliosis. Paper presented at: Scoliosis Research Society annual meeting, Dublin, Ireland, September 1993
7. Fisk JR, Peterson HA, Laughlin R, Lutz R. Spontaneous fusion in scoliosis after instrumentation without arthrodesis. J Pediatr Orthop 1995;15:182–186
8. Cahill PJ, Marvil SC, Schutt C, et al. Autofusion of the skeletally immature spine after growing rod instrumentation. Spine, In press
9. Smith JT, Smart MP. Bilateral rib to pelvis VEPTR technique for treatment of progressive spinal deformity in children. Paper presented at: International Meeting on Advanced Spine Techniques, Paradise Island, Bahamas, July 2007
10. Carrier J, Aubin CE, Villemure I, Labelle H. Biomechanical modelling of growth modulation following rib shortening or lengthening in adolescent idiopathic scoliosis. Med Biol Eng Comput 2004;42: 541–548
11. Xiong B, Sevastik JA. A physiological approach to surgical treatment of progressive early idiopathic scoliosis. Eur Spine J 1998;7:505–508
12. Zhang H, Sucato DJ. Unilateral pedicle screw epiphysiodesis of the neurocentral synchondrosis. Production of idiopathic-like scoliosis in an immature animal model. J Bone Joint Surg Am 2008;90:2460–2469
13. Huynh AM, Aubin CE, Rajwani T, Bagnall KM, Villemure I. Pedicle growth asymmetry as a cause of adolescent idiopathic scoliosis: A biomechanical study. Eur Spine J 2007;16:523–529
14. Zhang H, Sucato DJ, Nurenberg P, McClung A. Pedicle and neurocentral synchondrosis development in infantile and juvenile idiopathic scoliosis. Paper presented at: American Academy of Orthopaedic Surgeons annual meeting, Las Vegas, NV, Feb. 25–28, 2009.
15. Blount WP, Clarke GR. The classic. Control of bone growth by epiphyseal stapling. A preliminary report. Journal of Bone and Joint Surgery, July, 1949. Clin Orthop Relat Res 1971;77:4–17
16. Iatridis JC, Mente PL, Stokes IA, Aronsson DD, Alini M. Compression-induced changes in intervertebral disc properties in a rat tail model. Spine 1999;24:996–1002
17. MacEwen GD, Kirsch P. Factors affecting the growth of the vertebral bodies and invertebral discs. Scoliosis and growth, proceedings of a third symposium held at the Institute of Diseases of the chest, Brampton Hospital, London on 13th November, 1970. Edited by PA Zorab. Edinburgh: Churchill Livingstone, 1971.
18. Mente PL, Stokes IA, Spence H, Aronsson DD. Progression of vertebral wedging in an asymmetrically loaded rat tail model. Spine 1997;22:1292–1296
19. Stokes IA, Aronsson DD, Spence H, Iatridis JC. Mechanical modulation of intervertebral disc thickness in growing rat tails. J Spinal Disord 1998;11:261–265
20. Wall EJ, Bylski-Austrow DI, Kolata RJ, Crawford AH. Endoscopic mechanical spinal hemiepiphysiodesis modifies spine growth. Spine 2005;30:1148–1153
21. Nachemson AL, Peterson LE. Effectiveness of treatment with a brace in girls who have adolescent idiopathic scoliosis. A prospective, controlled study based on data from the Brace Study of the Scoliosis Research Society. J Bone Joint Surg Am 1995;77:815–822
22. Bengtsson G, Fällström K, Jansson B, Nachemson A. A psychological and psychiatric investigation of the adjustment of female scoliosis patients. Acta Psychiatr Scand 1974;50:50–59
23. Clayson D, Luz-Alterman S, Cataletto MM, Levine DB. Long-term psychological sequelae of surgically versus nonsurgically treated scoliosis. Spine 1987;12:983–986

24. Fällström K, Cochran T, Nachemson A. Long-term effects on personality development in patients with adolescent idiopathic scoliosis. Influence of type of treatment. Spine 1986;11:756–758
25. Nachlas IW, Borden JN. The cure of experimental scoliosis by directed growth control. J Bone Joint Surg Am 1951; 33(A:1, A:1)24–34
26. Smith AD, Von Lackum WH, Wylie R. An operation for stapling vertebral bodies in congenital scoliosis. J Bone Joint Surg Am 1954; 36(A:2, A:2)342–348
27. Akyuz E, Braun JT, Brown NA, Bachus KN. Static versus dynamic loading in the mechanical modulation of vertebral growth. Spine 2006;31:E952–E958
28. Aronsson DD, Stokes IA, Rosovsky J, Spence H. Mechanical modulation of calf tail vertebral growth: Implications for scoliosis progression. J Spinal Disord 1999;12:141–146
29. Braun JT, Ogilvie JW, Akyuz E, Brodke DS, Bachus KN, Stefko RM. Experimental scoliosis in an immature goat model: A method that creates idiopathic-type deformity with minimal violation of the spinal elements along the curve. Spine 2003;28: 2198–2203
30. Braun JT, Ogilvie JW, Akyuz E, Brodke DS, Bachus KN. Fusionless scoliosis correction using a shape memory alloy staple in the anterior thoracic spine of the immature goat. Spine 2004;29: 1980–1989
31. Qiu Y, Zhu F. [Anterior and posterior spinal growth plates in adolescent idiopathic scoliosis: A histological study]. Zhongguo Yi Xue Ke Xue Yuan Xue Bao 2005;27:148–152
32. Dickson RA. The etiology and pathogenesis of idiopathic scoliosis. Acta Orthop Belg 1992;52 (suppl 1):21–25
33. Betz RR, Ranade A, Samdani AF, et al. Vertebral body stapling: A fusionless treatment option for a growing child with moderate idiopathic scoliosis. Spine 2010;35(2):169–176
34. Weis JC, Betz RR, Clements DH III, Balsara RK. Prevalence of perioperative complications after anterior spinal fusion for patients with idiopathic scoliosis. J Spinal Disord 1997;10:371–375
35. Guo X, Chau WW, Chan YL, Cheng JC. Relative anterior spinal overgrowth in adolescent idiopathic scoliosis. Results of disproportionate endochondral-membranous bone growth. J Bone Joint Surg Br 2003;85:1026–1031
36. Braun JT, Akyuz E, Ogilvie JW, Bachus KN. The efficacy and integrity of shape memory alloy staples and bone anchors with ligament tethers in the fusionless treatment of experimental scoliosis. J Bone Joint Surg Am 2005;87:2038–2051
37. Newton PO, Fricka KB, Lee SS, Farnsworth CL, Cox TG, Mahar AT. Asymmetrical flexible tethering of spine growth in an immature bovine model. Spine 2002;27:689–693
38. Newton PO, Upasani VV, Farnsworth CL, et al. Spinal growth modulation with use of a tether in an immature porcine model. J Bone Joint Surg Am 2008;90:2695–2706
39. Crawford CH III, Lenke LG. Growth modulation by means of anterior tethering resulting in progressive correction of juvenile idiopathic scoliosis: A case report. J Bone Joint Surg Am 2010;92(1): 202–209
40. Parent S, Labelle H, Skalli W, de Guise J. Vertebral wedging characteristic changes in scoliotic spines. Spine 2004;29: E455–E462
41. Didelot WP, Kling TF, Jr., Lindseth RE. Technique of anterior vertebral osteotomy designed to preserve lumbar motion and correct idiopathic lumbar scoliosis. Paper presented at: Scoliosis Research Society Annual Meeting, Cairns, Australia, October 18–21, 2000
42. Guille JT, Betz RR, Balsara RK, Mulcahey MJ, D'Andrea LP, Clements DH. The feasibility, safety, and utility of vertebral wedge osteotomies for the fusionless treatment of paralytic scoliosis. Spine 2003;28:S266–S274
43. McCarthy KP, Chafetz RS, Mulcahey MJ, Frisch RF, D'Andrea LP, Betz RR. Clinical efficacy of the vertebral wedge osteotomy for the fusionless treatment of paralytic scoliosis, Spine 2010;35(4):403–410
44. Maruyama T, Kitagawa T, Takeshita K, et al. Fusionless surgery for scoliosis: 2-17 year radiographic and clinical follow-up. Spine 2006;31:2310–2315
45. Lowe TG, Wilson L, Chien JT, et al. A posterior tether for fusionless modulation of sagittal plane growth in a sheep model. Spine 2005; 30(17, suppl)S69–S74
46. Thompson GH, Akbarnia BA, Campbell RM Jr. Growing rod techniques in early-onset scoliosis. J Pediatr Orthop 2007;27:354–361
47. Thompson GH, Akbarnia BA, Kostial P, et al. Comparison of single and dual growing rod techniques followed through definitive surgery: A preliminary study. Spine 2005;30(18): 2039–2044
48. Blakemore LC, Scoles PV, Poe-Kochert C, Thompson GH. Submuscular Isola rod with or without limited apical fusion in the management of severe spinal deformities in young children: Preliminary report. Spine 2001;26:2044–2048
49. Akbarnia BA, McCarthy R. Pediatric Isola Instrumentation Without Fusion for the Treatment of Progressive Early-onset Scoliosis. Chicago, IL: Scoliosis Research Society, 1998
50. Akbarnia BA, Marks DS. Instrumentation with limited arthrodesis for the treatment of progressive early-onset scoliosis. Spine 2000; 14:181–190
51. Akbarnia BA, Marks DS, Boachie-Adjei O, Thompson AG, Asher MA. Dual growing rod technique for the treatment of progressive early-onset scoliosis: A multicenter study. Spine 2005; 30(17, suppl) S46–S57
52. Akbarnia BA, Breakwell LM, Marks DS et al. Dual growing rod technique followed for 3 to 11 years until final fusion: The effect of frequency of lengthening. Spine 2008;33(9):984–990
53. Smith JT, Smart MP, Emans JB, et al. Results of surgical experience using the VEPTR device for the treatment of thoracic insufficiency syndrome: A multicenter study. Paper presented at: 13th International Meeting on Advanced Spine Techniques, Athens, Greece, July 12–15, 2006
54. Campbell RM Jr, Smith MD. Thoracic insufficiency syndrome and exotic scoliosis. J Bone Joint Surg Am 2007;89(suppl 1):108–122
55. Tello CA. Harrington instrumentation without arthrodesis and consecutive distraction program for young children with severe spinal deformities. Experience and technical details. Orthop Clin North Am 1994;25:333–351

# 28 The Impact of Genetics Research on Adolescent Idiopathic Scoliosis

*John T. Braun, William F. Lavelle, and James W. Ogilvie*

The optimal management of any condition necessitates not only a clear understanding of its etiology but also the ability to diagnose the condition early in its course, accurately determine its prognosis, and treat it definitively with minimal morbidity. Unfortunately, adolescent idiopathic scoliosis (AIS) presents challenges in all of these areas in that its etiology is unknown or at best ill-defined; its diagnosis is made *ex post facto*; determination of its prognosis is inaccurate; and the treatment options for it are limited.

Genetics research holds great promise for improving the management of AIS by targeting each of these challenging areas. However, there remains wide skepticism about its ever having any practical effect on the diagnosis or treatment of AIS. Although significant genetic discoveries have affected many other areas of medicine, genetics research in AIS has trailed behind, and despite a recent increase in genetics research in AIS and its discovery of much new and important information, it has not provided either a fully defined etiology of AIS or a practical application of the genetic findings made so far. This has led to questions about whether AIS may be too complex a condition to be affected in any real way by genetics research.

Despite its genetic complexity, however, AIS is not too complex for genetics research to influence its clinical care. In fact, the discovery of prognostic genetic markers that accurately predict the progression of spinal curvature has recently initiated a revolution in the management of AIS. At the outset, prognostic genetic testing will potentially allow the accurate identification of patients at high risk for progression of their spinal curvature. In contrast to current radiographic methods, the genetic identification of risk for curve progression will be possible before a curve becomes significant. With this genetic support and the confidence that a patient with scoliosis is at high risk for curve progression, the opportunity for earlier, more effective, and more physiological treatment will be substantial. Whether bracing with greater conviction at smaller curve magnitudes or pursuing novel fusionless procedures for treating scoliosis, more definitive treatment will be possible with probable reduced morbidity.

Conversely, prognostic genetic testing will also allow the accurate identification of patients at low risk for curve progression. Physicians will be able to reassure the majority of patients and their families at a single encounter, with a consequent reduction in the number of surveillance radiographs of AIS patients and a greater overall efficiency in their clinical monitoring. All of these represent significant improvements over current algorithms for managing AIS.

Additional opportunities for a clinical effect of genetics research on AIS are likely to present themselves as the genes associated with AIS and curve progression are mapped. Although this is a more involved undertaking than defining prognostic genetic markers, ongoing efforts in this area will probably result in more diagnostic and therapeutic options for AIS.

Before discussing the practical impact of prognostic genetic testing and the potential benefits of additional genetics research in AIS, it is important to review the substantial body of work that has served as a foundation for these recent discoveries. Because most of the genetics research in AIS has focused on defining its etiology, this chapter will first review the efforts made over the past century to establish the heredity of this condition, and will then discuss more contemporary work directed at locating and mapping the specific genes involved in its occurrence. The recent discovery of several prognostic genetic markers for AIS will then be discussed. In each of these sections, emphasis will be put on important advances that have not only improved the understanding of idiopathic scoliosis, but which also stand to affect its clinical care.

## Heritability

Although scoliosis has been recognized for centuries, its familial nature was not noted until the late nineteenth century.[1] The first credible evidence supporting a familial bias of scoliosis was reported in the 1930s.[2-4] Although not definitive, this early work was important because it initiated systematic investigation of the hereditary nature of AIS and established three general categories of its study that continue today: (1) studies of single, multigenerational families; (2) studies of relatives of index patients or probands; and (3) twin studies.

Perhaps the most significant early study of a single, multigenerational family with idiopathic scoliosis ("not due to neurological or congenital causes") was reported by Garland in 1934.[3] The mode of transmission of the disease in this five-generation family was described as father to son over the first three generations and then through both sexes over the last two generations. With approximately half of the offspring in the latter two generations being affected with scoliosis, a dominant Mendelian mode of inheritance was proposed. Faber, in 1936, published the first population study of scoliosis, involving 660 patients with what was initially thought to be rachitic scoliosis.[2] The patients included in this study, in the author's conclusion, probably had AIS. More than 200 of these patients were found to have family members with scoliosis, with 7% of siblings and 14% of parents affected. Faber also proposed a dominant mode of inheritance for scoliosis In the first twin study of the disease, described in 1933, Nitsche and Armknecht reported on several twin pairs, some of whom shared the diagnosis of scoliosis whereas others did not.[4]

Over the remainder of the twentieth century, the accumulation of data in each of the three study categories named above has led to general acceptance of the conept that hereditary factors contribute to the transmission of AIS. Family and population studies by Harrington,[5] Wynne-Davies,[6] Riseborough and Wynne-Davies,[7] Cowell et al[8] Filho and Thompson,[9] and others[10] support a greater incidence of idiopathic scoliosis in families than in the general population. These studies found that up to a third of the members of families in which the disease recurs are affected with scoliosis. These studies documented an increased incidence of scoliosis in first-degree relatives of index patients (up to 11%) as compared with second- and third-degree relatives (up to 3.7% and 1.6%, respectively), as is characteristic of polygenic traits. Although all of these studies support a genetic basis for idiopathic scoliosis, they are fraught with potential limitations including the size of the study population, family size, genealogical resources, false paternity, clinical and genetic heterogeneity, and diagnostic accuracy.

Our group sought to overcome many of these limitations by initially studying the heritability of AIS with a unique population database for Utah and the Intermountain West region of the United States. Known as GenDB, this database derives its power from multiple factors, including a massive size (21 million birth, death, and marriage records), a population that has been geographically stable for over 150 years, extensive genealogical resources, the largest families in the developed world over multiple generations, and low false-paternity rates. Furthermore, the database does not represent a population isolate but rather a group that is outbred and representative of the general population of the United States. Using GenDB, our group demonstrated that AIS had familiar origins for 97% of 145 patients or probands. Kinship coefficients for the scoliosis patients had standard deviations threefold greater than those of controls, and a substantial founder effect was demonstrated. More than 50% of probands or individual families were connected by a common ancestor in sixteenth-century England.[11] One group of 14 previously unconnected families created an extended pedigree with a common ancestor in Essex, England, ca. 1520 AD, and another 17-family group had a common ancestor in Kent, England, ca. 1560 AD (**Fig. 28.1**). This statistically well-powered study further supports the familial nature of AIS.

Twin studies have consistently supported the familial nature of AIS,[10,12,13] demonstrating higher concordance in monozygotic (up to 73%) than in dizygotic (up to 36%) twins. However, the usefulness of twin studies in distinguishing between environmental and heritable effects in complex disorders has recently been questioned. It is now apparent that many monozygotic twins are not identical, eitherphenotypically or genotypically, and have major differences often evident in birth weight, the presence of genetic disease, and congenital anomalies. Although certain postzygotic events that lead to discordance in monozygotic twins are well understood (e.g., mosaicism, X-chromosome inactivation),

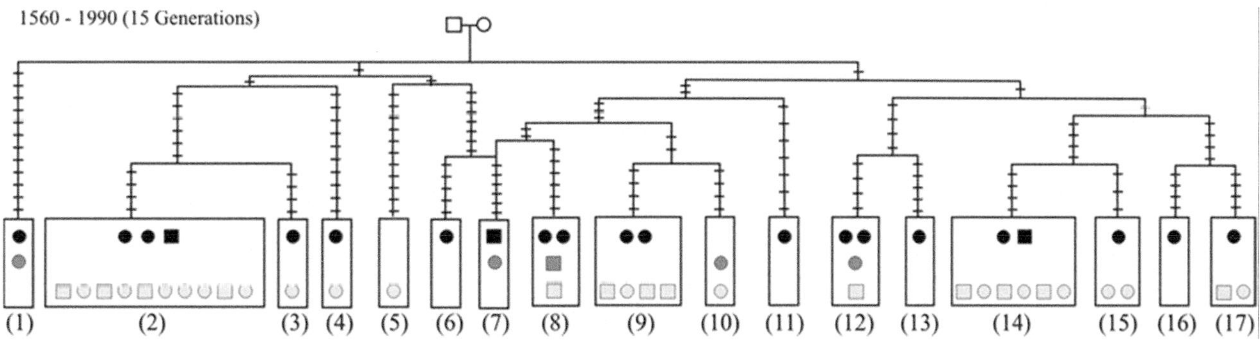


**Fig. 28.1** Pedigree of 17 families in which scoliosis has recurred and which are all linked to a single common ancestor in Kent, England, ca. 1560. The GenDB database uses unique numbers to identify relationships among families with scoliosis. (From Ogilvie JW, Braun J, Argyle V, Nelson L, Meade M, Ward K. The search for idiopathic scoliosis genes. Spine. Mar 15 2006;31(6):679-681. Reprinted with permission.)

other factors, resulting in discordance for lateral asymmetries (e.g., handedness, situs inversus), major malformations (e.g., vertebral anomalies alone or in combination with the VATER association of *v*ertebral abnormalities, an imperforate *a*nus, [cardiac anomalies], *t*rans*e*sophageal fistula, *r*enal anomalies, and *l*imb anomalies), and fetal growth (e.g., placental vascular anatomy) are poorly understood.[14,15] Thus, although twin studies are somewhat helpful in supporting the familial nature of AIS, the complexities of twinning make these types of studies less than ideal for defining the genetics of a structural asymmetry such as that in AIS.

Multiple modes of inheritance for AIS have been proposed over the years.[6–8,11,16–21] For example, in some families AIS follows simple mendelian inheritance patterns, whereas in others it folows more complex patterns. Still, most data suggest that the inheritance of AIS is polygenic and multifactorial.

Establishing the heritability of AIS has been an arduous process involving contributions from multiple investigators over the past century. Although the clinical impact of this body of work has been small, perhaps serving only to increase vigilance in screening patients' family members for scoliosis, the overall impact of this research has been substantial in that it has focused efforts at centers around the world on defining the genetic etiology of this condition.

## Gene Search

The search for specific genes associated with AIS has been greatly aided by recent advances in genetic technology, statistics, and computers, as well as by completion of the mapping of the human genome.[22,23] Whereas previous investigations of AIS had relied primarily on a candidate-gene approach alone, current investigations, using newer technologies, have used a genome-wide assessment based on linkage analysis, genetic association studies, or both. Multiple approaches are often combined in a complimentary fashion to improve the chance of success and validate the results with particular genetic techniques.

The standard candidate-gene approach is one way of identifying genes involved in a disease process. This type of analysis depends on genes with known protein products that appear relevant to the physiological basis of the disease and that may be investigated individually in patients or the families of patients with the disease. Through a process of trial and error, genes known to be associated with a specific disease process in animals or thought to be related to the underlying biology or physiology of the disease process can be individually evaluated to determine their association with the condition. Unfortunately, this approach has found limited success in defining genes for AIS,[17,18,20,21,24,25] probably because of poor understanding of the biology and physiology of this particular idiopathic source of spinal asymmetry and the lack of an animal model for it. However, a candidate-gene approach can be used in combination with other approaches that identify particular areas on the human genome that are associated with AIS.

The mapping of the human genome, as well as advances in genetic technology, now allow screening of the entire genome for one or more genes. In contrast to the more limited standard candidate-gene approach, both linkage analysis and genome-wide association studies (GWAS) allow screening of the full genome with known genetic markers. A genetic linkage occurs when a particular gene is inherited jointly. Specifically, genetic loci on the same chromosome are physically connected and tend to stay together during meiosis, and are thus genetically linked, as shown in **Fig. 28.2**. Within a linkage analysis, benign variations in the deoxyribonucleic acid (DNA) among different individuals are used as markers to identify regions or loci containing genes that predispose to a condition in related individuals. The algorithm used to study the linkage may be designated as parametric or nonparametric. A parametric linkage analysis is used to study major gene disorders, and assumes

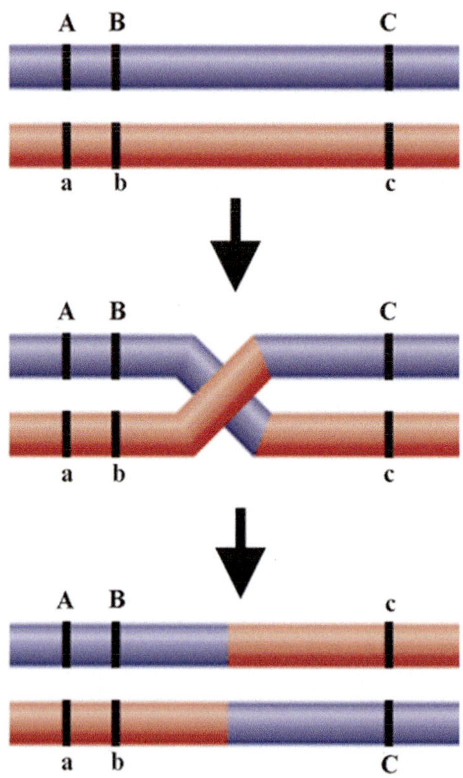


**Fig. 28.2** Genes located in close proximity to each other tend to be inherited together. This is referred to as genetic linkage. The process of meiosis is illustrated here. Genes A and B are located next to each other, whereas gene C is located farther away. As a result the particular traits associated with genes A and B tend to be inherited together, whereas the traits associated with gene C are inherited with little to no association with genes A and B.

that the inheritance of such a disorder follows a specific and known genetic model, such as mendelian inheritance. A nonparametric linkage analysis is used for more complex diseases and when the inheritance of a disease does not follow a specific genetic model. The results of a simple linkage analysis are expressed as a logarithm of the odds ( LOD) score, which compares the probability or odds of obtaining a particular test result when two genes are linked to one another with the probability or odds of obtaining the same score when the same two genes are not linked to one another.

The LOD score is calculated as follows:

[Equation 28.1]

where NR = the number of offspring with a nonrecombinant gene pattern or offspring that have a genotype identical to the parent's genotype

R = the number of offspring with a recombinant gene pattern or offspring that have a genotype that differs from the parent's genotype

$\theta$ or the recombinant fraction = R / (NR + R).

An LOD score >3.0 is considered evidence for linkage.

The techniques currently used for linkage analysis have become very robust; however, they must be applied to large families with reliable clinical- and family-history data if they are to yield significant findings. Furthermore, in complex genetic diseases such as AIS, linkage analysis is usually most efficient at discovering rare genes with very large effects.

The large-scale screening of the genome of an individual with a particular condition may be done through the use of known genetic markers or polymorphisms. Genetic polymorphisms are benign variations in the structure of DNA that may vary among individuals. In GWAS, single nucleotide polymorphisms, or SNPs, are used as the markers to detect an association with a disease or condition in the population as a whole. These studies are similar to epidemiological studies that often employ case-control or cohort designs to assess multiple risk factors for disease (e.g., smoking as one of many risk factors for lung cancer). In GWAS, SNP markers are analyzed as risk factors. Typical microarrays that are gene "chips" with a million or more genetic probes attached to them are used to rapidly and systematically analyze a patient's genetic makeup (**Fig. 28.3**). A GWAS is done over short region of the genome and may help target discrete regions of the genome for fine mapping, defining them as regions of interest (ROIs).

Several recent studies have used linkage analysis in an effort to identify specific regions of human chromosomes that may be associated with AIS. Wise et al[20] identified potential linkage regions on chromosomes 3, 6, 10, 12, and 18 in a single family with scoliosis, with the 18q and 6p regions being the most significant. Chan et al[25] subsequently evaluated the regions that Wise et al identified as most significant (6p, 10q, and 18q) but found no evidence of linkage in a single family with scoliosis. In the same family, Chan et al went on to identify linkage regions 19p13.3 and 2q as potentially important. In another single family with scoliosis, Salehi et al[24] identified a region on 17p11 as potentially important. Miller, reporting on a large group of 202 families with scoliosis, noted multiple areas of linkage in two different subgroups. In a subgroup that demonstrated an X-linked dominant mode of inheritance, linkage region Xq 23–26 was found to be important. However, in the subgroup, which demonstrated an autosomal dominant mode of inheritance, five primary (6p, 6q, 9, 16, and 17) and eight secondary (1, 3, 5, 7, 8, 11, 12, and 19) regions of possible linkage were identified.

Although it has been suggested that the multiple locations identified in these sophisticated genetic studies of AIS represent conflicting results,[17,18,20,24–26] it has also been suggested that this great variability merely reflects the polygenic nature of the heritability of scoliosis. It is likely that multiple factors contributed to the wide variability of

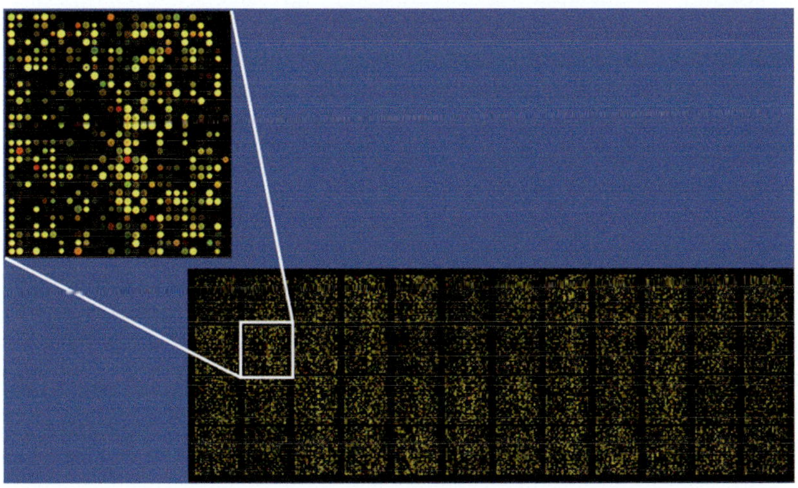

**Fig. 28.3** Example of a 37,500-probe spotted microarray with an enlarged inset. The chip contains thousands of small DNA sequences that can probe or hybridize to cDNA or cRNA in a patient sample. Chips like this may be used to detect SNPs.

results in these studies. Certainly the small size of many of the studies was a factor in this variability. But perhaps the most significant issue relates to the quality of the populations studied. The quality of any population used in a genetic study is directly proportional to the genetic informativeness of the families selected for study. Informativeness can be adversely affected by small family size, poor genealogical resources, high false-paternity rates, significant clinical and genetic heterogeneity, and low diagnostic accuracy. Linkage-analysis studies that are substantially compromised in one or more of these areas will yield inconsistent results of questionable significance.

In a preliminary investigation, our group reported on 500 probands with AIS and identified regions on chromosomes 3 and 7 that were more statistically significant in terms of linkage to the condition than were regions found in any previous study (with LOD scores of 7.0 and 7.3, respectively).[27] The significance of these markers was ~10,000 greater than that of regions found in the next largest study. We then conducted an additional case–control genetic association analysis to confirm the significance of these loci with regard to AIS. The high level of significance in our study was probably related to the informativeness of the families studied. Use of the GenDB database minimized or eliminated many of the limitations evident in previous studies. Work is underway to further validate these two linkage regions and identify possible additional markers associated with AIS.

Once areas or regions on the human genome are identified as being highly linked or associated with AIS, these loci can be further investigated with a positional-candidate approach. The ROI in a positional-candidate approach is relatively small as compared with that in candidate-gene analysis, and the association with AIS is clearer (**Fig. 28.4**). Several studies have employed linkage analysis in an attempt to target specific regions of the human genome for subsequent positional-candidate-gene analysis. Although several investigators have targeted linkage regions containing the genes for melatonin, aggrecan, and other genes related to the structure of the extracellular fluid matrix, they have yet to reveal any specific association with idiopathic scoliosis.[24,28–30]

The search for specific genes associated with AIS represents an ongoing effort at multiple centers throughout the world. Although great progress has been made, the ultimate goal of fully understanding the molecular basis of this unique deformity has yet to be achieved. Once the genes responsible for AIS are mapped, substantial opportunities will become available for improving the management of this disease. These include the potential for early diagnosis through broad population screening and novel treatment options using cellular, molecular, or pharmacological strategies alone or in combination. Two-thirds of disease-gene discoveries made today are exploitable, allowing the targeting of related proteins or biochemical pathways for diagnosis or treatment. AIS may eventually evolve from a condition treated mechanically (either with a brace or surgery) to one treated medically. At present, the greatest clinical effect of the search for genes involved in AIS has not come from the mapping of genes themselves but through the related discovery of prognostic genetic markers.

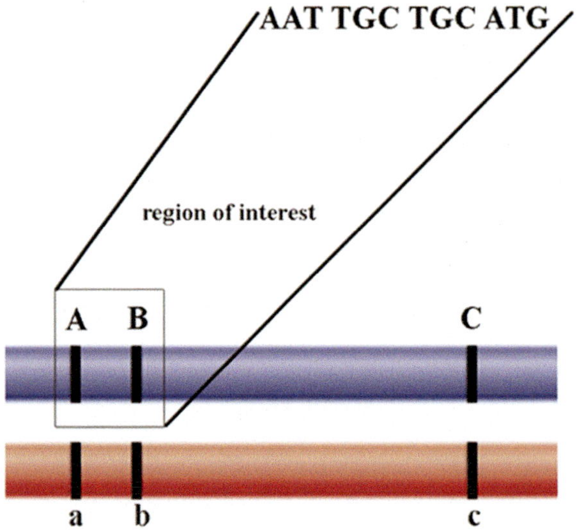


**Fig. 28.4** Once areas or regions on the human genome are identified as being strongly linked to or associated with AIS through a linkage analysis or a genome-wide association study, an ROI is defined that can be further investigated with a positional-candidate-gene approach, as shown here.

## Prognostics

Genome-wide linkage analysis and genetic association studies commonly use genetic markers merely as means to the ends of identifying genes associated with a particular condition. Yet genetic markers can also be used as ends in themselves. As an interim result in our quest to fully understand the molecular basis of AIS and fine map the genes responsible for this condition, we have identified genetic markers associated with severe and progressive scoliosis. An initial panel of markers associated with surgical-grade scoliosis (defined as spinal deformity progressing to 40 degrees or more before skeletal maturity) has proven highly accurate in identifying such deformity at an early stage. In an early study, involving 675 skeletally mature Caucasian subjects with AIS at centers across the United States, our group identified 12 SNP markers as having prognostic utility. Using an additive model involving both genetic and clinical risk factors (which had weights of ~90% and 10%, respectively), we obtained a summed risk score that correctly identified 97% of patients at low risk and 92% of those at high risk for progressive AIS, for an overall sensitivity of 93% and specificity of 90% ($P < 2.2 \times 10^{-16}$).[26]

The inclusion in this early work of >5000 patients from across the United States has allowed additional refinement of the initial marker panel. With the goal of improving the accuracy of genetic analysis in the prognosis of AIS, and including multiple races and ethnicities in such analysis, we have identified a panel of 53 genetic markers that now allows the prediction of progression of scoliosis to severe curvature with a range of accuracy of 90%. Although a highly accurate assessment of such risk can be achieved with these markers alone, the addition of clinical parameters, such as curve magnitude and skeletal maturity, further improves the sensitivity and specificity of this assessment, minimizing the frequency of false-positive and false-negative results.

Because most AIS is diagnosed at an early stage, either through school screening efforts or awareness among pediatricians, methods for predicting its progression have been sought for some time. However, accurate determination of the prognosis in individual cases of AIS has been elusive, perhaps because of a reliance on clinical variables that change with time. Lonstein and Carlson described the most widely accepted current method for clinically assessing the risk of progression of AIS in 1984.[31] With this method, the magnitude of a patient's curve and the patient's skeletal maturity (Risser grade) are used to estimate the risk of progression. Yet these radiographic parameters are accurate only in cases of extreme curve magnitude and skeletal maturity, in which there is little question about the decision to treat. For example, a large curve in a skeletally immature patient (e.g., 39 degrees and Risser grade 0) is at high risk for continued progression and is likely to require treatment, whereas a small curve in a skeletally mature patient (e.g., 11 degrees and Risser grade 4) is unlikely to progress or ever require treatment.

For the majority of skeletally immature patients who present with AIS in the mild to moderate range, the current clinical methods of diagnosis of AIS provide significantly less ability to predict outcome than do prognostic genetic markers. To demonstrate the substantial differences in sensitivity and specificity in assessing the risk of progression of AIS with these two methods, we compared the Lonstein and Carlson method with the use of prognostic genetic markers in a cohort of our patients. Using radiographs from a patient's initial presentation to determine the risk of progression with the Lonstein and Carlson method, we found that it had 60% sensitivity and 55% specificity in predicting outcome at skeletal maturity, whereas the prognostic genetic markers had a 95% and 93% sensitivity and specificity, respectively.

The uncertainty created by the radiographic methods for assessing the risk of progression of AIS has led to great inefficiencies in management of this disease. Patients with a mild scoliosis, at least 90% of whom are unlikely to experience progression of their curvature to a grade of surgical severity, are observed for years with serial X-rays at 4- to 6-month intervals until skeletal maturity. For patients who present with a moderate curve or whose curves progress into a moderate range, bracing is often recommended. Yet bracing is probably unnecessary in some such patients and ineffective in others, even with good compliance. For those whose curves progress beyond 40 degrees during skeletal immaturity, fusion surgery is often considered. However, fusion surgery essentially represents a nonphysiological salvage procedure that eliminates growth, motion, and function of the spine, and is justifiable only for curves of large magnitude. Whenever possible, avoidance of such a procedure would be ideal.

The discovery of prognostic genetic markers will profoundly affect the management of AIS by providing powerful information that accurately defines the risk of its progression at the earliest possible stage (**Fig. 28.5**). For patients with a low risk of curve progression, the use of such markers may

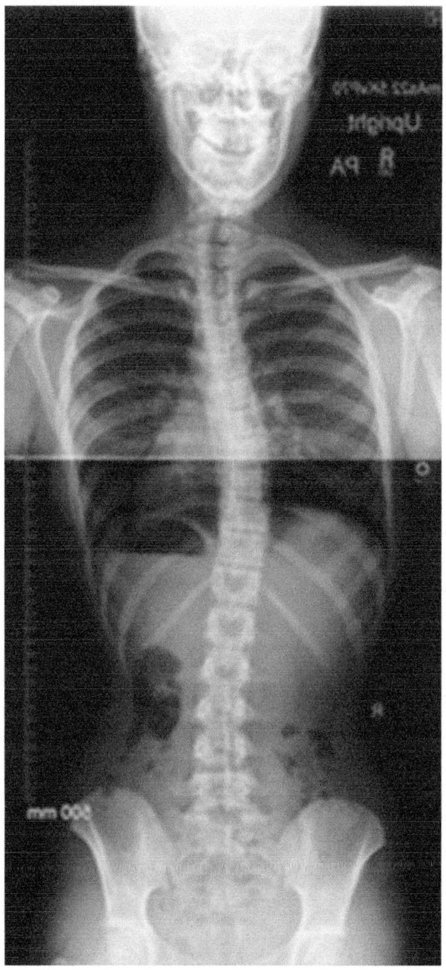

**Fig. 28.5** Using standard radiographic methods, the risk of curve progression for this 12-year-old girl of Risser grade 0, with AIS and a 20-degree curve is roughly in the 20 to 70% range, leaving great uncertainty about the potential need for her future treatment. Prognostic genetic testing of this child will allow an accurate determination, at a probability of 93 to 97%, of the risk of progression of her curve to a surgical-grade curve, providing the opportunity to reduce or eliminate the need for observation in the case of a low- risk test result or to intervene early, with greater conviction, if the test demonstrates a high risk of progression.

permit their reassurance and the reassurance of their families at a single encounter, eliminating years of uncertainty and serial radiographic evaluation. This will result in great individual and aggregate savings. For patients at high risk of curve progression, early intervention with standard bracing treatment or more novel procedures of fusionless scoliosis surgery will be possible. For patients thought to be reasonable candidates for bracing, it could be offered at an earlier stage and undertaken with conviction. For patients for whom bracing is not optimal (because of anticipated or evident compliance issues or psychological factors or both), or is contraindicated (thoracic lordosis, pulmonary issues), unwanted, or likely to fail (high-risk prognostic markers), novel, more physiological treatment options may be possible. These include fusionless scoliosis surgery on the convexity or concavity of a curve, anteriorly or posteriorly, with the goal of guiding growth for the correction of deformity while preserving motion and function of the spine.

## ■ Conclusion

The genetics of AIS is complex. Consequently, establishing the familial nature of this condition and confirming a genetic basis for it has been a slow and painstaking process that has continued throughout the past century. These achievements represent important steps. The search for the genes responsible for AIS with fine mapping of the genetic mutations involved in its causation will continue until these genes are fully characterized, when additional options for the diagnosis and treatment of AIS may be possible, ranging from broad population screening for idiopathic scoliosis to cellular, molecular, or pharmacological interventions that target the biochemical pathways involved it its occurrence.

Although there is great promise of achieving these goals in the near future, the recent discovery of prognostic genetic markers for AIS will have an immediate impact. Because progressive scoliosis appears to have a greater genetic component than does scoliosis generally, specific prognostic genetic markers should allow its early and accurate diagnosis and the identification of patients whose idiopathic curves are at low risk and high risk of progressing. Given the limitations currently faced by clinicians attempting to gauge the risk of progression of scoliosis on the basis of radiographic variables that change over time, prognostic genetic markers provide new and powerful tools for accurate and definitive decision-making about the treatment of scoliosis, with an emphasis on individualizing a given patient's care. Genetic research will improve all aspects of the care of scoliosis, providing greater efficiency both in managing patients at low risk for its progression and in treating those at high risk.

### References


1. Robin GC. The Aetiology of Idiopathic Scoliosis: A Review of a Century of Research. Boca Raton, FL: CRC Press; 1990
2. Faber A. Untersuchungen uber die Erblichkeit der Skoliosie. Arch Orthop Trauma Surg 1935;36:217–296
3. Garland H. Hereditary scoliosis. Br Med J 1934;1:686
4. Nitsche F, Armknecht P. Orthopaedische Leiden bei Zwilligen. Z Orthop Chir 1933;58:528–537
5. Harrington PR. The etiology of idiopathic scoliosis. Clin Orthop Relat Res 1977;(126):17–25
6. Wynne-Davies R. Familial (idiopathic) scoliosis. A family survey. J Bone Joint Surg Br 1968;50:24–30
7. Riseborough EJ, Wynne-Davies R. A genetic survey of idiopathic scoliosis in Boston, Massachusetts. J Bone Joint Surg Am 1973;55:974–982
8. Cowell HR, Hall JN, MacEwen GD. Genetic aspects of idiopathic scoliosis. A Nicholas Andry Award essay, 1970. Clin Orthop Relat Res 1972;86:121–131
9. Filho N, Thompson M. Genetic studies in scoliosis. J Bone Joint Surg Am 1971;53:199
10. van Rhijn LW, Jansen EJ, Plasmans CM, Veraart BE. Curve characteristics in monozygotic twins with adolescent idiopathic scoliosis: 3 new twin pairs and a review of the literature. Acta Orthop Scand 2001;72:621–625
11. Ogilvie JW, Braun J, Argyle V, Nelson L, Meade M, Ward K. The search for idiopathic scoliosis genes. Spine 2006; 31:679–681
12. Carr AJ. Adolescent idiopathic scoliosis in identical twins. J Bone Joint Surg Br 1990;72:1077
13. Kesling KL, Reinker KA. Scoliosis in twins. A meta-analysis of the literature and report of six cases. Spine 1997;22:2009–2014, discussion 2015
14. Hall JG. Twins and twinning. Am J Med Genet 1996;61:202–204
15. Machin GA. Some causes of genotypic and phenotypic discordance in monozygotic twin pairs. Am J Med Genet 1996;61:216–228
16. Aksenovich TI, Semenov IR, Ginzburg EKh, Zaĭdman AM. [Preliminary analysis of inheritance of scoliosis]. Genetika 1988;24:2056–2063
17. Miller NH, Justice CM, Marosy B, et al. Identification of candidate regions for familial idiopathic scoliosis. Spine 2005;30:1181–1187
18. Justice CM, Miller NH, Marosy B, Zhang J, Wilson AF. Familial idiopathic scoliosis: Evidence of an X-linked susceptibility locus. Spine 2003;28:589–594
19. Czeizel A, Bellyei A, Barta O, Magda T, Molnár L. Genetics of adolescent idiopathic scoliosis. J Med Genet 1978;15:424–427
20. Wise CA, Barnes R, Gillum J, Herring JA, Bowcock AM, Lovett M. Localization of susceptibility to familial idiopathic scoliosis. Spine 2000;25:2372–2380
21. Miller NH. Genetics of familial idiopathic scoliosis. Clin Orthop Relat Res 2007;462:6–10
22. Lander ES, Linton LM, Birren B, et al; International Human Genome Sequencing Consortium. Initial sequencing and analysis of the human genome. Nature 2001;409:860–921

23. McPherson JD, Marra M, Hillier L, et al; International Human Genome Mapping Consortium. A physical map of the human genome. Nature 2001;409:934–941
24. Salehi LB, Mangino M, De Serio S, et al. Assignment of a locus for autosomal dominant idiopathic scoliosis (IS) to human chromosome 17p11. Hum Genet 2002;111:401–404
25. Chan V, Fong GC, Luk KD, et al. A genetic locus for adolescent idiopathic scoliosis linked to chromosome 19p13.3. Am J Hum Genet 2002;71:401–406
26. Braun JT, Nelson L, Ogilvie JW, Ward K. Twelve DNA markers accurately assess risk of progression in adolescent idiopathic scoliosis. Paper presented at: 42nd Annual Meeting of the Scoliosis Research Society. Edinburgh, Scotland, 2007
27. Ogilvie JW, Braun JT, Nelson L, Ward K. Identification of 2 new genetic markers for idiopathic scoliosis. Scoliosis Research Society 41st Annual Meeting. Monterey, California, 2006
28. Morcuende JA, Minhas R, Dolan L, et al. Allelic variants of human melatonin 1A receptor in patients with familial adolescent idiopathic scoliosis. Spine 2003;28:2025–2028, discussion 2029
29. Marosy B, Justice CM, Nzegwu N, Kumar G, Wilson AF, Miller NH. Lack of association between the aggrecan gene and familial idiopathic scoliosis. Spine 2006;31:1420–1425
30. Bashiardes S, Veile R, Allen M, et al. SNTG1, the gene encoding gamma1-syntrophin: A candidate gene for idiopathic scoliosis. Hum Genet 2004;115:81–89
31. Lonstein JE, Carlson JM. The prediction of curve progression in untreated idiopathic scoliosis during growth. J Bone Joint Surg Am 1984;66:1061–1071

# Index

Note: Page numbers followed by *f* and *t* indicate figures and tables, respectively.

## B



## C

**N**

## O



## P

## Q



## R

**S**

## T